Prioritization, Delegation, and Assignment

Practice Exercises
for the NCLEX-RN® Examination

5th EDITION

Prioritization, Delegation, *and* Assignment

Practice Exercises
for the NCLEX-RN® Examination

Linda A. LaCharity, PhD, RN
Formerly, Accelerated Program Director
Assistant Professor
College of Nursing
University of Cincinnati
Cincinnati, Ohio

Shirley M. Hosler, MSN, RN
Formerly, Nursing Instructor
School of Nursing
National American University
Albuquerque, New Mexico

Candice K. Kumagai, MSN, RN
Formerly, Clinical Instructor
School of Nursing
University of Texas at Austin
Austin, Texas

With an introduction by
Ruth Hansten, MBA, PhD, RN, FACHE
Principal Consultant and CEO
Hansten Healthcare
Santa Rosa, California

ELSEVIER

Elsevier
3251 Riverport Lane
St. Louis, Missouri 63043

PRIORITIZATION, DELEGATION, AND ASSIGNMENT: PRACTICE EXERCISES
FOR THE NCLEX-RN® EXAMINATION, FIFTH EDITION

ISBN: 978-0-323-68316-6

Copyright © 2022 by Elsevier, Inc. All rights reserved.

Notice

Practitioners and researchers must always rely on their own experience and knowledge in evaluating and using any information, methods, compounds or experiments described herein. Because of rapid advances in the medical sciences, in particular, independent verification of diagnoses and drug dosages should be made. To the fullest extent of the law, no responsibility is assumed by Elsevier, authors, editors or contributors for any injury and/or damage to persons or property as a matter of products liability, negligence or otherwise, or from any use or operation of any methods, products, instructions, or ideas contained in the material herein.

Previous editions copyrighted 2019, 2014, 2011, and 2006.

Library of Congress Control Number: 2021936204

Executive Content Strategist: Lee Henderson
Senior Content Development Manager: Lisa Newton
Senior Content Development Specialist: Tina Kaemmerer
Publishing Services Manager: Julie Eddy
Senior Project Manager: Abigail Bradberry
Design Direction: Margaret Reid

Printed in Canada

Last digit is the print number: 9 8 7 6 5 4 3 2 1

Working together
to grow libraries in
developing countries

www.elsevier.com • www.bookaid.org

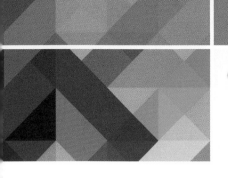

Contributors and Reviewers

CONTRIBUTORS

Martha Barry, MS, RN, APN, CNM
Certified Nurse Midwife
OB Faculty Practice
Advocate Medical Group
Chicago, Illinois;
Adjunct Clinical Instructor
College of Nursing
University of Illinois at Chicago
Chicago, Illinois

Mary Tedesco-Schneck, PhD, RN, CPNP
Assistant Professor
School of Nursing
University of Maine
Orono, Maine

REVIEWERS

Amber Ballard, MSN, RN
Registered Nurse
Emergency Department
Sparrow Health System
Lansing, Michigan

Angela McConachie, DNP, MSN-FNP, RN
Director, BSN Program Accelerated Option
Associate Professor
Goldfarb School of Nursing at Barnes Jewish College
St. Louis, Missouri

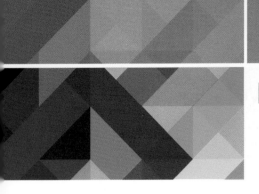

Preface

Prioritization, Delegation, and Assignment: Practice Exercises for the NCLEX-RN® Examination has evolved since its first edition from a medical-surgical nursing–focused test preparation workbook to a resource that spans general nursing knowledge while emphasizing management of care to assist students in preparing for the NCLEX® Examination. Our fifth edition includes many examples of new question types that will be included in the forthcoming Next-Generation NCLEX® Examination (NGN). A second and equally important purpose of the book continues to be assisting students, novice nurses, and seasoned nurses in applying concepts of prioritization, delegation, and assignment to nursing practice in today's patient care settings.

TO FACULTY AND OTHER USERS

Patient care acuity continues to be higher than ever with the essential added care of COVID-19 patients, while staffing shortages remain very real. Nurses must use all available patient care personnel and resources competently and efficiently and be familiar with variations in state laws governing the practice of nursing, as well as differences in scopes of practice and facility-specific job descriptions. Nurses must also be aware of the different skill and experience levels of the health care professionals with whom they work on a daily basis. Which nursing actions can be assigned to an experienced versus a new graduate RN or LPN/LVN? What forms of patient care can the nurse delegate to assistive personnel (AP)? Who should help the postoperative patient who has had a total hip replacement get out of bed and ambulate to the bathroom? Can the nurse ask APs such as nursing assistants to check a patient's oxygen saturation using pulse oximetry or check a diabetic patient's glucose level? What reporting parameters should the nurse give to an LPN/LVN who is monitoring a patient after cardiac catheterization or to the AP checking patients' vital signs? What patient care interventions and actions should not be delegated by the nurse? The answers to these and many other questions should be much clearer after completion of the exercises in this book.

Exercises in this book range from simple to complex and use various patient care scenarios. The purpose of the chapters and case studies is to encourage the student or new graduate nurse to conceptualize using the skills

of prioritization, delegation, and assignment, as well as supervision in many different settings. Our goal is to make these concepts tangible to our readers.

The questions are written in NCLEX® Examination formats, including new NGN styles to help faculty as they teach student nurses how to prepare for licensure examination. The chapters and case studies focus on real and hypothetical patient care situations to challenge nurses and nursing students to develop the skills necessary to apply these concepts in practice. The exercises are also useful to nurse educators as they discuss, teach, and test their students and nurses for understanding and application of these concepts in nursing programs, examination preparations, and facility orientations. Correct answers, along with in-depth rationales, are provided at the end of each chapter and case study to facilitate the learning process, along with the focus/foci for each item. The faculty exercise keys include QSEN (Quality and Safety Education for Nurses) categories, concepts, and cognitive levels for each question, as well as IPEC (Interprofessional Education Collaborative) competencies where appropriate.

TO STUDENTS

Prioritization, delegation, and assignment are essential concepts and skills for nursing practice. Our students and graduate nurses have repeatedly told us of their difficulties with the application of these principles when taking program exit and licensure examinations. Nurse managers have told us many times that novice nurses and even some experienced nurses lack the expertise to effectively and safely practice these skills in real-world settings.

Although several excellent resources deal with these issues, there is still a need for a book that incorporates management of these care concepts into real-world practice scenarios. Our goal in writing the fifth edition of *Prioritization, Delegation, and Assignment: Practice Exercises for the NCLEX-RN® Examination* is to provide a resource that challenges nursing students, as well as novice and experienced nurses, to develop the knowledge and understanding necessary to effectively apply these important nursing skills: examination preparation and real-world practice. From the original focus on medical-surgical nursing, subsequent editions have expanded to include pediatrics, labor and delivery, psychiatric nursing, and long-term care as well as the role of the nurse in a variety of nonacute care settings. Additionally, we have made changes that reflect the current focus on evidence-based best practices, fundamentals of safe practice, and expansion of diabetes care. For the fifth edition, we responded to requests for more questions, especially about medications. New questions, including drug-related questions, have been added to each chapter. We also added questions specific to the needs of the lesbian, gay, bisexual, transgender, queer, intersexual, and asexual (LGBTQIA) community. New questions were added and revised throughout the book to broaden comprehension of key concepts and knowledge areas and to update current knowledge levels. Our fifth edition expands on all of these topics and incorporates examples of Next-Generation NCLEX® Examination (NGN) question formats to prepare students for the upcoming NCLEX® changes.

Each new copy of the book comes with a fully interactive version of the book content, with scoring, on Evolve at http://evolve.elsevier.com/LaCharity/prioritization. This interactive version of the book helps to simulate the experience of taking the NCLEX® Examination. Students can use this interactive option to create multiple different test versions for practice and self-assessment.

ACKNOWLEDGMENTS

We would like to thank the many people whose support and assistance made the creation of the fifth edition of this book possible. Thanks to our families, colleagues, and friends for listening, reading, encouraging, and making sure we had the time to research, write, and review this book. We truly appreciate the expertise of our two contributing authors, Martha Barry (reproductive health) and Mary Tedesco-Schneck (pediatrics), who each contributed an excellent chapter and case study related to their areas of expertise. Very special thanks to Ruth Hansten, whose expertise in the area of clinical prioritization, delegation, and assignment skills continues to keep us on track. Many thanks to the faculty reviewers, whose expertise helped us keep the scenarios accurate and realistic. Finally, we wish to acknowledge our faculty, students, graduates, and readers who have taken the time to keep in touch and let us know about their needs for additional assistance in developing the skills to practice the arts of prioritization, delegation, and assignment.

Linda A. LaCharity
Candice K. Kumagai
Shirley M. Hosler

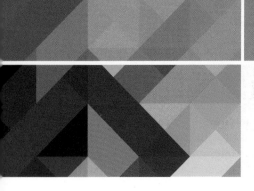

Contents

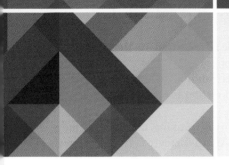

Guidelines for Prioritization, Delegation, and Assignment Decisions

Ruth Hansten, PhD, MBA, BSN, RN, FACHE

OUTCOMES FOCUS

Expert nurses have discovered that the most successful method of approaching their practice is to maintain a laser-like focus on the outcomes that the patients and their families want to achieve. To attempt to prioritize, delegate, or assign care without understanding the patient's preferred results is like trying to put together a jigsaw puzzle without the top of the puzzle box that shows the puzzle picture. Not only does the puzzle player pick up random pieces that don't fit well together, wasting time and increasing frustration, but also the process of puzzle assembly is fraught with inefficiencies and wrong choices. In the same way, a nurse who scurries haphazardly without a plan, unsure of what could be the most important, life-saving task to be done first or which person should do which tasks for this group of patients, is not fulfilling his or her potential to be a channel for healing.

Let's visit a change-of-shift report in which a group of nurses receives information about two patients whose blood pressure is plummeting at the same rate. How would one determine which nurse would be best to assign to care for these patients, which patient needs to be seen first, and which tasks could be delegated to assistive personnel (APs), if none of the nurses is aware of each patient's preferred outcomes? Patient A is a young mother who has been receiving chemotherapy for breast cancer; she has been admitted this shift because of dehydration from uncontrolled emesis. She is expecting to regain her normally robust good health and watch her children graduate from college. Everyone on the health care team would concur with her long-term goals. Patient Z is an elderly gentleman, 92 years of age, whose wife recently died from complications of repeated cerebrovascular events and dementia. Yesterday while in the emergency department (ED), he was given the diagnosis of acute myocardial infarction and preexisting severe heart failure. He would like to die and join his wife, has requested a "do not resuscitate" order, and is awaiting transfer to a hospice. These two patients share critical clinical data but require widely different prioritization, delegation, and assignment. A savvy charge RN would make the obvious decisions: to assign the most skilled RN to the young mother and to ask APs to function in a supportive role to the primary care RN.

The elderly gentleman needs palliative care and would be best cared for by an RN and care team with excellent people skills. Even a novice nursing assistant could be delegated tasks to help keep Mr. Z and his family comfortable and emotionally supported. The big picture on the puzzle box for these two patients ranges from long-term "robust good health" requiring immediate emergency assessment and treatment to "a supported and comfortable death" requiring timely palliative care, including supportive emotional and physical care. Without envisioning these patients' pictures and knowing their preferred outcomes, the RNs cannot prioritize, delegate, or assign appropriately.

There are many times in nursing practice, however, when correct choices are not so apparent. Patients in all care settings today are often complex, and many have preexisting comorbidities that may stump the expert practitioners and clinical specialists planning their care. Care delivery systems must flex on a moment's notice as an AP arrives in place of a scheduled LPN/LVN and agency, float, or traveling nurses fill vacancies, while new patients, waiting to be admitted, accumulate in the ED or wait to be transferred to another setting. APs arrive with varying educational preparation and dissimilar levels of motivation and skill. Critical thinking and complex clinical judgment are required from the minute the shift begins until the nurse clocks out.

In this book, the authors have filled an educational need for students and practicing nurses who wish to hone their skills in prioritizing, assigning, and delegating. The scenarios and patient problems presented in this workbook are practical, challenging, and complex learning tools. Quality and Safety Education for Nurses (QSEN) competencies are incorporated into this chapter and throughout the questions to highlight patient- and family-centered care, quality and safety improvement, and teamwork and collaboration concepts and skills (QSEN Institute, 2019). Patient stories will stimulate thought and discussion and help polish the higher-order intellectual skills necessary to practice as a successful, safe, and effective nurse. The Interprofessional Collaboration Competency Community and Population Oriented Domains from the Interprofessional Education Collaborative (IPEC) are applied to the questions in this book as appropriate (Interprofessional Education Collaborative, 2016, https://ipecollaborative.org). Domains include Interprofessional Teamwork and Team-Based Practices, Interprofessional Teamwork Practices,

Roles and Responsibilities for Collaborative Practice, and Values/Ethics for Interprofessional Practice. As reflected in the IPEC sub-competencies, especially crucial for patient outcomes is the role of the RN, armed with knowledge of scopes of practice, successfully communicating with team members to delegate, assign, and supervise (IPEC, 2016).

DEFINITION OF TERMS

The intellectual functions of prioritization, delegation, and assignment engage the nurse in projecting into the future from the present state. Thinking about what impact might occur if competing decisions are chosen, weighing options, and making split-second decisions, given the available data, is not an easy process. Unless resources in terms of staffing, budget, time, or supplies are unlimited, nurses must relentlessly focus on choosing which issues or concerns must take precedence.

Prioritization

Prioritization is defined as "ranking problems in order of importance" or "deciding which needs or problems require immediate action and which ones could tolerate a delay in action until a later time because they are not urgent" (Silvestri, 2018). Prioritization in a clinical setting is a process that involves clearly envisioning patient outcomes but also includes predicting possible problems if another task is performed first. One also must weigh potential future events if the task is not completed, the time it would take to accomplish it, and the relationship of the tasks and outcomes. New nurses often struggle with prioritization because they have not yet worked with typical patient progressions through care pathways and have not experienced the complications that may emerge in association with a particular clinical condition. In short, knowing the patient's **purpose for care, current clinical picture,** and **picture of the outcome or result** is necessary to be able to plan priorities. The part played by each team member is designated as the RN assigns or delegates. The "four Ps"—purpose, picture, plan, and part—become a guidepost for appropriately navigating these processes (Hansten, 2008a, 2011, 2014b; Hansten and Jackson, 2009). The four Ps will be referred to throughout this introduction because these concepts are the framework on which RNs base decisions about supporting patients and families toward their preferred outcomes, whether RNs provide the care themselves or work closely with assistive team members.

Prioritization includes evaluating and weighing each competing task or process using the following criteria (Hansten and Jackson, 2009, pp. 194–196):

- Is it life threatening or potentially life threatening if the task is not done? Would another patient be endangered if this task is done now or the task is left for later?

- Is this task or process essential to patient or staff safety?
- Is this task or process essential to the medical or nursing plan of care?

In each case, an understanding of the overall patient goals and the context and setting is essential.

1. In her book on critical thinking and clinical judgment, Rosalinda Alfaro-Lefevre (2017) suggests three levels of priority setting: The first level is **a**irway, **b**reathing, **c**ardiac status and circulation, and **v**ital signs and **l**ab values that could be life threatening ("ABCs plus V and L").
2. The second level is immediately subsequent to the first level and includes concerns such as mental status changes, untreated medical issues, acute pain, acute elimination problems, and imminent risks.
3. The third level comprises health problems other than those at the first two levels, such as more long-term issues in health education, rest, coping, and so on (p. 171).

Maslow's hierarchy of needs can be used to prioritize from the most crucial survival needs to needs related to safety and security, affiliation (love, relationships), self-esteem, and self-actualization (Alfaro-Lefevre, 2017, p. 170).

Delegation and Assignment

The official definitions of **assignment** have been altered through ongoing dialogue among nursing leaders in various states and nursing organizations, and terminology distinctions such as *observation* versus *assessment, critical thinking* versus *clinical reasoning,* and *delegation* versus *assignment* continue to be discussed as nursing leaders attempt to describe complex thinking processes that occur in various levels of nursing practice. Assignment has been defined as **"the distribution of work that each staff member is responsible for during a given work period"** (American Nurses Association [ANA], Duffy & McCoy, 2014, p. 22). In 2016, the National Council of State Boards of Nursing (NCSBN) published the results of two expert panels to clarify that **assignment** includes **"the routine care, activities, and procedures that are within the authorized scope of practice of the RN or LPN/LVN or part of the routine functions of the UAP (Unlicensed Assistive Personnel)"** (NCSBN, 2016b, pp. 6–7), and this definition was adopted by the ANA in 2019 in a joint statement with the NCSBN with the addition of the acronym **AP (assistive personnel)** (ANA & NCSBN 2019 National Guidelines for Nursing Delegation, p. 2). **Delegation** was defined traditionally as **"transferring to a competent individual the authority to perform a selected nursing task in a selected situation"** (NCSBN, 1995), and similar definitions are used by some nurse practice statutes or regulations. Both the ANA and the NCSBN describe delegation as **"allowing a delegate** to perform a specific nursing activity, skill, or procedure **that is beyond the delegatee's traditional role and is not routinely performed**" (ANA & NCSBN 2019, p. 2). Nevertheless, the delegatee must be competent to perform that delegated task as a result of extra training and skill validation. The ANA specifies that delegation is a transfer of responsibility or assignment of an activity while retaining the accountability for the outcome and the overall care (ANA, 2014; Duffy & McCoy, p. 22).

Some state boards have argued that assignment is the process of directing a nursing assistant to perform a task such as taking blood pressure, a task on which nursing assistants are tested in the certified nursing assistant examination and that would commonly appear in a job description. Others contend that all nursing care is part of the RN scope of practice and therefore that such a task would be delegated rather than assigned. Other nursing leaders argue that only when a task is clearly within the RN's scope of practice, and not included in the role of an AP, is the task delegated. Regardless of whether the allocation of tasks to be done is based on assignment or delegation, in this book, assignment means the "work plan" and connotes the nursing leadership role of human resources deployment in a manner that most wisely promotes the patient's and family's preferred outcome.

Although states vary in their definitions of the functions and processes in professional nursing practice, including that of delegation, the authors use the NCSBN and ANA's definition, including the caveat present in the sentence following the definition: delegation is "transferring to a competent individual the authority to perform a selected nursing task in a selected situation. The nurse retains the accountability for the delegation" (NCSBN, 1995, p. 2). Assignments are work plans that would include tasks the delegatee would have been trained to do in their basic educational program; the nurse "assigns" or distributes work and also "delegates" nursing care as she or he works through others. In advanced personnel roles, such as when certified medication aides are taught to administer medications or when certified medical assistants give injections, the NCSBN (2016) asserts that because of the extensive responsibilities involved, the employers and nurse leaders in the settings where certified medication aides are employed, such as ambulatory care, skilled nursing homes, or home health settings, should regard these procedures as being delegated and AP competencies must be assured (NCSBN, 2016b, p. 7). ANA designates these certified but unlicensed individuals as APs rather than UAPs (ANA & NSCBN 2019). The differences in definitions among states and the differentiation between delegation and assignment are perplexing to nurses. Because both processes are similar in terms of the actions and thinking processes of the RN from a practical standpoint, this workbook will merge the definitions to mean that RNs delegate or assign tasks when they are allocating work to competent trained individuals, keeping within each state's scope of practice, rules, and organizational job descriptions. Whether assigning or

delegating, the RN is accountable for the total nursing care of the patient and for making choices about which competent person is permitted to perform each task successfully. Whether the RN is delegating or assigning, depending on their state regulations, the expert RN will not ask a team member to perform a task that is beyond the RN's own scope of practice or job description, or a task outside of any person's competencies. In all cases the choices made to allocate work must prioritize which allocation of work is optimal for the patient's safe and effective care (Hansten 2020, in Kelly Vana and Tazbir).

Delegation or Assignment and Supervision

The definitions of delegation and assignment offer some important clues to nursing practice and to the composition of an effective patient care team. The person who makes the decision to ask a person to do something (a task or assignment) must know that the chosen person is competent to perform that task. The RN selects the particular task, given his or her knowledge of the individual patient's condition and that particular circumstance. Because of the nurse's preparation, knowledge, and skill, the RN chooses to render judgments of this kind and stands by the choices made. According to licensure and statute, the nurse is obligated to delegate or assign based on the unique situation, patients, and personnel involved and to provide ongoing follow-up.

Supervision

Whenever nurses delegate or assign, they must also supervise. **Supervision** is defined by the NCSBN as **"the provision of guidance and direction, oversight, evaluation, and follow up by the licensed nurse for accomplishment of a nursing task delegated to nursing assistive personnel"** and by the ANA as **"the active process of directing, guiding, and influencing the outcome of an individual's performance of a task"** (ANA, 2014; Duffy & McCoy, p. 23). Each state may use a different explanation, such as Washington State's supervision definition: **"initial direction… periodic inspection… and the authority to require corrective action"** (Washington Administrative Code 246-840-010 Definitions, https://app.leg.wa.gov/wac/default.aspx?cite=246-840-010). The act of delegating or assigning is just the beginning of the RN's responsibility. As for the accountability of the delegatees (or people given the task duty), these individuals are accountable for a) accepting only the responsibilities that they know they are competent to complete, b) maintaining their skill proficiency, c) pursuing ongoing communication with the team's leader, and d) completing and documenting the task appropriately (ANA and NCSBN, 2019, p. 9). For example, nursing assistants who are unprepared or untrained to complete a task should say as much when asked and can then decline to perform that particular duty. In such a situation, the RN would determine whether to allocate time to train the AP and review the skill as it is learned, to delegate the task to another competent person, to do it herself or himself, or to make arrangements for later skill training. The RN's job continues throughout the performance and results of task completion, evaluation of the care, and ongoing feedback to the delegatees.

Scope of Practice for RNs, LPNs/LVNs, and APs

Heretofore this text has discussed national recommendations for definitions. National trends suggest that nursing is moving toward standardized licensure through mutual recognition compacts and multistate licensure, and as of April 2019, 31 states had adopted the nurse license compact allowing a nurse in a member state to possess one state's license and practice in another member state, with several states pending (NCSBN, 2019a). Standardized and multistate licensure supports electronic practice and promotes improved practice flexibility. Each RN must know his or her own state's regulations, however. Definitions still differ from state to state, as do regulations about the tasks that nursing assistants or other APs are allowed to perform in various settings.

For example, APs are delegated tasks for which they have been trained and that they are currently competent to perform for stable patients in uncomplicated circumstances; these are routine, simple, repetitive, common activities not requiring nursing judgment, such as activities of daily living, hygiene, feeding, and ambulation. Some states have generated statutes and/or rules that list specific tasks that can or cannot be delegated. Nevertheless, trends indicate that more tasks will be delegated as research supports such delegation through evidence of positive outcomes. Acute care hospital nursing assistants have not historically been authorized to administer medications. In some states, specially certified medication assistants administer oral medications in the community (group homes) and in some long-term care facilities, although there is substantial variability in state-designated certified nursing assistant (CNA) duties (McMullen et al., 2015). More states are employing specially trained nursing assistants as CMAs (certified medication assistants) or MA-Cs (medication assistants-certified) to administer routine, nonparenteral medications in long-term care or community settings with training as recommended by the NCSBN's Model Curriculum (NCSBN, 2016, p. 7). For over a decade, Washington state has altered the statute and related administrative codes to allow trained nursing assistants in home or community-based settings, such as boarding homes and adult family homes, to administer insulin if the patient is an appropriate candidate (in a stable and predictable condition) and if the nursing assistant has been appropriately trained and supervised for the first 4 weeks of performing this task (Revised Code of Washington, 2012). Nationally, consistency of state regulation of AP medication administration in residential care and adult day-care settings has been stated to be inadequate to ensure RN oversight of APs (Carder & O'Keeffe, 2016).

This research finding should serve as a caution for all practicing in these settings. Other studies of nursing homes and assisted living facilities show evidence of role confusion among RNs, LPN/LVNs, and APs (Mueller et al., 2018; Dyck & Novotny, 2018). In ambulatory care settings, medical assistants (MAs) are being used extensively, supervised by RNs, LPNs (depending on the state), physicians, or other providers, and nurses are cautioned to know both the state nursing and medical regulations. In some cases (Maryland, for example), a physician could delegate peripheral IV initiation to an MA with on-site supervision, but in some states an LPN is prohibited from this same task (Maningo and Panthofer, 2018, p.2).

In all states, nursing judgment is used to delegate tasks that fall within, but never exceed, the nurse's legal scope of practice, and an RN always makes decisions based on the individual patient situation. An RN may decide not to delegate the task of feeding a patient if the patient is dysphagic and the nursing assistant is not familiar with feeding techniques. A "Lessons Learned from Litigation" article in the *American Journal of Nursing* in May 2014 describes the hazards of improper RN assignment, delegation, and supervision of patient feeding, resulting in a patient's death and licensure sanctions (Brous, 2014).

The scope of practice for LPNs or LVNs also differs from state to state and is continually evolving. For example, in Texas, LPNs are prohibited from delegating nursing tasks; only RNs are allowed to delegate (Texas Board of Nursing, 2019, http://www.bon.texas.gov/faq_delegati on.asp#t6), whereas in Washington state an LPN could delegate to nursing assistants in some settings (listed as hospitals, nursing homes, clinics, and ambulatory surgery centers) (Washington Nursing Care Quality Assurance Commission 2019, https://www.doh.wa.gov/Portals/1/ Documents/6000/NCAO13.pdf). Although practicing nurses know that LPNs often review a patient's condition and perform data-gathering tasks such as observation and auscultation, RNs remain accountable for the total assessment of a patient, including the synthesis and analysis of reported and reviewed information to lead care planning based on the nursing diagnosis. In their periodic review of actual practice by LPNs, the NCSBN found that assigning client care or related tasks to other LPNs or APs was ranked sixth in frequency, with monitoring activities of APs ranked seventh (NCSBN, 2019, p. 156). IV therapy and administration of blood products or total parenteral nutrition by LPNs/LVNs also vary widely. Even in states where regulations allow LPNs/LVNs to administer blood products, a given health care organization's policies or job descriptions may limit practice and place additional safeguards because of the life-threatening risk involved in the administration of blood products and other medications. The RN must review the agency's job descriptions as well as the state regulations because either is changeable.

LPN/LVN practice continues to evolve, and in any state, tasks to support the assessment, planning, intervention, and evaluation phases of the nursing process can be allocated. When it is clear that a task could possibly be delegated to a skilled delegatee according to your state's scope of practice rules and is not prohibited by the organization policies, the principles of delegation and/or assignment remain the same. The totality of the nursing process remains the responsibility of the RN. Also, the total nursing care of the patient rests squarely on the RN's shoulders, no matter which competent and skilled individual is asked to perform care activities. To obtain more information about the statute and rules in a given state and to access decision trees and other helpful aides to delegation and supervision, visit the NCSBN website at http://www.ncsbn.org. The state practice act for each state is linked at that site.

ASSIGNMENT PROCESS

In current hospital environments, the process of assigning or creating a work plan is dependent on who is available, present, and accounted for and what their roles and competencies are for each shift. Assignment has been understood to be the "work plan" or **"the distribution of work that each staff member is responsible for during a given work period"** (American Nurses Association (ANA), Duffy & McCoy, 2014, p. 22). Classical care delivery models once known as *total patient care* have been transformed into a combination of team, functional, and primary care nursing, depending on the projected patient outcomes, the present patient state, and the available staff. Assignments must be created with knowledge of the following issues (Hansten and Jackson, 2009, pp. 207–208, Hansten, 2020 in Kelly Vana and Tazbir):

- How complex is the patient's required care?
- What are the dynamics of the patient's status and their stability?
- How complex is the assessment and ongoing evaluation?
- What kind of infection control is necessary?
- Are there any individual safety precautions?
- Is there special technology involved in the care, and who is skilled in its use?
- How much supervision and oversight will be needed based on the staff's numbers and expertise?
- How available are the supervising RNs?
- How will the physical location of patients affect the time and availability of care?
- Can continuity of care be maintained?
- Are there any personal reasons to allocate duties for a particular patient, or are there nurse or patient preferences that should be taken into account? Factors such as staff difficulties with a particular diagnosis, patient preferences for an employee's care on a previous admission, or a staff member's need for a particular learning experience will be taken into account.
- Is there an acuity rating system that will help distribute care based on a point or number system?

For more information on care delivery modalities, refer to the texts by Hansten and Jackson (2009) or access Hansten's webinars related to assignment and care delivery models at http://learning.hansten.com/ and Alfaro-LeFevre (2017) listed in the References section. Whichever type of care delivery plan is chosen for each particular shift or within your practice arena, the relationship with the patient and the results that the patient wants to achieve must be foremost, followed by the placing together of the right pieces in the form of competent team members, to compose the complete picture (Hansten, 2019).

DELEGATION AND ASSIGNMENT: THE FIVE RIGHTS

As you contemplate the questions in this workbook, you can use mnemonic devices to order your thinking process, such as the "five rights." The right task is assigned to the right person in the right circumstances. The RN then offers the right direction and communication and the right supervision and evaluation (Hansten and Jackson, 2009, pp. 205–206; NCSBN, 1995, pp. 2–3; Hansten, 2014a, p. 70; NCSBN, 2016b, p. 8; ANA & NCSBN, 2019, p. 4).

Right Task

Returning to the guideposts for navigating care, the patient's four Ps (purpose, picture, plan, and part), the right task is a task that, in the nurse's best judgment, is one that can be safely delegated for this patient, given the patient's current condition (picture) and future preferred outcomes (purpose, picture), if the nurse has a competent willing individual available to perform it. Although the RN may believe that he or she personally would be the best person to accomplish this task, the nurse must prioritize the best use of his or her time given a myriad of factors, such as: What other tasks and processes must I do because I am the only RN on this team? Which tasks can be delegated based on state regulations and my thorough knowledge of job descriptions here in this facility? How skilled are the personnel working here today? Who else could be available to help if necessary?

In its draft model language for nursing APs, the NCSBN lists criteria for determining nursing activities that can be delegated. The following are recommended for the nurse's consideration. It should be kept in mind that the nursing process and nursing judgment cannot be delegated.

- Knowledge and skills of the delegatee
- Verification of clinical competence by the employer
- Stability of the patient's condition
- Service setting variables such as available resources (including the nurse's accessibility) and methods of communication, complexity and frequency of care, and proximity and numbers of patients relative to staff

APs are not to be allocated the duties of the nursing process of assessment (except gathering data), nursing diagnosis, planning, implementation (except those tasks delegated/assigned), or evaluation. Professional clinical judgment or reasoning and decision making related to the manner in which the RN makes sense of the patient's data and clinical progress cannot be delegated or assigned (ANA & NCSBN, 2019, p. 3).

Right Circumstances

Recall the importance of the context in clinical decision making. Not only do rules and regulations adjust based on the area of practice (i.e., home health care, acute care, schools, ambulatory clinics, long-term care), but patient conditions and the preferred patient results must also be considered. If information is not available, a best judgment must be made. Often RNs must balance the need to know as much as possible and the time available to obtain the information. The instability of patients immediately postoperatively or in the intensive care unit (ICU) means that a student nurse will have to be closely supervised and partnered with an experienced RN. The questions in this workbook give direction as to context and offer hints to the circumstances.

For example, in long-term care skilled nursing facilities, LPNs/LVNs often function as "team leaders" with ongoing care planning and oversight by a smaller number of on-site RNs. Some EDs use paramedics, who may be regulated by the state emergency system statutes, in different roles in hospitals. Medical clinics often employ "medical assistants" who function under the direction and supervision of physicians, other providers, and RNs. Community group homes, assisted living facilities, and other health care providers beyond acute care hospitals seek to create safe and effective care delivery systems for the growing number of older adults. Whatever the setting or circumstance, the nurse is accountable to know the specific laws and regulations that apply.

Right Person

Licensure, Certification, and Role Description

One of the most commonly voiced concerns during workshops with staff nurses across the nation is, "How can I trust the delegatees?" Knowing the licensure, role, and preparation of each member of the team is the first step in determining competency. What tasks does a patient care technician (PCT) perform in this facility? What is the role of an LPN/LVN? Are different levels of LPN/LVN designated here (LPN I or II)? Nearly 100 different titles for APs have been developed in care settings across the country. To effectively assign or delegate, the RN must know the role descriptions of co-workers as well as his or her own.

Strengths and Weaknesses

The personal strengths and weaknesses of everyday team members are no mystery. Their skills are discovered through practice, positive and negative experiences, and an ever-present but unreliable rumor mill. An expert RN helps create better team results by using strengths in assigning personnel to make the most of their gifts. The most compassionate team members will be assigned work with the hospice patient and his or her family. The supervising nurse helps identify performance flaws and develops staff by providing judicious use of learning assignments. For example, a novice nursing assistant can be partnered with an experienced oncology RN during the assistant's first experiences with a terminally ill patient.

When working with students, float nurses, or other temporary personnel, nurses sometimes forget that the assigning RN has the duty to determine competency. Asking personnel about their previous experiences and about their understanding of the work duties, as well as pairing them with a strong unit staff member, is as essential as providing the ongoing support and supervision needed throughout the shift. If your mother was an ICU patient and her nurse was an inexperienced float from the rehabilitation unit, what level of leadership and direction would that nurse need from an experienced ICU RN? Many hospitals delegate only tasks and not overall patient responsibility, a functional form of assignment, to temporary personnel who are unfamiliar with the clinical area.

Right Direction and Communication

Now that the right staff member is being delegated the right task for each particular situation and setting, team members must find out what they need to do and how the tasks must be done. Relaying instructions about the plan for the shift or even for a specific task is not as simple as it seems. Some RNs believe that a written assignment board provides enough information to proceed because "everyone knows his or her job," but others spend copious amounts of time giving overly detailed directions to bored staff. The "four Cs" of initial direction will help clarify the salient points of this process (Hansten and Jackson, 2009, pp. 287–288; Hansten, 2021 in Zerwekh and Garneau, p. 316). Instructions and ongoing direction must be clear, concise, correct, and complete.

Clear communication is information that is understood by the listener. An ambiguous question such as: "Can you get the new patient?" is not helpful when there are several new patients and returning surgical patients, and "getting" could mean transporting, admitting, or taking full responsibility for the care of the patient. Asking the delegatee to restate the instructions and work plan can be helpful to determine whether the communication is clear.

Concise statements are those that give enough but not too much additional information. The student nurse who merely wants to know how to turn on the chemical strip analyzer machine does not need a full treatise on the transit of potassium and glucose through the cell membrane. Too much or irrelevant information confuses the listener and wastes precious time.

Correct communication is that which is accurate and is aligned to rules, regulations, or job descriptions. Are the room number, patient name, and other identifiers correct? Are there two patients with similar last names? Can this task be delegated to this individual? Correct communication is not cloudy or confusing (Hansten and Jackson, 2009, pp. 287–288; Hansten, 2021 in Zerwekh and Garneau, p. 318).

Complete communication leaves no room for doubt on the part of supervisor or delegatees. Staff members often say, "I would do whatever the RNs want if they would just tell me what they want me to do and how to do it." Incomplete communication wins the top prize for creating team strife and substandard work. Assuming that staff "know" what to do and how to do it, along with what information to report and when, creates havoc, rework, and frustration for patients and staff alike. Each staff member should have in mind a clear map or plan for the day, what to do and why, and what and when to report to the team leader. Parameters for reporting and the results that should be expected are often left in the team leader's brain rather than being discussed and spelled out in sufficient detail. RNs are accountable for clear, concise, correct, and complete initial and ongoing direction.

Right Supervision and Evaluation

After prioritization, assignment, and delegation have been considered, determined, and communicated, the RN remains accountable for the total care of the patients throughout the tour of duty. Recall that the definition of **supervision** includes not only initial direction but also that "supervision is the active process of directing, guiding, and influencing the outcome of an individual's performance of a task. Similarly, NCSBN defines supervision as "the provision of guidance or direction, oversight, evaluation and follow-up by the licensed nurse for the accomplishment of a delegated nursing task by assistive personnel" (ANA, 2014, in Duffy and McCoy, p. 23). RNs may not actually perform each task of care, but they must oversee the ongoing progress and results obtained, reviewing staff performance. Evaluation of the care provided, and adequate documentation of the tasks and outcomes, must be included in this last of the five rights. On a typical unit in an acute care facility, assisted living, or long-term care setting, the RN can ensure optimal performance as the RN begins the shift by holding a short "second report" meeting with APs, outlining the day's plan and the plan for each patient, and giving initial direction at that time. Subsequent short team update or "checkpoint" meetings should be held before and after breaks and meals and before the end of the shift (Hansten, 2005, 2008a, 2008b, 2019). During each short update, feedback is often offered, and plans are altered. The last checkpoint presents all team members with an opportunity to give feedback to one another using the step-by-step feedback process (Hansten, 2008a, pp. 79–84; Hansten, 2021, in Zerweck and Garneau, pp. 301–302).

This step is often called the "debriefing" checkpoint or huddle, in which the team's processes are also examined. In ambulatory care settings, this checkpoint may be toward the end of each patient's visit or the end of the shift; in home health care, these conversations are often conducted on a weekly basis. Questions such as, "What would you recommend I do differently if we worked together tomorrow on the same group of patients?" and "What can we do better as a team to help us navigate the patients toward their preferred results?" will help the team function more effectively in the future.

1. **The team member's input should be solicited first.** "I noted that the vital signs for the first four patients aren't yet on the electronic record. Do you know what's been done?" rather than "WHY haven't those vital signs been recorded yet?" At the end of the shift, the questions might be global, as in "How did we do today?" "What would you do differently if we had it to do over?" "What should I do differently tomorrow?"

2. **Credit should be given for all that has been accomplished.** "Oh, so you have the vital signs done, but they aren't recorded? Great, I'm so glad they are done so I can find out about Ms. Johnson's temperature before I call Dr. Smith." "You did a fantastic job with cleaning Mr. Hu after his incontinence episodes; his family is very appreciative of our respect for his dignity."

3. **Observations or concerns should be offered.** "The vital signs are routinely recorded on the electronic medical record (EMR) before patients are sent for surgery and procedures and before the doctor's round so that we can see the big picture of patients' progress before they leave the unit and to make sure they are stable for their procedures." Or, "I think I should have assigned another RN to Ms. A. I had no idea that your mother recently died of breast cancer."

4. **The delegatee should be asked for ideas on how to resolve the issue.** "What are your thoughts on how you could order your work to get the vital signs on the EMR before 8:30 AM?" Or, "What would you like to do with your work plan for tomorrow? Should we change Ms. A.'s team?"

5. **A course of action and plan for the future should be agreed upon.** "That sounds great. Practice use of the handheld computers today before you leave, and that should resolve the issue. When we work together tomorrow, let me know whether that resolves the time issue for recording; if not, we will go to another plan." Or, "If you still feel that you want to stay with this assignment tomorrow after you've slept on it, we will keep it as is. If not, please let me know first thing tomorrow morning when you awaken so we can change all the assignments before the staff arrive."

PRACTICE BASED ON RESEARCH EVIDENCE

Rationale for Maximizing Nursing Leadership Skills at the Point of Care

If the skills presented in this book are used to save lives by providing care prioritized to attend to the most unstable patients first, optimally delegated to be delivered by the right personnel, and assigned using appropriate language with the most motivational and conscientious supervisory follow-up, then clinical outcomes should be optimal and work satisfaction should flourish. Solid correlational research evidence has been lacking related to "the best use of personnel to multiply the RN's ability to remain vigilant over patient progress and avoid failures to rescue, but common sense would advise that better delegation and supervision skills would prevent errors and omissions as well as unobserved patient decline" (Hansten, 2008b, 2019).

In an era of value-based purchasing and health care reimbursement based on clinical results with linkages for care along the continuum from site to site, an RN's accountability has irrevocably moved beyond task orientation to leadership practices that ensure better outcomes for patients, families, and populations. The necessity of efficiency and effectiveness in health care means that RNs must delegate and supervise appropriately so that all tasks that can be safely assigned to APs are completed flawlessly. Patient safety experts have linked interpersonal communication errors and teamwork communication gaps as major sources of medical errors and The Joint Commission associated these as root causes of 70% or more of serious reportable events (Grant, 2016, p. 11). Severe events that harm patients (sentinel events) can occur through inadequate hand-offs between caregivers and along the health care continuum as patients are transferred (The Joint Commission, 2017).

Nurses are accountable for processes as well as outcomes measures so that insurers will reimburse health care organizations. If hospital-acquired conditions occur, such as pressure injuries falls with injury, and some infections, reimbursement for the care of that condition will be negatively impacted.

- Nurses have been reported to spend more than half their time on tasks other than patient care, including searching for team members and internal communications (Voalte Special Report, 2013). Shift report at the bedside, along with better initial direction and a plan for supervision during the day, all ultimately decrease time wasted when nurses must attempt to connect with team members when delegation and assignment processes do not include the five rights. At one facility in the Midwest, shift hand-offs were reduced to 10 to 15 minutes per shift per RN as a result of a planned approach to initial direction and care planning, which thus saved each RN 30 to 45 minutes per day (Hansten, 2008a, p. 34). Better

use of nursing and AP time can result in more time to care for patients, giving RNs the opportunity to teach patients self-care or to maintain functional status.

- When nurses did not appropriately implement the five rights of delegation and supervision with assistive personnel, errors occurred that potentially could have been avoided with better RN leadership behaviors. Early research about the impact of supervision on errors showed that about 14% of task errors or care omissions related to teamwork were because of lack of RN direction or communication, and approximately 12% of the issues stemmed from lack of supervision or follow-up (Standing, Anthony, & Hertz, 2001). Lack of communication among staff members has been an international issue leading to care that is not completed appropriately (Diab & Ebrahim, 2019). Errors can result in uncompensated conditions or readmissions; unhappy patients and providers; disgruntled health care purchasers; and a disloyal, anxious patient community (Hansten, 2019).

- Teamwork and job satisfaction have been found to be negatively correlated with over-delegation and a hierarchical relationship between nurses and assistive personnel (Kalisch 2015, p. 266–227), but offering feedback effectively has been shown to improve team thinking and performance (Mizne, D., 2018, https://www.15five.com/blog/7-employee-engagement-trends-2018/). Workplace injuries, expensive employee turnover, and patient safety have been linked with employee morale. Daily or weekly feedback has been requested by a majority of teams and this could be achieved by excellent delegation, assignment, and supervision shift routines (McNee, 2017, https://www.mcknights.com/blogs/guest-columns/nurse-morale-and-its-impact-on-ltc/). Best practices for deployment of personnel include a connection to patient outcomes, which can occur during initial direction and debriefing supervision checkpoints (Hansten, 2021 in LaCharity and Garneau).

- Unplanned readmissions to acute care within 30 days of discharge are linked to potential penalties and reduced reimbursement. Inadequate RN initial direction and supervision of APs can lead to missed mobilization, hydration, and nutrition of patients, thereby discharging deconditioned patients, and can be traced to ED visits and subsequent readmissions. Reimbursement bundling for specific care pathways such as total joint replacements or acute exacerbation of chronic obstructive pulmonary disease requires that team communication and RN supervision of coworkers along the full continuum must be seamless from ambulatory care to acute care, rehabilitation, and home settings (Kalisch, 2015; Hansten, 2019).

- As public quality transparency and competition for best value become the norm, ineffective delegation has been a significant source of missed care, such as lack of care planning, lack of turning or ambulation, delayed or missed nutrition, and lack of hygiene (Bittner et al., 2011; Kalisch, 2015, pp. 266–270). These care omissions can be contributing factors for the occurrence of unreimbursed "never events" (events that should never occur), such as pressure ulcers and pneumonia, as well as prolonged lengths of stay. Other nurse-sensitive quality indicators such as catheter-associated urinary tract infections could be correlated to omitted perineal hygiene and inattention to discontinuation of catheters. Useful models that link delegation with care omissions and ensuing care hazards such as thrombosis, pressure injuries, constipation, and infection, combined with a Swiss Cheese Safety Model showing defensive steps against health care–acquired conditions and errors through excellence in RN leadership, can be accessed in the August 2014 *Nurse Leader* at https://doi.org/10.1016/j.mnl.2013.10.007 (Hansten, 2014a; Hansten, 2020 in Kelly Vana and Tazbir).

- In perioperative nursing, such omissions as lack of warming, oral care, head elevation and deep breathing, can lead to postoperative pneumonia and lack of optimal healing (Ralph and Viljoen, 2018). Many of these interventions could be delegated or assigned.

Evidence does indicate that appropriate nursing judgment in prioritization, delegation, and supervision can save time and improve communication and thereby improve care, patient safety, clinical outcomes, and job satisfaction, potentially saving patient-days and absenteeism and recruitment costs. Patient satisfaction, staff satisfaction, and clinical results decline when nursing care is poor. Potential reimbursement is lost, patients and families suffer, and the health of our communities decays when RNs do not assume the leadership necessary to work effectively with all team members (Bittner et al., 2011, Kalisch, 2015, Hansten, 2019).

PRINCIPLES FOR IMPLEMENTATION OF PRIORITIZATION, DELEGATION, AND ASSIGNMENT

Return to our goalposts of the four Ps (purpose, picture, plan, and part) as a framework as you answer the questions in this workbook and further develop your own expertise and recall the following principles:

- The RN should always start with the patient's and family's preferred outcomes in mind. The RN is first clear about the patient's purpose for accessing care and his or her picture for a successful outcome.
- The RN should refer to the applicable state nursing practice statute and rules as well as the organization's job descriptions for current information about roles and responsibilities of RNs, LPNs/LVNs, and APs. (These are the roles or the parts that people play.)

- Student nurses, novices, float nurses, and other infrequent workers also require variable levels of supervision, guidance, or support (The workers' abilities and roles become a piece of the plan.) (NCSBN, 2016b).
- The RN is accountable for nursing judgment decisions and for ongoing supervision of any care that is delegated or assigned.
- The RN cannot delegate the nursing process (in particular the assessment, planning, and evaluation phases) or clinical judgment to a non-RN. Some interventions or data-gathering activities may be delegated based on the circumstances.
- The RN must know as much as practical about the patients and their conditions, as well as the skills and competency of team members, to prioritize, delegate, and assign. Decisions must be specifically individualized to the patient, the delegatees, and the situation.
- In a clinical situation, everything is fluid and shifting. No priority, assignment, or delegation is written indelibly and cannot be altered. The RN in charge of a unit, a team, or one patient is accountable to choose the best course to achieve the patient's and family's preferred results.

Best wishes in completing this workbook! The authors invite you to use the questions as an exercise in assembling the pieces to the puzzle that will become a picture of health-promoting practice.

REFERENCES

Alfaro-Lefevre R: *Critical thinking, clinical reasoning, and clinical judgment: a practical approach*, ed 6, St Louis, 2017, Saunders.

American Nurses Association. National Guidelines for Nursing Delegation. Effective 4/1/2019, by ANA Board of Directors/NCSBN Board of Directors. Retrieved April 12, 2019 from https://www.nursingworld.org/practice-policy/nursing-excellence/official-position-statements/id/joint-statement-on-delegation-by-ANA-and-NCSBN/ [file available to members only at https://www.nursingworld.org/globalassets/practiceandpolicy/nursing-excellence/ana-position-statements-secure/ana-ncsbn-joint-statement-on-delegation.pdf, accessed April 12, 2019.]

American Nurses Association, Duffy M, Fields McCoy S: *Delegation and YOU: when to delegate and to whom*, Silver Springs, MD, 2015. ANA.

Bittner N, Gravlin G, Hansten R, Kalisch B: Unraveling care omissions, *J Nurs Adm* 41(12):510–512, 2011.

Brous E: Lessons learned from litigation: the case of Bernard Travaglini, *Am J Nurs* (114):5:68–70, 2014 5.

Carder PC, O'Keeffe J: State regulation of medication administration by unlicensed assistive personnel in residential care and adult day services settings, *Res Gerontol Nurs* 7:1–14, 2016.

Diab G, Ebrahim R: Factors leading to missed nursing care among nurses at selected hospitals, *Am J Nurs Res* 7 (2): 136-147, 2019.

Dyck M, Novotny N: Exploring reported practice habits of registered nurses and licensed practical nurses at Illinois nursing homes, *J Nurs Reg* 9 (2): 18-30, 2018.

Grant V: Sharpening your legal IQ: safeguarding your license, *Viewpoint* 38(3):10–12, 2016.

Hansten R: Relationship and results-oriented healthcare: evaluate the basics, *J Nurs Adm* 35(12):522–524, 2005.

Hansten R: Leadership at the point of care: nursing delegation, 2011. Retrieved May 31, 2012, from http://www.MyFreeCE.com.

Hansten R: *Relationship and results oriented healthcare™ planning and implementation manual*, Port Ludlow, Wash, 2008a, Hansten Healthcare PLLC.

Hansten R: Why nurses still must learn to delegate, *Nurse Leader* 6(5):19–26, 2008b.

Hansten R, Jackson M: *Clinical delegation skills: a handbook for professional practice*, ed 4, Sudbury, Mass, 2009, Jones & Bartlett.

Hansten R: *The master coach manual for the relationship & results oriented healthcare program*, Port Ludlow, Wash, 2014b, Hansten Healthcare PLLC.

Hansten R: Coach as chief correlator of tasks to results through delegation skill and teamwork development, *Nurse Leader*, 12 (4):69–73, 2014a.

Hansten R: Another Look at RN leadership skill level and patient outcomes. *LinkedIn Pulse*. Retrieved April 21, 2019 from https://www.linkedin.com/pulse/another-look-rn-leadership-skill-level-patient-hansten-rn-mba-phd.

Hansten R: Delegation, assignment, and supervision in Kelly Vana P & Tazbir J, ed. *Nursing leadership and management*, 4th Ed. Hoboken, NJ. 2020 (in press), Wiley.

Hansten R: Delegation in the clinical setting. In Zerwekh J, Garneau A, editors: *Nursing today: transitions and trends*, ed 10, St Louis, 2021, Elsevier.

Interprofessional Education Collaborative. Core competencies for interprofessional collaborative practice: 2016 update. Washington, DC: Interprofessional Education Collaborative. Retrieved April 16, 2019 from 780E69ED19E2B3A5&disposition=0&alloworigin=1.

Kalisch B: *Errors of Omission: How missed nursing care imperils patents*. Silver Springs, MD., 2015, ANA.

Kalisch B: Missed nursing care, *J Nurs Care Qual* 21(4):306–313, 2006.

Maningo MJ, Panthofer N: Appropriate delegation in an ambulatory care setting AAACN *Viewpoint* 40 (1): 1-2, 2018.

McMullen TL, Resnick B, Chin-Hansen J, et al: Certified nurse aide scope of practice: state-by-state differences in allowable delegated activities, *J Am Med Dir Assoc* 6(1):20–24, 2015.

Mizne D. 7 fascinating employee engagement trends for 2018. 15Five.com. Retrieved April 21, 2019 from https://www.15five.com/blog/7-employee-engagement-trends-2018/, pp. 1-11, 2018.

McNee B. Nurse morale and its impact on LTC, McKnights Long-Term Care News, June 28, 2017. Retrieved April 21, 2019 from https://www.mcknights.com/blogs/guest-columns/nurse-morale-and-its-impact-on-ltc/, pp. 1-2, 2017

Mueller C, Vogelsmeier A, Anderson R, McConnell E, & Corazzini K. Interchangeability of licensed nurses in nursing homes: perspective of directors of nursing. *The End to End Journal*, 1, 1-27, 2018.

National Council of State Boards of Nursing: *Delegation: concepts and decision-making process*, Issues December:1–4, 1995.

National Council of State Boards of Nursing. 2018 LPN/VN Practice Analysis: Linking the NCLEX-PN Examination to Practice. NCSBN Research Brief vol. 75: March 2019. Retrieved April 17, 2019 from https://www.ncsbn.org/13443.htm.m 2019.

National Council of State Boards of Nursing: National guidelines for nursing delegation. *J Nurs Reg* 7(1):5–14, 2016b. Accessed April 21, 2019 at https://www.ncsbn.org/NCSBN_Delegation_Guidelines.pdf

National Council of State Boards of Nursing: Participating states in the nurse licensure compact implementation. Retrieved April 17, 2019 from https://www.ncsbn.org/compacts.htm., 2019.

QSEN Institute: QSEN Institute Website: QSEN Competencies. Retrieved April 19, 2019 from http://qsen.org/competencies/graduate-ksas/.

Ralph N, Viljoen B. Fundamentals of missed care: Implications for the perioperative environment, *ACORN Journal of Perioperative Nursing* 31 (3): Spring, 3-4, 2018.

Revised Code of Washington, Title 18, Chapter 18.79, Section 18.79.260, Registered nurse—activities allowed—delegation of tasks. Retrieved April 18, 2019 from http://apps.leg.wa.gov/RCW/default.aspx?cite=18.79.260.

Silvestri L, Silvestri A. Saunders 2018-2019 Strategies for Test Success: p. 63. St Louis, 2018, Elsevier.

Standing T, Anthony M, Hertz J: Nurses' narratives of outcomes after delegation to unlicensed assistive personnel, *Outcomes Manag Nurs Pract* 5(1):18–23, 2001.

The Joint Commission. Inadequate hand-off communication. *Sentinel Event Alert Issue* 58, September 12, 2017.

Texas Board of Nursing 2013. "Frequently Asked Questions: Delegation:" P. 2 (1-7), 2013. Retrieved April 21, 2019 from http://www.bon.texas.gov/faq_delegation.asp#t6.

Voalte: Special Report top 10 clinical communication trends 2013 pp. 1-16. Retrieved April 24, 2019 from https://www.voalte.com/press-releases/new-survey-finds-hospital-nurses-spend-half-shift-tasks-patient-care.

Washington State Administrative Code 246-840-010 Definitions. Retrieved April 19, 2019 from https://app.leg.wa.gov/wac/default.aspx?cite=246-840-010, 2019.

Washington State Department of Health Nursing Care Quality Assurance Commission Advisory Opinion 13.01 2019 Registered Nurse and Licensed Practical Nurse Scope of Practice, 3-8-2019: p. 4 (1-12). Retrieved April 25, 2019 from https://www.doh.wa.gov/Portals/1/Documents/6000/NCAO13.pdf.

RECOMMENDED RESOURCES

Alfaro-Lefevre R: *Critical thinking, clinical reasoning, and clinical judgment: a practical approach*, ed 6, St Louis, 2017, Saunders.

Hansten R: *The master coach manual for the relationship & results oriented healthcare program*, Port Ludlow, Wash, 2014, Hansten Healthcare PLLC.

Hansten R: *Relationship and results oriented healthcare™ planning and implementation manual*, Port Ludlow, Wash, 2008, Hansten Healthcare PLLC.

Hansten R, Jackson M: *Clinical delegation skills: a handbook for professional practice*, ed 4, Sudbury, Mass, 2009, Jones & Bartlett.

Hansten R. Coach as chief correlator of tasks to results through delegation skill and teamwork development. *Nurse Leader* 12(4): 69–73.

Hansten Healthcare PLLC website, http://www.Hansten.com or http://www.RROHC.com. Check for new delegation/supervision resources, online delegation, and assignment education modules at http://learning.Hansten.com/.

National Council of State Boards of Nursing website, http://www.ncsbn.org. Contains links to state boards and abundant resources relating to delegation and supervision. Also download the ANA and NCSBN Joint Statement on Delegation. The decision trees and step-by-step process through the five rights are exceptionally clear and a great review to prepare for the NCLEX at https://www.ncsbn.org/NCSBN_Delegation_Guidelines.pdf and https://www.ncsbn.org/Delegation_joint_statement_NCSBN-ANA.pdf

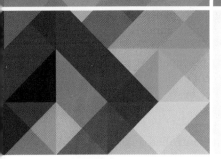

Questions

1. Based on the principles of pain treatment, which consideration comes **first**?
   1. Treatment is based on patient goals.
   2. A multidisciplinary approach is needed.
   3. Patient's perception of pain must be accepted.
   4. Drug side effects must be prevented and managed.

2. According to Centers for Disease Control and Prevention (CDC) guidelines for opioid use for patients with chronic pain, which actions are part of the nurse's responsibility related to the current opioid crisis? **Select all that apply.**
   1. Recognize that negative attitudes toward substance abusers is a barrier to patient compliance.
   2. Access electronic prescription drug monitoring program whenever patients receive an opioid prescription.
   3. Learn to recognize the signs and symptoms of opioid overdose and the proper use of naloxone.
   4. Use a tone of voice and facial expression that convey acceptance and understanding of patients who are addicted.
   5. Report health care providers who fail to safely prescribe opioids according to the guidelines.

3. On the first day after surgery, a patient who is on a patient-controlled analgesia pump reports that the pain control is inadequate. Which action would the nurse take **first**?
   1. Deliver the bolus dose per standing order.
   2. Contact the health care provider (HCP) to increase the dose.
   3. Try nonpharmacologic comfort measures.
   4. Assess the pain for location, quality, and intensity.

4. The team is providing emergency care to a patient who received an excessive dose of opioid pain medication. Which task is **best** to assign to the LPN/LVN?
   1. Calling the health care provider (HCP) to report SBAR (situation, background, assessment, recommendation)
   2. Giving naloxone and evaluating response to therapy

3. Monitoring the respiratory status for the first 30 minutes
4. Applying oxygen per nasal cannula as ordered

5. What is the **best** way to schedule medication for a patient with constant pain?
   1. As needed at the patient's request
   2. Before painful procedures
   3. IV bolus after pain assessment
   4. Around-the-clock

6. Which patient is at **greatest** risk for respiratory depression when receiving opioids for analgesia?
   1. Older adult patient with chronic pain related to joint immobility
   2. Patient with a heroin addiction and back pain
   3. Young female patient with advanced multiple myeloma
   4. Opioid-naïve adolescent with an arm fracture and cystic fibrosis

7. The home health nurse is interviewing an older patient with a history of rheumatoid arthritis who reports "feeling pretty good, except for the pain and stiffness in my joints when I first get out of bed." Which member of the health care team would be notified to aid in the patient's pain?
   1. Health care provider to review the dosage and frequency of pain medication
   2. Physical therapist for evaluation of function and possible exercise therapy
   3. Social worker to locate community resources for complementary therapy
   4. Home health aide to help patient with a warm shower in the morning

8. A patient with diabetic neuropathy reports a burning, electrical-type pain in the lower extremities that is worse at night and not responding to nonsteroidal antiinflammatory drugs. Which medication will the nurse advocate for **first**?
   1. Gabapentin

2. Corticosteroids
3. Hydromorphone
4. Lorazepam

9. When an analgesic is titrated to manage pain, what is the **priority** goal?
   1. Titrate to the smallest dose that provides relief with the fewest side effects.
   2. Titrate upward until the patient is pain free or an acceptable level is reached.
   3. Titrate downward to prevent toxicity, overdose, and adverse effects.
   4. Titrate to a dosage that is adequate to meet the patient's subjective needs.

10. According to recent guidelines from the American Pain Society in collaboration with the American Society of Anesthesiologists, which pain management strategies are **important** for postsurgical patients? **Select all that apply.**
    1. Acetaminophen and/or nonsteroidal anti-inflammatory drugs (NSAIDs) for management of postoperative pain in adults and children without contraindications
    2. Surgical site–specific peripheral regional anesthetic techniques in adults and children for procedures
    3. Neuraxial (epidural) analgesia for major thoracic and abdominal procedures if the patient has risk for cardiac complications or prolonged ileus
    4. Multimodal therapy that could include opioids and nonopioid therapies, regional anesthetic techniques, and nonpharmacologic therapies
    5. IV administration of opioids, rather than oral opioids, for postoperative analgesia
    6. Pain specialists to manage the postoperative pain for all surgical patients

11. When a patient stoically abides with his parent's encouragement to "tough out the pain" rather than risk an addiction to opioids, the nurse recognizes that the sociocultural dimension of pain is the current **priority** for the patient. Which question will the nurse ask?
    1. "Where is the pain located, and does it radiate to other parts of your body?"
    2. "How would you describe the pain, and how is it affecting you?"
    3. "What do you believe about pain medication and drug addiction?"
    4. "How is the pain affecting your activity level and your ability to function?"

12. Which patient is **most** likely to receive opioids for extended periods of time?
    1. A patient with fibromyalgia
    2. A patient with phantom limb pain in the leg

3. A patient with progressive pancreatic cancer
4. A patient with trigeminal neuralgia

13. The nurse is caring for a postoperative patient who reports pain. Based on recent evidence-based guidelines, which approach would be **best**?
    1. Multimodal strategies
    2. Standing orders by protocol
    3. Intravenous patient-controlled analgesia (PCA)
    4. Opioid dosage based on valid numerical scale

14. A newly graduated RN has correctly documented dose and time of medication, but there is no documentation regarding nonpharmaceutical measures. What action should the charge nurse take **first**?
    1. Make a note in the nurse's file and continue to observe clinical performance.
    2. Refer the new nurse to the in-service education department.
    3. Quiz the nurse about knowledge of pain management and pharmacology.
    4. Give praise for documenting dose and time and discuss documentation deficits.

15. Which patients must be assigned to an experienced RN? **Select all that apply.**
    1. Patient who was in an automobile crash and sustained multiple injuries
    2. Patient with chronic back pain related to a workplace injury
    3. Patient who has returned from surgery and has a chest tube in place
    4. Patient with abdominal cramps related to food poisoning
    5. Patient with a severe headache of unknown origin
    6. Patient with chest pain who has a history of arteriosclerosis

16. Which postoperative patient is manifesting the **most** serious negative effect of inadequate pain management?
    1. Demonstrates continuous use of call bell related to unsatisfied needs and discomfort
    2. Develops venous thromboembolism because of immobility caused by pain and discomfort
    3. Refuses to participate in physical therapy because of fear of pain caused by exercises
    4. Feels depressed about loss of function and hopeless about getting relief from pain

17. The nurse is considering seeking clarification for several prescriptions of pain medication. Which patient circumstance is the **priority** concern?
    1. A 35-year-old opioid-naïve adult will receive a basal dose of morphine via IV patient-controlled analgesia.

2. A 65-year-old adult will be discharged with a prescription for nonsteroidal antiinflammatory drugs (NSAIDs).
3. A 25-year-old adult is prescribed as-needed intramuscular (IM) analgesic for pain.
4. A 45-year-old adult is taking oral fluids and foods and has orders for IV morphine.

18. Which patient has the **most** immediate need for IV access to deliver analgesia with rapid titration?
    1. Patient who has sharp chest pain that increases with cough and shortness of breath
    2. Patient who reports excruciating lower back pain with hematuria
    3. Patient who is having an acute myocardial infarction with severe chest pain
    4. Patient who is having a severe migraine with an elevated blood pressure

19. A patient received as-needed morphine, lorazepam, and cyclobenzaprine. The unlicensed assistive personnel (AP) reports that the patient has a respiratory rate of 10 breaths/min. Which action is the **priority**?
    1. Call the health care provider to obtain a prescription for naloxone.
    2. Assess the patient's responsiveness and respiratory status.
    3. Obtain a bag-valve mask and deliver breaths at 20 breaths/min.
    4. Double-check the prescription to see which drugs were prescribed.

20. The patient is diagnosed with an acute migraine by the health care provider (HCP). For which situation is it **most** important to have a discussion with the HCP before medication is prescribed?
    1. The HCP is considering dexamethasone, and the patient has type 2 diabetes.
    2. The HCP is considering subcutaneous sumatriptan, and the patient took ergotamine 3 hours ago.
    3. The HCP is considering valproate sodium, and the patient recently started birth control pills.
    4. The HCP is considering prochlorperazine, and the patient drove himself to the hospital.

21. A patient is crying and grimacing but denies pain and refuses opioid medication because "my brother is a drug addict and has ruined our lives." Which intervention is the **priority** for this patient?
    1. Encourage expression of fears and past experiences.
    2. Respect the patient's wishes and use nonpharmacologic therapies.
    3. Explain that addiction is unlikely when opioids are used for acute pain.
    4. Seek family assistance to support the prescribed therapy.

22. A patient's opioid therapy is being tapered off, and the nurse is watchful for signs of withdrawal. What is one of the **first** signs of withdrawal?
    1. Fever
    2. Nausea
    3. Diaphoresis
    4. Abdominal cramps

23. In the care of patients with pain and discomfort, which task is **most** appropriate to delegate to unlicensed assistive personnel (AP)?
    1. Assisting the patient with preparation of a sitz bath
    2. Monitoring the patient for signs of discomfort while ambulating
    3. Coaching the patient to deep breathe during painful procedures
    4. Evaluating relief after applying a cold compress

24. The health care provider (HCP) prescribed a placebo for a patient with chronic pain. The newly hired nurse feels very uncomfortable administering a placebo. Which action would the new nurse take **first**?
    1. Prepare the prescribed placebo and hand it to the HCP.
    2. Check the hospital policy regarding the use of a placebo.
    3. Follow a personal code of ethics and refuse to participate.
    4. Contact the charge nurse for advice and suggestions.

25. For a cognitively impaired patient who cannot accurately report pain, which action would the nurse take **first**?
    1. Closely assess for nonverbal signs such as grimacing or rocking.
    2. Obtain baseline behavioral indicators from family members.
    3. Note the time of and patient's response to the last dose of analgesic.
    4. Give the maximum as-needed dose within the minimum time frame for relief.

26. A patient with chronic pain reports to the charge nurse that the other nurses have not been responding to requests for pain medication. What is the charge nurse's **initial** action?
    1. Check the medication administration records for the past several days.
    2. Ask the nurse educator to provide in-service training about pain management.
    3. Perform a complete pain assessment on the patient and take a pain history.
    4. Have a conference with the staff nurses to assess their care of this patient.

Answer Key for this chapter begins on p. 19

27. According to recent guidelines from the Center for Disease Control and Prevention for prescribing/using opioid medication for chronic pain, which prescriptions would the nurse question because of the increased risk for opioid overdose? **Select all that apply.**
    1. Extended-release/long-acting (ER/LA) transdermal fentanyl for a patient with fibromyalgia
    2. Time-scheduled ER/LA oxycodone for a patient with chronic low back pain
    3. As-needed (PRN) morphine for arthritis pain for an elderly patient with sleep apnea
    4. 90 morphine milligram equivalents/day for a patient who has a hip fracture
    5. ER/LA methadone PRN for a patient with headache pain
    6. Patient-controlled analgesia (PCA) morphine for a patient with postsurgical abdominal pain

28. Which patients can be appropriately assigned to a newly graduated RN who has recently completed orientation? **Select all that apply.**
    1. Anxious patient with chronic pain who frequently uses the call button
    2. Patient on the second postoperative day who needs pain medication before dressing changes
    3. Patient with acquired immune deficiency syndrome who reports headache and abdominal and pleuritic chest pain
    4. Patient with chronic pain who is to be discharged with a new surgically implanted catheter
    5. Patient who is reporting pain at the site of a peripheral IV line
    6. Patient with a kidney stone who needs frequent as-needed pain medication

29. A patient's spouse comes to the nurse's station and says, "He needs more pain medicine. He is still having a lot of pain." Which response is **best**?
    1. "The medication is prescribed to be given every 4 hours."
    2. "If medication is given too frequently, there are ill effects."
    3. "Please tell him that I will be right there to check on him."
    4. "Let's wait 40 minutes. If he still hurts, I'll call the health care provider."

30. A patient with pain disorder and depression has chronic low back pain. He states, "None of these doctors has done anything to help." Which patient statement is cause for **greatest** concern?
    1. "I twisted my back last night, and now the pain is a lot worse."
    2. "I'm so sick of this pain. I think I'm going to find a way to end it."

    3. "Occasionally, I buy pain killers from a guy in my neighborhood."
    4. "I'm going to sue you and the doctor; you aren't doing anything for me."

31. A patient has severe pain and bladder distention related to urinary retention and possible obstruction; insertion of an indwelling catheter is prescribed. An experienced unlicensed assistive personnel (AP) states that she is trained to do this procedure. Which task can be delegated to this AP?
    1. Assessing the bladder distention and the pain associated with urinary retention
    2. Inserting the indwelling catheter after verifying her knowledge of sterile technique
    3. Evaluating the relief of pain and bladder distention after the catheter is inserted
    4. Measuring the urine output after the catheter is inserted and obtaining a specimen

32. The nurse is caring for a young man with a history of substance abuse who had exploratory abdominal surgery 4 days ago for a knife wound. There is a prescription to discontinue the morphine via patient-controlled analgesia and to start oral pain medication. The patient begs, "Please don't stop the morphine. My pain is really a lot worse today than it was yesterday." Which response is **best**?
    1. "Let me stop the pump; we can try oral pain medication to see if it gives relief."
    2. "I realize that you are scared of the pain, but we must try to wean you off the pump."
    3. "Show me where your pain is and describe how it feels compared with yesterday."
    4. "Let's take your vital signs; then I will call the health care provider."

33. The nurse is working with a health care provider who prescribes opioid doses based on a specific pain intensity rating (dosing to the numbers). Which patient circumstance is cause for **greatest** concern?
    1. A 73-year-old frail female patient with a history of chronic obstructive pulmonary disease is prescribed 4 mg IV morphine for pain of 1 to 3 on a scale of 0 to 10.
    2. A 25-year-old postoperative male patient with a history of opioid addiction is prescribed one tablet of oxycodone and acetaminophen for pain of 4 to 5 on a scale of 0 to 10.
    3. A 33-year-old opioid-naïve female patient who has a severe migraine headache is prescribed 5 mg IV morphine for pain of 7 to 8 on a scale of 0 to 10.
    4. A 60-year-old male with a history of rheumatoid arthritis is prescribed one tablet of hydromorphone for pain of 5 to 6 on scale of 0 to 10.

34. Which nursing action is the **best** example of the principle of nonmaleficence as an ethical consideration in pain management?
    1. Patient seems excessively sedated but continues to ask for morphine, so the nurse conducts further assessment and seeks alternatives to opioid medication.
    2. Patient has no known disease disorders and no objective signs of poor health or injury, but reports severe pain, so nurse advocates for pain medicine.
    3. Patient is older, but he is mentally alert and demonstrates good judgment, so the nurse encourages the patient to verbalize personal goals for pain management.
    4. Patient repeatedly refuses pain medication but shows grimacing and reluctance to move, so the nurse explains the benefits of taking pain medication.

35. The nurse is assessing a patient who has been receiving opioid medication via patient-controlled analgesia. Which **early** sign alerts the nurse to a possible adverse opioid reaction?
    1. Patient reports shortness of breath.
    2. Patient is more difficult to arouse.
    3. Patient is more anxious and nervous.
    4. Patient reports pain is worsening.

36. The charge nurse of a long-term care facility is reviewing the methods and assessment tools that are being used to assess the residents' pain. Which nurse is using the **best** method to assess pain?
    1. Nurse A uses a behavioral assessment tool when the resident is engaged in activities.
    2. Nurse B asks a resident who doesn't speak English to point to the location of pain.
    3. Nurse C uses the same numerical rating scale every day for the same resident.
    4. Nurse D asks the daughter of a confused patient to describe the resident's pain.

37. For which of these patients is IV morphine the first-line choice for pain management?
    1. A 33-year-old intrapartum patient needs pain relief for labor contractions.
    2. A 24-year-old patient reports severe headache related to being hit in the head.
    3. A 56-year-old patient reports breakthrough bone pain related to multiple myeloma.
    4. A 73-year-old patient reports chronic pain associated with hip replacement surgery.

38. The patient is prescribed a fentanyl patch for persistent severe pain. Which patient behavior **most** urgently requires correction?

    1. Frequently likes to sit in the hot tub to reduce joint stiffness
    2. Prefers to place the patch only on the upper anterior chest wall
    3. Saves and reuses the old patches when he can't afford new ones
    4. Changes the patch every 4 days rather than the prescribed 72 hours

39. The home health nurse discovers that an older adult patient has been sharing his pain medication with his daughter. He acknowledges the dangers of sharing, but states, "My daughter can't afford to see a doctor or buy medicine, so I must give her a few of my pain pills." Which member of the health care team would the nurse consult **first**?
    1. Health care provider to renew the prescription so that the patient has enough medicine
    2. Pharmacist to monitor the frequency of the prescription refills
    3. Social worker to help the family locate resources for health care
    4. Home health aide to watch for inappropriate medication usage by family

40. For a postoperative patient, the health care provider (HCP) prescribed multimodal therapy, which includes acetaminophen, nonsteroidal antiinflammatory drugs, as-needed (PRN) opioids, and nonpharmaceutical interventions. The patient continuously asks for the PRN opioid, and the nurse suspects that the patient may have a drug abuse problem. Which action by the nurse is **best**?
    1. Administer acetaminophen and spend extra time with the patient.
    2. Explain that opioid medication is reserved for moderate to severe pain.
    3. Give the opioid because the patient deserves relief and drug abuse is unconfirmed.
    4. Ask the HCP to validate suspicions of drug abuse and alter the opioid prescription.

41. An inexperienced new nurse compares the medication administration record (MAR) and the health care provider's (HCP's) prescription for a patient who has a patient-controlled analgesia (PCA) pump for pain management. Both the MAR and prescription indicate that larger doses are prescribed at night compared with doses throughout the day. Who would the new nurse consult **first**?
    1. Ask the patient if he typically needs extra medication in the evening.
    2. Ask the HCP to verify that the larger amount is the correct dose.
    3. Ask the pharmacist to confirm the dosage on the original prescription.
    4. Ask the charge nurse if this is a typical dosage for nighttime PCA.

 Answer Key for this chapter begins on p. 19

42. Which instruction would the nurse give to the unlicensed assistive personnel (AP) related to the care of a patient who has received ketamine for analgesia?
    1. Keep the environment calm and quiet.
    2. Watch for and report respiratory depression.
    3. Offer frequent sips of noncaffeinated fluids.
    4. Keep the bed flat and frequently turn patient.

43. The health care provider (HCP) prescribes 7 mg morphine IV as needed. The nursing student prepares the medication and shows the syringe (see figures below) to the nursing instructor. Which action would the nursing instructor take **first?**

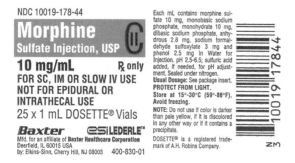

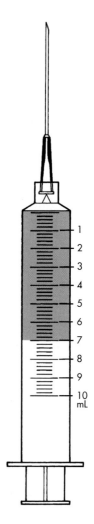

1. Tell the student to review the HCP's prescription before administering medication.
2. Waste the medication and tell the student that remediation is required for serious error.
3. Ask the student to demonstrate the calculations and steps required to prepare the dose.
4. Accompany the student to the patient's room and observe as the medication is administered.

44. Expanded Hot Spot _____

Scenario: The nurse is caring for a patient who had abdominal surgery yesterday. The patient is restless and anxious and reports that the pain is getting worse (8 out of 10) despite morphine via patient-controlled analgesia. Physical assessment findings include: T 100.3°F (37.9°C), P 110 beats/min, R 24 breaths/min, and BP 110/70 mmHg. The abdomen is rigid and tender to the touch with hypoactive bowel sounds. The nurse tries to make the patient comfortable, and he is willing to wait until the next scheduled dose of pain medication. However, the nurse decides to notify the patient's health care provider (HCP) because the pain warrants evaluation, possible diagnostic testing, and additional therapies.

Which information would the nurse include in the assessment component of the SBAR (situation, background, assessment, recommendation) report to the HCP?

Instructions: Underline or highlight the information the nurse would include in the assessment component of the SBAR report.

45. Extended Multiple Response _____

Question: Based on the American Society for Pain Management Nursing recommendations for "As needed" (PRN) range prescriptions for opioid analgesics, for which prescriptions, does the nurse need to seek clarification from the health care provider?

Instructions: Place an X in the space provided or highlight each patient situation where the nurse would seek clarification for the prescrip-tion. **Select all that apply.**

The nurse is reviewing the PRN (as-needed) pain prescriptions for the following patients:

1. _____ Ms. A is a 35-year old female admitted for an acute episode of cholelithiasis. Prescribed: Morphine 1 to 15 mg IV every 2 hours PRN pain

2. _____ Mr. B is a 75-year old male who had hip surgery yesterday. He has chronic obstructive pulmonary disease. Prescribed: Morphine 2 to 3 mg IV every 2 hours PRN pain

3. _____ Mr. C is a 55-year old male with acute pancreatitis. He has a history of alcohol and substance abuse. Prescribed: Morphine 1 to 3 mg IV every 4 hours PRN pain

4. _____ Mrs. D is an 83-year old female with an ankle fracture. She has dementia and is unable to maintain elevation of the ankle. Prescribed: Meperidine 25 to 50 mg PO PRN pain

5. _____ Mr. E is a 46-year old male admitted for bacterial meningitis. He reports severe headaches. Prescribed: Codeine 15 mg PO 1-2 tablets every 4 to 6 hours PRN pain

6. _____ Mr. F is a 25-year old male. He has extensive abrasions on the left side of the body sustained in a motorcycle accident. No other obvious trauma detected in the emergency department. Prescribed: Oxycodone 9 mg PO every 12 hours; Hydrocodone with acetaminophen 5/325 PO 1 to 2 tablets every 4 to 6 hours PRN pain; acetaminophen 500 mg 2 tablets PO every 6 to 8 hours PRN pain

7. _____ Ms. G is a 57-year old female who had a hysterectomy yesterday for uterine prolapse. She is opioid naive and has no preexisting health conditions other than prolapse of the uterus. Prescribed: Fentanyl 50 to 100 mcg IV every 2 hours PRN for severe pain

8. _____ Mr. H is a 68-year old male; he has pain associated with postherpetic neuralgia. Prescribed: Morphine 2 to 3 mg IV every 4 hours PRN pain

PART 2 Common Health Scenarios

46. Matrix _____

Scenario: The nurse is caring for a 73-year old patient who was admitted for dehydration and observation for compartment injury. The patient fell between the toilet and the wall. His right arm was pinned underneath his body, for several hours before he was discovered by a neighbor. Fractures and other obvious injuries were ruled out in the emergency department. Patient received 400 mg ibuprofen for pain in the right arm.

Which nursing actions would the nurse take for suspicion of compartment syndrome?

Instructions: For each potential nursing action listed below, check to specify whether the action is anticipated, nonessential or contraindicated.

Vital signs:
Temperature 98.7F° (37°C)
Pulse 120 beats/min
Respirations 24 breaths/min
Blood pressure 140/70 mmHg
Oxygen saturation 95% (on room air)
Body Mass Index (BMI) 30

Assessment findings: Patient is anxious and tearful. He reports stiffness and soreness in his right leg, but "My leg is okay compared to my arm. My arm really hurts (9/10 on pain scale). Stretching makes the pain worse and there is burning and tingling in my fingers. When is that pain medication supposed to start working?"

Potential Nursing Actions	Anticipated	Nonessential	Contraindicated
Assess the location, quality, and intensity of pain			
Assess for 5Ps (pain, pallor, pulselessness, paralysis, paresthesia)			
Elevate right arm above the level of the heart			
Apply an ice pack wrapped in a towel			
Assess urine color and output			
Wrap the forearm with an elastic bandage			
Obtain an order for an x-ray of the arm			
Notify health care provider for unrelieved pain and paresthesia			

47. Drag and Drop

Scenario: The oncoming day shift nurse has received the shift report from the night nurse. The day shift nurse has done a quick check on all of the patients and has determined that all are stable and not in acute distress.

In which order would the nurse care for these patients?

Instructions: Patients are listed in the left-hand column. In the right- hand column write in the number to indicate the order of priority for care; 1 being the first and 5 being the last.

Patients	Order of priority
1. 17-year-old adolescent who is alert and oriented. He was admitted 2 days ago for treatment of meningitis. He reports a continuous headache that is partially relieved by medication.	
2. 65-year-old man who underwent total knee replacement surgery 2 days ago. He is using the patient-controlled analgesia (PCA) pump frequently and occasionally asks for a bolus dose.	
3. 53-year-old woman who is demanding and frequently calls for assistance. She was admitted for investigation of functional abdominal pain and is scheduled for diagnostic testing this morning.	
4. 82-year-old woman with advanced Alzheimer disease who requires total care for all activities of daily living. She will be transferred to a long-term care facility in a few days after arrangements are finalized.	
5. 26-year-old man who was admitted with chest pain secondary to a spontaneous pneumothorax. Today, the chest tube will be removed and the PCA pump will be discontinued.	

Answers

1. **Ans: 3** The patient must be believed, and his or her experience of pain must be acknowledged as valid. The data gathered via patient reports can then be applied to the other options in developing the treatment plan. **Focus:** Prioritization.

2. **Ans: 1, 3, 4** The widespread use of opioids and the increase in mortality and morbidity make it essential for nurses to recognize any personal negative bias and work toward conveying acceptance and understanding. This increases the likelihood of patient engagement and success in treatment programs. Learning about the signs and symptoms of an opioid overdose and the proper use of naloxone is also a nursing responsibility. Electronic prescription drug monitoring programs show promise but are not currently available nationwide and checking the database for all opioid prescriptions may be time-consuming and unnecessary (short-term opioid prescriptions for acute pain are less problematic). The nurse would question a health care provider if an opioid prescription did not seem safe; however, the CDC recommendations are not legally binding and deviations are not reportable. **Focus:** Prioritization.

3. **Ans: 4** Assess the pain for changes in location, quality, and intensity, as well as changes in response to medication. This assessment will guide the next steps. **Focus:** Prioritization. **Test-Taking Tip:** During clinical rotations, you may observe nurses giving pain medication without performing an adequate pain assessment. This is an error in clinical performance. In postoperative patients, pain could signal complications, such as hemorrhage, infection, or decreased perfusion related to tissue swelling. Always assess pain first, then make a decision about giving medication, using nonpharmacologic methods, or contacting the HCP.

4. **Ans: 4** The LPN/LVN is well trained to administer oxygen per nasal cannula. This patient is considered unstable; therefore the RN should take responsibility for administering drugs and monitoring the response to therapy, which includes the effects on the respiratory system. The RN should also take responsibility to communicate with the HCP for ongoing treatment and therapy. **Focus:** Assignment.

5. **Ans: 4** If the pain is constant, the best schedule is around-the-clock to provide steady analgesia and pain control. The other options may require higher dosages to achieve control. **Focus:** Prioritization.

6. **Ans: 4** At greatest risk are older adult patients, opioid-naïve patients, and those with underlying pulmonary disease. The adolescent has two of the three risk factors. **Focus:** Prioritization.

7. **Ans: 4** One of the common features of rheumatoid arthritis is joint pain and stiffness when first rising. This usually resolves over the course of the day. A non-pharmaceutical measure is to take a warm shower (or apply warm packs to joints if pain is limited to one or two joints). If pain worsens, then the nurse may elect to contact other members of the health care team for additional interventions. **Focus:** Delegation.

8. **Ans: 1** Gabapentin is an antiepileptic drug, but it is also used to treat diabetic neuropathy. Corticosteroids are for pain associated with inflammation. Hydromorphone is a stronger opioid, and it is not the first choice for chronic pain that can be managed with other drugs. Lorazepam is an anxiolytic that may be prescribed as an adjuvant medication. **Focus:** Prioritization.

9. **Ans: 1** The goal is to control pain while minimizing side effects. For severe pain, the medication can be titrated upward until the pain is controlled. Downward titration occurs when the pain begins to subside. **Focus:** Prioritization.

10. **Ans: 1, 2, 3, 4** The recommendations of the American Pain Society, in collaboration with the American Society of Anesthesiologists, for postoperative patients include: acetaminophen and/or NSAIDs if there are no contraindications; surgical site–specific peripheral regional anesthetic for procedures; neuraxial analgesia (also known as epidural analgesia) for major thoracic and abdominal procedures, if patient has risk for cardiac complications or prolonged ileus; and multimodal therapy, which includes use of different types of medications and other therapies. Oral opioids are preferred in the postoperative period. Pain specialists should be consulted if patients have inadequately controlled postoperative pain. **Focus:** Prioritization. **Test-Taking Tip:** Passing a test and working as a competent nurse requires keeping up to date with current practice guidelines.

11. **Ans: 3** Beliefs, attitudes, and familial influence are part of the sociocultural dimension of pain. Location and radiation of pain address the sensory dimension. Describing pain and its effects addresses the affective dimension. Activity level and function address the behavioral dimension. Asking about knowledge addresses the cognitive dimension. **Focus:** Prioritization.

12. **Ans: 3** Cancer pain generally worsens with disease progression, and the use of opioids is more generous. Fibromyalgia is more likely to be treated with non-opioid and adjuvant medications. Trigeminal neuralgia is treated with antiseizure medications such as carbamazepine. Phantom limb pain usually subsides after ambulation begins. **Focus:** Prioritization.

13. **Ans: 1** Multimodal therapies for postoperative patients include opioids and nonopioid therapies, regional anesthetic techniques, and nonpharmacologic therapies. This approach is thought to be the most important strategy for pain management for most postoperative patients. Standing orders are less optimal because there is no consideration of individual needs or characteristics. PCA is one important element, but not all patients can manage PCA devices. Assessment tools are an important part of overall management, but basing opioid dose on a numerical scale does not consider individual patient circumstances. **Focus:** Prioritization.

14. **Ans: 4** When supervising a new RN, good performance should be reinforced first and then areas of improvement can be addressed. Asking the nurse about knowledge of pain management is also an option; however, it would be a more indirect and time-consuming approach. Making a note and watching does not help the nurse to correct the immediate problem. In-service training might be considered if the problem persists. **Focus:** Supervision.

15. **Ans: 1, 3, 5, 6** Patients with acute conditions that require close monitoring for complications should be assigned to an experienced RN. Abdominal cramps secondary to food poisoning is an acute condition; however, cramping, vomiting, and diarrhea are usually self-limiting. The patient with chronic back pain would be considered physically stable. Although all patients will benefit from care provided by an experienced RN, the patient with abdominal cramps and the patient with back pain could be assigned to a new RN, an LPN/LVN, or a float nurse. **Focus:** Assignment. **Test Taking Tip:** To determine acuity of patients, use nursing concepts, such as gas exchange and perfusion. Patients 1, 3, 5, and 6 could have potential problems related to perfusion. The patient with the chest tube could also have a potential problem related to gas exchange.

16. **Ans: 2** Inadequate pain management for postsurgical patients can affect quality of life, function, recovery, and postsurgical complication; thus all the manifestations are examples of negative results. Nevertheless, venous thromboembolism is the most serious because it can lead to pulmonary embolism, which is an immediate life-threatening concern. The nurse also needs to implement interventions to resolve unsatisfied needs, fear of pain, and hopelessness related to pain and function. **Focus:** Prioritization. **Test-Taking Tip:** Physiologic needs are the first concern. In this case, venous thromboembolism is the most serious physiologic outcome secondary to inadequate pain management.

17. **Ans: 1** The nurse would consider questioning all of the medication prescriptions, but the opioid-naïve adult has the greatest immediate risk because use of a basal dose has been associated with an increased incidence of respiratory depression in opioid-naïve patients. Older adults are frequently prescribed NSAIDs; however, they are used with caution, and the patient's history should be reviewed for potential problems, such as a history of gastrointestinal bleeding, cardiac disease, or renal dysfunction. Many medications such as anticoagulants, oral hypoglycemics, diuretics, and antihypertensives can also cause adverse drug–drug interactions with NSAIDs. IM injections cause pain, absorption is unreliable, and there are no advantages over other routes of administration. If a patient is able to tolerate oral foods and fluids, oral medications are preferred because the efficacy of the oral route is equal to the IV route. **Focus:** Prioritization. **Test-Taking Tip:** It is worthwhile to study the purposes, pharmacologic actions, and side effects of commonly used medications. Morphine is considered the prototype of the opioid medications. For opioid-naïve patients, the priority concern is respiratory depression. For patients who need opioids for long-term pain management, the primary side effect is constipation.

18. **Ans: 3** The patient with an acute myocardial infarction has the greatest need for IV access and is likely to receive morphine, which will relieve pain and increase venous capacitance. The other patients may also need IV access for delivery of pain medication, other drugs, or IV fluids, but the need is less urgent. **Focus:** Prioritization.

19. **Ans: 2** The AP has correctly reported findings, but the nurse is ultimately responsible to assess first and then determine the correct action. Based on assessment findings, the other options may also be appropriate. **Focus:** Prioritization.

20. **Ans: 2** The American Headache Society has guidelines for the treatment of acute migraines. Migraines may be treated with nonsteroidal antiinflammatory drugs (including aspirin), nonopioid analgesics, acetaminophen, caffeinated analgesic combinations or migraine-specific agents (triptans, dihydroergotamine), corticosteroids, antiemetics, or anticonvulsants (e.g., valproate sodium and topiramate, except in women of childbearing age who are not using reliable birth control). Sumatriptan should not be used if ergotamine, dihydroergotamine, or another triptan medication has been used in the past 24 hours because of the additive effect of narrowing of the blood vessels that could result in damage to major organs (e.g., stroke or myocardial infarction). Thus it is most important for the nurse to have a conversation with the HCP about the sumatriptan. The other options are concerning but not to the same degree. Dexamethasone may cause increased glucose levels. If the patient recently started birth control pills, pregnancy should be ruled out before prescribing valproate sodium. Prochlorperazine can cause drowsiness. **Focus:** Prioritization.

21. **Ans: 1** This patient has strong beliefs and emotions related to the issue of the brother's addiction. First,

encourage expression. This indicates to the patient that the feelings are real and valid. Listening is respectful and increases the likelihood of compliance with prescribed therapies. It is also an opportunity to assess beliefs and fears. Giving facts and information is appropriate at the right time. Family involvement is important, and their beliefs about drug addiction may be similar to those of the patient. **Focus:** Prioritization.

22. **Ans: 3** Diaphoresis is one of the early signs that occurs between 6 and 12 hours after withdrawal. Fever, nausea, and abdominal cramps are late signs that occur between 48 and 72 hours after withdrawal. **Focus:** Prioritization. **Test-Taking Tip:** In studying for the NCLEX®, pay attention to early signs of disease processes. Early detection is considered a safety measure; therefore NCLEX® tests to determine if you can perform early identification of potential problems.

23. **Ans: 1** The AP can assist the patient with hygiene issues and knows the principles of safety and comfort for the sitz bath. Monitoring the patient, teaching techniques, and evaluating outcomes are nursing responsibilities. **Focus:** Delegation.

24. **Ans: 4** Administering placebos is generally considered unethical. (There are circumstances, such as clinical drug research, where placebos are used, but patients are aware of that possibility.) The charge nurse is a resource person who can help clarify the situation and locate and review the hospital policy. If the HCP is insistent, suggest that he or she could give the placebo. Although following a personal ethical code is correct, the nurse must ensure that the patient is not abandoned and that care continues. **Focus:** Prioritization.

25. **Ans: 2** Complete information should be obtained from the family during the initial comprehensive history taking and assessment. If this information is not obtained, the nursing staff must rely on observation of nonverbal behavior and careful documentation to determine pain and relief patterns. **Focus:** Prioritization.

26. **Ans: 4** The charge nurse must assess the performance and attitude of the staff in relation to this patient. After data are gathered from the nurses, additional information can be obtained from the records and the patient as necessary. The educator may be of assistance if a knowledge deficit or need for performance improvement is the problem. **Focus:** Supervision, Prioritization. **Test-Taking Tip:** The first step of the nursing process is assessment. In this case, the charge nurse applies the nursing process to assess the nursing staff's performance and attitudes.

27. **Ans 1, 2, 3, 4, 5** In general, opioids are not the first-line choice for fibromyalgia, chronic low back pain, arthritis, or headache. There are other therapies that are safer for long-term use. ER/LA opioids increase the risk for overdose and are not recommended for chronic pain; time scheduling does not reduce the risk of harm. Age and sleep apnea increase the risk

for respiratory depression. Morphine for hip fracture would be acceptable, but 90 morphine milligram equivalents would be considered a high dose, and high doses are associated with greater risk for overdose. Headaches are treated with nonsteroidal anti-inflammatory drugs (NSAIDs), nonopioid analgesics, acetaminophen, caffeinated analgesic combinations (triptans, dihydroergotamine), anticonvulsants (e.g., valproate sodium and topiramate), or corticosteroids. Methadone is prescribed with caution because of the cardiotoxic effects. PCA morphine for postsurgical pain is common and acceptable because of the acute nature of the pain, the low dose, and the controlled delivery. **Focus:** Prioritization.

28. **Ans: 2, 5, 6** The patient who is on the second postoperative day, the patient who has pain at the IV site, and the patient with the kidney stone have predictable needs and require routine care that a new nurse can manage. The anxious patient with chronic pain needs an in-depth assessment of the psychological and emotional components of pain and expert intervention. The patient with acquired immune deficiency syndrome has complex issues that require expert assessment skills. The patient pending discharge will need special and detailed instructions for the implanted catheter. **Focus:** Assignment. **Test-Taking Tip:** "Select all that apply" questions are particularly challenging. At least two options must be correct; it is likely that three or more are correct. Read each option carefully and try to exclude incorrect options.

29. **Ans: 3** Responding to the patient and family in a timely fashion is important. Next, directly ask the patient about the pain and perform a complete pain assessment. This information will determine which action to take next. **Focus:** Prioritization.

30. **Ans: 2** This statement could be a veiled suicide threat, and patients with pain disorder and depression have a high risk for suicide. New injuries must be evaluated, but this type of pain report is not uncommon for patients with pain disorder. Risk for substance abuse is very high and should eventually be addressed. The patient can always threaten to sue, but the nurse must remain calm and continue to provide care with professional courtesy. **Focus:** Prioritization.

31. **Ans: 4** Measuring output and obtaining a specimen are within the scope of practice of the AP. Insertion of the indwelling catheter in this patient should be done by an experienced RN because patients with obstruction and retention are usually very difficult to catheterize, and the nurse must evaluate the pain response during the procedure. The AP's knowledge of sterile technique or catheter insertion is not the issue. **Focus:** Delegation.

32. **Ans: 3** Assessing the pain is the priority in this acute care setting because there is a risk of infection or hemorrhage. The other options might be appropriate based on the assessment findings. **Focus:** Prioritization.

PART 2 Common Health Scenarios

33. **Ans: 1**   According to the American Society for Pain Management Nursing, prescribing opioid medication based solely on pain intensity should be prohibited because there are many other factors to consider (e.g., age, health conditions, medication history, respiratory status). Age, small body mass, and underlying respiratory disease put the 73-year-old patient at greatest risk for overmedication and respiratory depression. Patients with a history of opioid addiction will have a different response to medication and may need higher doses to achieve relief. IV morphine may actually worsen migraine headaches, and other first-line drugs (e.g., nonsteroidal antiinflammatory drugs, nonopioid analgesics, acetaminophen, sumatriptan, corticosteroids) are more effective. Hydromorphone is a potent opioid that is not typically prescribed for the pain associated with chronic rheumatoid arthritis. **Focus:** Prioritization.

34. **Ans: 1**   Nonmaleficence is to prevent harm. If the patient is excessively sedated, the nurse knows that giving additional opioid medication could do more harm than good, so the nurse would conduct further assessments and seek alternative options for pain relief. The patient's report of pain should be believed, so based on the principle of justice, the nurse advocates for pain medication even though an organic cause of disease is not identified. By encouraging the patient to have a voice in his or her own pain management goals, the nurse is applying the principle of autonomy. By explaining the benefits of pain medication, the nurse is applying the principle of beneficence to help the patient recognize the balance between pain control and safety. **Focus:** Prioritization.

35. **Ans: 2**   Most adverse opioid events are preceded by an increased level of sedation. **Focus:** Prioritization.

36. **Ans: 3**   Pain assessment is very complex, but the consistent use of the same assessment tool is the best method. All tools are used in conjunction with observation, self-report, and other assessment skills. When a person is engaged in an activity, behavior may not accurately reflect pain. Asking someone to point to the pain is only one part of the total pain assessment. Relatives of confused residents can assist the nurse to recognize the meaning of behaviors, but they are not able to describe pain sensations for the resident. **Focus:** Prioritization, Supervision

37. **Ans: 3**   The patient with cancer needs morphine for symptom relief. For obstetric patients, morphine can suppress fetal respiration and uterine contractions, so regional or epidural methods are preferred. For head injuries, morphine could make evaluation of mental status more difficult. In addition, if respirations are depressed, intracranial pressure could increase. Opioids are usually not the first-line choice for chronic pain, and opioids must be used with caution in older adult patients because of changes related to aging, such as renal clearance. In addition, use of

opioids increases the risk for falls and contributes to constipation. **Focus:** Prioritization.

38. **Ans: 1**   All of these behaviors require correction; however, heat can increase the release of medication from the patch and result in a sudden overdose. The patient should be urged to rotate sites to prevent irritation of the skin. Reusing old patches and delaying the patch changes are likely to give less than optimal pain relief. Based on assessment of behaviors, the nurse would reeducate about use of the patch, help the patient seek financial resources, or develop a reminder system for patch change intervals. **Focus:** Prioritization.

39. **Ans: 3**   If the social worker can help the family to find affordable alternatives, then the father is more likely to stop giving his medication to the daughter. **Focus:** Prioritization.

40. **Ans: 3**   The nurse is weighing benefit against harm. If the patient is a drug abuser, the medication given in the hospital is not harming him. If the patient is not a drug abuser, then withholding the medication causes him to suffer pain because of unconfirmed suspicions. Administration of correctly prescribed opioids does not cause addiction, and for patients who are addicted, withholding medication in the hospital setting does not resolve the addictive behavior. **Focus:** Prioritization.

41. **Ans: 4**   The nurse has taken the first correct step and compared the MAR to the HCP's original prescription. Because the nurse is new, the charge nurse would be the best resource. In fact, larger PCA doses are given at night to increase the interval between doses. This helps the patient to rest and sleep. The nurse can contact the other members of the health care team at any time if the charge nurse is unable to help. **Focus:** Prioritization.

42. **Ans: 1**   A calm and quiet environment helps to reduce the psychomimetic effects (e.g., hallucinations/delusions, anxiety). Other side effects of ketamine include nausea, vomiting, and headaches; therefore giving fluids, keeping the patient flat, and frequent turning would not be advised. Ketamine is not associated with respiratory depression or sedation. **Focus:** Prioritization.

43. **Ans: 3** $\dfrac{10 \text{ mg}}{1 \text{ mL}} : \dfrac{7 \text{ mg}}{x} = 7 \div 10 = 0.7 \text{ mL}$. The student has made an error. The syringe contains 7 mL, which yields 70 mg of medication. The student should have obtained a tuberculin syringe and drawn up 0.7 mL. First, the nursing instructor would assess the student's knowledge and understanding of the calculations and method of preparing the medication. The instructor would use this approach to help the student self-identify errors, which might include misinterpreting the original prescription, misreading the label, or misreading the syringe markings. **Focus:** Prioritization,

Supervision. **Test Taking Tip:** This is a basic ratio and proportion method that is very useful in calculating doses. If you had trouble understanding the math in this question, ask your instructor for assistance. One resource is: Calculation of Drug Dosages, 11th Edition by Sheila J. Ogden, RN, MSN and Linda Fluharty, RN, MSN.

44. **Ans:** The nurse is caring for a patient who had abdominal surgery yesterday. The **patient is restless and anxious** and says that the **pain is getting worse (8 out of 10) despite morphine via patient-controlled analgesia.** Physical assessment findings include: **T 100.3°F (37.9°C), P 110 beats/min, R 24 breaths/min, and BP 110/70 mm Hg. The abdomen is rigid and tender to the touch with hypoactive bowel sounds.** The nurse tries to make the patient comfortable, and he is willing to wait until the next scheduled dose of pain medication. Escalating or unrelieved pain and a rigid, tender abdomen could signal hemorrhage or infection. A slightly elevated temperature is normal after surgery because of the body's response to tissue damage, however, the nurse would monitor for an upward trend that could indicate infection. A pulse rate of 110 beats/min could be caused by pain, postoperative dehydration, elevated temperature, or blood loss (initially the pulse increases to compensate for blood loss). A blood pressure of 110/70 mm Hg would be compared to baseline and examined for trends; 110/70 mmHg suggests blood loss if patient's BP is generally higher. **Focus:** Prioritization.

45. **Ans: 1, 3, 4, 6, 7, 8** According to the American Society for Pain Management Nursing recommendations for "As needed" (PRN) range prescriptions for opioid analgesics, the commonly prescribed range for morphine is 2 to 6 mg IV every 2 hours PRN for pain. Broad ranges, such as 1 to 15 mg morphine prescribed for Ms. A should be avoided. Patients with a history of alcohol or substance abuse may need larger or more frequent doses; therefore morphine 1 to 3 mg IV every 4 hours PRN pain for Mr. C is likely to be ineffective. In addition, the pain associated with pancreatitis is usually severe. Meperidine is usually not prescribed for older patients; there is a high risk for respiratory depression and other side effects and there

are other pain medications that have fewer risks. For Mr. F, the provider has ordered several PO medications with overlapping times and pharmacologic action (maximum dose of acetaminophen in 24 hours is 4000 mg; some sources recommend 3000 mg/24 hours as the limit). Fentanyl is a very potent opioid (100 mcg is approximately equivalent in analgesic activity to 10 mg of morphine) that would not be used for opioid naïve patients such as Ms. G. For Mr. H, postherpetic neuralgia is considered a chronic condition and antiseizure medications are more likely to be prescribed. The nurse will closely monitor Mr. B because of the underlying respiratory disease, but morphine 2 to 3 mg is within the recommended range of 2-3 times the lower dose. For Mr. E, codeine 15 mg PO 1 to 2 tablets every 4 to 6 hours is within the recommended dosage; however, the nurse would evaluate the efficacy after each dose. Headaches related to meningitis can be severe. **Focus:** Prioritization.

46. **Ans:** Compartment syndrome occurs when blood flow to the arm is constricted. As pressure in the muscle rises, muscle and surrounding tissues are deprived of oxygen and nutrients. Compartment syndrome is accompanied by pain that is disproportionate to an injury or pain that is unrelieved by prescribed medication and worsens with stretching of the muscles. The nurse must monitor the 5Ps and compare the affected side to nonaffected side for subtle changes. Pain and paresthesia (numbness, tingling, or burning sensation) are the early signs that would be reported. Pulselessness and paralysis are considered late signs and permanent damage may have already occurred. Elevating the arm above the level of the heart, applying an ice pack, or wrapping the arm with an elastic bandage are contraindicated because these measures would contribute to decreased perfusion of the extremity. Dark urine is important to note because muscle damage can cause creatine kinase and myoglobin to enter the blood circulation (rhabdomyolysis); this can lead to acute kidney failure. An x-ray is not used to confirm compartment syndrome. To diagnose compartment syndrome, a pressure measurement test is done. A fasciotomy is performed to relieve the pressure. **Focus:** Prioritization.

Potential Nursing Actions	Anticipated	Nonessential	Contraindicated
Assess the location, quality, and intensity of pain	X		
Assess for 5Ps (pain, pallor, pulselessness, paralysis, paresthesia)	X		
Elevate right arm above the level of the heart			X
Apply an ice pack wrapped in a towel			X
Assess urine color and output	X		
Wrap the forearm with an elastic bandage			X
Obtain an order for an x-ray of the arm		X	
Notify health care provider for unrelieved pain and paresthesia	X		

PART 2 Common Health Scenarios

47. Ans: 5, 3, 1, 2, 4 All of the patients are in relatively stable condition. The patient with the pneumothorax has priority because chest tubes can leak or become dislodged or blocked. Lung sounds and respiratory effort should be evaluated before and after removal of the chest tube. The woman who will be leaving the unit for diagnostic testing should be assessed and prepared, as needed, before she leaves for the procedure. For a patient with meningitis, a headache is not unexpected, but neurologic status and pain should be assessed. Postoperative pain from knee surgery is expected, but this patient is getting reasonable relief most of the time. Caring for and assessing the patient with Alzheimer disease is likely to be very time consuming; caring for her last prevents delaying care for all the others. In addition, older patients with dementia benefit if the caregiver does not act rushed or hurried. **Focus:** Prioritization.

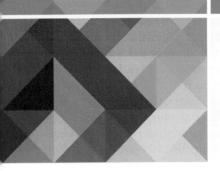

CHAPTER 2
Cancer

1. The patient who is receiving chemotherapy describes a burning sensation in the leg, which the health care provider diagnoses as neuropathic pain secondary to the therapy. The nurse is **most** likely to question the prescription of which drug?
   1. Imipramine
   2. Carbamazepine
   3. Gabapentin
   4. Morphine

2. A patient who has cancer will need ongoing treatment for pain. Which brochure is the nurse **most** likely to prepare that addresses questions related to the first-line treatment of cancer pain?
   1. "An Illustrated Guide to the Analgesic Ladder"
   2. "Common Questions About Radiation Therapy"
   3. "How to Make Preparations for Your Cancer Surgery"
   4. "How Nerve Blocks Can Help to Manage Cancer Pain"

3. A person who is receiving chemotherapy is approaching the nadir period. Which instruction will the team leader give to the LPN/LVN?
   1. Monitor the neutrophil count; be vigilant for signs/symptoms of infection.
   2. Expect nausea and vomiting; give antiemetics as prescribed.
   3. Observe for breakthrough pain; report frequency of bolus doses of opioids.
   4. Monitor for anorexia; initiate daily weights as needed.

4. After assessing the patient's pain patterns, the nurse determines that frequent breakthrough cancer pain is occurring. Which member of the health care team is the nurse most likely to contact **first**?
   1. Physical therapist to reevaluate physical therapy routines
   2. Health care provider (HCP) to review medication, dosage, and frequency
   3. Assistive personnel to increase help with activities of daily living
   4. Psychiatric clinical nurse specialist to evaluate psychogenic pain

5. During the handoff report, the oncoming day shift nurse hears that the cancer patient is on around-the-clock dosing of morphine but that end-of-dose pain might be occurring. Which question is the **most** important to ask the night shift nurse?
   1. "How many times did you have to give a bolus dose of morphine?"
   2. "Did the patient tell you that the pain was greater than a 5 out of 10?"
   3. "Did you notify the health care provider (HCP) and were changes prescribed?"
   4. "Did you try any nonpharmaceutical therapies or adjuvant medications?"

6. The nurse is caring for a patient with esophageal cancer. Which task could be delegated to assistive personnel (AP)?
   1. Assisting with oral hygiene
   2. Observing response to feedings
   3. Evaluating risk for aspiration
   4. Initiating weight measurements, as needed

7. A patient had radiation therapy 3 months ago and recently the health care provider prescribed epoetin. Which instruction will the home health nurse give to the home health aide related to this new therapy?
   1. Encourage the patient to eat smaller amounts until nausea subsides.
   2. Allow the patient to rest between care activities until energy improves.
   3. Help the patient to stand up slowly until orthostatic hypotension resolves.
   4. Frequently cleanse the mouth with clear water until mucositis abates.

8. Which patient is at **greatest** risk for pancreatic cancer?
   1. An older African-American man who smokes
   2. A young obese Asian woman with gallbladder disease
   3. A young African-American man with type 1 diabetes
   4. An elderly white woman who has pancreatitis

9. Patients receiving chemotherapy are at risk for thrombocytopenia related to the therapy or cancer disease process. Which actions for bleeding precautions can be delegated to assistive personnel? **Select all that apply.**
   1. Provide mouthwash with alcohol for oral rinsing.
   2. Use paper tape on fragile skin, if tape is needed.
   3. Use a soft toothbrush or oral sponge.
   4. Gently insert the rectal thermometer.
   5. Handle gently to reduce bruising.
   6. Avoid overinflation of blood pressure cuffs.

10. Which patient with a health problem related to gastrointestinal (GI) cancer would be the **most** appropriate to assign to an LPN/LVN under the supervision of a team leader RN?
   1. A patient who needs a blood transfusion secondary to GI bleeding
   2. A patient who needs enemas and antibiotics to control GI bacteria
   3. A patient who needs preoperative teaching for bowel resection surgery
   4. A patient who needs central line insertion for chemotherapy

11. A community health center is preparing a presentation on the prevention and detection of cancer. Which task would be **best** to assign to the LPN/LVN?
   1. Explain screening examinations and diagnostic testing for common cancers.
   2. Discuss how to plan a balanced diet and reduce fats and preservatives.
   3. Prepare a poster on the seven warning signs of cancer.
   4. Describe strategies for reducing risk factors such as smoking and obesity.

12. The patient with cancer needs an initial course of treatment with continued maintenance treatments and ongoing observation for signs and symptoms over a prolonged period of time. Which patient statement is cause for **greatest** concern?
   1. "My symptoms will eventually be cured; I'm so happy that I don't have to worry any longer."
   2. "My doctor is trying to help me control the symptoms; I am grateful for the extension of time with my family."
   3. "My pain will be relieved, but I am going to die soon; I would like to have control over my own life and death."
   4. "Initially, I may have to take some time off work for my treatments; I can probably work full time in the future."

13. For a patient who is experiencing side effects of radiation therapy, which task would be the **most** appropriate to delegate to assistive personnel (AP)?
   1. Helping the patient to cope with fatigue and lack of energy
   2. Encouraging participation in a walking program
   3. Reporting the amount and type of food consumed from the tray
   4. Checking the skin for redness and irritation after the treatment

14. An older patient needs treatment for severe localized pain related to postherpetic neuralgia secondary to chemotherapy. The nurse is **most** likely to question the prescription of which type of medication?
   1. Lidocaine patch
   2. Gabapentinoid
   3. Capsaicin patch
   4. Tricyclic antidepressant

15. For a patient receiving the chemotherapeutic drug vincristine, which side effect would be reported to the health care provider (HCP)?
   1. Fatigue
   2. Nausea
   3. Paresthesia
   4. Anorexia

16. A newly hired nurse, who has 2 years of medical-surgical experience but limited experience caring for patients with cancer, seems to be consistently undermedicating the patients' pain. What would the supervising nurse do **first**?
   1. Reassess all of the patients and administer additional pain medication as needed.
   2. Write an incident report and inform the nurse manager about the nurse's performance.
   3. Assess the new hire's understanding and beliefs about cancer pain and treatments.
   4. Ask the nurse about past experience in administering pain medications.

17. For a patient who is receiving chemotherapy, which laboratory result is of particular importance?
    1. White blood cell count (WBC): 3000/mm^3 (3 × 10^9/L)
    2. Serum potassium (K$^+$): 3.4 mEq/L (3.4 mmol/L)
    3. Prealbumin (PAB): 14 mg/dL (140 mg/L)
    4. Blood urea nitrogen (BUN): 9 mg/dL (3.21 mmol/L)

18. For care of a patient who has oral cancer, which task would be appropriate to assign to an LPN/LVN?
    1. Assisting the patient to perform oral hygiene
    2. Explaining when brushing and flossing are contraindicated
    3. Giving antacids and sucralfate suspension as prescribed
    4. Recommending saliva substitutes

19. When staff assignments are made for the care of patients who are receiving chemotherapy, which consideration related to chemotherapeutic drugs is the **most** important?
    1. Administration of chemotherapy requires precautions to protect self and others.
    2. Many chemotherapeutic drugs are vesicants.
    3. Chemotherapeutic drugs are frequently given through central venous access devices.
    4. Oral and intravenous routes of administration are the most common.

20. The oncoming day shift nurse has just received the handoff report from the night shift nurse. List the order of priority for assessing and caring for the following patients, with 1 being first and 4 being last.
    1. A patient who developed tumor lysis syndrome around 5:00 AM
    2. A patient who is currently pain free but had breakthrough pain during the night
    3. A patient scheduled for exploratory laparotomy this morning
    4. A patient with anticipatory nausea and vomiting for the past 24 hours
    _____, _____, _____, _____

21. The nurse is monitoring a patient who is at risk for spinal cord compression related to tumor growth. Which patient statement is **most** likely to suggest an **early** manifestation?
    1. "Last night my back really hurt, and I had trouble sleeping."
    2. "My leg has been giving out when I try to stand."
    3. "My bowels are just not moving like they usually do."
    4. "When I try to pass urine, I have difficulty starting the stream."

22. Which instruction would the nurse give to the assistive personnel (AP) about caring for a patient who is experiencing "chemo brain"?
    1. "The patient can understand you but cannot speak clearly."
    2. "Be cautious; the patient may be unpredictably aggressive."
    3. "Calmly give explanations if the patient seems forgetful."
    4. "Report immediately if the patient complains of a headache."

23. A patient who has breast cancer is receiving immunotherapy in the form of trastuzumab, a monoclonal antibody (MoAb). Which medication side effect is the patient **most** likely to experience?
    1. Capillary leak syndrome
    2. Hepatotoxicity
    3. Flu-like symptoms
    4. Memory loss

24. For a patient with osteogenic sarcoma, which laboratory value causes the **most** concern?
    1. Sodium level of 135 mEq/L (135 mmol/L)
    2. Calcium level of 13 mg/dL (3.25 mmol/L)
    3. Potassium level of 4.9 mEq/L (4.9 mmol/L)
    4. Blood urea nitrogen (BUN) of 10 mg/dL (3.6 mmol/L)

25. Drag and Drop

Case Study and Question

The nursing supervisor has advised the charge nurse that there is a new admission who needs a private room. The charge nurse must review the conditions and statuses of patients who are currently on the unit to determine who could be moved and placed the same room.

Which two cancer patients could be cohorted?.

Instructions: Patients are listed in the left-hand column. In the right- hand column, use an X to indicate which two patients could be cohorted.

Patients who are currently on the unit	Two patients for cohorting
1. Patient A has a neutrophil count of 1000/mm³ (1 × 10⁹/L)	
2. Patient B underwent debulking of a tumor to relieve pressure	
3. Patient C just underwent a bone marrow transplantation	
4. Patient D had a laminectomy for spinal cord compression	
5. Patient E is undergoing brachytherapy for prostate cancer	
6. Patient F has terminal cancer and is receiving end-of-life care	
7. Patient G is approaching the nadir associated with the chemotherapy treatment	

26. An athletic young man with pain, a low-grade fever, and anemia was recently diagnosed with Ewing sarcoma. The surgeon recommended amputation of the right lower leg for an operable tumor. The nurse discovers the patient preparing to leave the hospital "to go on a long hiking trip." What is the **priority** nursing concept to consider at this time?
1. Pain
2. Cellular regulation
3. Stress and coping
4. Adherence

27. After chemotherapy, a patient is being closely monitored for tumor lysis syndrome. Which laboratory result requires particular attention?
1. Platelet count
2. Electrolyte levels
3. Red blood cell count
4. White blood cell count

28. People at risk are the target populations for cancer screening programs. According to the latest screening recommendations from the American Cancer Society, which of these asymptomatic patients need extra encouragement to participate in cancer screening? **Select all that apply.**
1. A 25-year-old African-American woman who is sexually inactive, for a Pap test
2. A 30-year-old Asian-American woman, for an annual mammogram
3. A 45-year-old African-American man, to talk with the health care provider (HCP) about prostate cancer
4. A 55-year-old white American man who smokes, to talk with the HCP about a lung cancer screening
5. A 50-year-old white American woman, for colon cancer screening
6. A 70-year-old Asian-American woman who had a total hysterectomy 15 years ago (not for cancer reasons), for a Pap test

29. A patient with lung cancer develops syndrome of inappropriate antidiuretic hormone secretion (SIADH). Which treatment does the nurse anticipate that the health care provider will prescribe **first**?
    1. A fluid bolus
    2. Fluid restrictions
    3. A urinalysis
    4. A sodium-restricted diet

30. In the care of a patient with neutropenia, what tasks would the nurse delegate to assistive personnel (AP) to perform? **Select all that apply.**
    1. Taking vital signs every 4 hours
    2. Reporting temperature of more than 100.4°F (38°C)
    3. Assessing for sore throat, cough, or burning with urination
    4. Gathering the supplies to prepare the room for protective isolation
    5. Reporting superinfections, such as candidiasis
    6. Practicing good hand-washing technique

31. A primary nursing responsibility is the prevention of lung cancer by assisting patients in the cessation of smoking or other tobacco use. Which task would be appropriate to assign to an LPN/LVN?
    1. Develop a "quit plan"
    2. Explain how to apply a nicotine patch
    3. Discuss strategies to avoid relapse
    4. Suggest ways to deal with urges for tobacco

32. A patient with terminal liver cancer is receiving end-of-life-care. The patient is weak and restless and her skin is mottled and cool. Dyspnea develops, and she appears anxious and frightened. What would the nurse do **first**?
    1. Administer an as needed dose of morphine elixir.
    2. Alert the rapid response team and call the health care provider.
    3. Deliver breaths at 20 breaths/min with a bag-valve mask and prepare for intubation.
    4. Sit quietly with the patient and offer emotional support and comfort.

33. During report, the float nurse hears that the patient is receiving IV vincristine that will finish within the next 15 minutes. The IV site is intact, and the patient is not having any problems with the infusion. The float nurse is not certified in chemotherapy administration. What is the **priority** action?
    1. Ask the off-going nurse to stay until the vincristine infusion is finished.
    2. Ask the off-going nurse about problems to expect with vincristine infusions.
    3. Contact the charge nurse and discuss the lack of chemotherapy certification.
    4. Look up drug side effects and monitor because the infusion is almost complete.

34. A patient with uterine cancer is being treated with intracavitary radiation therapy. The assistive personnel (AP) reports that the patient insisted on ambulating to the bathroom and now "something feels like it is coming out." What is the **priority** action?
    1. Assess the AP's knowledge; explain the rationale for strict bed rest.
    2. Assess for dislodgment; use forceps and a lead container to retrieve and store as needed.
    3. Assess the patient's knowledge of the treatment plan and her willingness to participate.
    4. Notify the health care provider about dislodgment of the radiation implant.

35. The charge nurse discovers that two nurses have switched patient assignments because Nurse A does "not like to take care of patients with prostate cancer." Which action would the charge nurse take **first**?
    1. Insist that they switch back to the original patient assignments and talk to each of them at the end of the shift.
    2. Allow them this flexibility; as long as the patients are well cared for, it doesn't matter if the assignments are changed.
    3. Ask Nurse A to explain her position regarding prostate cancer patients and seek alternatives to prevent future issues.
    4. Explain to Nurse A and Nurse B that all patients deserve kindness and care regardless of their condition or the nurses' personal feelings.

36. Which assessment finding strongly suggests that the patient with cancer is having incident pain?
    1. Frequently reports pain about 30 to 35 minutes before the next scheduled dose
    2. Demonstrates protectiveness of right arm whenever moving or standing up
    3. Reports a continuous burning and tingling sensation in left lower leg
    4. Appears quiet, withdrawn, and depressed when family leaves after visiting

37. Which question is the home health nurse **most** likely to ask to evaluate the efficacy of a bisphosphonate medication that was prescribed for a patient with cancer?
    1. "Has the medication helped relieve the discomfort in your mouth?"
    2. "Have you noticed any increase or changes in your energy level?"
    3. "Has the medication helped to stop the nausea and vomiting?"
    4. "Has the medication relieved the bone pain that you reported?"

 Answer Key for this chapter begins on p. 33

Common Health Scenarios   PART 2

38. The oncoming nurse hears in the handoff report that the patient with cancer received an as needed oral dose of lorazepam. Which question is the oncoming nurse **most** likely to ask the off-going nurse in relation to the medication?
    1. "What did the patient say about the location and level of the pain?"
    2. "Were you able to determine what was making the patient so anxious?"
    3. "When is the patient allowed to have another dose of lorazepam?"
    4. "Did the patient have a normal bowel movement after the medication?"

39. The nurse is interviewing a patient who was treated several months ago for breast cancer. The patient reports taking nonsteroidal anti-inflammatory drugs (NSAIDs) for back pain. Which patient comment is cause for **greatest** concern?

1. "The NSAIDs are really not relieving the back pain."
2. "The NSAID tablets are too large, and they are hard to swallow."
3. "I gained weight because I eat a lot before taking NSAIDs."
4. "The NSAIDs are upsetting my stomach in the morning."

40. Which assessment finding is the **most** critical and needs to be addressed **first**?
    1. A patient with small cell lung cancer has tracheal deviation after a pulmonary resection.
    2. A patient with bladder cancer has decreased urination after intravesical chemotherapy.
    3. A patient with non-Hodgkin lymphoma has cardiac dysrhythmias after chemotherapy
    4. A patient has severe abdominal pain after a bowel resection for colon cancer.

41. Cloze _____

Scenario: The nurse is performing the morning assessment on a patient who has breast cancer. Patient says her gown feels tight and uncomfortable at the neckline. She also reports feeling uneasy and having a restless night with mild shortness of breath and a dry cough.

Instructions: Complete the sentences by choosing the most probable option for the omitted information that corresponds with the same numbered list of options provided.

Vital signs:
Temperature 98.6°F (37°C)
Pulse 110 beats/min
Respirations 30 breaths/minute Oxygen
Saturation 92% on room air

Assessment findings: Alert and oriented. Facial and periorbital edema and jugular vein distention are noted and are more pronounced in the supine position.

The nurse suspects an oncology emergency and assesses the patient for additional signs and symptoms of ___1___. The priority nursing assessment is ___2___. ___3___ would be an ominous sign for this oncology emergency. The first nursing action is to ___4___.

Option 1	Option 2	Option 3	Option 4
Third space syndrome	Progression of edema in the extremities	Electrocardiogram changes	Establish IV access
Superior vena cava syndrome	Auscultation of breath sounds	Hypotension	Alert the rapid response team
Tumor lysis syndrome	Patency of airway	Stridor	Place patient in a Fowler's position
Cardiac tamponade	Auscultation of heart sounds	Chest pain	Obtain order for an IV diuretic
Cardiac artery rupture	Assess for headache	Intense back pain	Oxygenate using a bag-valve mask

On the figure below, insert an arrow to point to the superior vena cava.

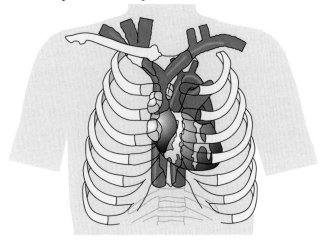

PART 2   Common Health Scenarios

42. Expanded Drag and Drop

Scenario: At 8:00 am the patient, a 63-year-old woman with liver cancer, is alert and conversant. She is weak, but able to sit up in bed with minimal assistance. Glasgow Coma Scale (GCS) score is 15.

Vital signs:
Temperature 98.3° F (36.8°C)
Pulse 110 beats/min
Respirations 30 breaths/minute Oxygen
Saturation 92% on room air
Respirations 30 breaths/minute Oxygen

Laboratory results:
Blood glucose (fingerstick) 70mg/dL (3.9 mmol/L)
Potassium 3.5 mEq/L (3.5 mmol/L)
Sodium 136 mEq/L (136mmol/L)
Ammonia 80 mcg/dl (47µmol/L)

Assessment findings: At 11:00 am arousable, but lethargic and confused. Follows simple commands with repetitive encouragement.

Instructions: Nursing actions are listed in the left-hand column. In the right- hand column, indicate the order in which the nurse will perform the nursing actions.

Nursing actions to perform at 11:	Order of Priority
1. Assess vital signs, including pulse, respirations, blood pressure, and temperature.	
2. Assess responsiveness and level of consciousness.	
3. Obtain a blood glucose reading; give glucose as needed per protocol.	
4. Assess previous electrolyte values and ammonia level; analyze need for repeat laboratory tests.	
5. Notify health care provider using SBAR.	
6. Apply pulse oximeter assess oxygen saturation; administer oxygen as needed.	
7. Attach patient to the cardiac monitor; observe for cardiac dysrhythmias.	
8. Examine for signs of trauma, particularly head injury.	
9. Assess for neurologic changes, repeat Glasgow Coma and compare findings to baseline.	

    Answer Key for this chapter begins on p. 33

43. Expanded Hot Spot _____

Case Study and Question

A 56-year-old patient comes to the clinic for scant rectal bleeding and intermittent diarrhea and constipation, cramping, and fatigue for the past several months. Despite an unintentional weight loss of 20 lb in the past month, his body mass index (BMI) is 31. He reports a chronic "smoker's cough" and shortness of breath with minor exertion, that influences his desire to exercise. He reports, "My father was an alcoholic, so I limit myself to an occasional social drink." He has a history of appendectomy as a child and a gunshot wound to the abdomen sustained in military service. His mother died from colorectal cancer at age 45. His father died of complications related to alcoholism at age 63.

Which factors would the nurse identify as increasing the patient's risk for colon cancer?

Instructions: Underline or highlight the factors that increase the patient's risk for colon cancer.

Common Health Scenarios   PART 2

Answers

PART 2

Common Health Scenarios

1. **Ans: 4**   Morphine is usually not prescribed for neuropathic pain because pain relief response is poor. Other medications, such as some antidepressants (e.g., imipramine) and some anticonvulsants (e.g., carbamazepine and gabapentin), provide better relief. **Focus:** Prioritization.

2. **Ans: 1**   Analgesic drugs are the first-line treatment for cancer pain management. If pain is not controlled by medication, other options are available, including radiation, surgery, and nerve blocks. **Focus:** Prioritization.

3. **Ans: 1**   The nadir, usually 7 to 10 days after the start of therapy, is the point where blood cell counts are the lowest; therefore the LPN/LVN would be instructed to monitor the neutrophil count and watch for signs of infection. Low platelet count could also result in spontaneous bleeding, and low red cell count would contribute to anemia and fatigue. Nausea and vomiting, breakthrough pain, and anorexia are side effects of chemotherapy but are not necessarily linked to the nadir. **Focus:** Supervision.

4. **Ans: 2**   Breakthrough pain is defined as being of rapid onset, short duration, and moderate to severe intensity; it is a temporary exacerbation related to poorly controlled around-the-clock dosing of background pain. Frequent breakthrough pain suggests that the around-the-clock dosing needs reevaluation, so the nurse would contact the HCP and advocate for a change of medication or dose or frequency. **Focus:** Prioritization.

5. **Ans: 3**   The most important question is whether the HCP was notified and if any changes were made to address the patient's pain. If the HCP was not called during the night (which is often the case), the nurse would also ask the other questions. The patient's current pain, pattern of last night's pain, data about the frequency of bolus doses, and data about other options that were tried need to be communicated to the HCP. **Focus:** Prioritization.

6. **Ans: 1**   Oral hygiene is within the scope of duties of the AP. The nurse would give the AP specific instructions related to the esophageal cancer. It is the responsibility of the nurse to observe the response to treatments and evaluate the risk of aspiration. The AP can be directed to weigh the patient but would not be expected to know when to initiate the measurements. **Focus:** Delegation.

7. **Ans: 2**   The patient needs to rest between activities because of fatigue caused by anemia. This can show up 3 to 4 months after radiation therapy. Epoetin is given to improve low hemoglobin and red cell factors. It is the nurse's responsibility to determine resolution of nausea, energy loss, orthostatic hypotension, and mucositis, but giving information to the home health aide helps him or her to understand the relevance and parameters of care actions. **Focus:** Supervision, Delegation.

8. **Ans: 1**   Pancreatic cancer is more common in African-Americans, men, and smokers. Other associated factors include older age, alcohol use, diabetes, obesity, history of pancreatitis, exposure to organic chemicals, consumption of a high-fat diet, and previous abdominal irradiation. **Focus:** Prioritization.

9. **Ans: 2, 3, 5, 6**   Mouthwash should not include alcohol because it has a drying action that leaves the mucous membranes more vulnerable. Insertion of suppositories, probes, or tampons into the rectal or vaginal cavity is not recommended. All other options are appropriate. **Focus:** Delegation.

10. **Ans: 2**   Administering enemas and antibiotics is within the scope of practice of LPNs/LVNs. Although some states and facilities may allow the LPN/LVN to administer blood, in general, administering blood, providing preoperative teaching, and assisting with central line insertion are the responsibilities of the RN. **Focus:** Assignment.

11. **Ans: 3**   The LPN/LVN will know the standard seven warning signs and can educate through standard teaching programs. The health care provider performs the physical examinations and recommends diagnostic testing. The nutritionist can give information about diet. The RN has the primary responsibility for educating people about risk factors. **Focus:** Assignment.

12. **Ans: 3**   The nurse would assess what the patient means by having "control over my own life and death." This could be an indirect statement of suicidal intent. A patient who believes he will be cured would also be assessed for misunderstanding the plan and outcomes; however, denial can also be used as a temporary defense mechanism. Acknowledgment that the treatments are for control of symptoms and plans for the immediate future suggest an understanding of treatment goals. **Focus:** Prioritization.

13. **Ans: 3**   The AP can observe the amount that the patient eats (or what is gone from the tray) and report to the nurse. Helping the patient to cope with fatigue and assessing skin reactions are the responsibilities of the RN. The initial recommendation for exercise would come from the health care provider. **Focus:** Delegation.

14. **Ans: 4**   The American Geriatrics Society recommends that tricyclics should be avoided for older adults because of side effects, such as confusion or orthostatic hypotension. Lidocaine patches, gabapentinoids (e.g.,

gabapentin), and tricyclic antidepressants (e.g., imipramine) are first-line choices for postherpetic neuralgia, which can be a long-term sequela to herpes zoster. Capsaicin patches are considered a second-line option. A lidocaine patch would be a good choice for this patient because it can be applied to the local area with limited systemic effects. **Focus:** Prioritization. **Test-Taking Tip:** Recall that age, malignancy, immunocompromised conditions (e.g., human immunodeficiency virus), and immunosuppressive medications increase the risk for herpes zoster.

15. **Ans: 3** Paresthesia is a side effect associated with some chemotherapy drugs, such as vincristine. The HCP can modify the dosage or discontinue the drug. Fatigue, nausea, vomiting, and anorexia are common side effects of many chemotherapy medications. The nurse can assist the patient by planning for rest periods, giving antiemetics as prescribed, and encouraging small meals containing high-protein and high-calorie foods. **Focus:** Prioritization. **Test-Taking Tip:** In caring for patients with cancer, many nursing interventions target the common side effects of chemotherapy, including fatigue, nausea, vomiting, and anorexia.

16. **Ans: 3** First, the supervising nurse assesses the newly hired nurse's knowledge and beliefs about cancer pain and treatment. The nurse has experience, but that past experience may be related to caring for patients with acute pain, such as postoperative pain or acute exacerbations of disease. After assessing knowledge, the supervising nurse can then correct misconceptions or make suggestions for further study. Reassessing the patients together could be a learning opportunity. Writing an incident report and going to the nurse manager might occur if the new nurse is unable to adapt and correct the behavior. **Focus:** Prioritization. **Test-Taking Tip:** Recall that the first step in the nursing process is always assessment. In this case, the newly hired nurse's performance is the focus of the assessment.

17. **Ans: 1** Chemotherapy can decrease WBCs, particularly neutrophils (known as neutropenia). This leaves the patient vulnerable to infection. Normal range for WBC is 5000 to 10,000/mm³ ($5-10 \times 10^9$ /L). The other tests are important in the total management but are less directly specific to chemotherapy. Normal range for K^+ is 3.5 to 5.0 mEq/L (3.5 to 5.0 mmol/L). Low K^+ could be associated with vomiting secondary to chemotherapy. Normal range for PAB is 15 to 36 mg/dL (150 to 360 mg/L); for BUN the range is 10 to 20 mg/dL (3.6 to 7.1 mmol/L) ; lower values for PAB or BUN could reflect malnutrition in a cancer patient. **Focus:** Prioritization.

18. **Ans: 3** Giving medications is within the scope of practice of the LPN/LVN. Assisting the patient with oral hygiene would be delegated to assistive personnel; the nurse would give specific instructions related to the condition of the patient's mouth. Explaining contraindications is the responsibility of the RN.

Recommendations for saliva substitutes would come from the health care provider or pharmacist. **Focus:** Assignment.

19. **Ans: 1** Chemotherapy drugs would be given by nurses who have received additional training in how to safely prepare and deliver the drugs and protect themselves and others from potential toxic exposure. All nurses are trained to use the general principles of drug administration in dealing with vesicant medications, using central lines, and administering medications via intravenous or oral routes; however, chemotherapy medications require specialized knowledge. **Focus:** Prioritization.

20. **Ans: 1, 3, 2, 4** Tumor lysis syndrome is an emergency involving electrolyte imbalances and potential renal failure. A patient scheduled for surgery would be assessed before leaving the unit, and any final preparations for surgery would be completed. A patient with breakthrough pain needs a thorough pain assessment, an investigation of pain patterns, and a chart review of all attempted pharmaceutical and nonpharmaceutical interventions; the health care provider may need to be contacted for a change of dosage or medication. Anticipatory nausea and vomiting have a psychogenic component that requires assessment, teaching, reassurance, and administration of antiemetics. **Focus:** Prioritization.

21. **Ans: 1** Back pain is an early sign of spinal cord compression occurring in 95% of patients. The other symptoms are later signs. **Focus:** Prioritization.

22. **Ans: 3** The AP would be instructed to remain calm and give clear and simple directions. In chemo brain, patients experience mental cloudiness with memory problems. This is usually temporary, but this condition can potentially last for years and impair ability to return to work or other social activities. **Focus:** Supervision, Delegation.

23. **Ans 3:** Flu-like symptoms are the most common side effects of the MoAbs. Acetaminophen may be given prophylactically to reduce these symptoms. Capillary leak syndrome (a dangerous side effect that may lead to pulmonary edema), confusion, and hepatoxicity may also occur but are less common. **Focus:** Prioritization. **Test-Taking Tip:** All medications have numerous side effects. For test-taking and for clinical practice, start your study by focusing on the most common side effects and the side effects that are the most dangerous.

24. **Ans: 2** The normal range for calcium is 9.0 to 10.5 mg/dL (2.25 to 2.75 mmol/L). Potentially life-threatening hypercalcemia can occur in cancers with destruction of bone. Other laboratory values are pertinent for overall patient management but are less specific to bone cancers. Normal ranges are: sodium 136 to 145 mEq/L (136 to 145 mmol/L); potassium 3.5 to 5.0 mEq/L (3.5 to 5.0 mmol/L); and BUN 10 to 20 mg/dL (3.6 to 7.1 mmol/L). **Focus:** Prioritization. **Test-Taking Tip:** For test-taking and for clinical

practice, memorizing normal ranges for common laboratory tests can help you to quickly identify potential problems.

25. **Ans: 2, 4**   Patient B underwent debulking of tumor and Patient D had a laminectomy require postoperative care and pain management for these palliative procedures; they can be placed in the same room. Patients who have low neutrophil counts (normal range: 2500-8000/mm^3 [5-10 x 10^9 /L]) or those with recent bone marrow transplantation require protective isolation. The patient who is undergoing brachytherapy needs a private room because radiation is being emitted while the implant is in place. The patient with terminal cancer needs comfort measures, such as privacy, family members at the bedside, and symptom relief. In addition, observing a roommate who has end-of-life symptoms could be very stressful for other patients who have cancer. The nadir represents the point of the lowest white blood cell count following chemotherapy. This condition may also require protective isolation. **Focus:** Assignment.

26. **Ans: 3**   The patient is not coping with the recent diagnosis of cancer and stressful prospect of losing his leg. His decision to go hiking may be a form of denial or possibly a veiled suicide threat. It is also possible that he has decided not to have any treatment; however, the nurse needs to make an additional assessment about his decision and actions and help him to discuss alternatives and consequences. This situation is complex, but if he leaves the hospital, there may be no chance to address any other issues. **Focus:** Prioritization.

27. **Ans: 2**   Tumor lysis syndrome can result in severe electrolyte imbalances and potential kidney failure. The other laboratory values are important to identify general chemotherapy side effects but are less pertinent to tumor lysis syndrome. **Focus:** Prioritization.

28. **Ans: 1, 3, 4, 5**   At 25 years of age, women should have a Pap smear, regardless of sexual activity. Annual mammograms are recommended for women with average risk starting at age 45. African-American men with average risk starting at age 45 years should talk to their HCPs about prostate cancer and risk versus benefits of prostate-specific antigen testing. Men aged 55 years or older who smoke should be advised to talk to their provider about lung cancer screening. Colon cancer screening tests are recommended for those with average risk starting at age 45 years. Women who have had a total hysterectomy for reasons other than cancer do not need a Pap test. **Focus:** Prioritization. **Test-Taking Tip:** Cancer screening guidelines are constantly being updated and revised. The American Cancer Society is a good resource for this information (http://www.cancer.org/healthy/findcancerearly/cancerscreeningguidelines/american-cancer-society-guidelines-for-the-early-detection-of-cancer).

29. **Ans: 2**   Hyponatremia is a concern; therefore fluid restrictions would be prescribed. Urinalysis is less pertinent; however, the nurse would monitor for changes in urine specific gravity. The diet may need to include sodium supplements. Fluid bolus is unlikely for patients with SIADH; however, IV normal saline or hypertonic saline solutions may be given very cautiously. **Focus:** Prioritization.

30. **Ans: 1, 2, 4, 6**   Measuring vital signs and reporting on specific parameters, practicing good hand washing, and gathering equipment are within the scope of duties for an AP. Assessing for symptoms of infections and superinfections is the responsibility of the RN. **Focus:** Delegation.

31. **Ans: 2**   An LPN/LVN is versed in medication administration and able to teach patients standardized information. The other options require more in-depth assessment, planning, and teaching, which would be performed by the RN. Helping patients with smoking cessation is a Core Measure. **Focus:** Assignment.

32. **Ans: 1**   Morphine elixir is the therapy of choice because it is thought to reduce anxiety and the subjective sensation of air hunger. End-of-life care would not include aggressive measures such as intubation or resuscitation. Support and comfort are always welcome, but in this case, there is an option that would offer some physical relief for the patient. **Focus:** Prioritization.

33. **Ans: 3**   Contact the charge nurse about the patient assignment. All nurses can assess patients, IV sites, and infusions; however, chemotherapy medications require special expertise. Asking the nurse to stay is not the best solution because the care of the patient and the effects of the medication continue after the infusion has been completed. Asking about or looking up the side effects of the drug is okay for personal information, but lack of chemotherapy certification is still an issue. In addition, knowing how to properly discontinue the infusion and dispose of the equipment are essential for personal safety and the safety of others. (Note to students: Facility policies may vary regarding chemotherapy certification. In your future career, for your safety and the safety of your patients, find out what the facility policy is and pursue certification as needed.) **Focus:** Prioritization.

34. **Ans: 2**   If the radiation implant has obviously been expelled (e.g., is on the bed linens), use a pair of forceps to place the radiation source in a lead container. The other options would be appropriate after safety of the patient and personnel are ensured. **Focus:** Prioritization.

35. **Ans: 3**   First, the charge nurse identifies the reason for the switch. After the underlying issue is discovered, a plan can be made to assist Nurse A (e.g., referral to counseling or in-service training). The charge nurse should avoid being too draconian or condescending. Nurses frequently switch patients to help one another out, but the charge nurse should always be informed

before changing assignments. **Focus:** Assignment, Supervision.

36. **Ans: 2** Incident pain is pain that is associated with an event, such as walking, position change, or coughing. In this case, movement is the incident that causes pain and the patient's reaction to protect the arm. Pain 30 to 45 minutes before the next scheduled dose is breakout pain. Burning and tingling are descriptors of neuropathic pain. Depression and withdrawal could occur with all types of pain, especially severe chronic pain. When friends and family are not available, the nurse could try other forms of distraction. **Focus:** Prioritization.

37. **Ans: 4** Bisphosphonate medications are used for patients with cancer to relieve bone pain associated with primary bone cancer or metastasis and to reduce the risk of fractures. They also lower the calcium level in the blood. **Focus:** Prioritization.

38. **Ans: 2** If the trigger factors for anxiety are identified, the nursing staff can plan nonpharmaceutical interventions. Lorazepam is a benzodiazepine, and it is not a first-line drug for cancer pain. It can be used for anxiety, insomnia, alcohol withdrawal, and muscle spasms and may be used in combination with antiemetics for cancer-induced nausea and vomiting. **Focus:** Prioritization.

39. **Ans: 1** Primary cancers (lung, prostate, breast, and colon) may metastasize to the spine. In spinal cord compression, back pain is a common early symptom. Later symptoms include weakness, loss of sensation, urinary retention or incontinence, and constipation. **Focus:** Prioritization. **Test-Taking Tip:** Reports of pain in distal areas, worsening pain, or difficulty controlling pain can signal metastasis or reoccurrence, which is always a concern for cancer patients. Pain would be reported to the health care provider for evaluation.

40. **Ans: 1** All of these conditions warrant calling the health care provider (HCP). Nevertheless, tracheal deviation is a symptom of tension pneumothorax, which is a medical emergency, and the nurse may have to intervene before the rapid response team or the HCP can arrive. Decreased urinary output for a patient with cancer is probably related to an obstruction, but other causes would be investigated. Dysrhythmias are one sign of tumor lysis syndrome secondary to hyperkalemia. After bowel resection, patients are at risk for hemorrhage or peritonitis. **Focus:** Prioritization.

41. **Ans: Option 1, superior vena cava syndrome; Option 2, patency of airway; Option 3, Stridor; Option 4, place patient in a Fowler's position.** Superior vena cava syndrome is a compression or obstruction of the vessel that leads to congestion of the blood. Early manifestations include edema in the face, periorbital edema, and tightness around the neck of the gown. Other symptoms include cough, dyspnea, orthopnea, headache, upper extremity swelling, and distended chest veins.

Stridor caused by narrowing of the pharynx or larynx is an ominous sign. Late symptoms include hemorrhage, cyanosis, mental status changes, decreased cardiac output, and hypotension. Elevation of the head of bed or placing the patient in a high Fowler's position immediately helps to relieve the symptoms. Nasal cannula or a simple face mask would be used to increase oxygen saturation level. **Focus:** Prioritization; **QSEN:** S; **Concept:** Perfusion, Cellular Regulation; **Cognitive Level:** Analyzing; **Cognitive Skill:** Recognize Cues, Take Action.

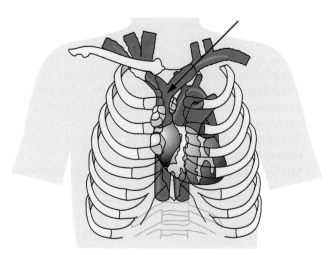

42. **Ans: 2, 6, 1, 3, 7, 9, 8, 4, 5** Level of consciousness and responsiveness are assessed and compared to baseline and 8:00 am status. Oxygen is administered immediately for respiratory distress or risk for decreased oxygenation and perfusion. Pulse oximeter is secured for continuous monitoring. Adequate pulse, blood pressure, and respirations are required for cerebral perfusion. Increased temperature may signal infection or sepsis. Blood glucose levels would be checked even if the patient does not have diabetes. Severe hypoglycemia would be immediately treated per protocol. Cardiac dysthymias can alter cerebral perfusion. Glasgow Coma Scale and neurological changes are assessed because change of mental status could be related to stroke or injury. Trauma may seem unlikely for a hospitalized patient but falls that result in head injury are a possibility, especially for older adults or confused patients. The liver plays a key role in blood clotting; liver cell dysfunction associated with the cancer increases the risk for bleeding even with minor injury. At 08:00 am, the sodium, potassium and blood glucose are in the lower range of normal and the ammonia level is in the upper range of normal. (Normal ranges: blood glucose, 70-110mg/dL (3.9-6.1 mmol/L); Potassium, 3.5-5.0 mEq/L (3.5-5.0 mmol/L); Sodium 136-145 mEq/L (136-145 mmol/L); Ammonia 10-80 mcg/dl (6-47μmol/L). With change in mental status, repeating laboratory tests is considered because cancer

increases risk for hyponatremia. Liver cell dysfunction increases the risk for hypokalemia, hypoglycemia and elevated ammonia. Assessment findings and response to oxygen and glucose (if administered) are reported using SBAR. **Focus:** Prioritization; **Test Taking Tip:** For patients who have a sudden change in mental status or a decreased level of consciousness, assume that the brain is experiencing decreased perfusion, decreased oxygenation, or both until proven otherwise. Administering oxygen and glucose are braincell–preserving interventions that must occur within several minutes.

43. **Ans:** A **56-year-old** patient comes to the clinic for scant **rectal bleeding** and intermittent **diarrhea and constipation, cramping, and fatigue** for the past several months. Despite an **unintentional weight loss** of 20lbs in the past month, his **body mass index (BMI) is 31.** He reports a chronic **"smoker's** cough" and shortness of breath with minor exertion, that **influences his desire to exercise.** He reports "My father was an alcoholic, so I limit myself to an occasional social drink." He has a history of appendectomy as a child and a gunshot wound to the abdomen sustained in military service. His **mother died from colorectal cancer at age 43** and his father died of complications related to alcoholism at age 63.

Signs and symptoms may not appear in the early stages of colon cancer. When signs/symptoms finally appear, they will include: change in bowel habits, such as diarrhea, constipation, change in consistency of stool, rectal bleeding or blood in stool; abdominal discomfort, such as cramps, gas, or a feeling that the bowel doesn't empty completely; weakness; fatigue; or unexplained weight loss. Modifiable risk factors include: obesity, lack of physical exercise, smoking, diet high in red meats, and heavy alcohol consumption. Non-modifiable factors include: age over 50; family history, especially if a first degree relative is less than 45 years old when colorectal cancer develops; inherited syndromes, such as Lynch syndrome or familial adenomatous polyposis; and ethnicity, such as, African American.   Personal history includes: inflammatory bowel disease, such as ulcerative colitis, Crohn's disease; polyps; previous episode of colorectal cancer and type 2 diabetes. **Focus:** Prioritization.

PART 2   Common Health Scenarios

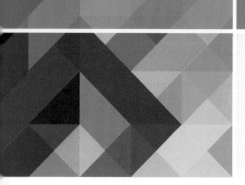

CHAPTER 3
Immunologic Problems

Questions

1. When scheduling a patient for skin testing for allergies, which information is **most** important for the allergy clinic nurse to include in patient teaching?
   1. Avoid taking antihistamines or antihistamine containing medications for 5 to 7 days before the skin testing.
   2. You may need to wear a patch for 48 hours in case of delayed reaction.
   3. Swelling and itching may occur at the site of the skin testing.
   4. Patient will need to wait in the clinic for 20 minutes after the testing.

2. Which finding will be **most** important for the nurse to report to the health care provider about a patient who is taking prednisone chronically after an organ transplant?
   1. Multiple arm bruises
   2. Sodium level of 146 mEq/dL (146 mmol/L)
   3. Blood glucose of 110 mg/dL (6.1 mmol/L)
   4. Black-colored stools

3. When the occupational health nurse is teaching assistive personnel about bloodborne pathogen exposure and human immunodeficiency virus (HIV) risk, which information is **most** important to emphasize?
   1. Occupational transmission of HIV from patients to health care workers is relatively rare.
   2. Occupational exposure to HIV-containing fluids should be reported immediately to the supervisor.
   3. Treatment for occupational exposure to HIV may include use of antiretroviral medications.
   4. Postexposure treatment will include HIV testing at baseline and at several intervals after the exposure.

4. A patient in the allergy clinic who has a rash has received diphenhydramine 50 mg PO. Which patient information is **most** indicative of a need for action by the nurse?
   1. The patient is preparing to drive home.
   2. The patient reports itching at the site of the rash.
   3. The patient has a history of constipation.
   4. The patient states, "My mouth feels so very dry!"

5. After a change-of-shift report, which newly admitted patient should the nurse assess **first**?
   1. A patient with human immunodeficiency virus whose CD4 count is 45 mm^3 (45 cells/mcL)
   2. A patient with acute kidney transplant rejection who has a scheduled dose of prednisone due
   3. A patient with graft-versus-host disease who has frequent liquid stools
   4. A patient with hypertension who has angioedema after receiving lisinopril

6. A few minutes after the nurse has given an intradermal injection of an allergen to a patient who is undergoing skin testing for allergies, the patient reports feeling anxious, short of breath, and dizzy. Which action included in the emergency protocol should the nurse take **first**?
   1. Start oxygen at 6 L/min using a face mask
   2. Obtain IV access with a large-bore IV catheter
   3. Give epinephrine 0.5 mg intramuscularly
   4. Administer albuterol per nebulizer mask

7. The nurse manager in a public health department is implementing a plan to reduce the incidence of infection with human immunodeficiency virus (HIV) in the community. Which nursing action will be delegated to assistive personnel (AP) working for the agency?
   1. Supplying injection drug users with sterile injection equipment such as needles and syringes
   2. Interviewing patients about behaviors that indicate a need for annual HIV testing
   3. Teaching high-risk community members about the use of condoms in preventing HIV infection
   4. Assessing the community to determine which population groups to target for education

Common Health Scenarios

8. The nurse is supervising a student nurse who is caring for a patient with human immunodeficiency virus (HIV). The patient has severe esophagitis caused by *Candida albicans*. Which action by the student requires the **most** rapid intervention by the nurse?
   1. Putting on a mask and gown before entering the patient's room
   2. Giving the patient a glass of water after administering the prescribed oral nystatin suspension
   3. Suggesting that the patient should order chili con carne or chicken soup for the next meal
   4. Placing a "No Visitors" sign on the door of the patient's room

9. The nurse is evaluating a patient with human immunodeficiency virus who is receiving trimethoprim-sulfamethoxazole (TMP-SMX) as a treatment for *Pneumocystis jiroveci* pneumonia. Which information is **most** important to communicate to the health care provider?
   1. The patient reports a blistering rash.
   2. The patient's fluid intake is 2 L/day.
   3. The patient's potassium is 3.4 mg/dL (3.4 mmol/L).
   4. The patient enjoys spending time outside in the sun.

10. A nursing student is helping the precepting nurse work through a preoperative checklist for a patient with rheumatoid arthritis who is scheduled to have an arthrodesis. The student asks the nurse what an arthrodesis is so she can explain the procedure and the risks to the patient before having the permit signed. What is the **best** response by the nurse?
    1. "A student nurse is not allowed to teach a patient without a preceptor present. We can do it together."
    2. "This surgery involves removing the affected joint and fusing the adjacent bones together."
    3. "Don't worry about it; the surgeon will explain the procedure and all the potential risks."
    4. "We'll discuss arthrodesis but the surgeon will explain the procedure and risks; we witness the patient's signature."

11. A patient with newly diagnosed acquired immunodeficiency syndrome has a 6-mm induration at 48 hours after a skin test for tuberculosis (TB). Which action will the nurse anticipate taking **next**?
    1. Arrange for a chest x-ray to check for active TB.
    2. Tell the patient that the TB test results are negative.
    3. Teach the patient about multidrug treatment for TB.
    4. Schedule TB skin testing again in 12 months.

12. The nurse is working in a hospice facility for patients with acquired immunodeficiency syndrome. The facility is staffed with LPNs/LVNs and assistive personnel (AP). Which action will the nurse assign to the LPN/LVN?
    1. Assessing patients' nutritional needs and individualizing diet plans to improve nutrition
    2. Collecting data about the patients' responses to medications used for pain and anorexia
    3. Developing AP training programs about how to lower the risk for spreading infections
    4. Assisting patients with personal hygiene and other activities of daily living as needed

13. A patient who has received a kidney transplant has been admitted to the medical unit with acute rejection and is receiving IV cyclosporine and methylprednisolone. Which staff member is **best** to assign to care for this patient?
    1. RN who floated to the medical unit from the coronary care unit for the day
    2. RN with 3 years of experience in the operating room who is orienting to the medical unit
    3. RN who has worked on the medical unit for 5 years and is working a double shift today
    4. Newly graduated RN who needs experience with IV medication administration

14. The nurse is caring for a patient with rheumatoid arthritis who is taking naproxen twice a day to reduce inflammation and joint pain. Which symptom is **most** important to communicate to the health care provider?
    1. Joint pain worse in the morning
    2. Dry eyes bilaterally
    3. Round and moveable nodules under the skin
    4. Dark-colored stools

15. Which of these patients cared for by the nurse in the clinic presents the **highest** risk for infection with human immunodeficiency virus (HIV) during sexual intercourse?
    1. Uninfected man who reports performing oral intercourse with an HIV-infected woman
    2. Uninfected man who is the receiver during anal intercourse with an HIV-infected man
    3. Uninfected woman who has had vaginal intercourse with an HIV-infected man
    4. Uninfected woman who has performed oral intercourse with an HIV-infected woman

16. A patient with a history of liver transplantation is receiving cyclosporine, prednisone, and mycophenolate. Which finding is of **most** concern?
    1. Gums that appear very pink and swollen
    2. Blood glucose level of 162 mg/dL (9 mmol/L)
    3. Nontender lump above the clavicle
    4. Grade 1 + pitting edema in the feet and ankles

 Answer Key for this chapter begins on p. 43

Common Health Scenarios
PART 2

17. A patient with human immunodeficiency virus (HIV) who has been started on antiretroviral therapy is seen in the clinic for follow-up. Which test will be **best** to monitor when determining the response to therapy?
    1. CD4 level
    2. Complete blood count
    3. Total lymphocyte percent
    4. Viral load

18. A hospitalized patient with acquired immunodeficiency syndrome has wasting syndrome. Which nursing action is appropriate to assign to an LPN/LVN who is providing care to this patient?
    1. Administering oxandrolone 5 mg/day
    2. Assessing the patient for other nutritional risk factors
    3. Developing a plan of care to improve the patient's appetite
    4. Providing instructions about a high-calorie, high-protein diet

19. The nurse assesses a 24-year-old patient with rheumatoid arthritis who is considering using methotrexate for treatment. Which patient information is **most** important to communicate to the health care provider?
    1. The patient has many concerns about the safety of the drug.
    2. The patient has been trying to get pregnant.
    3. The patient takes a daily multivitamin tablet.
    4. The patient says that she has taken methotrexate in the past.

20. An 18-year-old college student with an exacerbation of systemic lupus erythematosus (SLE) has been receiving prednisone 20 mg/day for 4 days. Which action prescribed by the health care provider is **most** important for the nurse to question?
    1. Discontinue prednisone after today's dose.
    2. Give a "catch-up" dose of varicella vaccine.
    3. Check the patient's C-reactive protein level.
    4. Administer ibuprofen 800 mg PO TID.

21. A patient with wheezing and coughing caused by an allergic reaction is admitted to the emergency department. Which medication will the nurse anticipate administering **first**?
    1. Methylprednisolone 100 mg IV
    2. Cromolyn 20 mg via nebulizer
    3. Albuterol 2.5mg/3 mL via nebulizer
    4. Aminophylline 500 mg IV

22. A patient with systemic lupus erythematosus (SLE) is admitted to the hospital with acute joint inflammation. Which information obtained in the laboratory testing will be of **highest** concern to the nurse?
    1. Elevated blood urea nitrogen (BUN) level
    2. Increased C-reactive protein level

    3. Positive antinuclear antibody test result
    4. Positive lupus erythematosus cell preparation

23. The nurse obtains this information when assessing a patient with human immunodeficiency virus who is taking antiretroviral therapy. Which finding is **most** important to report to the health care provider?
    1. The blood glucose level is 144 mg/dL (8 mmol/L).
    2. The hemoglobin level is 10.9 g/dL (109 g/L).
    3. The patient reports frequent nausea.
    4. The patient's viral load has increased.

24. Initiation of subcutaneous etanercept for a patient with rheumatoid arthritis is being considered. Which patient information is **most** important for the nurse to communicate with the health care provider?
    1. The patient is currently taking methotrexate.
    2. The patient has a positive tuberculin skin test result.
    3. The patient has had type 2 diabetes for 5 years.
    4. The patient is anxious about having to self-inject.

25. The hospital employee health nurse is completing a health history for a newly hired staff member. Which information given by the new employee **most** indicates the need for further nursing action before the new employee begins orientation to patient care?
    1. The employee takes enalapril for hypertension.
    2. The employee has allergies to bananas, avocados, and papayas.
    3. The employee received a tetanus vaccination 3 years ago.
    4. The employee's tuberculin skin test has a 5-mm induration at 48 hours.

26. A patient who has human immunodeficiency virus and is taking nucleoside reverse transcriptase inhibitors and a protease inhibitor is admitted to the psychiatric unit with a panic attack. Which information about the patient is **most** important to discuss with the health care provider?
    1. The patient exclaims, "I'm afraid I'm going to die right here!"
    2. The prescribed patient medications include midazolam 2 mg IV immediately.
    3. The patient is diaphoretic and tremulous and reports dizziness.
    4. The symptoms occurred suddenly while the patient was driving to work.

27. A patient seen in the sexually transmitted disease clinic has just tested positive for human immunodeficiency virus (HIV) with a rapid HIV test. Which action will the nurse take **next**?
    1. Ask about patient risk factors for HIV infection.
    2. Send a blood specimen for Western blot testing.
    3. Provide information about antiretroviral therapy.
    4. Discuss the positive test results with the patient.

28. Cloze _____

Scenario: A patient with a history of heart failure and rheumatoid arthritis is on a daily dose of prednisone 5 mg to decrease __1__ and __2__.
The health care provider has increased the daily dose of prednisone to 20 mg every day and added a non-steroidal anti-inflammatory to be taken every day with meals for increased pain relief. The next day the patient reports swollen legs and feet.
Based on the patient's history and report of swollen legs and feet what nursing intervention should be initiated __3__?

Instructions: Complete the sentences by choosing the most probable option for the omitted information that corresponds with the same numbered list of options provided.

Option 1	Option 2	Option 3
Swelling	Bone erosion	Administer furosemide
Immunity	Heart rate	Daily weights
Heart failure	Synovial fluid	Increase trans fats in diet
Inflammation	Joint movement	Limit fluids

29. A patient diagnosed with systemic erythematosus lupus (SLE) is being seen in the clinic for a follow-up appointment. She is prescribed cyclosporine and indomethacin. Which statement made by the patient should the nurse assess **first**?
1. "My feet are swollen."
2. "I have a paper cut on my index finger and it's red and painful."
3. "It seems like I'm always so tired."
4. "I'm using a vitamin C cream to minimize the rash on my face."

30. Drag and Drop _____

Instructions: Indicate which staff member listed in the second and third columns are most appropriate to be assigned to the patient scenario listed in the first column.

Patient Scenario	Assign to RN	Assign to LPN/LVN
1. Perform assessment on a patient with dementia.		
2. Administer rilpivirine and cabotegravir by way of intramuscular injection to a patient in a phase 3 trial.		
3. Collect a sterile urine specimen using a urinary catheter.		
4. Provide discharge teaching to a patient waiting for discharge.		
5. Flushing a peripherally inserted central line with normal saline.		
6. Assisting the health care provider with debridement of a third degree wound.		
7. Obtain a routine 12-lead electrocardiogram on a new admission		

Answer Key for this chapter begins on p. 43

PART 2 Common Health Scenarios

31. Matrix

Scenario: The nurse is caring for a patient with a diagnosis of human immunodeficiency virus (HIV). He reports that he is currently using injectable heroin and methamphetamine.

Vital signs:
Temperature 99°F (37.2°C)
Blood pressure 100/90 mm Hg
Pulse 100 beats/min
Respirations 24 breaths/min

Labs:
CD4 600 cells/mm^3
WBC: 9000/mm.
Viral load 30,000

Medications:
bictegravir 50mg
emtricitabine 200mg
tenofovir alafenamide 25mg

Instructions: For each potential Health Care Provider (HCP) request, place an X in the box to indicate whether it is indicated, contraindicated, or non-essential.

HCP Requests	Indicated	Contraindicated	Non-essential
1. Referral to substance treatment program			
2. Enroll patient in a needle exchange program.			
3. Directly observe antiretroviral drug treatment.			
4. Chest x-ray			
5. Prescription for Rifampin 300mg orally twice day			
6. Prescription for buprenorphine/naloxone			
7. Transthoracic echocardiogram			

Answer Key for this chapter begins on p. 43

Answers

1. **Ans: 1** Because antihistamine use before skin testing may prevent a reaction to an allergen, it is important that no antihistamine be taken before arriving for the skin testing, or the testing will have to be rescheduled. The other information may also be included, but it is not as important as avoiding any antihistamine before the skin testing takes place. **Focus:** Prioritization.

2. **Ans: 4** Dark green or black stools may indicate gastrointestinal bleeding, a possible adverse effect of oral steroid use, and further assessment and treatment are needed. Although thinning of the skin, electrolyte disturbances, and changes in glucose metabolism also occur with steroids, bruising and mild changes in sodium or glucose level do not require treatment. **Focus:** Prioritization.

3. **Ans: 2** The Centers for Disease Control and Prevention guidelines indicate that if postexposure prophylaxis is to be used, antiretroviral drugs should be started as soon as possible, preferably within hours of the exposure. It is important that staff understand that reporting the possible exposure is a priority so that rapid assessment and treatment can be initiated. The other statements are also true but will not impact the efficacy of any needed treatment. **Focus:** Prioritization.

4. **Ans: 1** Sedation is a common effect of the first-generation antihistamines, and patients should be cautioned against driving when taking medications such as diphenhydramine. Itching of the rash is expected with an allergic reaction. The patient should be taught how to manage common antihistamine side effects such as constipation and oral dryness, but these side effects are not safety concerns. **Focus:** Prioritization.

5. **Ans: 4** Because angioedema may cause airway obstruction, this patient should be assessed for any difficulty breathing, and treatment should be started immediately. The other patients also will need to be assessed as quickly as possible, but the patient with potential airway difficulty will need the most rapid care. **Focus:** Prioritization.

6. **Ans: 3** The World Allergy Organization guidelines indicate that intramuscular epinephrine should be the initial drug for treatment of anaphylaxis. Giving epinephrine rapidly at the onset of an anaphylactic reaction may prevent or reverse cardiovascular collapse as well as airway narrowing caused by bronchospasm and inflammation. Oxygen use is also appropriate, but oxygen delivery will be effective only if airways are open. Albuterol may also be administered to decrease airway narrowing but would not be the first therapy used for anaphylaxis. IV access will take longer to establish and should not be the first intervention. **Focus:** Prioritization.

7. **Ans: 1** Supplying sterile injection supplies to patients who are at risk for HIV infection can be done by staff members with AP education. Assessing for high-risk behaviors, education, and community assessment are RN-level skills. **Focus:** Delegation.

8. **Ans: 2** Nystatin should be in contact with the oral and esophageal tissues as long as possible for maximum effect. The other actions are also inappropriate and should be discussed with the student but do not require action as quickly. HIV-positive patients do not require droplet or contact precautions or visitor restrictions to prevent opportunistic infections. Hot or spicy foods are not usually well tolerated by patients with oral or esophageal fungal infections. **Focus:** Prioritization.

9. **Ans: 1** Because TMP-SMX can cause Stevens-Johnson syndrome (a life-threatening skin condition), a blistering rash indicates a need to discontinue the medication immediately. Meanwhile, 2 L/day of fluid is adequate to prevent crystalluria and renal damage associated with TMP-SMX. TMP-SMX can cause hyperkalemia; the nurse will report the potassium level to the provider, but the low potassium level is not caused by the medication. Patient teaching about photosensitivity is needed, but the nurse does not need guidance from the provider to implement this action. **Focus:** Prioritization.

10. **Ans: 4** The surgeon is responsible for explaining the procedure and the potential risks. The nurse is responsible for explaining the postoperative nursing care. The only role that the nurse has regarding the permit is to witness that the signature is that of the patient, guardian, or durable attorney. If the patient has further questions, the nurse acts as an advocate and calls the surgeon to return and clarify for the patient before the permit is signed. **Focus:** Supervision.

11. **Ans: 1** According to the National Institutes of Health guidelines, an induration of 5 mm or greater indicates TB infection in patients with HIV and a chest radiograph will be needed to determine whether the patient has active or latent TB infection. Teaching about multidrug therapy is needed if the patient has active TB, but latent TB is treated with a single drug (usually isoniazid) only. Positive skin test results generally persist throughout the patient's lifetime and will not be repeated, although other tests such as follow-up chest radiographs and sputum testing may be used to evaluate for effective TB treatment. **Focus:** Prioritization.

12. **Ans: 2** The collection of data used to evaluate the therapeutic and adverse effects of medications is included in LPN/LVN education and scope of practice. Assessment, planning, and developing teaching programs are more complex skills that require RN education. Assistance with hygiene and activities of daily living should be delegated to the AP. **Focus:** Assignment, Delegation.

PART 2 Common Health Scenarios

13. **Ans: 3** To be most effective, cyclosporine must be mixed and administered in accordance with the manufacturer's instructions, so the RN who is likely to have the most experience with the medication should care for this patient or monitor the new graduate carefully during medication preparation and administration. The coronary care unit float nurse and the nurse who is new to the unit would not have experience with this medication. **Focus:** Assignment.

14. **Ans: 4** Naproxen, a nonsteroidal anti-inflammatory drug, can cause gastrointestinal bleeding, and the stool appearance indicates that blood may be present in the stool. The health care provider should be notified so that actions such as testing a stool specimen for occult blood and administering proton pump inhibitors can be prescribed. The other symptoms are common in patients with rheumatoid arthritis and require further assessment or intervention, but they do not indicate that the patient is experiencing adverse effects from the medications. **Focus:** Prioritization.

15. **Ans: 2** Because anal intercourse allows contact of the infected semen with mucous membrane and causes tearing of mucous membrane, there is a high risk of transmission of HIV. HIV can be transmitted through oral or vaginal intercourse as well but not as easily. **Focus:** Prioritization.

16. **Ans: 3** Patients taking immunosuppressive medications are at increased risk for development of cancer. A nontender swelling or lump may signify that the patient has lymphoma. The other data indicate that the patient is experiencing common side effects of the immunosuppressive medications. **Focus:** Prioritization.

17. **Ans: 4** Viral load testing measures the amount of HIV genetic material in the blood, so a decrease in viral load indicates that the antiretroviral therapy is effective. The CD4 level, total lymphocytes, and complete blood count will also be used to assess the impact of HIV on immune function but will not directly measure the effectiveness of antiretroviral therapy. **Focus:** Prioritization.

18. **Ans: 1** Administration of oral medication is included in LPN/LVN education and scope of practice. Assessment, planning of care, and teaching are more complex RN-level interventions. **Focus:** Assignment.

19. **Ans: 2** Methotrexate is teratogenic and should not be used by patients who are pregnant. The health care provider will need to discuss the use of contraception during the time the patient is taking methotrexate. The other patient information may require further patient assessment or teaching but does not indicate that methotrexate may be contraindicated for the patient. **Focus:** Prioritization.

20. **Ans: 2** The varicella (chicken pox) vaccine is a live-virus vaccine and should not be administered to patients who are receiving immunosuppressive medications such as prednisone. The other medical actions may need some further clarification by the nurse.

Prednisone doses should be tapered gradually when patients have received long-term steroid therapy, but tapering is not usually necessary for short-term prednisone use. Measurement of C-reactive protein level is not the most specific test for monitoring treatment, but the test is inexpensive and frequently used. High doses of nonsteroidal anti-inflammatory drugs such as ibuprofen are more likely to cause side effects such as gastrointestinal bleeding but are useful in treating the joint pain associated with exacerbations of SLE. **Focus:** Prioritization. **Test-Taking Tip:** Because even an attenuated virus may lead to serious infection in patients with inadequate immune function, think about the patient's immune status whenever administering an attenuated live-virus vaccine such as measles, mumps, and rubella; varicella; or rotavirus.

21. **Ans: 3** Albuterol is the most rapidly acting of the medications listed. Corticosteroids are helpful in preventing and treating allergic reactions but do not act rapidly. Cromolyn is used as a prophylactic medication to prevent asthma attacks but not to treat acute attacks. Aminophylline is not a first-line treatment for bronchospasm. **Focus:** Prioritization.

22. **Ans: 1** A high number of patients with SLE develop nephropathy, so an increase in the BUN level may indicate a need for a change in therapy or for further diagnostic testing, such as a creatinine clearance test or renal biopsy. The other laboratory results are expected in patients with SLE. **Focus:** Prioritization. **Test-Taking Tip:** When prioritizing which information to discuss with a provider, consider which patient signs and symptoms are typical of the patient's disease and which findings may indicate complications. New findings that may indicate disease complications should be reported, but symptoms that are frequently seen as a part of the disease process are not usually a priority to report unless further treatment is necessary.

23. **Ans: 4** The increase in viral load indicates ineffective therapy, which will require further evaluation and treatment. The patient may not be adhering to the prescribed regimen, or resistance to the antiviral medications may have developed. Nausea, anemia, and hyperglycemia are common adverse effects with antiretroviral therapy and may require further evaluation, but the most concerning finding is the lack of effectiveness of the medications. **Focus:** Prioritization.

24. **Ans: 2** Tumor necrosis factor antagonists such as etanercept suppress immune function and increase the risk for reactivation of latent tuberculosis (TB). Further assessment for and possible treatment of TB will be needed before starting etanercept therapy. The other data will be communicated and may require patient monitoring or teaching but are not contraindications to starting etanercept. **Focus:** Prioritization.

25. **Ans: 2** A high incidence of latex allergy in seen in individuals with allergic reactions to these fruits. More information or testing is needed to determine whether

the new employee has a latex allergy, which might affect the ability to provide direct patient care. The other findings are important to include in documenting the employee's health history but do not affect the ability to provide patient care. **Focus:** Prioritization.

26. **Ans: 2** Because protease inhibitors decrease the metabolism of many drugs, including midazolam, serious toxicity can develop when protease inhibitors are given with other medications. Midazolam should not be given to this patient. The other patient data are consistent with the patient's diagnosis of panic attack and do not indicate an urgent need to communicate with the provider. **Focus:** Prioritization. **Test-Taking Tip:** Because the antiretroviral drug combinations used to treat HIV infection affect the metabolism of many other medications, investigate for possible drug interactions before administering any new medications in patients who are taking antiretrovirals.

27. **Ans: 4** A major purpose of HIV testing for asymptomatic patients is to ensure that HIV-positive individuals are aware of their HIV status, take actions to prevent HIV transmission, and effectively treat the HIV infection. According to current national guidelines, the other actions are also appropriate, but the initial action will be to communicate the test results to the patient. Rapid HIV testing must be confirmed by another test, usually the Western blot test. Antiretroviral therapy is recommended for all HIV-positive patients. Risk factor information will be used in tracking patient contacts and in teaching the patient how to reduce the risk for transmission to others. **Focus:** Prioritization.

28. **Ans: Option 1, Inflammation; Option 2, Bone erosion; Option 3, Daily weights.** The purpose of prednisone when given for rheumatoid arthritis, an autoimmune inflammatory disease, is to decrease the chronic inflammation in the joints that eventually causes cartilage and bone erosion from thickening of the synovium. Prednisone is a cortisone and like the cortisone normally produced in the body, affects the body's balance of water and sodium. Prednisone can cause fluid retention for this reason. Furosemide must be ordered by the health care provider (HCP) so it is considered a medical intervention rather than a nursing intervention. Increasing trans fats promotes weight gain. The health care provider (HCP) should be notified of a 2 pound weight gain in one day or 5 or more pounds in one week. This may indicate worsening heart failure in this patient. **Focus:** Prioritization.

29. **Ans: 2** Swollen feet and hands, a facial rash, and fatigue are symptoms normally associated with SLE. Vitamin C cream won't harm the patient but an infection in her left index finger could cause sepsis because cyclosporine suppresses the immune system. **Focus:** Prioritization.

30. **Ans:** LPN/LVN'S can perform skills such as administering an Intramuscular injection as well as duties on stable patients that do not require advanced procedures such as flushing a central line with normal saline. LPN/LVN's with addition training and certification may be able to perform advanced procedures in some states. Assessment and patient education are under the purview of the RN. **Focus:** Assignment.

Patient Scenario	Assign to RN	Assign to LPN/LVN
1. Perform assessment on a patient with dementia.	X	
2. Administer rilpivirine and cabotegravir by way of intramuscular injection to a patient in a phase 3 trial.		X
3. Collect a sterile urine specimen using a urinary catheter.		X
4. Provide discharge teaching to a patient waiting for discharge.	X	
5. Flushing a peripherally inserted central line with normal saline.	X	
6. Assisting the health care provider with debridement of a third degree wound.		X
7. Obtain a routine 12-lead electrocardiogram on a new admission		X

31. Ans: Ongoing substance abuse is a risk factor for poor adherence to antiretroviral therapy. Strategies to improve adherence include directly observing patients taking medications, needle exchange programs, and referral to substance treatment programs. Buprenorphine/naloxone can be used in combination with counseling. A chest x-ray is non-essential as the patient's vital signs and lab work do not indicate any pulmonary problems. Rifampin is an antibiotic whose use is contraindicated with bictegravir 50mg/ emtricitabine 200mg/ tenofovir alafenamide 25mg. A transthoracic echocardiogram is indicated as the patient states he is injecting methamphetamine which is known to interfere with cardiac valvular function. **Focus:** Prioritization.

HCP Requests	Indicated	Contraindicated	Non-essential
1. Referral to substance treatment program	X		
2. Enroll patient in a needle exchange program.	X		
3. Directly observe antiretroviral drug treatment.	X		
4. Chest x-ray			X
5. Prescription for Rifampin 300mg orally twice day		X	
6. Prescription for buprenorphine/naloxone	X		
7. Transthoracic echocardiogram	X		

Common Health Scenarios   PART 2

CHAPTER 4

Fluid, Electrolyte, and Acid-Base Balance Problems

Questions

1. A patient is receiving IV fluid of normal saline (0.9%) at a rate of 100 mL per hour. Which effect on red blood cells shown in the figures below would the nurse expect?
   1. _____
   2. _____
   3. _____
   4. _____

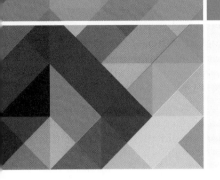

2. The RN is admitting a patient with benign prostatic hyperplasia to an acute care unit. The patient describes an oral intake of about 1400 mL/day. What is the RN's **priority** concern?
   1. Ask the patient about his bowel movements.
   2. Have the patient complete a diet diary for the past 2 days.
   3. Instruct the patient to increase oral intake to 2 to 3 L/day.
   4. Ask the patient to describe his urine output.

3. The patient has fluid volume deficit related to excessive fluid loss. Which action related to fluid management should be delegated by the RN to the assistive personnel (AP)?

1. Administering IV fluids as prescribed by the health care provider
2. Providing straws and offering fluids between meals
3. Developing a plan for added fluid intake over 24 hours
4. Teaching family members to assist the patient with fluid intake

4. The assistive personnel (AP) reports to the nurse that a patient's urine output for the past 24 hours has been only 360 mL. What is the nurse's **priority** action at this time?
   1. Place an 18-gauge IV in the nondominant arm.
   2. Elevate the patient's head of bed at least 45 degrees.
   3. Instruct the AP to provide the patient with a pitcher of ice water.
   4. Contact and notify the health care provider immediately.

5. The patient is at risk for poor perfusion related to decreased plasma volume. Which assessment finding supports this risk?
   1. Flattened neck veins when the patient is in the supine position
   2. Full and bounding pedal and post-tibial pulses
   3. Pitting edema located in the feet, ankles, and calves
   4. Shallow respirations with crackles on auscultation

6. The nursing plan of care for an older patient with dehydration includes interventions for oral health. Which interventions are within the scope of practice for an LPN/LVN being supervised by an RN? **Select all that apply.**
   1. Reminding the patient to avoid commercial mouthwashes
   2. Encouraging mouth rinsing with warm saline
   3. Assessing skin turgor by pinching the skin over the back of the hand
   4. Observing the lips, tongue, and mucous membranes
   5. Providing mouth care every 2 hours while the patient is awake
   6. Seeking a dietary consult to increase fluids on meal trays

Common Health Scenarios   PART 2

7. The health care provider has written these orders for a patient with a diagnosis of pulmonary edema. The patient's morning assessment reveals bounding peripheral pulses, a weight gain of 2 lb, pitting ankle edema, and moist crackles bilaterally. Which order takes **priority** at this time?
   1. Weigh the patient every morning.
   2. Maintain accurate intake and output records.
   3. Restrict fluids to 1500 mL/day.
   4. Administer furosemide 40 mg IV push.

8. Which statement related to dehydration made by a patient with hypovolemia is the **best** indicator to the nurse of the need for additional teaching?
   1. "I will drink 2 to 3 L of fluids every day."
   2. "I will drink a glass of water whenever I feel thirsty."
   3. "I will drink coffee and cola drinks throughout the day."
   4. "I will avoid drinks containing alcohol."

9. The nurse has been floated to the telemetry unit for the day. The monitor technician informs the nurse that the patient has developed prominent U waves. Which laboratory value should be checked **immediately**?
   1. Sodium
   2. Potassium
   3. Magnesium
   4. Calcium

10. A patient's potassium level is 6.7 mEq/L (6.7 mmol/L). Which intervention should the nurse delegate to the first-year student nurse under his or her supervision?
   1. Administer sodium polystyrene sulfonate 15 g orally.
   2. Administer spironolactone 25 mg orally.
   3. Assess the electrocardiogram (ECG) strip for tall T waves.
   4. Administer potassium 10 mEq (10 mmol/L) orally.

11. A patient is admitted to the unit with a diagnosis of syndrome of inappropriate antidiuretic hormone secretion (SIADH). For which electrolyte abnormality would the nurse be sure to monitor?
   1. Hypokalemia
   2. Hyperkalemia
   3. Hyponatremia
   4. Hypernatremia

12. The charge nurse assigned the care of a patient with acute kidney failure and hypernatremia to a newly graduated RN. Which actions can the new RN delegate to the assistive personnel (AP)? **Select all that apply.**
   1. Providing oral care every 3 to 4 hours
   2. Monitoring for indications of dehydration
   3. Administering 0.45% saline by IV line
   4. Recording urine output when patient voids
   5. Assessing daily weights for trends
   6. Helping the patient change position every 2 hours

13. An experienced LPN/LVN reports to the RN that a patient's blood pressure and heart rate have decreased and that when his face was assessed, one side twitched. What action should the RN take at this time?
   1. Reassess the patient's blood pressure and heart rate.
   2. Review the patient's morning calcium level.
   3. Request a neurologic consult today.
   4. Check the patient's pupillary reaction to light.

14. The nurse is preparing to discharge a patient whose calcium level was low but is now just barely within the normal range (9 to 10.5 mg/dL [2.25 to 2.63 mmol/L]). Which statement by the patient indicates the need for additional teaching?
   1. "I will call my doctor if I experience muscle twitching or seizures."
   2. "I will make sure to take my vitamin D with my calcium each day."
   3. "I will take my calcium citrate pill every morning before breakfast."
   4. "I will avoid dairy products, broccoli, and spinach when I eat."

15. Which prescription for a patient with hypercalcemia would the nurse question?
   1. 0.9% saline at 50 mL/hr IV
   2. Furosemide 20 mg orally each morning
   3. Apply cardiac telemetry monitoring.
   4. Hydrochlorothiazide (HCTZ) 25 mg orally each morning

16. The assistive personnel (AP) asks the nurse why the patient with a chronically low phosphorus level needs so much assistance with activities of daily living. What is the RN's **best** response?
   1. "The patient's low phosphorus is probably because of malnutrition."
   2. "The patient is just worn out from not getting enough rest."
   3. "The patient's skeletal muscles are weak because of the low phosphorus."
   4. "The patient will do more for himself when his phosphorus level is normal."

17. The RN is reviewing the patient's morning laboratory results. Which of these results is of **most** concern?
   1. Serum potassium level of 5.2 mEq/L (5.2 mmol/L)
   2. Serum sodium level of 134 mEq/L (134 mmol/L)
   3. Serum calcium level of 10.6 mg/dL (2.65 mmol/L)
   4. Serum magnesium level of 0.8 mEq/L (0.4 mmol/L)

18. Which patient would the charge nurse assign to the step-down unit nurse who was floated to the intensive care unit for the day?
    1. A 68-year-old patient on a ventilator with acute respiratory failure and respiratory acidosis
    2. A 72-year-old patient with chronic obstructive pulmonary disease (COPD) and normal blood gas values who is ventilator dependent
    3. A newly admitted 56-year-old patient with diabetic ketoacidosis receiving an insulin drip
    4. A 38-year-old patient on a ventilator with narcotic overdose and respiratory alkalosis

19. The patient with respiratory failure is receiving mechanical ventilation and continues to produce arterial blood gas results indicating respiratory acidosis. Which change in ventilator setting should the nurse expect to correct this problem?
    1. Increase in ventilator rate from 6 to 10 breaths/min
    2. Decrease in ventilator rate from 10 to 6 breaths/min
    3. Increase in oxygen concentration from 30% to 40%
    4. Decrease in oxygen concentration from 40% to 30%

20. Which actions should the nurse delegate to an assistive personnel (AP) for the patient with diabetic ketoacidosis? **Select all that apply.**
    1. Checking fingerstick glucose results every hour
    2. Recording intake and output every hour
    3. Measuring vital signs every 15 minutes
    4. Assessing for indicators of fluid imbalance
    5. Notifying the health care provider of changes in glucose level
    6. Assisting the patient to reposition every 2 hours

21. The nurse is admitting an older adult patient to the acute care medical unit. Which assessment factor alerts the nurse that this patient has a risk for acid-base imbalances?
    1. History of myocardial infarction (MI) 1 year ago
    2. Antacid use for occasional indigestion
    3. Shortness of breath with extreme exertion
    4. Chronic renal insufficiency

22. A patient with lung cancer has received oxycodone 10 mg orally for pain. When the student nurse assesses the patient, which finding would the nurse instruct the student nurse to report **immediately**?
    1. Respiratory rate of 8 to 10 breaths/min
    2. Decrease in pain level from 6 to 2 (on a scale of 1 to 10)
    3. Request by the patient that the room door be closed
    4. Heart rate of 90 to 100 beats/min

23. The assistive personnel (AP) reports to the nurse that a patient seems very anxious, and vital sign measurement included a respiratory rate of 38 breaths/min. Which acid-base imbalance should the nurse suspect?
    1. Respiratory acidosis
    2. Respiratory alkalosis
    3. Metabolic acidosis
    4. Metabolic alkalosis

24. A patient is admitted to the oncology unit for chemotherapy. To prevent an acid-base problem, which finding would the nurse instruct the assistive personnel to report?
    1. Repeated episodes of nausea and vomiting
    2. Reports of pain associated with exertion
    3. Failure to eat all the food on the breakfast tray
    4. Patient hair loss during the morning bath

25. The patient has a nasogastric (NG) tube connected to intermittent wall suction. The student nurse asks why the patient's respiratory rate and depth has decreased. What is the nurse's **best** response?
    1. "It's common for patients with uncomfortable equipment such as NG tubes to have a lower rate of breathing."
    2. "The patient may have a metabolic alkalosis because of the NG suctioning, and the decreased respiratory rate is a compensatory mechanism."
    3. "Whenever a patient develops a respiratory acid-base problem, decreasing the respiratory rate helps correct the problem."
    4. "The patient is hypoventilating because of anxiety, and we will have to stay alert for the development of respiratory acidosis."

26. The patient has an order for hydrochlorothiazide (HCTZ) 10 mg orally every day. What should the nurse be sure to include in a teaching plan for this drug? **Select all that apply.**
    1. "Take this medication in the morning."
    2. "This medication should be taken in two divided doses: half when you get up and half when you go to bed."
    3. "Eat foods with extra sodium every day."
    4. "Inform your health care provider (HCP) if you notice weight gain or increased swelling."
    5. "You should expect your urine output to increase."
    6. "Your HCP may also prescribe a potassium supplement."

27. Which blood test result would the nurse be sure to monitor for the patient taking hydrochlorothiazide (HCTZ)?
    1. Sodium level
    2. Potassium level
    3. Chloride level
    4. Calcium level

    Answer Key for this chapter begins on p. 51

28. The RN is providing care for a patient diagnosed with dehydration and hypovolemic shock. Which prescribed intervention from the health care provider should the RN question?
    1. Blood pressure every 15 minutes
    2. Place two 18-gauge IV lines.
    3. Oxygen at 3 L via nasal cannula
    4. IV 5% dextrose in water (D_5W) to run at 250 mL/hr

29. The student nurse, under the supervision of an RN, is reviewing a patient's arterial blood gas results and notes an acute increase in arterial partial pressure of carbon dioxide ($Paco_2$) to 51 mm Hg compared with the previous results. Which statement by the student nurse indicates an accurate understanding of the acid-base balance for this patient?
    1. "When the $Paco_2$ is acutely elevated, the blood pH should be lower than normal."
    2. "This patient should be taught to breathe and re-breathe in a paper bag."
    3. "An elevated $Paco_2$ always means that a patient has an acidosis."
    4. "When a patient's $Paco_2$ is increased, the respiratory rate should decrease to compensate."

30. The nurse is providing care for several patients who are at risk for acid-base imbalance. Which patient is **most** at risk for respiratory acidosis?
    1. A 68-year-old patient with chronic emphysema
    2. A 58-year-old patient who uses antacids every day
    3. A 48-year-old patient with an anxiety disorder
    4. A 28-year-old patient with salicylate intoxication

31. The nurse is caring for a patient who experiences frequent generalized tonic-clonic seizures associated with periods of apnea. The nurse must be alert for which acid-base imbalance?
    1. Respiratory alkalosis
    2. Respiratory acidosis
    3. Metabolic alkalosis
    4. Metabolic acidosis

32. The nurse is completing a history for an older patient at risk for an acidosis imbalance. Which questions would the nurse be sure to ask? **Select all that apply.**
    1. "Which drugs do you take on a daily basis?"
    2. "Do you have any problems with breathing?"
    3. "When was your last bowel movement?"
    4. "Have you experienced any activity intolerance or fatigue in the past 24 hours?"
    5. "Over the past month have you had any dizziness or tinnitus?"
    6. "Do you have episodes of drowsiness or decreased alertness?"

33. Which specific instruction does the charge nurse give the assistive personnel helping to provide care for a patient who is at risk for metabolic acidosis?
    1. Check to see that the patient keeps his oxygen in place at all times.
    2. Inform the nurse immediately if the patient's respiratory rate and depth increases.
    3. Record any episodes of reflux or constipation.
    4. Keep the patient's ice water pitcher filled at all times.

34. Enhanced Multiple Response

Case Study and Question

The nurse is admitting a 72-year-old patient from the health care provider's office to the medical/surgical unit. The patient was alert until recently and has become confused. Over the past 36 hours the patient developed signs and symptoms of fluid overload.

On admission assessment which manifestations would the RN expect to assess?

Vital Signs:
Pulse 112 beats/min
Respiration 34 breaths/min
Blood Pressure 168/94 mmHg

Instructions: Read the case study on the left and circle the numbers that best answer the question.
1. Increased heart rate
2. Weak, thready pulse
3. Alert and oriented
4. Pitting edema of lower extremities
5. Deep respirations
6. Distended neck veins
7. Bilateral rhonchi
8. Hyperactive bowel sounds
9. Weight loss
10. Pale, cool skin

Answers

1. **Ans: 4** The first circle depicts sickled red blood cells (cells become sickle-shaped and inflexible and may occlude blood flow). The second shows what happens when a patient receives hypertonic solutions (water leaves the cells and cells shrink), and the third circle shows what happens with hypotonic fluids (water moves into cells causing them to swell and possibly burst). Normal saline (0.9%) is an isotonic fluid with the same tonicity as the body; thus these fluids do not affect red blood cells, and the nurse would expect normal-appearing red blood cells. **Focus:** Prioritization.

2. **Ans: 3** An adult should take in about 2 to 3 L of fluid daily from food and liquids. Although the RN would want to know about bowel movements, dietary intake, and urine output, in this case the priority concern is that the patient is not taking in enough oral fluids. **Focus:** Prioritization.

3. **Ans: 2** APs can reinforce additional fluid intake when it is part of the care plan. Administering IV fluids, developing plans, and teaching families require additional education and skills that are within the scope of practice of an RN. **Focus:** Delegation, Supervision. **Test-Taking Tip:** The nurse must be familiar with the scope of practice for APs before delegating patient care tasks. AP scope of practice includes checking vital signs and performing tasks associated with activities of daily living such as bathing and oral care, feeding, and recording intake and output. APs can provide items such as drinking straws and can encourage and remind patients about instructions from the nurse such as increasing fluid intake.

4. **Ans: 4** The minimum amount of urine per day needed to excrete toxic waste products is 400 to 600 mL. This minimum volume is called the obligatory urine output. If the 24-hour urine output falls below the obligatory output amount, wastes are retained and can cause lethal electrolyte imbalances, acidosis, and a toxic buildup of nitrogen. The patient may need additional fluids (IV or oral) after the cause of the low urine output is determined. Elevating the head of the bed will not help with urine output. Notifying the health care provider is the first priority in this case. **Focus:** Prioritization.

5. **Ans: 1** Normally, neck veins are distended when the patient is in the supine position. These veins flatten as the patient moves to a sitting position. The other three responses are characteristic of excess fluid volume. **Focus:** Prioritization.

6. **Ans: 1, 2, 4, 5** The LPN/LVN scope of practice and educational preparation includes oral care and routine observation. State practice acts vary as to whether LPNs/LVNs are permitted to perform assessments. The patient should be reminded to avoid most commercial mouthwashes, which contain agents such as

alcohol. To assess skin turgor in an older adult, skin tenting is best checked by pinching the skin over the sternum or on the forehead rather than over the back of the hand. With aging, the skin loses elasticity and tents on hands and arms even when the adult is well hydrated. Initiating a dietary consult is within the purview of the RN or health care provider. **Focus:** Supervision.

7. **Ans: 4** Bilateral moist crackles indicate fluid-filled alveoli, which interferes with gas exchange. Furosemide is a potent loop diuretic that will help mobilize the fluid in the lungs. The other orders are important but are not urgent. **Focus:** Prioritization. **Test-Taking Tip:** When asked a question like this, the student must consider which action is most urgent. With fluid-filled lungs, gas exchange is at risk. Think ABCs!

8. **Ans: 3** Mild dehydration is very common among healthy adults and is corrected or prevented easily by matching fluid intake with fluid output. Teach all adults to drink more fluids, especially water. Beverages with caffeine can increase fluid loss, as can drinks containing alcohol. These beverages should not be used to prevent or treat dehydration. **Focus:** Prioritization.

9. **Ans: 2** Suspect hypokalemia and check the patient's potassium level. Common electrocardiogram changes with hypokalemia include ST-segment depression, inverted T waves, and prominent U waves. Patients with hypokalemia may also develop heart block. Other abnormal electrolyte levels can affect cardiac rhythms, but the occurrence of U waves is associated with low potassium levels. **Focus:** Prioritization.

10. **Ans: 1** The patient's potassium level is high (normal range is 3.5 to 5 mEq/L or 3.5 to 5 mmol/L). Sodium polystyrene sulfonate removes potassium from the body through the gastrointestinal system. Spironolactone is a potassium-sparing diuretic that may cause the patient's potassium level to go even higher. A potassium chloride supplement can also raise the potassium level even higher. The beginning nursing student does not have the skill to assess ECG strips. **Focus:** Delegation, Supervision.

11. **Ans: 3** SIADH results in a relative sodium deficit caused by excessive retention of water. Thus the nurse should monitor the patient with SIADH for hyponatremia. **Focus:** Prioritization.

12. **Ans: 1, 4, 6** Providing oral care, assisting patients to reposition, and recording urine output are within the scope of practice of the AP. Monitoring or assessing patients, as well as administering IV fluids, requires the additional education and skills of the RN. **Focus:** Assignment, Delegation, Supervision.

13. **Ans: 2** A positive Chvostek sign (facial twitching of one side of the mouth, nose, and cheek in response to

tapping the face just below and in front of the ear) is a neurologic manifestation of hypocalcemia. The heart rate may be slower or slightly faster than normal, with a weak, thready pulse. Severe hypocalcemia causes severe hypotension. The LPN/LVN is experienced and possesses the skills to accurately measure vital signs. **Focus:** Prioritization.

14. **Ans: 4**   Patients with low calcium levels should be encouraged to consume dairy products, seafood, nuts, broccoli, and spinach, which are all good sources of dietary calcium. The other three options indicate a correct understanding of calcium therapy. **Focus:** Prioritization.

15. **Ans: 4**   Calcium excretion is decreased with thiazide diuretics (e.g., HCTZ), so the calcium level is at risk for going even higher. Loop diuretics (e.g., furosemide) increase calcium excretion. The addition of IV fluids and cardiac monitoring are appropriate actions for monitoring and treating a patient with hypercalcemia. **Focus:** Prioritization.

16. **Ans: 3**   A musculoskeletal manifestation of low phosphorus levels is generalized muscle weakness, which may lead to acute muscle breakdown (rhabdomyolysis). Phosphate is necessary for energy production in the form of adenosine triphosphate, and when not produced, it leads to generalized muscle weakness. Although the other statements are true, they do not answer the AP's question. **Focus:** Delegation, Supervision.

17. **Ans: 4**   Although all of these laboratory values are outside of the normal range, the magnesium level is the furthest from normal. With a magnesium level this low, the patient is at risk for electrocardiogram changes and life-threatening ventricular dysrhythmias. **Focus:** Prioritization.

18. **Ans: 2**   The patient with COPD, although ventilator dependent, is in the most stable condition of the patients in this group and should be assigned to the float nurse from the step-down unit. Patients with acid-base imbalances often require frequent laboratory assessment and changes in therapy to correct their disorders. In addition, the patient with diabetic ketoacidosis is a new admission and requires an in-depth admission assessment. All three of these other patients need care from an experienced critical care nurse. **Focus:** Assignment.

19. **Ans: 1**   The blood gas component responsible for respiratory acidosis is carbon dioxide, thus increasing the ventilator rate will blow off more carbon dioxide and decrease or correct the acidosis. Changes in the oxygen setting may improve oxygenation but will not affect respiratory acidosis. **Focus:** Prioritization.

20. **Ans: 2, 3, 6**   The AP's training and education includes how to measure vital signs, record intake and output, and reposition patients. Performing fingerstick glucose checks or assessing patients requires additional education and skill, as possessed by licensed nurses. Notifying the health care provider of glucose changes is within the scope of practice for licensed nurses. Some facilities may train experienced APs to perform fingerstick glucose checks and change their role descriptions to designate their new skills, but this task is beyond the normal scope of practice of an AP. **Focus:** Delegation, Supervision.

21. **Ans: 4**   Risk factors for acid-base imbalances in older adults include chronic kidney disease and pulmonary disease. Occasional antacid use will not cause imbalances, although antacid abuse is a risk factor for metabolic alkalosis. The MI occurred 1 year ago and is no longer a risk factor. **Focus:** Prioritization.

22. **Ans: 1**   A decreased respiratory rate indicates respiratory depression, which also puts the patient at risk for respiratory acidosis. All of the other findings are important and should be reported to the RN, but the respiratory rate demands urgent attention. **Focus:** Delegation, Supervision.

23. **Ans: 2**   The patient is most likely hyperventilating and blowing off carbon dioxide. This decrease in carbon dioxide will lead to an increase in pH and cause respiratory alkalosis. Eliminating carbon dioxide would lead to an alkalosis. Metabolic imbalances would be related to renal changes. **Focus:** Prioritization, Supervision.

24. **Ans: 1**   Prolonged nausea and vomiting can result in acid deficit that can lead to metabolic alkalosis. The other findings are important and need to be assessed but are not related to acid-base imbalances. **Focus:** Prioritization, Supervision.

25. **Ans: 2**   NG suctioning can result in a decrease in acid components and metabolic alkalosis. The patient's decrease in rate and depth of ventilation is an attempt to compensate by retaining carbon dioxide. The first response may be true, but it does not address all the components of the question. The third and fourth answers are inaccurate. **Focus:** Supervision, Prioritization.

26. **Ans: 1, 4, 5, 6**   HCTZ is a thiazide diuretic. It should not be taken at night because it will cause the patient to wake up to urinate. This type of diuretic causes a loss of potassium, so the nurse should teach the patient about eating foods rich in potassium and should inform the patient that the HCP may prescribe a potassium supplement. Weight gain and increased edema should not occur while the patient is taking this drug, so these should be reported to the HCP. **Focus:** Prioritization.

27. **Ans: 2**   Potassium is lost when a patient is taking HCTZ, and so the patient's potassium level should be monitored regularly. **Focus:** Prioritization.

28. **Ans: 4**   To correct hypovolemic shock with dehydration, the patient needs IV fluids that are isotonic and will increase intravascular volume, such as normal saline. With D_5W, the body rapidly metabolizes the dextrose, and the solution becomes hypotonic. All of the other interventions are appropriate for a patient with shock. **Focus:** Prioritization.

29. **Ans: 1** This patient's $Paco_2$ is elevated (normal is 35 to 45 mm Hg). Whenever the $Paco_2$ level changes acutely, the pH changes to the same degree but in the opposite direction. As the amount of CO_2 begins to rise above normal in the brain's blood and tissues, these central receptors trigger the neurons to increase the rate and depth of breathing (hyperventilation). For these reasons, answers 2, 3, and 4 are inaccurate. **Focus:** Supervision, Prioritization.

30. **Ans: 1** Patients at greatest risk for acute acidosis are those with problems that impair breathing. Older adults with chronic health problems are at greater risk for developing acidosis. Whereas a patient who misuses antacids is at risk for metabolic alkalosis, a patient with anxiety is at risk for respiratory alkalosis. A patient with salicylate intoxication is at risk for metabolic acidosis. **Focus:** Prioritization. **Test-Taking Tip:** Respiratory acid-base disorders are related to respiratory function. When a patient has a chronic respiratory illness, he or she is at risk for a respiratory acid-base imbalance.

31. **Ans: 4** Seizures may be associated with apnea and thus hypoxemia and lactic acidosis. Lactic acidosis, a form of metabolic acidosis, occurs when cells use glucose without adequate oxygen (anaerobic metabolism); glucose then is incompletely broken down and forms lactic acid. This acid releases hydrogen ions, causing acidosis. Lactic acidosis occurs whenever the body has too little oxygen to meet metabolic oxygen demands (e.g., heavy exercise, seizure activity, reduced oxygen). **Focus:** Prioritization.

32. **Ans: 1, 2, 4, 6** Collect data about risk factors related to the development of acidosis. Older adults may be taking drugs that disrupt acid-base balance, especially diuretics and aspirin. Ask about specific risk factors, such as any type of breathing problem. Also ask about headaches, behavior changes, increased drowsiness, reduced alertness, reduced attention span, lethargy, anorexia, abdominal distention, nausea or vomiting, muscle weakness, and increased fatigue. Ask the patient to relate activities of the previous 24 hours to identify activity intolerance, behavior changes, and fatigue. Answers 3 and 5 are not common concerns with acidosis. **Focus:** Prioritization.

33. **Ans: 2** If acidosis is metabolic in origin, the rate and depth of breathing increase as the hydrogen ion level rises. Breaths are deep and rapid and not under voluntary control, a pattern called Kussmaul respiration. The patient may not require oxygen. Although it's important to record reflux and constipation, this is not related to metabolic acidosis, nor is keeping the water pitcher full specific to this condition. **Focus:** Supervision, Delegation.

34. **Ans: 1, 4, 6, 8, 10** The patient would also be likely to have pale dry skin, a bounding pulse, altered level of consciousness, shallow and increased respirations, moist crackles, and weight gain. Hyperactive bowel sounds are the result of increased motility. **Focus:** Prioritization.

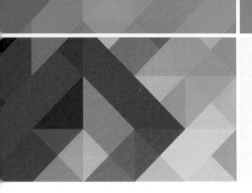

CHAPTER 5

Safety and Infection Control

Questions

1. The nurse is caring for a patient with intractable nausea and vomiting. The patient has a temperature of 99°F, a pulse of 100, a respiratory rate of 24, a blood pressure of 90/60, and oxygen saturation of 91%. What is the **first** action the nurse should take?
   1. Start an IV of normal saline.
   2. Administer ondansetron 4 mg IV.
   3. Apply oxygen at 2 L/min per nasal cannula.
   4. Make sure the wall suction is fully functioning.

2. The charge nurse is making patient assignments for the day shift. Which patient should be assigned to an RN who is pregnant?
   1. A 32-year-old male with coccidiomycosis
   2. A 67-year-old female with shingles
   3. A 42-year-old female with vancomycin resistant enterococcus (VRE)
   4. A 24-year-old male with chicken pox

3. The nurse is caring for a newly admitted patient with increasing dyspnea, hypoxia, and dehydration who has possible avian influenza ("bird flu"). Which of these prescribed actions will the nurse implement **first**?
   1. Start oxygen using a nonrebreather mask.
   2. Infuse 5% dextrose in water at 100 mL/hr.
   3. Administer the first dose of oral oseltamivir.
   4. Obtain blood and sputum specimens for testing.

4. A patient has been diagnosed with disseminated herpes zoster. Which personal protective equipment will the nurse need to put on when preparing to assess the patient? **Select all that apply.**
   1. Surgical face mask
   2. N95 respirator
   3. Gown
   4. Gloves
   5. Goggles
   6. Shoe covers

5. Four patients arrive simultaneously at the emergency department. Which patient requires the **most** rapid action by the triage nurse to protect other patients from infection?
   1. A 3-year-old patient who has paroxysmal coughing and whose sibling has pertussis
   2. A 5-year-old patient who has a new pruritic rash and possible measles
   3. A 62-year-old patient who has an ongoing methicillin-resistant *Staphylococcus aureus* (MRSA) abdominal wound infection
   4. A 74-year-old patient who needs tuberculosis (TB) testing after being exposed to TB during a recent international airplane flight

6. The nurse is caring for four patients who are receiving IV infusions of normal saline. Which patient is at **highest** risk for bloodstream infection?
   1. The patient with an implanted port in the right subclavian vein
   2. The patient who has a midline IV catheter in the left antecubital fossa
   3. The patient who has a nontunneled central line in the left internal jugular vein
   4. The patient with a peripherally inserted central catheter (PICC) line in the right upper arm

7. The nurse is caring for a patient who has been admitted to the hospital with a leg ulcer that is infected with vancomycin-resistant *Staphylococcus aureus.* Which nursing action can be assigned to an LPN/LVN?
   1. Planning ways to improve the patient's oral protein intake
   2. Teaching the patient about home care of the leg ulcer
   3. Obtaining wound cultures during dressing changes
   4. Assessing the risk for further skin breakdown

8. A hospitalized 88-year-old patient who has been receiving antibiotics for 10 days tells the nurse about having frequent watery stools. Which action will the nurse take **first**?
   1. Notify the health care provider about the stools.
   2. Obtain stool specimens for culture.
   3. Instruct the patient about correct hand washing.
   4. Place the patient on contact precautions.

9. The nurse notes white powder on the arms and chest of a patient who arrives at the emergency department and reports possible anthrax contamination. Which action included in the hospital protocol for a possible anthrax exposure will the nurse take **first**?
   1. Notify hospital security personnel about the patient.
   2. Escort the patient to a decontamination room.
   3. Give ciprofloxacin 500 mg PO.
   4. Assess the patient for signs of infection.

10. A pregnant patient in the first trimester tells the nurse that she was recently exposed to the Zika virus while traveling in Southeast Asia. Which action by the nurse is **most** important?
    1. Arrange for testing for the Zika virus infection.
    2. Discuss need for multiple fetal ultrasounds during pregnancy.
    3. Describe potential impact of Zika infection on fetal development.
    4. Assess for symptoms such as rash, joint pain, conjunctivitis, and fever.

11. The nurse at the infectious disease clinic has four patients waiting to be seen. Which patient should the nurse see **first**?
    1. Patient who has a 16-mm induration after a tuberculosis skin test
    2. Patient who has human immunodeficiency virus and a low CD4 count
    3. Patient who has swine influenza and reports increased dyspnea
    4. Patient who has been exposed to Zika virus and has a rash and joint pain

12. The nurse notices that the health care provider (HCP) omits hand hygiene after leaving a patient's hospital room. Which action by the nurse is **best** at this time?
    1. Report the HCP to the infection control department.
    2. Offer the HCP an alcohol-based hand sanitizing fluid.
    3. Provide the HCP with a list of upcoming in-services on hand hygiene.
    4. Remind the HCP about the importance of minimizing infection spread.

13. A patient with a vancomycin-resistant enterococcus (VRE) infection is admitted to the medical unit. Which action can be delegated to the assistive personnel who is assisting with the patient's care?
    1. Teaching the patient and family members about ways to prevent transmission of VRE
    2. Communicating with other departments when the patient is transported for ordered tests
    3. Implementing contact precautions when providing care for the patient
    4. Monitoring the results of ordered laboratory culture and sensitivity tests

14. A patient who has been diagnosed with possible avian influenza is admitted to the medical unit. Which prescribed action will the nurse take **first**?
    1. Place the patient in an airborne isolation room.
    2. Initiate infusion of 500 mL of normal saline bolus.
    3. Ask the patient about any recent travel to Asia.
    4. Obtain sputum specimen and nasal cultures.

15. Which infection control activity should the charge nurse delegate to an experienced assistive personnel (AP)?
    1. Screening patients for upper respiratory tract symptoms
    2. Asking patients about the use of immunosuppressant medications
    3. Demonstrating correct hand washing to the patients' visitors
    4. Disinfecting blood pressure cuffs after patients are discharged

16. The nurse is preparing to change the linens on the bed of a patient who has a sacral wound infected by methicillin-resistant *Staphylococcus aureus*. Which personal protective equipment (PPE) items will be used? **Select all that apply.**
    1. Gown
    2. Gloves
    3. Goggles
    4. Surgical mask
    5. N95 respirator

17. A patient who has frequent watery stools and a possible *Clostridium difficile* infection is hospitalized with dehydration. Which nursing action should the charge nurse assign to an LPN/LVN?
    1. Performing ongoing assessments to determine the patient's hydration status
    2. Explaining the purpose of ordered stool cultures to the patient and family
    3. Administering the prescribed metronidazole 500 mg PO to the patient
    4. Reviewing the patient's medical history for any risk factors for diarrhea

 Answer Key for this chapter begins on p. 59

18. Which action by the infection control nurse in an acute care hospital will be **most** effective in reducing the incidence of health care–associated infections?
    1. Requiring nursing staff to don gowns to change wound dressings for all patients
    2. Ensuring that dispensers for alcohol-based hand rubs are available in all patient care areas
    3. Screening all newly admitted patients for colonization or infection with methicillin-resistant *Staphylococcus aureus* (MRSA)
    4. Developing policies that automatically start antibiotic therapy for patients colonized by multidrug-resistant organisms

19. The nurse manager is preparing for another community surge of Covid-19. Personal protective equipment (PPE) is in short supply at the hospital. Which methods are approved by the Center for Disease Control (CDC) for optimizing the supply of PPE during the surge? **Select all that apply.**
    1. Wear a single pair of gloves between patients who have the same illness.
    2. Disinfect gloves between patients to prevent cross contamination.
    3. Wear the same N95 mask when in close contact with numerous patients.
    4. Continuously wear the N95 mask between cohort patient encounters.
    5. Use disposable patient isolation gowns for routine covid-19 patient care.
    6. Use of cotton masks is acceptable if changed after every patient encounter.

20. When the community health nurse is counseling a patient who has an acute Zika virus infection, which information is **most** important to include?
    1. Drink fluids to prevent dehydration.
    2. Use acetaminophen to reduce pain and fever.
    3. Apply insect repellant frequently to prevent mosquito bites.
    4. Symptoms of Zika infection include fever, red eyes, rash, and joint pain.

21. Which policy implemented by the infection control nurse will **most** effectively reduce the incidence of catheter-associated urinary tract infections (CAUTIs)?
    1. Limit the use of indwelling urinary catheters in all hospitalized patients.
    2. Ensure that patients with catheters have at least a 1500-mL fluid intake daily.
    3. Use urine dipstick testing to screen catheterized patients for asymptomatic bacteria.
    4. Require the use of antimicrobial/antiseptic-impregnated catheters for catheterization.

22. The nurse admits four patients with infections to the medical unit, but only one private room is available. Which patient is **most** appropriate to assign to the private room?
    1. The patient with diarrhea caused by *Clostridium difficile*
    2. The patient with vancomycin-resistant enterococcus (VRE) infection
    3. The patient with a cough who may have active tuberculosis (TB)
    4. The patient with toxic shock syndrome and fever

23. Which information about a patient who has meningococcal meningitis is the **best** indicator that the nurse can discontinue droplet precautions?
    1. Pupils are equal and reactive to light.
    2. Appropriate antibiotics have been given for 24 hours.
    3. Cough is productive of clear, nonpurulent mucus.
    4. Temperature is lower than 100°F (37.8°C).

24. While administering vancomycin 500 mg IV to a patient with a methicillin-resistant *Staphylococcus aureus* (MRSA) wound infection, the nurse notices that the patient's neck and face are becoming flushed. Which action should the nurse take **next**?
    1. Discontinue the vancomycin infusion.
    2. Slow the rate of the vancomycin infusion.
    3. Obtain an order for an antihistamine.
    4. Check the patient's temperature.

25. A healthy 65-year-old patient who cares for a newborn grandchild has a clinic appointment in May. The patient needs several immunizations but tells the nurse, "I hate shots! I will only take one today." Which immunization is **most** important to give?
    1. Influenza
    2. Herpes zoster
    3. Pneumococcal
    4. Tetanus, diphtheria, pertussis

26. The nurse is caring for a patient who is intubated and receiving mechanical ventilation. Which nursing actions are **most** essential in reducing the patient's risk for ventilator-associated pneumonia (VAP)? **Select all that apply.**
    1. Keep the head of the patient's bed elevated to at least 30 degrees.
    2. Assess the patient's readiness for extubation at least daily.
    3. Ensure that the pneumococcal vaccine is administered.
    4. Use a kinetic bed to continuously change the patient's position.
    5. Provide oral care with chlorhexidine solution at least daily.
    6. Perform inline sterile suctioning via endotracheal tube every 2 hours.

27. The nurse is preparing to insert a peripherally inserted central catheter (PICC) in a patient's left forearm. Which solution will be **best** for cleaning the skin before the PICC insertion?
    1. 70% isopropyl alcohol
    2. Povidone-iodine solution
    3. 0.5% chlorhexidine in alcohol
    4. Betadine followed by 70% isopropyl alcohol

28. The nurse has received a needlestick injury after giving a patient an intramuscular injection but has no information about whether the patient has human immunodeficiency virus (HIV) infection. What is the **most** appropriate method of obtaining this information about the patient?
    1. The nurse should personally ask the patient to authorize HIV testing.
    2. The charge nurse should tell the patient about the need for HIV testing.
    3. The occupational health nurse should discuss HIV status with the patient.
    4. HIV testing should be performed the next time blood is drawn for other tests.

29. Which medication order for a patient with a pulmonary embolism is **most** important to clarify with the prescribing health care provider before administration?
    1. Warfarin 1.0 mg PO
    2. Morphine 2 to 4 mg IV
    3. Cephalexin 250 mg PO
    4. Heparin infusion at 900 units/hr

30. A patient with atrial fibrillation is ambulating in the hallway on the coronary step-down unit and suddenly tells the nurse, "I feel really dizzy." Which action should the nurse take **first**?
    1. Help the patient to sit down.
    2. Check the patient's apical pulse.
    3. Take the patient's blood pressure.
    4. Have the patient breathe deeply.

31. The nurse is supervising an LPN/LVN who says, "I gave the patient with myasthenia gravis 90 mg of neostigmine instead of the ordered 45 mg!" In which order should the nurse perform the following actions?
    1. Assess the patient's heart rate.
    2. Complete a medication error report.
    3. Ask the LPN/LVN to explain how the error occurred.
    4. Notify the health care provider of the incorrect medication dose.

    _____, _____, _____, _____

32. The nurse is caring for a confused and agitated patient who has wrist restraints in place on both arms. Which action included in the patient plan of care can be assigned to an LPN/LVN?
    1. Determining whether the patient's mental status justifies the continued use of restraints
    2. Undoing and retying the restraints to improve patient comfort
    3. Reporting the patient's status and continued need for restraints to the health care provider
    4. Explaining the purpose of the restraints to the patient's family members

33. The nurse is checking medication prescriptions that were received by telephone for a patient with hypertensive crisis and tachycardia. Which medication is **most** important to clarify with the health care provider (HCP)?
    1. Carvedilol 12.5 mg PO BID daily
    2. Hydrochlorothiazide 25 mg PO daily
    3. Labetalol 20 mg IV over a 2-min time period now
    4. Hydroxyzine 50 mg PO as needed systolic blood pressure greater than 160 mm Hg

34. A 70-kg patient who has had unprotected sexual intercourse with a partner who has hepatitis B is to receive 0.06 mL/kg of hepatitis B immune globulin. The immune globulin is available in a 5-mL vial. The nurse will plan to administer _____ mL.

35. An 88-year-old patient who has not yet had the influenza vaccine is admitted after reporting symptoms of generalized muscle aching, cough, and runny nose starting about 24 hours previously. Which of these prescribed medications is **most** important for the nurse to administer at this time?
    1. Oseltamivir 75 mg PO
    2. Guaifenesin 600 mg PO
    3. Acetaminophen 650 mg PO
    4. Influenza vaccine 180 mcg IM

36. The nurse is admitting an 80-year-old female patient who has mild dementia and is incontinent. Which is the **best** way to assess the patient's pressure injury risk?
    1. Conduct a full head to toe physical assessment.
    2. Rely on empirical knowledge gained by caring for other patients with pressure ulcers.
    3. Utilize the Braden Scale.
    4. Consult with the wound care nurse specialist.

PART 2 Common Health Scenarios

 Answer Key for this chapter begins on p. 59

37. A patient who has had recent exposure to Ebola while traveling in Africa arrives in the emergency department with fever, headache, vomiting, and multiple ecchymoses. Which action should the nurse take **first**?
1. Place the patient in a private room.
2. Obtain heart rate and blood pressure.
3. Notify the hospital infection control nurse.
4. Start a large bore IV with normal saline.

38. A patient who has been infected with the Ebola virus has an emesis of 750 mL of bloody fluid and complains of headache, nausea, and severe lightheadedness. Which action included in the treatment protocol should the nurse take **first**?
1. Give acetaminophen 650 mg PO.
2. Administer ondansetron 4 mg IV.
3. Infuse normal saline at 500 mL/hr.
4. Increase oxygen flow rate to 6 L/min.

39. Drag and Drop

Instructions: Place the letter of the unit personnel in the right column who will be assigned to the nursing actions listed in the left column.

Nursing Action	RN	LPN/LVN	AP
1. Culture a wound on an infected leg			
2. Chart vital signs and weight on an admission assessment			
3. Administer a disposable saline enema to a patient with an infected sacral wound			
4. Perform range of motion and walk a patient with severe osteoporosis and septic arthritis			
5. Apply an antifungal cream to the groin a comatose MRSA positive patient during morning care.			
6. Rearrange an oxygen cannula from behind the ears back into the nostrils of a demented patient.			
7. Apply a clear dressing to a reddened area on the sacrum after RN assessment.			

40. Instructions: In the right column indicate which is the correct order to safely don the personal protective equipment listed below.

Personal Protective Equipment	Order
1. Don gloves	
2. Put on gown	
3. Wash hands	
4. Place goggles over eyes	
5. Put on a mask to cover nose and mouth	

41. Drag and Drop

Instructions: In the right column indicate which is the correct order to safely remove the personal protective equipment listed below

Personal Protective Equipment	Order
1. Remove N95 respirator	
2. Take off goggles	
3. Remove gloves	
4. Take off gown	
5. Wash hands	

Answers

1. **Ans: 4** Airway patency is the priority for this patient and the first thing the nurse should do is take measures to ensure the airway will be patent by making sure suction is readily available. Intractable nausea and vomiting pose a safety risk for aspiration. The other choices are all acceptable actions, but ensuring there is a patent airway is the first thing the nurse should do. **Focus:** Prioritization.

2. **Ans: 3** The National Institute for Occupational Safety and Health (NIOSH) lists 17 diseases that pregnant nurses should not be in contact with. These include airborne diseases such as chicken pox, shingles, and coccidiomycosis, as well as other airborne diseases like tuberculosis, measles, and influenza. Vancomycin-resistant *Staphylococcus aureus* (VRSA), VRE, and methicillin-resistant *S. aureus* (MRSA) are spread by direct contact and standard precautions taken by all nurses are sufficient in preventing transmission; thus patients with these diseases are considered safe for a pregnant nurse to take care of. **Focus:** Assignment.

3. **Ans: 1** Because the respiratory manifestations associated with avian influenza are potentially life threatening, the nurse's initial action should be to start oxygen therapy. The other interventions should be implemented after addressing the patient's respiratory problems. **Focus:** Prioritization.

4. **Ans: 2, 3, 4** Because herpes zoster (shingles) is spread through airborne means and by direct contact with the lesions, the nurse should wear an N95 respirator or high-efficiency particulate air filter respirator, a gown, and gloves. Surgical face masks filter only large particles and do not provide protection from herpes zoster. Goggles and shoe covers are not needed for airborne or contact precautions. **Focus:** Prioritization.

5. **Ans: 2** Measles is spread by airborne means and could be rapidly transmitted to other patients in the emergency department. The child with the rash should be quickly isolated from the other patients through placement in a negative-pressure room. Droplet or contact precautions (or both) should be instituted for the patients with possible pertussis and MRSA infection, but this can be done after isolating the child with possible measles. The patient who has been exposed to TB does not place other patients at risk for infection because there are no symptoms of active TB. **Focus:** Prioritization.

6. **Ans: 3** According to the Centers for Disease Control and Prevention guidelines, several factors increase the risk for infection for this patient. Central lines are associated with a higher infection risk, jugular vein lines are more prone to infection, and the line is nontunneled. Peripherally inserted IV lines such as PICC lines and midline catheters are associated with a lower

incidence of infection. Implanted ports are placed under the skin and are the least likely central line to be associated with catheter infection. **Focus:** Prioritization.

7. **Ans: 3** LPN/LVN education and scope of practice include performing dressing changes and obtaining specimens for wound culture. Teaching, assessment, and planning of care are complex actions that should be carried out by the RN. **Focus:** Assignment.

8. **Ans: 4** The patient's age, history of antibiotic therapy, and watery stools suggest that he may have *Clostridium difficile* infection. The initial action should be to place him on contact precautions to prevent the spread of *C. difficile* to other patients. The other actions are also needed and should be taken after placing the patient on contact precautions. **Focus:** Prioritization. **Test-Taking Tip**: Remember that implementation of infection control policies and precautions is an independent nursing action, and it is your responsibility to promptly implement appropriate precautions and use of personal protective equipment to prevent disease transmission.

9. **Ans: 2** To prevent contamination of staff or other patients by anthrax, decontamination of the patient by removal and disposal of clothing and showering are the initial actions in possible anthrax exposure. Assessment of the patient for signs of infection should be performed after decontamination. Notification of security personnel (and local and regional law enforcement agencies) is necessary in the case of possible bioterrorism, but this should occur after decontaminating and caring for the patient. According to the Centers for Disease Control and Prevention guidelines, antibiotics should be administered only if there are signs of infection or the contaminating substance tests positive for anthrax. **Focus:** Prioritization.

10. **Ans: 1** Current guidelines recommend that pregnant women who are exposed to Zika virus be tested for infection. Fetal ultrasonography is recommended for any pregnant woman who has had possible Zika virus exposure, but multiple ultrasound studies will not be needed unless test results are positive. Education about the effects of Zika infection on fetal development may be needed, but this is not the highest priority at this time. The nurse will assess for Zika symptoms, but testing for the virus will be done even if the patient is asymptomatic. **Focus:** Prioritization.

11. **Ans: 3** The patient with increased dyspnea should be seen first because rapid actions such as oxygen administration and IV fluids may be needed. The other patients will require further assessment, counseling, or treatment, but they do not have potentially life-threatening symptoms or diagnoses. **Focus:** Prioritization.

12. **Ans: 2** Because the most immediate need is to ensure that hand hygiene is accomplished, the nurse

should offer an alcohol-based cleanser to the health care provider. The other actions may also be needed, especially if there is a pattern of nonadherence to hand hygiene, but further assessment is necessary before these actions are taken. **Focus:** Prioritization.

13. **Ans: 3** All hospital personnel who care for the patient are responsible for correct implementation of contact precautions. The other actions should be carried out by licensed nurses, whose education covers monitoring of laboratory results, patient teaching, and communication with other departments about essential patient data. **Focus:** Delegation.

14. **Ans: 1** The initial action should be to prevent transmission of avian influenza to other patients, visitors, or health care personnel through the use of airborne, contact, and standard isolation precautions. Initiating IV fluids, determining whether the patient has been exposed to avian influenza through travel, and obtaining cultures are also appropriate, but the highest priority is to prevent spread of infection. **Focus:** Prioritization.

15. **Ans: 4** The AP can follow agency policy to disinfect items that come in contact with intact skin (e.g., blood pressure cuffs) by cleaning with chemicals such as alcohol. Teaching and assessment for upper respiratory tract symptoms or use of immunosuppressants require more education and a broader scope of practice, and these tasks should be performed by licensed nurses. **Focus:** Delegation.

16. **Ans: 1, 2** A gown and gloves should be used when coming in contact with linens that may be contaminated by the patient's wound secretions. The other PPE items are not necessary because transmission by splashes, droplets, or airborne means will not occur when the bed is changed. **Focus:** Prioritization.

17. **Ans: 3** LPN/LVN scope of practice and education include the administration of medications. Assessment of hydration status, patient and family education, and assessment of patient risk factors for diarrhea should be done by the RN. **Focus:** Assignment.

18. **Ans: 2** Because the hands of health care workers are the most common means of transmission of infection from one patient to another, the most effective method of preventing the spread of infection is to make supplies for hand hygiene readily available for staff to use. Wearing a gown to care for patients who are not on contact precautions is not necessary. Although some hospitals have started screening newly admitted patients for MRSA, this is not considered a priority action according to current national guidelines. Because administration of antibiotics to individuals who are colonized by bacteria may promote the development of antibiotic resistance, antibiotic use should be restricted to patients who have clinical manifestations of infection. **Focus:** Prioritization.

19. **Ans: 1, 2, 4, 5** The CDC has recommended all the above methods besides wearing an N95 mask between numerous patients and cotton masks. Disposable latex and nitrile gloves can be disinfected up to 6 times

using alcohol based hand sanitizer. If N95 masks are unavailable then the recommendation is to utilize goggles, a surgical facemask and a facial shield. N95 masks should not be continuously worn for more than 8 hours and only between a cohort of covid-19 patients. Disposable isolation patient gowns are fluid resistant. Surgical gowns may be used as well but are sterile so they are not as cost efficient. **Focus:** Prioritization.

20. **Ans: 3** Prevention of Zika transmission is the priority because Zika infection usually causes a relatively mild and short-duration illness. Because mosquitos spread Zika infection from infected individuals to others, it is essential that the patient use insect repellant consistently during the active infection. The other information is correct but will not assist in decreasing the risk to the community. **Focus:** Prioritization. **Test-Taking Tip:** The essential service of public health is to identify community health problems and take actions to prevent or solve those problems.

21. **Ans: 1** According to the Centers for Disease Control and Prevention (CDC), CAUTIs are the most common health care–acquired infection in the United States. Recommendations include avoiding the use of indwelling catheters and removing catheters as soon as possible. Although a high fluid intake will also help to reduce the risk for CAUTIs, 1500 mL may be excessive for some patients. The CDC recommends against routine screening for asymptomatic bacteriuria. Antimicrobial catheters are a secondary recommendation and may be appropriate if other measures are not effective in reducing the incidence of CAUTIs. **Focus:** Prioritization.

22. **Ans: 3** Patients with infections that require airborne precautions (e.g., TB) need to be in private rooms. Patients with infections that require contact precautions (e.g., those with *C. difficile* or VRE infections) should ideally be placed in private rooms; however, they can be placed in rooms with other patients with the same diagnosis. Standard precautions are required for the patient with toxic shock syndrome. **Focus:** Prioritization.

23. **Ans: 2** Current Centers for Disease Control and Prevention evidence-based guidelines indicate that droplet precautions for patients with meningococcal meningitis can be discontinued when the patient has received antibiotic therapy (with drugs that are effective against *Neisseria meningitidis*) for 24 hours. The other information may indicate that the patient's condition is improving but does not indicate that droplet precautions should be discontinued. **Focus:** Prioritization.

24. **Ans: 2** "Red man" syndrome occurs when vancomycin is infused too quickly. Because the patient needs the medication to treat the infection, vancomycin should not be discontinued. Antihistamines may help decrease the flushing, but vancomycin should be administered over at least 60 minutes to avoid vasodilation. Although the patient's temperature will be monitored, a temperature elevation is not the most likely cause of the patient's flushing. **Focus:** Prioritization.

25. **Ans: 4** Individuals who have contact with infants should be immunized against pertussis to avoid infection and to prevent transmission to the infant. The influenza and pneumococcal vaccines can be administered later in the year, before the influenza season. The herpes zoster vaccine is important to prevent shingles in the patient but does not need to be administered today. **Focus:** Prioritization.

26. **Ans: 1, 2, 5** The ventilator bundle developed by the Institute for Healthcare Improvement includes recommendations for continuous elevation of the head of the bed, daily assessment for extubation readiness, and daily oral care with chlorhexidine solution. Pneumococcal immunization will prevent pneumococcal pneumonia, but it is not designed to prevent VAP. The use of a kinetic bed may also be of benefit to the patient, but it is not considered essential. Routine suctioning is no longer recommended. **Focus:** Prioritization.

27. **Ans: 3** Current Institute for Healthcare Improvement guidelines indicate that chlorhexidine is more effective than the other options at reducing the risk for central line–associated bloodstream infections. The other solutions provide some decrease in the number of microorganisms on the skin but are not as effective as chlorhexidine. **Focus:** Prioritization.

28. **Ans: 3** The staff member who is most knowledgeable about the regulations regarding HIV prophylaxis and about how to obtain a patient's HIV status and order HIV testing is the occupational health nurse. It is unethical for the nurse to personally ask the patient to consent to HIV testing or to perform unauthorized HIV testing. The charge nurse is not responsible for obtaining this information (unless the charge nurse is also in charge of occupational health). **Focus:** Prioritization.

29. **Ans: 1** The Institute for Safe Medication Practices guidelines indicate that the use of a trailing zero is not appropriate when writing medication orders because the order can easily be mistaken for a larger dose (in this case, 10 mg). The order should be clarified before administration. The other orders are appropriate based on the patient's diagnosis. **Focus:** Prioritization.

30. **Ans: 1** The first priority for an ambulating patient who is dizzy is to prevent falls, which could lead to serious injury. The other actions are also appropriate but are not as high a priority. **Focus:** Prioritization.

31. **Ans: 1, 4, 3, 2** The first action after a medication error should be to assess the patient for adverse outcomes. The nurse should evaluate this patient for symptoms such as bradycardia and excessive salivation, which indicate cholinergic crisis, a possible effect of excessive doses of anticholinesterase medications such as neostigmine. The health care provider should be rapidly notified so that treatment with atropine can be ordered to counteract the effects of the neostigmine, if necessary. Determining the circumstances that led to the error will help decrease the risk for future errors

and will be needed to complete the medication error report. **Focus:** Prioritization.

32. **Ans: 2** Hospital staff who have been trained in the appropriate application of restraints may reposition the restraints. Evaluation of the continued need for restraints, communication with the provider about the patient status, and teaching of the family require RN-level education and scope of practice. **Focus:** Assignment.

33. **Ans: 4** Hydroxyzine is a first-generation antihistamine that is used to treat patients with anxiety and pruritus. It is likely that the correct medication is hydralazine, a vasodilator that is used to treat hypertension. Hydroxyzine and hydralazine are "look-alike, sound-alike" drugs that have been identified by the Institute for Safe Medication Practices (ISMP) as being at high risk for involvement in medication errors. All treatment prescriptions that are communicated by telephone should be reconfirmed with the health care provider; however, the most important order to clarify is the hydroxyzine, which is likely an error. **Focus:** Prioritization.

34. **Ans: 4.2 mL** 0.06 mL × 70 kg = 4.2 mL. **Focus:** Prioritization.

35. **Ans: 1** Because antivirals are most effective when used early in influenza infection, the nurse should administer the oseltamivir as soon as possible to decrease the severity of the infection and risk of transmission to others. Guaifenesin and acetaminophen will help with the symptoms of cough and muscle aching but will not shorten the course of the patient's illness or decrease risk of transmission. The influenza vaccine may still help in preventing future influenza caused by another virus. **Focus:** Prioritization.

36. **Ans: 3** The Braden Scale for Predicting Pressure Sore Risk is the best way to predict the patient's risk for developing an injury. The scale measures sensory perception, skin moisture, activity, mobility, nutrition, friction, and shear. Conducting a full head to toe assessment would not predict an ulcer. There is no wound, so consulting with the wound care nurse specialist would not be useful. Empirical knowledge is subjective and not evidenced based. **Focus:** Prioritization.

37. **Ans: 1** The Centers for Disease Control and Prevention guidelines recommend that the initial action be to place the patient in a private room and implement standard, contact, and droplet precautions. Further assessment of the type of possible Ebola exposure, obtaining vital signs, and notification of the infection control nurse will also be needed but should be done after measures to minimize transmission of Ebola are implemented. **Focus:** Prioritization. **Test-Taking Tip:** When caring for a patient with a communicable disease, consider that prevention of disease transmission to other patients, staff, and visitors is usually the highest priority, even when the patient is critically ill and needs rapid implementation of other actions.

38. **Ans: 3** Because hypovolemia is a major concern with Ebola infection and IV fluid infusion has been demonstrated to improve outcomes, the nurse's first action will be to infuse normal saline. Treatment of nausea and headache is appropriate and should be implemented next. There is no indication that this patient is hypoxemic, although patients with Ebola may develop multiorgan failure and require respiratory support. **Focus:** Prioritization.

39. **Ans:** Obtaining a wound culture is within their scope of LPN/LVN practice. The AP is able to take vital signs and weights, as well as chart the results on an admission assessment. The LPN/LVN should administer the disposable saline enema because this is considered a medication. An RN can also administer medications; however, using an RN to do a task that an LPN can accomplish is less efficient. The RN should do ROM and walk the severely osteoporotic patient. The RN has additional knowledge in the pathology of disease processes and is better able to prevent a fracture from occurring. An antifungal cream is considered a medication and should be administered by the LPN. The AP can rearrange the oxygen cannula. The AP can apply a dressing to the sacrum previously assessed by the RN. Focus: Delegation. **Focus:** Delegation.

40. **Ans: 3, 2, 5, 4, 1** The Centers for Disease Control and Prevention guidelines recommend starting with hand hygiene and then donning gown, mask, goggles, and finally gloves to protect staff members and limit the spread of contamination. Goggles and a mask (or use of a face shield) will be needed with this dressing change because of the possibility of splashing during wound irrigation. **Focus:** Prioritization.

41. **Ans: 3, 2, 4, 1, 5** This sequence will prevent contact of the contaminated gloves and gown with areas (e.g., the hair) that cannot be easily cleaned after patient contact and stop transmission of microorganisms to the nurse and to other patients. If the nurse is wearing a disposable gown, the gown and gloves can be removed simultaneously by grasping the front of the gown and breaking the ties and then peeling the gloves off while removing the gown. The correct method for donning and removing PPE has been standardized by agencies such as the Centers for Disease Control and Prevention and the Occupational Safety and Health Administration. **Focus:** Prioritization.

Nursing Action	RN	LPN/LVN	AP
1. Culture a wound on an infected leg		X	
2. Chart vital signs and weight on an admission assessment			X
3. Administer a disposable saline enema to a patient with an infected sacral wound		X	
4. Perform range of motion and walk a patient with severe osteoporosis and septic arthritis	X		
5. Apply an antifungal cream to the groin a comatose MRSA positive patient during morning care.		X	
6. Rearrange an oxygen cannula from behind the ears back into the nostrils of a demented patient.			X
7. Apply a clear dressing to a reddened area on the sacrum after RN assessment.			X

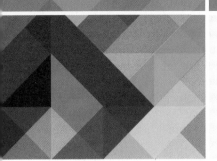

CHAPTER 6

Respiratory Problems

Questions

1. The nurse is providing care for a patient diagnosed with laryngeal cancer who is receiving radiation therapy. The patient tells the nurse that he is experiencing hoarseness and difficulty with speaking. What is the nurse's **best** response?
   1. "Let's elevate the head of your bed and see if that helps."
   2. "Your voice should improve in 6 to 8 weeks after completion of the radiation."
   3. "Sometimes patients also experience dry mouth and difficulty with swallowing."
   4. "I will call your health care provider and let him know about this."

2. Enhanced Multiple Response

Case Study and Question

The nurse is supervising a nursing student providing care for a patient with shortness of breath who has expressed interest in smoking cessation.

Which questions would the nurse suggest the student ask to determine nicotine dependence?

Instructions: Read the case study on the left and circle the numbers that best answer the question.
1. How soon after you wake up in the morning do you smoke?
2. Do other members of your family smoke?
3. Do you smoke when you are ill?
4. Do you wake up in the middle of your sleep time to smoke?
5. Do you smoke indoors or only outside?
6. Do you have a difficult time not smoking in places where it is not allowed?
7. Have you tried e-cigarettes?
8. Has anyone in your family developed lung cancer?
9. Have you ever tried to quit smoking?

3. The RN clinical instructor is discussing a patient's oxygen-hemoglobin dissociation curve with a student (Figure 6.1). The student states that the patient's oral body temperature is elevated at 100.8°F (38.2°C). Which statement by the student indicates correct understanding of this patient's curve shift?
   1. "When a patient's body temperature is elevated, there is no change in the oxygen-hemoglobin dissociation curve."
   2. "When a patient's body temperature is elevated, there is a shift to the left because the oxygen tension level is lower."
   3. "When a patient's body temperature is elevated, there is no shift in the curve because the patient is using less oxygen."
   4. "When the patient's body temperature is elevated, there is a shift to the right so that hemoglobin will dissociate oxygen faster."

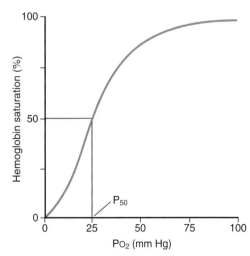

FIGURE 6.1

Common Health Scenarios

PART 2

4. An experienced LPN/LVN, under the supervision of the team leader RN, is assigned to provide nursing care for a patient with a respiratory problem. Which actions are appropriate to the scope of practice of an experienced LPN/LVN? **Select all that apply.**
   1. Auscultating breath sounds
   2. Administering medications via metered-dose inhaler (MDI)
   3. Completing an in-depth admission assessment
   4. Checking oxygen saturation using pulse oximetry
   5. Developing the nursing care plan
   6. Evaluating the patient's technique for using MDIs

5. The nurse is evaluating and assessing a patient with a diagnosis of chronic emphysema. The patient is receiving oxygen at a flow rate of 5 L/min by nasal cannula. Which finding concerns the nurse **immediately**?
   1. Fine bibasilar crackles
   2. Respiratory rate of 8 breaths/min
   3. Patient sitting up and leaning over the nightstand
   4. A large barrel chest

6. The assistive personnel (AP) tells the nurse that a patient who is receiving oxygen at a flow rate of 6 L/min by nasal cannula is reporting nasal passage discomfort. What intervention should the nurse suggest to the AP to improve the patient's comfort?
   1. Apply water-soluble jelly to the nares.
   2. Use a simple face mask instead of a nasal cannula.
   3. Provide the patient with an extra pillow.
   4. Have the patient sit up in a chair at the bedside.

7. The RN is teaching an assistive personnel (AP) to check oxygen saturation by pulse oximetry. What will the nurse be sure to tell the AP about patients with darker skin?
   1. "Be aware that patients with darker skin usually show a 3% to 5% higher oxygen saturation compared with light-skinned patients."
   2. "Usually dark-skinned patients show a 3% to 5% lower oxygen saturation by pulse oximetry than light-skinned patients."
   3. "With a dark-skinned patient, you may get more accurate results by measuring pulse oximetry on the patient's toes."
   4. "More accurate results may result from continuous pulse oximetry monitoring than spot checking when a patient has darker skin."

8. The nurse is caring for a patient after thoracentesis. Which actions can be delegated by the nurse to the assistive personnel (AP)? **Select all that apply.**
   1. Assess puncture site and dressing for leakage.
   2. Check vital signs every 15 minutes for 1 hour.
   3. Auscultate for absent or reduced lung sounds.
   4. Remind the patient to take deep breaths.
   5. Take the specimens to the laboratory.
   6. Teach the patient the symptoms of pneumothorax.

9. The nurse is supervising a student nurse who is performing tracheostomy care for a patient. Which action by the student would cause the nurse to intervene?
   1. Suctioning the tracheostomy tube before performing tracheostomy care
   2. Removing old dressings and cleaning off excess secretions
   3. Removing the inner cannula and cleaning using standard precautions
   4. Replacing the inner cannula and cleaning the stoma site

10. The nurse is supervising an RN who floated from the medical-surgical unit to the emergency department. The float nurse is providing care for a patient admitted with anterior epistaxis (nosebleed). Which directions would the supervising nurse clearly provide to the RN? **Select all that apply.**
    1. Position the patient supine and turned on his side.
    2. Apply direct lateral pressure to the nose for 5 minutes.
    3. Maintain standard body substance precautions.
    4. Apply ice or cool compresses to the nose.
    5. Instruct the patient not to blow the nose for several hours.
    6. Teach the patient to avoid vigorous nose blowing.

11. A patient with a diagnosis of sleep apnea has a problem with sleep deprivation related to a disrupted sleep cycle. Which action should the nurse delegate to the assistive personnel (AP)?
    1. Discussing weight-loss strategies such as diet and exercise with the patient
    2. Teaching the patient how to set up the bilevel positive airway pressure machine before sleeping
    3. Reminding the patient to sleep on his side instead of his back
    4. Administering modafinil to promote daytime wakefulness

12. The nurse is acting as preceptor for a newly graduated RN during the second week of orientation. The nurse would assign and supervise the new RN to provide nursing care for which patients? **Select all that apply.**
    1. A 38-year-old patient with moderate persistent asthma awaiting discharge
    2. A 63-year-old patient with a tracheostomy needing tracheostomy care every shift
    3. A 56-year-old patient with lung cancer who has just undergone left lower lobectomy
    4. A 49-year-old patient just admitted with a new diagnosis of esophageal cancer
    5. A 76-year-old patient newly diagnosed with type 2 diabetes
    6. A 69-year-old patient with emphysema to be discharged tomorrow

13. The nurse is providing care for a patient with recently diagnosed asthma. Which key points would the nurse be sure to include in the teaching plan for this patient? **Select all that apply.**
    1. Avoid potential environmental asthma triggers such as smoke.
    2. Use the inhaler 30 minutes before exercising to prevent bronchospasm.
    3. Wash all bedding in cold water to reduce and destroy dust mites.
    4. Be sure to get at least 8 hours of rest and sleep every night.
    5. Avoid foods prepared with monosodium glutamate.
    6. Keep a symptom and intervention diary to learn specific triggers for your asthma.

14. The nurse is the team leader RN working with a student nurse. The student nurse is teaching a patient how to use a metered-dose inhaler (MDI) without a spacer. Put in the correct order the steps that the student nurse should teach the patient.
    1. Remove the inhaler cap and shake the inhaler.
    2. Open your mouth and place the mouthpiece 1 to 2 inches (2.5 to 5.0 cm) away.
    3. Breathe out completely.
    4. Hold your breath for at least 10 seconds.
    5. Press down firmly on the canister and breathe deeply through your mouth.
    6. Wait at least 1 minute between puffs.

    _____, _____, _____, _____, _____, _____

15. A patient has chronic obstructive pulmonary disease. Which intervention for airway management should the nurse delegate to the assistive personnel (AP)?
    1. Assisting the patient to sit up on the side of the bed
    2. Instructing the patient to cough effectively
    3. Teaching the patient to use incentive spirometry
    4. Auscultating breath sounds every 4 hours

16. A patient with chronic obstructive pulmonary disease has rapid shallow respirations. Which is an appropriate action to assign to the experienced LPN/LVN under RN supervision?
    1. Observing how well the patient performs pursed-lip breathing
    2. Planning a nursing care regimen that gradually increases activity tolerance
    3. Assisting the patient with basic activities of daily living (ADLs)
    4. Consulting with the physical therapy department about reconditioning exercises

17. A patient with chronic obstructive pulmonary disease tells the assistive personnel (AP) that he did not get his annual flu shot this year and has not had a pneumonia vaccination. Which vital sign reported by the AP is **most** important for the nurse to report to the health care provider?
    1. Blood pressure of 152/84 mm Hg
    2. Respiratory rate of 27 breaths/min
    3. Heart rate of 92 beats/min
    4. Oral temperature of 101.2°F (38.4°C)

18. The nurse is responsible for the care of a postoperative patient with a thoracotomy. Which action should the nurse delegate to the assistive personnel (AP)?
    1. Instructing the patient to alternate rest and activity periods
    2. Encouraging, monitoring, and recording nutritional intake
    3. Monitoring cardiorespiratory response to activity
    4. Planning activities for periods when the patient has the most energy

19. The nurse is supervising a nursing student who is providing care for a thoracotomy patient with a chest tube. What finding would the nurse instruct the nursing student to report **immediately**?
    1. Chest tube drainage of 10 to 15 mL/hr
    2. Continuous bubbling in the water-seal chamber
    3. Reports of pain at the chest tube site
    4. Chest tube dressing dated yesterday

20. After the change of shift, the nurse is assigned to care for the following patients. Which patient should the nurse assess **first**?
    1. A 68-year-old patient on a ventilator whose sterile sputum specimen must be sent to the laboratory
    2. A 57-year-old patient with chronic obstructive pulmonary disease (COPD) and a pulse oximetry reading from the previous shift of 90% saturation
    3. A 72-year-old patient with pneumonia who needs to be started on IV antibiotics
    4. A 51-year-old patient with asthma who reports shortness of breath after using a bronchodilator inhaler

21. The nurse is initiating a nursing care plan for a patient with pneumonia. Which intervention for cough enhancement should the nurse delegate to the assistive personnel (AP)?
    1. Teaching the patient about the importance of adequate fluid intake and hydration
    2. Assisting the patient to a sitting position with neck flexed, shoulders relaxed, and knees flexed
    3. Reminding the patient to use an incentive spirometer every 1 to 2 hours while awake
    4. Encouraging the patient to take a deep breath, hold it for 2 seconds, and then cough two or three times in succession

Answer Key for this chapter begins on p. 69

PART 2 Common Health Scenarios

22. The assistive personnel (AP) is helping with feeding for a patient with severe end-stage chronic obstructive pulmonary disease (COPD). Which instruction will the nurse provide the AP?
    1. Encourage the patient to eat foods that are high in calories and protein.
    2. Feed the patient as quickly as possible to prevent early satiety.
    3. Offer lots of fluids between bites of food.
    4. Try to get the patient to eat everything on the tray.

23. The charge nurse is making assignments for the next shift. Which patient should be assigned to the fairly new nurse (6 months of experience) floated from the surgical unit to the medical unit?
    1. A 58-year-old patient on airborne precautions for tuberculosis (TB)
    2. A 65-year-old patient who just returned from bronchoscopy and biopsy
    3. A 72-year-old patient who needs teaching about the use of incentive spirometry
    4. A 69-year-old patient with chronic obstructive pulmonary disease who is ventilator dependent

24. When a patient with tuberculosis (TB) is being prepared for discharge, which statement by the patient indicates a need for further teaching?
    1. "Everyone in my family needs to go and see the doctor for TB testing."
    2. "I will continue to take my isoniazid until I am feeling completely well."
    3. "I will cover my mouth and nose when I sneeze or cough and put my used tissues in a plastic bag."
    4. "I will change my diet to include more foods rich in iron, protein, and vitamin C."

25. The nurse is admitting a patient for whom a diagnosis of pulmonary embolus (PE) must be ruled out. The patient's history and assessment reveal all of these findings. Which finding supports the diagnosis of PE?
    1. The patient was recently in a motor vehicle crash.
    2. The patient participated in an aerobic exercise program for 6 months.
    3. The patient gave birth to her youngest child 1 year ago.
    4. The patient was on bed rest for 6 hours after a diagnostic procedure.

26. Which intervention for a patient with a pulmonary embolus would the RN assign to the LPN/LVN on the patient care team?
    1. Evaluating the patient's reports of chest pain
    2. Monitoring laboratory values for changes in oxygenation
    3. Assessing for symptoms of respiratory failure
    4. Auscultating the lungs for crackles

27. A patient with a pulmonary embolus is receiving anticoagulation with IV heparin. What instructions would the nurse give the assistive personnel (AP) who will help the patient with activities of daily living? **Select all that apply.**
    1. Use a lift sheet when moving and positioning the patient in bed.
    2. Use an electric razor when shaving the patient each day.
    3. Use a soft-bristled toothbrush or tooth sponge for oral care.
    4. Use a rectal thermometer to obtain a more accurate body temperature.
    5. Be sure the patient's footwear has a firm sole when the patient ambulates.
    6. Assess the patient for any signs or symptoms of bleeding.

28. A patient with chronic obstructive pulmonary disease (COPD) tells the nurse that he is always tired. What advice would the nurse give this patient to cope with his fatigue? **Select all that apply.**
    1. Do not rush through your morning activities of daily living.
    2. Avoid working with your arms raised.
    3. Eat three large meals every day focusing on calories and protein.
    4. Organize your work area so that what you use most is easy to reach.
    5. Get all of your activities accomplished then take a nap.
    6. Don't hold your breath while performing any activities.

29. A patient with acute respiratory distress syndrome (ARDS) is receiving oxygen by nonrebreather mask, but arterial blood gas measurements continue to show poor oxygenation. Which action does the nurse anticipate that the health care provider (HCP) will prescribe?
    1. Perform endotracheal intubation and initiate mechanical ventilation.
    2. Begin IV normal saline at a high rate up to 250 mL per hour.
    3. Administer furosemide (Lasix) 100 mg IV push immediately.
    4. Call a code for respiratory arrest.

30. The nurse is the preceptor for an RN who is undergoing orientation to the intensive care unit. The RN is providing care for a patient with acute respiratory distress syndrome who has just been intubated in preparation for mechanical ventilation. The preceptor observes the RN performing all of these actions. For which action must the preceptor intervene **immediately**?
    1. Assesses for bilateral breath sounds and symmetrical chest movement
    2. Uses an end-tidal carbon dioxide detector to confirm endotracheal tube (ET) position
    3. Marks the tube 1 cm from where it touches the incisor tooth or nares
    4. Orders chest radiography to verify that tube placement is correct

31. The nurse is assigned to provide nursing care for a patient receiving mechanical ventilation. Which action should the nurse delegate to an experienced assistive personnel (AP)?
    1. Assessing the patient's respiratory status every 4 hours
    2. Taking vital signs and pulse oximetry readings every 4 hours
    3. Checking the ventilator settings to make sure they are as prescribed
    4. Observing whether the patient's tube needs suctioning every 2 hours

32. After the respiratory therapist performs suctioning on a patient who is intubated, the assistive personnel (AP) measures vital signs for the patient. Which vital sign value should the AP be instructed to report to the RN immediately?
    1. Heart rate of 98 beats/min
    2. Respiratory rate of 24 breaths/min
    3. Blood pressure of 168/90 mm Hg
    4. Tympanic temperature of 101.4°F (38.6°C)

33. The nurse is making a home visit to a 50-year-old patient who was recently hospitalized with a right leg deep vein thrombosis and a pulmonary embolism (venous thromboembolism). The patient's only medication is enoxaparin subcutaneously. Which assessment information will the nurse need to communicate to the health care provider (HCP)?
    1. The patient says that her right leg aches all night.
    2. The right calf is warm to the touch and is larger than the left calf.
    3. The patient is unable to remember her husband's first name.
    4. There are multiple ecchymotic areas on the patient's abdomen.

34. The high-pressure alarm on a patient's ventilator goes off. When the nurse enters the room to assess the patient, who has acute respiratory distress syndrome, the oxygen saturation monitor reads 87% and the patient is struggling to sit up. Which action should the nurse take **first**?
    1. Reassure the patient that the ventilator will do the work of breathing for him.
    2. Manually ventilate the patient while assessing possible reasons for the high-pressure alarm.
    3. Increase the fraction of inspired oxygen (F_{IO_2}) on the ventilator to 100% in preparation for endotracheal suctioning.
    4. Insert an oral airway to prevent the patient from biting on the endotracheal tube.

35. When assessing a 22-year-old patient who required emergency surgery and multiple transfusions 3 days ago, the nurse finds that the patient looks anxious and has labored respirations at a rate of 38 breaths/min. The oxygen saturation is 90% with the oxygen delivery at 6 L/min via nasal cannula. Which action is **most** appropriate?
    1. Increase the flow rate on the oxygen to 10 L/min and reassess the patient after about 10 minutes.
    2. Assist the patient in using the incentive spirometer and splint his chest with a pillow while he coughs.
    3. Administer the ordered morphine sulfate to the patient to decrease his anxiety and reduce the hyperventilation.
    4. Switch the patient to a nonrebreather mask at 95% to 100% fraction of inspired oxygen (F_{IO_2}) and call the health care provider (HCP) to discuss the patient's status.

36. The nurse has just finished assisting the health care provider (HCP) with a thoracentesis for a patient with recurrent left pleural effusion caused by lung cancer. The thoracentesis removed 1800 mL of fluid. Which patient assessment information is **most** important to report to the HCP?
    1. The patient starts crying and says she can't go on with treatment much longer.
    2. The patient reports sharp, stabbing chest pain with every deep breath.
    3. The blood pressure is 100/48 mm Hg, and the heart rate is 102 beats/min.
    4. The dressing at the thoracentesis site has 1 cm of bloody drainage.

   Answer Key for this chapter begins on p. 69

37. The nurse is caring for a patient with emphysema and respiratory failure who is receiving mechanical ventilation through an endotracheal tube. To prevent ventilator-associated pneumonia (VAP), which action is **most** important to include in the plan of care?
    1. Administer ordered antibiotics as scheduled.
    2. Hyperoxygenate the patient before suctioning.
    3. Maintain the head of bed at a 30- to 45-degree angle.
    4. Suction the airway when coarse crackles are audible.

38. The critical care charge nurse is responsible for the care of four patients receiving mechanical ventilation. Which patient is **most** at risk for failure to wean and ventilator dependence?
    1. A 68-year-old patient with a history of smoking and emphysema
    2. A 57-year-old patient who experienced a cardiac arrest
    3. A 49-year-old postoperative patient who had a colectomy
    4. A 29-year-old patient who is recovering from flail chest

39. After extubation of a patient, which finding would the nurse report to the health care provider **immediately**?
    1. Respiratory rate of 25 breaths/min
    2. Patient has difficulty speaking
    3. Oxygen saturation of 93%
    4. Crowing noise during inspiration

40. The RN is supervising a nursing student who will suction a patient on a mechanical ventilator. Which actions indicate that the student has a correct understanding of this procedure? **Select all that apply.**
    1. The student nurse uses a sterile catheter and glove.
    2. The student nurse applies suction while inserting the catheter.
    3. The student nurse applies suction during catheter removal.
    4. The student nurses uses a twirling motion when withdrawing the catheter.
    5. The student nurse uses a no. 12 French catheter.
    6. The student nurse applies suction for at least 20 seconds.

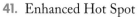

41. Enhanced Hot Spot

Case Study and Question

The nurse is orienting a new RN to the medical/surgical unit. They are providing care for a 58-year-old patient who is at risk for lung and breathing problems.

Which findings will the nurses recognize as factors that increase the patient's risk for development of lung and breathing problems?

Instructions: Read the case study on the left then refer to the findings below to answer the question. Underline or highlight the factors that increase the patient's risk for HHS.

Patient has a history of 40 pack-years smoking cigarettes. Patient states he would like to quit smoking. Patient was exposed to secondhand smoke during his childhood and teen years. Patient started smoking at age 13. Patient tried e-cigarettes, which were not successful. Most members of the patient's family are smokers. Patient's daughter does not want to be around smokers while she is pregnant.

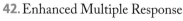

42. Enhanced Multiple Response

Case Study and Question

The nurse is caring for a 55-year-old female patient with chronic obstructive pulmonary disease (COPD) and hypertension. She has no known allergies. Albuterol and Symbicort inhalers are prescribed for COPD. Hydrochlorothiazide (HCTZ) and lisinopril are prescribed for hypertension.

Which of the following statements made by the patient are important with regard to her COPD?

Vital signs:
Pulse 68 beats/min
Respirations 32 breaths/min
Blood Pressure 164/90 mmHg
Oxygen Saturation 90%

Instructions: Read the case study on the left and circle the numbers that best answer the question.

1. I get short of breath when I walk more than 2 blocks.
2. My father died a year ago and I still grieve for having lost him.
3. I'm afraid that I'll need home oxygen soon and I still smoke 5 to 6 cigarettes a day.
4. I've had a cough for about 4 weeks now.
5. I use my inhalers just twice a day.
6. I rest better at night when I sleep in my recliner chair.
7. I often have to get up to urinate during the day and night.
8. I sometimes feel my heart race after I take my medicines.

Answers

1. **Ans: 2** Hoarseness often gets worse during treatment with radiation therapy. The nurse should reassure the patient that this usually improves within 6 to 8 weeks after therapy is completed. Strategies that may help during radiation therapy include voice rest with use of alternative means of communication, as well as saline gargles or sucking on ice chips. Elevating the head of the bed may help with oxygenation but will not help with hoarseness. Responses 3 and 4 are important but do not speak directly to the patient's concern. **Focus:** Prioritization.

2. **Ans: 1, 3, 4, 6** When a patient expresses interest in smoking cessation, this is an important teaching moment for the nurse. It is essential that the nurse first determine the patient's level of nicotine dependence by asking questions such as 1, 3, 4, and 6, which will give clues to this important information. Although it is important to know about other family smokers, whether the patient smokes inside or outside, and if a patient has tried e-cigarettes, this information does not necessarily help with determining nicotine dependence. **Focus:** Supervision, Prioritization.

3. **Ans: 4** When the need for oxygen is greater in the tissues, there is a curve shift to the right. This means that oxygen is dissociated from hemoglobin faster. Conditions that shift the curve to the right include increased body temperature, increased carbon dioxide concentration, and decreased pH or acidosis. This means that the hemoglobin unloads oxygen to the tissues because they need it to support the higher metabolism; this is a tissue protection that increases oxygen delivery to the tissues that need it the most. **Focus:** Prioritization, Supervision.

4. **Ans: 1, 2, 4** The experienced LPN/LVN is capable of gathering data and making observations, including noting breath sounds and performing pulse oximetry. Administering medications, such as those delivered via MDIs, is within the scope of practice of the LPN/LVN. Independently completing the admission assessment, developing the nursing care plan, or evaluating a patient's abilities requires additional education and skills within the scope of practice of the professional RN. **Focus:** Assignment, Supervision.

5. **Ans: 2** For patients with chronic emphysema, the stimulus to breathe is a low serum oxygen level (the normal stimulus is a high carbon dioxide level). This patient's oxygen flow is too high and is causing a high serum oxygen level, which results in a decreased respiratory rate. If the nurse does not intervene, the patient is at risk for respiratory arrest. Crackles, barrel chest, and assumption of a sitting position leaning over the nightstand are common in patients with chronic emphysema. **Focus:** Prioritization. **Test-Taking Tip:** Immediate or priority concerns are issues that can threaten life or limb. In this case, the nurse should remember the normal drive to breathe and recognize that this patient's drive is different. With a respiratory rate this low, the patient is at risk for respiratory arrest.

6. **Ans: 1** When the oxygen flow rate is higher than 4 L/min, the mucous membranes can become dried out. The best treatment is to add humidification to the oxygen delivery system by having the AP apply water-soluble jelly to the nares. Applying the jelly can also help decrease mucosal irritation. None of the other options will treat the problem. **Focus:** Prioritization.

7. **Ans: 2** Teach the AP that compared with light-skinned adults, adults with darker skin usually show a lower oxygen saturation (3% to 5% lower) as measured by pulse oximetry; this results from deeper coloration of the nail bed and does not reflect true oxygen status. None of the other responses are correct. **Focus:** Supervision.

8. **Ans: 2, 4, 5** Checking vital signs, carrying specimens to the lab, and reminding patients about what has already been taught are actions that are within the scope of practice for an AP. Assessing or teaching patients requires additional knowledge and training that is within the scope of practice for professional nurses. **Focus:** Delegation.

9. **Ans: 3** When tracheostomy care is performed, a sterile field is set up and sterile technique is used. Standard precautions such as washing hands must also be maintained but are not enough when performing tracheostomy care. The presence of a tracheostomy tube provides direct access to the lungs for organisms, so sterile technique is used to prevent infection. All of the other steps are correct and appropriate. **Focus:** Delegation, Supervision.

10. **Ans: 2, 3, 4, 5, 6** The correct position for a patient with an anterior nosebleed is upright and leaning forward to prevent blood from entering the stomach and to avoid aspiration. All of the other instructions are appropriate according to best practice for emergency care of a patient with an anterior nosebleed. **Focus:** Assignment, Supervision.

11. **Ans: 3** The AP can remind patients about actions that have already been taught by the nurse and are part of the patient's plan of care. Discussing and teaching require additional education and training. These actions are within the scope of practice of the RN. The RN can administer or assign medication administration to an LPN/LVN. **Focus:** Delegation, Supervision.

12. **Ans: 1, 2, 6** The new RN is at an early point in orientation. The most appropriate patients to assign to the new RN are those in stable condition who

require routine care. The patient with the lobectomy will require the care of an experienced nurse, who will perform frequent assessments and monitoring for postoperative complications. The patient admitted with newly diagnosed esophageal cancer will also benefit from care by an experienced nurse. This patient may have questions and needs a comprehensive admission assessment. The newly diagnosed diabetic patient will need much teaching as well as careful monitoring. As the new nurse advances through orientation, the preceptor will want to work with him or her in providing care for patients with more complex needs. **Focus:** Assignment, Supervision.

13. **Ans: 1, 2, 4, 5, 6**   Bedding should be washed in hot water to destroy dust mites. All of the other points are accurate and appropriate to a teaching plan for a patient with a new diagnosis of asthma. **Focus:** Prioritization.

14. **Ans: 1, 3, 2, 5, 4, 6**   Before each use, the cap is removed, and the inhaler is shaken according to the instructions in the package insert. Next the patient should breathe out completely. As the patient begins to breathe in deeply through the mouth, the canister should be pressed down to release 1 puff (dose) of the medication. The patient should continue to breathe in slowly over 3 to 5 seconds and then hold the breath for at least 10 seconds to allow the medication to reach deep into the lungs. The patient should wait at least 1 minute between puffs from the inhaler. **Focus:** Prioritization.

15. **Ans: 1**   Assisting patients with positioning and activities of daily living is within the educational preparation and scope of practice of APs. Teaching, instructing, and assessing patients all require additional education and skills and are more appropriate to the scope of practice of licensed nurses. **Focus:** Delegation, Supervision.

16. **Ans: 1**   Experienced LPNs/LVNs can use observation of patients to gather data regarding how well patients perform interventions that have already been taught. Assisting patients with ADLs is more appropriately delegated to APs. Planning and consulting require additional education and skills, appropriate to the RN's scope of practice. **Focus:** Assignment, Supervision.

17. **Ans: 4**   A patient who did not have the pneumonia vaccination or flu shot is at an increased risk for developing pneumonia or influenza. An elevated temperature indicates some form of infection, which may be respiratory in origin. All of the other vital sign values are slightly elevated and should be followed up on but are not a cause for immediate concern. **Focus:** Prioritization.

18. **Ans: 2**   The AP's training includes how to monitor and record intake and output. After the nurse has taught the patient about the importance of adequate nutritional intake for energy, the AP can remind and encourage the patient to take in adequate nutrition.

Instructing patients and planning activities require more education and skill and are appropriate to the RN's scope of practice. Monitoring the patient's cardiovascular response to activity is a complex process requiring additional education, training, and skill and falls within the RN's scope of practice. **Focus:** Delegation, Supervision.

19. **Ans: 2**   Continuous bubbling indicates an air leak that must be identified. With the health care provider's (HCP's) order, an RN can apply a padded clamp to the drainage tubing close to the occlusive dressing. If the bubbling stops, the air leak may be at the chest tube insertion, which will require the RN to notify the HCP. If the air bubbling does not stop when the RN applies the padded clamp, the air leak is between the clamp and the drainage system, and the RN must assess the system carefully to locate the leak. Chest tube drainage of 10 to 15 mL/hr is acceptable. Chest tube dressings are not changed daily but may be reinforced. The patient's reports of pain need to be assessed and treated. This is important but not as urgent as investigating a chest tube leak. **Focus:** Delegation, Supervision.

20. **Ans: 4**   The patient with asthma did not achieve relief from shortness of breath after using the bronchodilator and is at risk for respiratory complications. This patient's needs are urgent. The other patients need to be assessed as soon as possible, but none of their situations are urgent. In patients with COPD, pulse oximetry oxygen saturations of more than 90% are acceptable. **Focus:** Prioritization.

21. **Ans: 3**   APs can remind the patient to perform actions that are already part of the plan of care. Assisting the patient into the best position to facilitate coughing requires specialized knowledge and understanding that is beyond the scope of practice of the basic AP, but an experienced AP could assist the patient with positioning after the AP and the patient had been taught the proper technique. In that case, the AP would still be under the supervision of the RN. Teaching patients about adequate fluid intake and techniques that facilitate coughing requires additional education and skill and is within the scope of practice of the RN. **Focus:** Delegation, Supervision.

22. **Ans: 1**   Patients with COPD often have food intolerance, nausea, early satiety (feeling too "full" to eat), poor appetite, and meal-related dyspnea. The increased work of breathing raises calorie and protein needs, which can lead to protein-calorie malnutrition. Urging the patient to eat high-calorie, high-protein foods can be done by the AP after the nurse has taught the patient about the importance of this strategy to prevent weight loss. Feeding the patient too rapidly will tire him or her. If early satiety is a problem, avoid fluids before or during the meal or provide smaller, more frequent meals. **Focus:** Delegation, Supervision.

23. **Ans: 3** Many surgical patients are taught about coughing, deep breathing, and the use of incentive spirometry preoperatively. Also, a fairly new nurse should be assigned more stable and less complicated patients. To care for the patient with TB in isolation, the nurse must be fitted for a high-efficiency particulate air respirator mask. The bronchoscopy patient needs specialized and careful assessment and monitoring after the procedure, and the ventilator-dependent patient needs a nurse who is familiar with ventilator care. Both of these patients need experienced nurses. **Focus:** Assignment.

24. **Ans: 2** Patients taking isoniazid must continue taking the drug for 6 months. The other three statements are accurate and indicate an understanding of TB. Family members should be tested because of their repeated exposure to the patient. Covering the nose and mouth when sneezing or coughing and placing tissues in plastic bags help prevent transmission of the causative organism. The dietary changes are recommended for patients with TB. **Focus:** Prioritization.

25. **Ans: 1** Patients who have recently experienced trauma are at risk for deep vein thrombosis (DVT) and PE. None of the other options are risk factors for PE. Prolonged immobilization is also a risk factor for DVT and PE, but this period of bed rest was very short. **Focus:** Prioritization.

26. **Ans: 4** An LPN/LVN who has been trained to auscultate lung sounds can gather data by routine assessment and observation under the supervision of an RN. Independently evaluating patients, assessing for symptoms of respiratory failure, and monitoring and interpreting laboratory values require additional education and skill, appropriate to the scope of practice of the RN. **Focus:** Assignment, Supervision.

27. **Ans: 1, 2, 3, 5** When a patient is receiving anticoagulation therapy, it is important to avoid trauma to the rectal tissue, which could cause bleeding (e.g., avoid rectal thermometers and enemas). Assessment of patients is within the scope of practice for professional nurses. All of the other instructions are appropriate for the AP scope of practice when caring for a patient receiving anticoagulants. **Focus:** Delegation, Supervision.

28. **Ans: 1, 2, 4, 6** Patients with COPD often have chronic fatigue. Teach them to not rush through activities but to alternate activities with periods of rest. Encourage patients to avoid working with their arms raised. Activities involving the arms decrease exercise tolerance because the accessory muscles are used to stabilize the arms and shoulders rather than to assist breathing. Smaller, more frequent meals may be less tiring. Teach the patient to avoid holding their breath when performing any activity because this interferes with gas exchange. **Focus:** Prioritization.

29. **Ans: 1** A nonrebreather mask can deliver nearly 100% oxygen. When the patient's oxygenation status does not improve adequately in response to delivery of oxygen at this high concentration, refractory hypoxemia is present. Usually at this stage, the patient is working very hard to breathe and may go into respiratory arrest unless HCPs intervene by providing intubation and mechanical ventilation to decrease the patient's work of breathing. Research has shown that patients with ARDS who are treated with conservative amounts of IV fluids while ventilated have improved lung function and shorter intensive care unit stays. Furosemide is a loop diuretic, which will not help with oxygenation. **Focus:** Prioritization.

30. **Ans: 3** The ET should be marked at the level where it touches the incisor tooth or nares. This mark is used to verify that the tube has not shifted. The other three actions are appropriate after ET placement. The priority at this time is to verify that the tube has been correctly placed. Use of an end-tidal carbon dioxide detector is the gold standard for evaluating and confirming ET position in patients who have adequate tissue perfusion. **Focus:** Assignment, Supervision, Prioritization.

31. **Ans: 2** The AP's educational preparation includes measuring vital signs, and an experienced AP would have been taught and know how to check oxygen saturation by pulse oximetry. Assessing and observing the patient, as well as checking ventilator settings, require the additional education and skills of the RN. **Focus:** Delegation, Supervision.

32. **Ans: 4** Infections are always a threat for the patient receiving mechanical ventilation. The endotracheal tube bypasses the body's normal air-filtering mechanisms and provides a direct access route for bacteria or viruses to the lower parts of the respiratory system. The other vital signs are important and should be followed up on but are not of as urgent concern. **Focus:** Prioritization.

33. **Ans: 3** Confusion in a patient this age is unusual and may be an indication of intracerebral bleeding associated with enoxaparin use. The right leg symptoms are consistent with a resolving deep vein thrombosis; the patient may need teaching about keeping the right leg elevated above the heart to reduce swelling and pain. The presence of ecchymoses may point to a need to do more patient teaching about avoiding injury while taking anticoagulants but does not indicate that the HCP needs to be called. **Focus:** Prioritization.

34. **Ans: 2** Manual ventilation of the patient will allow the nurse to deliver an F_{IO_2} of 100% to the patient while attempting to determine the cause of the high-pressure alarm. The patient may need reassurance, suctioning, or insertion of an oral airway, but the first step should be assessing the reason for the high-pressure alarm and resolving the hypoxemia. **Focus:** Prioritization.

35. **Ans: 4** The patient's history and symptoms suggest the development of acute respiratory

PART 2 Common Health Scenarios

distress syndrome, which will require intubation and mechanical ventilation to maintain oxygenation and gas exchange. The HCP must be notified so that appropriate interventions can be taken. Application of a nonrebreather mask can improve oxygenation up to 95% to 100%. The maximum oxygen delivery with a nasal cannula is an F_{IO_2} of 44%. This is achieved with the oxygen flow at 6 L/min, so increasing the flow to 10 L/min will not be helpful. Helping the patient to cough and deep breathe will not improve the lung stiffness that is causing the respiratory distress. Morphine sulfate will only decrease the respiratory drive and further contribute to his hypoxemia. **Focus:** Prioritization.

36. **Ans: 3** Removal of large quantities of fluid from the pleural space can cause fluid to shift from the circulation into the pleural space, causing hypotension and tachycardia. The patient may need to receive IV fluids to correct this. The other data indicate that the patient needs ongoing monitoring or interventions but would not be unusual findings for a patient with this diagnosis or after this procedure. **Focus:** Prioritization.

37. **Ans: 3** Research indicates that nursing actions such as maintaining the head of the bed at 30 to 45 degrees decrease the incidence of VAP. These actions are part of the standard of care for patients who require mechanical ventilation. The other actions are also appropriate for this patient but will not decrease the incidence of VAP. **Test-Taking Tip:** Prevention of VAP has been a subject of research; as a result, a ventilator bundle order set has been developed to apply to patients placed on ventilators with the goal of preventing VAP. **Focus:** Prioritization.

38. **Ans: 1** Older patients, especially those who have smoked or who have chronic lung problems such as chronic obstructive pulmonary disease, are at risk for ventilator dependence and failure to wean. Age-related changes, such as chest wall stiffness, reduced ventilatory muscle strength, and decreased lung elasticity, reduce the likelihood of weaning. Younger patients without respiratory illnesses are likely to wean from the ventilator without difficulty. **Focus:** Prioritization.

39. **Ans: 4** Stridor is a high-pitched, crowing noise during inspiration caused by laryngospasm or edema around the glottis. It is a sign that the patient may need to be reintubated. When stridor or other symptoms of obstruction occur after extubation, respond by immediately calling the rapid response team before the airway becomes completely obstructed. It is common for patients to be hoarse and have a sore throat for a few days after extubation. A respiratory rate of 25 breaths/min should be rechecked but is not an immediate danger, and an oxygen saturation of 93% is low normal. **Focus:** Prioritization.

40. **Ans: 1, 3, 4, 5** The standard size catheter for an adult is a no. 12 or 14 French. Infection is possible because each catheter pass can introduce bacteria into the trachea. In the hospital, use the sterile technique for suctioning and for all suctioning equipment (e.g., suction catheters, gloves, saline or water). Apply suction only during catheter withdrawal and use a twirling motion to prevent the catheter from grabbing tracheal mucosa and leading to damage to tracheal tissue. Apply suction for no more than 10 seconds to minimize hypoxemia during suctioning. **Focus:** Prioritization.

41. **Ans:** Patient has a history of 40 pack-years smoking cigarettes. Patient states he would like to quit smoking. Patient was exposed to secondhand smoke during his childhood and teen years. Patient started smoking at age 13. Patient tried e-cigarettes, which were not successful. Most members of the patient's family are smokers. Patient's daughter does not want to be around smokers while she is pregnant. **Focus:** Prioritization.

42. **Ans: 1, 3, 5, 6, 8** The answers 1, 3, 5, 6, 8 are all related to the patient's COPD. Answer 2 is related to the psychosocial concerns of loss and grief. Answer 4 is significant for angiotensin-converting enzyme inhibitors (e.g. lisinopril). A nonproductive cough signals an adverse effect of these drugs so the drug needs to be discontinued and the patient started on a different cardiac drug class. Answer 7 relates to the patient's HCTZ, which is a thiazide diuretic, leading to increased urine output and lowered BP. **Focus:** Prioritization.

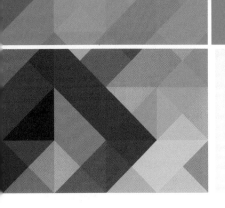

Questions

1. An RN is admitting a patient to the cardiac unit who has stable angina and a history of type 2 diabetes mellitus. The patient is scheduled for a cardiac catheterization the next day. Which medication would need to be withheld for 24 hours before the procedure and for 48 hours after the procedure?
   1. Glucophage
   2. Glimepiride
   3. Pravastatin
   4. Vitamin C

2. The clinic nurse is evaluating a patient who had coronary artery stenting through the right femoral artery a week previously and is taking metoprolol, clopidogrel, and aspirin. Which information reported by the patient is **most** important to report to the health care provider?
   1. Patient is experiencing shortness of breath and fatigue.
   2. Bruising is present at the right groin.
   3. Home blood pressure today was 104/52 mm Hg.
   4. Home radial pulse rate has been 55 to 60 beats/min.

3. Which topics will the nurse plan to include in discharge teaching for a patient who has been admitted with heart failure? **Select all that apply.**
   1. How to monitor and record daily weight
   2. Importance of stopping exercise if heart rate increases
   3. Symptoms of worsening heart failure
   4. Purpose of chronic antibiotic therapy
   5. How to read food labels for sodium content
   6. Date and time for follow-up appointments

4. The nurse is reviewing the laboratory results for a patient with an elevated cholesterol level who is taking atorvastatin. Which result is **most** important to discuss with the health care provider?
   1. Serum potassium is 3.4 mEq/L (3.4 mmol/L).
   2. Blood urea nitrogen (BUN) is 9 mg/dL (3.2 mmol/L).
   3. Aspartate aminotransferase (AST) is 30 units/L (0.5 μkat/L).
   4. Low-density lipoprotein (LDL) cholesterol is 170 mg/dL (4.4 mmol/L).

5. Which finding in a patient with aortic stenosis will be **most** important for the nurse to report to the health care provider?
   1. Temperature of 102.1°F (38.9°C)
   2. Loud systolic murmur over sternum
   3. Blood pressure of 110/88 mm Hg
   4. Weak radial and pedal pulses to palpation

6. A patient who has just arrived in the emergency department reports substernal and left arm discomfort that has been going on for about 3 hours. Which laboratory test will be **most** useful in determining whether the nurse should anticipate implementing the acute coronary syndrome standard protocol?
   1. Creatine kinase MB level
   2. Troponin I level
   3. Myoglobin level
   4. C-reactive protein level

7. When the nurse is monitoring a 53-year-old patient who is undergoing a treadmill stress test, which finding will require the **most** immediate action?
   1. Blood pressure of 152/88 mm Hg
   2. Heart rate of 134 beats/min
   3. Oxygen saturation of 91%
   4. Three premature ventricular contractions (PVCs) in a row

8. The health care provider prescribes these actions for a patient who was admitted with acute substernal chest pain. Which actions are appropriate to assign to an experienced LPN/LVN who is working in the emergency department? **Select all that apply.**
   1. Attaching cardiac monitor leads
   2. Giving heparin 5000 units IV push
   3. Administering morphine sulfate 4 mg IV
   4. Obtaining a 12-lead electrocardiogram (ECG)

5. Asking the patient about pertinent medical history
6. Having the patient chew and swallow aspirin 162 mg

9. Based on this information in a patient's medical record, which topic is the **highest priority** for the nurse to include in the initial teaching plan for a 26-year-old patient who has blood pressures ranging from 150/84 to 162/90 mm Hg?

Health History	Physical Exam	Social and Diet History
• Denies any chronic health problems • Takes no medications currently	• Height: 5 feet, 6 inches • Weight: 115 lb (52.2 kg) • Body mass index (BMI): 18.6	• Works as an accountant • 1 glass of wine once or twice weekly • Eats "fast food" frequently

1. Symptoms of acute stroke and myocardial infarction
2. Adverse effects of alcohol on blood pressure
3. Methods for decreasing dietary caloric intake
4. Low-sodium food choices when eating out

10. The nurse makes a home visit to evaluate a hypertensive patient who has been taking enalapril. Which finding is **most** important to report to the health care provider?
1. Patient reports frequent urination.
2. Patient's blood pressure is 138/86 mm Hg.
3. Patient complains about a frequent dry cough.
4. Patient says, "I get dizzy sometimes if I stand up fast."

11. While reviewing a hospitalized patient's medical record, the nurse obtains this information about cardiovascular risk factors. Which interventions will be important to include in the discharge plan for this patient? **Select all that apply.**

Health History	Family History	Social History
• Hypertension for 10 years • Takes hydrochlorothiazide 25 mg daily • Blood pressure range 110/60 to 132/72 mm Hg	• Patient's mother and two siblings have had myocardial infarctions	• 20 pack-year history of cigarette use • Walks 2 to 3 miles daily

1. Referral to community programs that assist in smoking cessation
2. Teaching about the impact of family history on cardiovascular risk
3. Education about the need for a change in antihypertensive therapy
4. Assistance in reducing emotional stress
5. Discussion of the risks associated with having a sedentary lifestyle
6. Teaching about the signs of hypokalemia and foods to supplement potassium loss

12. Which patient is **best** for the coronary care charge nurse to assign to a float RN who has come for the day from the general medical-surgical unit?
1. Patient requiring discharge teaching about coronary artery stenting before going home today
2. Patient receiving IV furosemide to treat acute left ventricular failure
3. Patient who just transferred in from the radiology department after a coronary angioplasty
4. Patient just admitted with unstable angina who has orders for a heparin infusion and aspirin

13. At 9:00 PM, the nurse admits a 63-year-old patient with a diagnosis of acute myocardial infarction. Which finding is **most** important to communicate to the health care provider who is considering the use of fibrinolytic therapy with tissue plasminogen activator (alteplase) for the patient?
1. The patient was treated with alteplase about 8 months ago.
2. The patient takes famotidine for gastroesophageal reflux disease.
3. The patient has ST-segment elevations on the electrocardiogram.
4. The patient reports having continuous chest pain since 8:00 AM.

14. The nurse is caring for a patient who has heart failure and a new prescription for sacubitril–valsartan. Which patient information is **most** important to discuss with the health care provider before administration of the medication?
1. The patient's oxygen saturation is 92%.
2. The patient receives lisinopril 10 mg/day.
3. The patient's blood pressure is 150/90 mm Hg.
4. The patient's potassium is 3.3 mEq/L (3.3 mmol/L).

15. A patient whose systolic blood pressure is always higher than 140 mm Hg in the clinic tells the nurse, "My blood pressure at home is always fine!" What action should the nurse take **next**?
1. Instruct the patient about the effects of untreated high blood pressure on the cardiovascular and cerebrovascular systems.

Answer Key for this chapter begins on p. 80

2. Educate the patient about lifestyle changes such as a low-sodium diet, daily exercise, and restricting alcohol use to no more than 2 beers per day.

3. Ask the patient to obtain blood pressures twice daily with an automatic blood pressure cuff at home and bring the results to the clinic in a week.

4. Provide the patient with a handout describing the various types of antihypertensive medications with the medication effects and adverse effects.

16. The nurse is working with an experienced assistive personnel (AP) and an LPN/LVN on the telemetry unit. A patient who had an acute myocardial infarction 3 days ago has been reporting fatigue and chest discomfort when ambulating. Which nursing activity included in the care plan is **best** assigned to the LPN/LVN?
    1. Administering nitroglycerin 0.4 mg sublingually if chest discomfort occurs during patient activities
    2. Taking pulse, blood pressure, and oxygen saturation before and after patient ambulation
    3. Teaching the patient energy conservation techniques to decrease myocardial oxygen demand
    4. Explaining the rationale for alternating rest periods with exercise to the patient and family

17. The emergency department nurse is caring for a patient who was just admitted with left anterior chest pain, suggesting possible acute myocardial infarction (MI). Which action will the nurse take **first**?
    1. Insert an IV catheter.
    2. Auscultate heart sounds.
    3. Administer sublingual nitroglycerin.
    4. Draw blood for troponin I measurement.

18. An 80-year-old patient on the coronary step-down unit tells the nurse, "I do not need to take that docusate. I never get constipated!" Which action by the nurse is **most** appropriate?
    1. Document the medication on the patient's chart as "refused."
    2. Mix the medication with food and administer it to the patient.
    3. Explain that his decreased activity level may cause constipation.
    4. Reinforce that the docusate has been prescribed for a good reason.

19. The nurse has given morphine sulfate 4 mg IV to a patient who is having an acute myocardial infarction. When evaluating the patient's response 5 minutes after giving the medication, which finding indicates a need for **immediate** further action?
    1. Blood pressure decrease from 114/65 to 106/58 mm Hg
    2. Respiratory rate drop from 18 to 12 breaths/min

3. Cardiac monitor indicating sinus rhythm at a rate of 96 beats/min
4. Persisting chest pain at a level of 1 (on a scale of 0 to 10)

20. The nurse is preparing to implement teaching about a heart-healthy diet and activity levels for a patient who has had a myocardial infarction and the patient's spouse. The patient says, "I don't see why I need any teaching. I don't think I need to change anything right now." Which response is **most** appropriate?
    1. "Do you think your family may want you to make some lifestyle changes?"
    2. "Can you tell me why you don't feel that you need to make any changes?"
    3. "You are still in the stage of denial, but you will want this information later on."
    4. "Even though you don't want to change, it's important that you have this teaching."

21. The nurse is caring for a hospitalized patient with heart failure who is receiving captopril and spironolactone. Which laboratory value will be **most** important to monitor?
    1. Sodium level
    2. Blood glucose level
    3. Potassium level
    4. Alkaline phosphatase level

22. The health care provider telephones the nurse with new prescriptions for a patient with angina who is already taking aspirin. Which medication is **most** important to clarify further with the health care provider?
    1. Clopidogrel 75 mg/day
    2. Ibuprofen 200 mg every 4 hours as needed
    3. Metoprolol succinate 50 mg/day
    4. Nitroglycerin patch 0.4 mg/hr

23. At 10:00 AM, a hospitalized patient receives a new order for transesophageal echocardiography as soon as possible. Which action will the nurse take **first**?
    1. Put the patient on NPO status.
    2. Teach the patient about the procedure.
    3. Insert an IV catheter in the patient's forearm.
    4. Attach the patient to a cardiac monitor.

24. A patient with stable angina has a prescription for ranolazine 500 mg twice a day. Which patient finding is **most** important for the nurse to discuss with the health care provider (HCP)?
    1. Heart rate is 52 beats/min.
    2. Patient is also taking carvedilol for angina.
    3. Patient reports having chronic constipation.
    4. Blood pressure is 106/56 mm Hg.

 Answer Key for this chapter begins on p. 80

25. The nurse assesses a patient who has just returned to the recovery area after undergoing coronary arteriography. Which information is of **most** concern?
    1. Blood pressure is 154/78 mm Hg.
    2. Pedal pulses are palpable at + 1.
    3. Left groin has a 3-cm bruised area.
    4. Apical pulse is 122 beats/min and regular.

26. The nurse is working in an outpatient clinic where many vascular diagnostic tests are performed. Which task associated with vascular testing is **most** appropriate to delegate to experienced assistive personnel (AP)?
    1. Measuring ankle and brachial pressures in a patient for whom the ankle-brachial index is to be calculated
    2. Checking blood pressure and pulse every 10 minutes in a patient who is undergoing exercise testing
    3. Obtaining information about allergies from a patient who is scheduled for left leg contrast venography
    4. Providing brief patient teaching for a patient who will undergo a right subclavian vein Doppler study

27. While working on the cardiac step-down unit, the nurse is precepting a newly graduated RN who has been in a 6-week orientation program. Which patient will be **best** to assign to the new graduate?
    1. A 19-year-old patient with rheumatic fever who needs discharge teaching before going home with a roommate today
    2. A 33-year-old patient admitted a week ago with endocarditis who will be receiving a scheduled dose of ceftriaxone 2 g IV
    3. A 50-year-old patient with newly diagnosed stable angina who has many questions about medications and nursing care
    4. A 75-year-old patient who has just been transferred to the unit after undergoing coronary artery bypass grafting yesterday

28. The nurse is monitoring the cardiac rhythms of patients in the coronary care unit. Which patient will need **immediate** intervention?
    1. Patient admitted with heart failure who has atrial fibrillation with a rate of 88 beats/min while at rest
    2. Patient with a newly implanted demand ventricular pacemaker who has occasional periods of sinus rhythm at a rate of 90 to 100 beats/min
    3. Patient who has had an acute myocardial infarction and has sinus rhythm at a rate of 76 beats/min with frequent premature ventricular contractions
    4. Patient who recently started taking atenolol and has a first-degree heart block, with a rate of 58 beats/min

29. A patient in the emergency department who is being monitored with a portable cardiac monitor/defibrillator develops this rhythm.

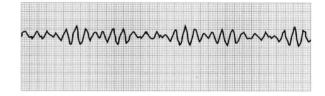

WHICH ACTION WILL THE NURSE TAKE FIRST?
    1. Defibrillate at 200 joules.
    2. Start cardiopulmonary resuscitation (CPR).
    3. Administer epinephrine 1 mg IV.
    4. Intubate and manually ventilate.

30. Two weeks ago, a patient with heart failure received a new prescription for carvedilol 12.5 mg orally. Which finding by the nurse who is evaluating the patient in the cardiology clinic is of **most** concern?
    1. Reports of increased fatigue and activity intolerance
    2. Weight increase of 0.5 kg over a 1-week period
    3. Sinus bradycardia at a rate of 48 beats/min
    4. Traces of edema noted over both ankles

31. The nurse has just received a change-of-shift report about these patients on the coronary step-down unit. Which one will the nurse assess **first**?
    1. A 26-year-old patient with heart failure caused by congenital mitral stenosis who is scheduled for balloon valvuloplasty later today
    2. A 45-year-old patient with constrictive cardiomyopathy who developed acute dyspnea and agitation about 1 hour before the shift change
    3. A 56-year-old patient who underwent coronary angioplasty and stent placement yesterday and has reported occasional chest pain since the procedure
    4. A 77-year-old patient who was transferred from the intensive care unit 2 days ago after coronary artery bypass grafting and has a temperature of 100.6°F (38.1°C)

32. The charge nurse in a long-term care facility that employs RNs, LPNs/LVNs, and assistive personnel (AP) has developed a plan for the ongoing assessment of all residents with a diagnosis of heart failure. Which activity included in the plan is **most** appropriate to assign to an LPN/LVN team member?
    1. Weighing all residents with heart failure each morning
    2. Listening to lung sounds and checking for edema each week

3. Reviewing all heart failure medications with residents every month
4. Updating activity plans for residents with heart failure every quarter

33. The nurse is participating as a team member in the resuscitation of a patient who has experienced a cardiac arrest. The health care provider who is directing the resuscitation asks the nurse to administer epinephrine 1 mg IV. After giving the medication, which action should the nurse take **next**?
1. Prepare to defibrillate the patient.
2. Offer to take over chest compressions.
3. State: "Epinephrine 1 mg IV has been given."
4. Continue to monitor the patient's responsiveness.

34. During a home visit to an 88-year-old patient who is taking digoxin 0.25 mg/day to treat heart failure and atrial fibrillation, the nurse obtains this assessment information. Which finding is **most** important to communicate to the health care provider?
1. Apical pulse 68 beats/min and irregular
2. Digoxin taken with meals
3. Vision that is becoming "fuzzy"
4. Lung crackles that clear after coughing

35. The nurse is ambulating a cardiac surgery patient whose heart rate suddenly increases to 146 beats/min. In which order will the nurse take the following actions?
_____, _____, _____, _____
1. Call the patient's health care provider.
2. Have the patient sit down.
3. Check the patient's blood pressure.
4. Administer as needed oxygen by nasal cannula.

36. A patient who has endocarditis with vegetation on the mitral valve suddenly reports severe left foot pain. The nurse notes that no pulse is palpable in the left foot and that it is cold and pale. Which action should the nurse take **next**?
1. Lower the patient's left foot below heart level.
2. Administer oxygen at 4 L/min to the patient.
3. Notify the health care provider about the change in status.
4. Reassure the patient that embolization is common in endocarditis.

37. A resident in a long-term care facility who has venous stasis ulcers is treated with an Unna boot. Which nursing activity included in the resident's care is **best** for the nurse to delegate to the assistive personnel (AP)?
1. Teaching family members the signs of infection
2. Monitoring capillary perfusion once every 8 hours
3. Evaluating foot sensation and movement each shift
4. Assisting the patient in cleaning around the Unna boot

38. A patient with acute coronary syndrome is receiving a continuous heparin infusion. The patient is to receive 700 units/hour.

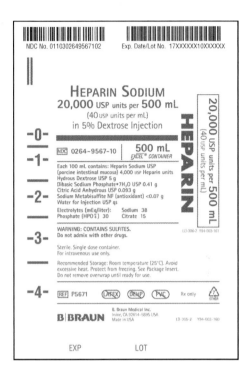

Based on the heparin concentration on the label, the nurse will set the infusion pump to deliver _____ mL/hr.

39. The clinic nurse obtains this information about a patient who is taking warfarin after having a deep vein thrombosis. Which finding is **most** indicative of a need for a change in therapy?
1. Blood pressure is 106/54 mm Hg.
2. International normalized ratio (INR) is 1.2.
3. Bruises are noted at sites where blood has been drawn.
4. Patient reports eating a green salad for lunch every day.

40. The nurse in the cardiovascular clinic receives telephone calls from four patients. Which patient should be scheduled to be seen **most** urgently?
1. Patient with peripheral arterial disease who complains of leg cramps when walking
2. Patient with atrial fibrillation who reports episodes of lightheadedness and syncope
3. Patient with a new permanent pacemaker who has severe itchiness at the wound site
4. Patient with angina who took nitroglycerin twice in the last week while exercising

 Answer Key for this chapter begins on p. 80

Common Health Scenarios

PART 2

41. During the initial postoperative assessment of a patient who has just been transferred to the postanesthesia care unit after repair of an abdominal aortic aneurysm, the nurse obtains these data. Which finding has the **most** immediate implications for the patient's care?
    1. Arterial line indicates a blood pressure of 190/112 mm Hg.
    2. Cardiac monitor shows frequent premature atrial contractions.
    3. There is no response to verbal stimulation.
    4. Urine output is 40 mL of amber urine.

42. The nurse is developing a standardized care plan for the postoperative care of patients undergoing cardiac surgery. The unit is staffed with RNs, LPN/LVNs, and assistive personnel. Which nursing activity will need to be performed by RN staff members?
    1. Removing chest and leg dressings on the second postoperative day and cleaning the incisions with antibacterial swabs
    2. Reinforcing patient and family teaching about the need to deep breathe and cough at least every 2 hours while awake
    3. Developing an individual plan for discharge teaching based on discharge medications and needed lifestyle changes
    4. Administering oral analgesic medications as needed before helping the patient out of bed on the first postoperative day

43. The nurse is preparing to administer the following medications to a patient with multiple health problems who has been hospitalized with deep vein thrombosis. Which medication is **most** important to double-check with another licensed nurse?
    1. Famotidine 20 mg IV
    2. Furosemide 40 mg IV
    3. Digoxin 0.25 mg PO
    4. Warfarin 2.5 mg PO

44. A patient seen in the clinic with shortness of breath and fatigue is being evaluated for a possible diagnosis of heart failure. Which laboratory result will be **most** useful to monitor?
    1. Serum potassium
    2. B-type natriuretic peptide
    3. Blood urea nitrogen
    4. Hematocrit

45. A patient who is scheduled for a coronary arteriogram is admitted to the hospital on the day of the procedure. Which patient information is **most** important for the nurse to communicate to the health care provider (HCP) before the procedure?
    1. Blood glucose level is 144 mg/dL (8 mmol/L).
    2. Cardiac monitor shows sinus bradycardia with a rate of 56 beats/min.
    3. Patient reports chest pain that occurred yesterday.
    4. Patient took metformin 500 mg this morning.

46. Enhanced Multiple Response

Case Study and Question

The nurse is caring for a female patient with coronary artery disease and hypertension. She has no known allergies and takes lisinopril for hypertension.

Which of the statements made by the patient are significant when considering a problem with perfusion?

Vital signs:
Temperature 36.6°C (98°F)
Pulse 82 beats/min
Blood Pressure 134/90 mmHg
Respirations 18 breaths/min
Oxygen Saturation 97%.

Instructions: Read the case study on the left and circle the numbers that best answer the question.

1. I get short of breath when I vacuum.
2. I sleep better since I started to use two pillows.
3. I had to buy new shoes because my old ones were getting too tight.
4. Many people in my family have pernicious anemia.
5. I feel lightheaded when I get up in the morning.
6. I have been so tired lately I worry I may be depressed.
7. I only smoke three cigarettes a day.
8. I recently developed a nonproductive cough.
9. When I get anxious, I can't seem to catch my breath.

47. The RN in an emergency room has triaged four patients who arrived simultaneously. List the order in which the patients should be seen.

1. A 14-year-old healthy male presenting with a swollen, discolored, and painful ankle (7 on a scale of 1-10). He reports he fell off his all-terrain vehicle. Vital signs are temperature (T) 37°C (98.6°F), pulse (P) 90 regular, respiratory rate (R) 20, oxygen saturation (O₂ Sat) 98% room air, and blood pressure (BP) 130/90.

2. A 24-year-old female with a history of mitral valve prolapse presenting with vomiting and diarrhea. She reports the symptoms started after breakfast 2 hours ago and complains of being somewhat lightheaded. Vital signs are T 39°C (102.2°F), P 110 regular, R 18, O₂ Sat 93% room air, and BP 94/62.

3. An 80-year-old female with a history of congestive heart failure presenting with constipation. She reports that she hasn't had a bowel movement in 2 weeks and is uncomfortable. Vital signs are T 36.4°C (97.5°F), P 77 irregular, R 16, O₂ Sat 95% on room air, and BP 120/70.

4. A 54-year-old obese male with a history of diabetes presenting with dyspnea, nausea, and indigestion. He reports that he has had the flu all week. Vital signs are T 38°C (100.4°F), P 84 irregular, R 22, O₂ Sat 95% on room air, and BP 140/92.

48. Cloze

Scenario: The nurse is caring for a patient who presents with chest pain. The patient is complaining of shortness of breath, nausea and level 10 chest pain, radiating down the left arm. Vital signs are T98° (36.6°C) P 68s R 24 Oxygen saturation 90% BP 88/60. Monitor shows a normal sinus rhythm with ST depression in lead II. Mild crackles are heard in both lung bases. He is not taking any medications and he has no known allergies. __1__ and __2__ are administered immediately followed by __3__.

Instructions: Complete the sentences by choosing the most probable option for the omitted information that corresponds with the same numbered list of options provided.

Options 1 and 2	Option 3
IV of normal saline	Heparin 5,000 units subcutaneous
Aspirin 650mg by mouth	Transesophageal echocardiogram
Oxygen 2 liters by nasal cannula	0.4mg sublingual nitroglycerine
Oxygen 100% nonrebreather mask	Percutaneous coronary intervention (PCI)
12 lead electrocardiogram	Morphine 2mg Intravenously
Chest x-ray	Fentanyl 1mcg/kg IV

Answer Key for this chapter begins on p. 80

Answers

1. **Ans: 1** Glucophage should be withheld 24 hours before and 48 hours after cardiac catheterization. Contrast medium is used during a cardiac catherization and can affect kidney function, leaving the patient at an increased risk for lactic acidosis. The rest of the medications do not need to be withheld for longer than the recommended time the patient would need to be NPO. **Focus:** Priority.

2. **Ans: 1** Shortness of breath and fatigue may indicate anemia from gastrointestinal bleeding, which is a possible adverse effect of both aspirin and clopidogrel. The patient will need to continue on the medications but may need treatment with proton pump inhibitors or histamine$_2$ blockers to decrease risk for gastrointestinal bleeding. The other findings will also be reported to the health care provider but will not require a change in the therapeutic plan for the patient. **Focus:** Prioritization.

3. **Ans: 1, 3, 5, 6** To avoid rehospitalization, topics that should be included when discharging a patient with heart failure include how to maintain a low-sodium diet, the purpose and common side effects of medications such as angiotensin-converting enzyme inhibitors and beta-blockers, what to do if symptoms of worsening heart failure occur, and the scheduling of follow-up appointments. The nurse will teach the patient that a moderate increase in heart rate and respiratory effort is normal with exercise. Antibiotics are not included in the treatment regimen for heart failure, which is not an infectious process. **Focus:** Prioritization.

4. **Ans: 4** The patient's LDL level continues to be elevated and indicates a need for further assessment (e.g., the patient may not be taking the atorvastatin), a change in medication, or both. Although statin medications may cause rhabdomyolysis, which could increase BUN and potassium, the patient's BUN and potassium levels are not elevated. Although ongoing monitoring of liver function is recommended when statins are used, this patient's AST is normal. **Focus:** Prioritization.

5. **Ans: 1** Because endocarditis is a concern with valvular disease, an elevated temperature indicates a need for further assessment and diagnostic testing (e.g., an echocardiogram and blood cultures). A systolic murmur, decreased pulse pressure, and weak pulses would be expected in a patient with aortic stenosis and would not indicate an immediate need for further evaluation or treatment. **Focus:** Prioritization.

6. **Ans: 2** Cardiac troponin levels are elevated 3 hours after the onset of myocardial infarction (MI) and are very specific to cardiac muscle injury or infarction. Creatine kinase MB and myoglobin levels also increase with MI, but creatine kinase levels take at least 6 hours to increase and myoglobin is nonspecific. Elevated C-reactive protein levels are a risk factor for coronary artery disease but are not useful in detecting acute injury or infarction. **Focus:** Prioritization.

7. **Ans: 4** Three premature ventricular contractions in a row indicate nonsustained ventricular tachycardia and are an indication to stop the testing to avoid a worsening dysrhythmia. Moderate elevations in blood pressure and heart rate and slight decreases in oxygen saturation are a normal response to exercise and are expected during stress testing. **Focus:** Prioritization.

8. **Ans: 1, 4, 6** Attaching cardiac monitor leads, obtaining an ECG, and administering oral medications are within the scope of practice for LPN/LVNs. An experienced LPN/LVN would be familiar with these activities. Although anticoagulants and narcotics may be administered by LPNs/LVNs to stable patients, these are high-alert medications that should be given by the RN to this unstable patient. Obtaining a pertinent medical history requires RN-level education and scope of practice. **Focus:** Assignment. **Test-Taking Tip:** Remember that the administration of "high-alert" medications (e.g., anticoagulants and narcotics) may require a higher level of knowledge and clinical judgment, especially when you are caring for an unstable patient.

9. **Ans: 4** Current guidelines recommend low sodium intake for lifestyle management of hypertension, and the nurse should teach the patient about the high sodium content in many fast foods and how to make low-sodium choices. A 26-year-old with this level of hypertension is not likely to have a stroke or myocardial infarction. Weight loss or changes in alcohol intake are not necessary. The patient's weight and BMI are normal. Alcohol intake of less than 1 or 2 glasses of wine daily is recommended to prevent hypertension. **Focus:** Prioritization.

10. **Ans: 3** A persistent and irritating cough (caused by accumulation of bradykinin) is a possible adverse effect of angiotensin-converting enzyme inhibitors such as enalapril and is a common reason for changing to another medication category such as the angiotensin II receptor blockers. The other assessment data indicate a need for more patient teaching and ongoing monitoring but would not require a change in therapy. **Focus:** Prioritization.

11. **Ans: 1, 2, 6** The patient's major modifiable risk factor is ongoing smoking. The family history is significant, and the patient should be aware that this increases cardiovascular risk. The blood pressure is well controlled on the current medication, and no change is needed. There is no indication that stress is a risk

factor for this patient, and the patient's activity level meets the American Heart Association recommendation for at least 150 minutes of moderate activity weekly. Hydrochlorothiazide can deplete potassium. Muscle weakness and cramping are signs of hypokalemia. Bananas, yogurt, spinach, and avocados are some foods that are high in potassium. **Focus:** Prioritization.

12. **Ans: 2** An RN who worked on a medical-surgical unit would be familiar with left ventricular failure, the administration of IV medications, and ongoing monitoring for therapeutic and adverse effects of furosemide. The other patients need to be cared for by RNs who are more familiar with the care of patients who have acute coronary syndrome and with collaborative treatments such as coronary angioplasty and coronary artery stenting. **Focus:** Assignment.

13. **Ans: 4** Because continuous chest pain lasting for more than 12 hours indicates that reversible myocardial injury has progressed to irreversible myocardial necrosis, fibrinolytic drugs are usually not recommended for patients with chest pain that has lasted for more than 12 hours. The other information is also important to communicate but would not impact the decision about alteplase use. **Focus:** Prioritization.

14. **Ans: 2** Because combination angiotensin receptor blocker–neprilysin blockers markedly increase the risk for angioedema in patients who are also taking angiotensin-converting enzyme inhibitors (e.g., lisinopril), the concomitant use of both lisinopril and sacubitril–valsartan is contraindicated. In addition, the risk for other adverse effects such as hyperkalemia and hypotension are increased. The other findings should be reported to the health care provider but do not indicate a need to withhold the sacubitril–valsartan. **Focus:** Prioritization.

15. **Ans: 3** The American Heart Association recommends home blood pressure monitoring for patients with hypertension or hypertension risk factors because home blood pressure monitoring provides more accurate data about usual blood pressure than periodic monitoring. The other actions may be necessary, but further assessment of the patient's usual blood pressure is needed before decisions about therapy can be made. **Focus:** Prioritization.

16. **Ans: 1** Administration of nitroglycerin and appropriate patient monitoring for therapeutic and adverse effects are included in LPN/LVN education and scope of practice. Taking of blood pressure, pulse, and oxygen saturation should be delegated to the AP. Patient teaching requires RN-level education and scope of practice. **Focus:** Delegation, Assignment.

17. **Ans: 3** The priority for a patient with unstable angina or MI is treatment of pain. It is important to remember to assess vital signs before administering sublingual nitroglycerin. The other activities also should be accomplished rapidly but are not as high a priority. **Focus:** Prioritization.

18. **Ans: 3** The best option in this situation is to educate the patient about the purpose of the docusate (to counteract the negative effects of immobility and opiate use on peristalsis). Charting the medication as "refused" or telling the patient that he should take the docusate simply because it was prescribed are possible actions but are not as appropriate as patient education. It is unethical to administer a medication to a patient who is unwilling to take it unless someone else has health care power of attorney and has authorized use of the medication. **Focus:** Prioritization.

19. **Ans: 4** The goal in pain management for the patient with an acute myocardial infarction is to completely eliminate the pain (because ongoing pain indicates cardiac ischemia). Even pain rated at a level of 1 out of 10 should be treated with additional morphine sulfate (although possibly a lower dose). The other data indicate a need for ongoing assessment for the possible adverse effects of hypotension, respiratory depression, and tachycardia but do not require further action at this time. **Focus:** Prioritization.

20. **Ans: 2** For behavior to change, the patient must be aware of the need to make changes. This response acknowledges the patient's statement and asks for further clarification. This will give the nurse more information about the patient's feelings, current diet, and activity levels and may increase the willingness to learn. The other responses (although possibly accurate) indicate an intention to teach whether the patient is ready or not and are not likely to lead to changes in lifestyle. **Focus:** Prioritization.

21. **Ans: 3** Hyperkalemia is a common adverse effect of both angiotensin-converting enzyme inhibitors and potassium-sparing diuretics. The other laboratory values may be affected by these medications but are not as likely or as potentially life threatening. **Focus:** Prioritization.

22. **Ans: 2** Nonsteroidal anti-inflammatory drugs (NSAIDs) other than aspirin inhibit the beneficial effect of aspirin in coronary artery disease. Current American Heart Association guidelines recommend against the use of other NSAIDs for patients with cardiovascular disease. Clopidogrel, metoprolol, and topical nitroglycerin are appropriate for the patient but should be verified because the prescriptions were received by telephone. **Focus:** Prioritization.

23. **Ans: 1** Because transesophageal echocardiography is performed after the throat is numbed using a topical anesthetic and with the use of IV sedation, it is important that the patient be placed on NPO status for several hours before the test. The other actions will also need to be accomplished before the echocardiogram but do not need to be implemented immediately. **Focus:** Prioritization.

24. **Ans: 3** Chronic constipation is a common adverse effect of ranolazine. Ranolazine does not impact heart rate or blood pressure and can be taken with beta-blockers or nitrates. The other information may also be reported to the HCP but does not require a change in the patient plan of care. **Focus:** Prioritization.

25. **Ans: 4**   The most common complication after coronary arteriography is hemorrhage, and the earliest indication of hemorrhage is an increase in heart rate. The other data may also indicate a need for ongoing assessment, but the increase in heart rate is of most concern. **Focus:** Prioritization.

26. **Ans: 1**   Measurement of ankle and brachial blood pressures for calculation is within the AP's scope of practice. Calculating the ankle-brachial index and any referrals or discussion with the patient are the responsibility of the supervising RN. The other patients require more complex assessments or patient teaching, which should be done by an experienced RN. **Focus:** Delegation.

27. **Ans: 2**   The new RN's education and hospital orientation would have included safe administration of IV medications. The preceptor will be responsible for the supervision of the new graduate in assessments and patient care. The other patients require more complex assessment or patient teaching by an RN with experience in caring for patients with these diagnoses. **Focus:** Assignment.

28. **Ans: 3**   Premature ventricular contractions occurring in the setting of acute myocardial injury or infarction can lead to ventricular tachycardia or ventricular fibrillation (cardiac arrest), so rapid treatment is necessary. The other patients also have dysrhythmias that will require further assessment, but these are not as immediately life threatening as the premature ventricular contractions in the setting of myocardial infarction. **Focus:** Prioritization.

29. **Ans: 1**   Research indicates that rapid defibrillation improves the success of resuscitation in cardiac arrest. If defibrillation is unsuccessful in converting the patient's rhythm into a perfusing rhythm, CPR should be initiated. Administration of medications and intubation are later interventions. Determining which of these interventions will be used first depends on other factors, such as whether IV access is available. **Focus:** Prioritization.

30. **Ans: 3**   Research indicates that mortality is decreased when patients with heart failure use beta-blocking medications such as carvedilol. When beta-blocker therapy is started for patients with heart failure, heart failure symptoms may initially become worse for a few weeks, so increased fatigue, activity intolerance, weight gain, and edema are not indicative of a need to discontinue the medication at this time. Nevertheless, a heart rate of 48 beats/min indicates a need to decrease the carvedilol dose. **Focus:** Prioritization.

31. **Ans: 2**   The patient's symptoms indicate acute hypoxia, so immediate further assessments (e.g., assessment of oxygen saturation, neurologic status, and breath sounds) are indicated. The other patients should also be assessed soon because they are likely to require nursing actions such as medication administration and teaching, but they are not as acutely ill as the dyspneic patient. **Focus:** Prioritization.

32. **Ans: 2**   LPN/LVN education and scope of practice include data collection such as listening to lung sounds and checking for peripheral edema when caring for stable patients. Weighing the residents should be delegated to an AP. Reviewing medications with residents and planning appropriate activity levels are nursing actions that require RN-level education and scope of practice. **Focus:** Delegation, Assignment.

33. **Ans: 3**   The American Heart Association recommends "closed loop" communication between team members who are involved in resuscitation of a patient. The other actions may also be needed, but the initial action after administering a medication is to ensure that the team leader knows that the prescribed medication has been administered. **Focus:** Prioritization.

34. **Ans: 3**   The patient's visual disturbances may be a sign of digoxin toxicity. The nurse should notify the health care provider and obtain an order to measure the digoxin level. An irregular pulse is expected with atrial fibrillation; there are no contraindications to taking digoxin with food; and crackles that clear with coughing are indicative of atelectasis, not worsening of heart failure. **Focus:** Prioritization.

35. **Ans: 2, 4, 3, 1**   Because the increased heart rate may be associated with a decrease in blood pressure and with lightheadedness, the nurse's first action should be to decrease risk for a fall by having the patient sit down. Cardiac ischemia may be causing the patient's tachycardia, and administration of supplemental oxygen should be the next action. Assessment of blood pressure should be done next. Finally, the health care provider should be notified about the patient's response to activity because changes in therapy may be indicated. **Focus:** Prioritization. **Test-Taking Tip:** Consider that safety concerns (e.g., fall prevention) are usually the highest priority when deciding the order in which to take listed actions.

36. **Ans: 3**   The patient's history and symptoms indicate that acute arterial occlusion has occurred. Because it is important to return blood flow to the foot rapidly, the health care provider should be notified immediately so that interventions such as balloon angioplasty or surgery can be initiated. Changing the position of the foot and improving blood oxygen saturation will not improve oxygen delivery to the foot. Telling the patient that embolization is a common complication of endocarditis will not reassure a patient who is experiencing acute pain. **Focus:** Prioritization.

37. **Ans: 4**   Assisting with hygiene is included in the role and education of the AP. Assessments and teaching are appropriate activities for licensed nursing staff members. **Focus:** Delegation.

38. **Ans: 17.5 mL/hr.**   Each mL of the solution contains heparin 40 units; 700 units/hour equals 17.5 mL/hr. **Focus:** Prioritization.

39. **Ans: 2**   An INR of 1.2 is not within the expected therapeutic range of 2 to 3 and indicates a need for an increase in the warfarin dose. The blood pressure is in the low to normal range. Although the patient will be encouraged to avoid injury, increased bruising is

common when patients are taking anticoagulants and not a reason to discontinue the medication. Although foods that are high in vitamin K will have an impact on INR, this is not a concern when these foods are eaten consistently because the warfarin dose will be adjusted accordingly. **Focus:** Prioritization.

40. **Ans: 2** Lightheadedness and syncope may indicate that the patient's heart rate is either too fast or too slow, affecting brain perfusion and causing risk for complications such as falls. The other patients will also need to be seen, but the data indicate that the symptoms of their diseases are relatively well controlled. **Focus:** Prioritization.

41. **Ans: 1** Elevated blood pressure in the immediate postoperative period puts stress on the graft suture line and could lead to graft rupture and hemorrhage, so it is important to lower blood pressure quickly. The other data also indicate the need for ongoing assessments and possible interventions but do not pose an immediate threat to the patient's hemodynamic stability. **Focus:** Prioritization. **Test-Taking Tip:** When deciding which patient findings are most important, think about which findings may lead quickly to a poor patient outcome and which data are normal for a given situation (such as nonresponsiveness in a patient who has just arrived in the recovery area after surgery).

42. **Ans: 3** Development of plans for patient care or teaching requires RN-level education and is the responsibility of the RN. Wound care, medication administration, assisting with ambulation, and reinforcing previously taught information are activities that can be assigned or delegated to other nursing personnel under the supervision of the RN. **Focus:** Assignment, Delegation.

43. **Ans: 4** Anticoagulant medications are high-alert medications and require special safeguards, such as the double-checking of medications by two nurses before administration. Although the other medications require the usual medication safety procedures, double-checking is not needed. **Focus:** Prioritization.

44. **Ans: 2** Research indicates that B-type natriuretic peptide levels increase in patients with poor left ventricular function and symptomatic heart failure and can be used to differentiate heart failure from other causes of dyspnea and fatigue such as pneumonia. The other values should also be monitored but do not indicate whether the patient has heart failure. **Focus:** Prioritization.

45. **Ans: 4** Because use of metformin may lead to acute lactic acidosis when patients undergo procedures that use iodine-based contrast dye, metformin should be held for 24 hours before and 48 hours after coronary arteriogram. The arteriogram will need to be rescheduled. The other information will also be reported to the HCP but would not be unusual in patients with coronary artery disease. **Focus:** Prioritization.

46. **Ans: 1, 2, 3, 5, 6** Perfusion refers to delivering nutrients and oxygen to the cells though blood flow. 1. Dyspnea on exertion indicates inadequate circulation interfering with oxygen transport to the tissues. 2. Orthopnea results from a buildup of pressure in the pulmonary circulation that can be caused by hypertension. 3. Excessive fluid in the interstitial spaces indicates fluid overload that can be caused by heart disease or renal disease. 5. Lightheadedness on arising indicates inadequate blood flow to the brain, 6. Fatigue is caused by inadequate blood flow through the coronary arteries. Answers 4, 7, 8, and 9 indicate problems with oxygenation. **Focus:** Priority.

47. **Ans: 4, 2, 1, 3** Patient #4 has symptoms of an ischemic pain pattern and has at least two risk factors for a myocardial infarction (diabetes and obesity). His temp of 38°C is an inflammatory reaction to myocardial damage that could have occurred earlier in the week (he complained of "flu" symptoms all week). Patient #2 should be seen next. Her symptoms started within hours of eating, which could indicate food poisoning. She is febrile, tachycardic, and her lightheadedness could be a result of dehydration. Patient #1 is stable, as is Patient #3; however, the 14-year-old is in pain and should have an x-ray as soon as possible to rule out a fracture. **Focus:** Prioritization.

48. **Ans: Option 1, Oxygen 2 liters by nasal cannula; Option 2, IV of normal saline; Option 3, Fentanyl 1mcg/kg IV.** Oxygen at 2 liters via nasal cannula is administered to maintain the oxygen saturation between 94% and 99%. High flow oxygen has been shown to reduce coronary blood flow and increase coronary vascular resistance. An IV of normal saline or a saline lock is needed for medication access or fluid resuscitation. A 12-lead ECG is performed to diagnose the location of the myocardial infarction and must be done but not until the patient has oxygen and an IV. The dose of aspirin to prevent platelet aggregation is 160mg to 325mg. A chest x-ray may also be ordered to show the heart size and pulmonary condition but is not done until the patient is stabilized. The patient's blood pressure is 88/60. Nitroglycerin and Morphine will cause further hypotension and possible reflex tachycardia from the hypotension so Fentanyl should be given for pain relief. The coronary catheterization lab should be notified immediately so the patient can be transferred for an atherectomy or balloon angioplasty within 90 minutes from entering the emergency department. Heparin is given before PCI. Transesophageal echocardiogram may be done before or after PCI. **Focus:** Priority.

PART 2   Common Health Scenarios

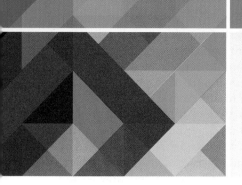

CHAPTER 8
Hematologic Problems

Questions

1. The RN is preparing to have a patient who has acute leukemia sign the permit for a bone marrow aspiration. The patient states that the oncologist has explained the procedure and the complications, and she has no further questions. What assessment is **most** important for the RN to complete before the procedure is carried out?
   1. Review the patient's do-not-resuscitate (DNR) status.
   2. Review the platelet count.
   3. Review the leukocyte count.
   4. Ask when the patient ate last.

2. A patient who has sickle cell disease is admitted with vaso-occlusive crisis and reports severe abdominal and flank pain. Which of the analgesic medications on the pain treatment protocol will be **best** for the nurse to administer initially?
   1. Ibuprofen 800 mg PO
   2. Morphine sulfate 4 mg IV
   3. Hydromorphone liquid 5 mg PO
   4. Fentanyl 25 mcg/hr transdermal patch

3. A patient with sickle cell disease is admitted with splenic sequestration. The blood pressure is 86/40 mm Hg, and heart rate is 124 beats/min. Which of these actions will the nurse take **first**?
   1. Complete a head-to-toe assessment.
   2. Draw blood for type and cross-match.
   3. Infuse normal saline at 250 mL/hr.
   4. Ask the patient about vaccination history.

4. When administering a blood transfusion to a patient, which action can the nurse delegate to the assistive personnel (AP)?
   1. Take the patient's vital signs before the transfusion is started.
   2. Ensure that the blood is infused within no more than 4 hours.
   3. Ask the patient at frequent intervals about the presence of chills or dyspnea.
   4. Assist with double-checking the patient's identification and blood bag number.

5. Which of these patients who have just arrived at the emergency department should the nurse assess **first**?
   1. Patient who reports several dark, tarry stools and a history of peptic ulcer disease
   2. Patient with hemophilia A who is experiencing thigh swelling after a fall
   3. Patient who has pernicious anemia and reports paresthesia of the hands and feet
   4. Patient with thalassemia major who needs a scheduled blood transfusion

6. A patient with chemotherapy-related neutropenia is receiving filgrastim injections. Which finding by the nurse is **most** important to report to the health care provider?
   1. The patient says, "My bones are aching."
   2. The patient's platelet count is 110,000 mm^3 (110 × 10^9/L).
   3. The patient's white blood cell count is 39,000 mm^3 (39.0 × 10^9/L).
   4. The patient reports that the medication stings when it is injected.

7. The nurse is reviewing the complete blood count for a patient who has been admitted for knee arthroscopy. Which value is **most** important to report to the health care provider before surgery?
   1. Hematocrit of 33% (0.33)
   2. Hemoglobin level of 10.9 g/dL (109 g/L)
   3. Platelet count of 426,000/mm^3 (426 × 10^9/L)
   4. White blood cell count of 16,000/mm^3 (16 × 10^9/L)

8. The nurse is providing orientation for a new RN who is preparing to administer packed red blood cells (PRBCs) to a patient who had blood loss during surgery. Which action by the new RN requires that the nurse intervene immediately?
   1. Waiting 20 minutes after obtaining the PRBCs before starting the infusion
   2. Starting an IV line for the transfusion using a 22-gauge catheter
   3. Priming the transfusion set using 5% dextrose in lactated Ringer's solution
   4. Telling the patient that the PRBCs may cause a serious transfusion reaction

9. A 32-year-old patient with sickle cell anemia is admitted to the hospital during a sickle cell crisis. Blood pressure is 104/62 mm Hg, oxygen saturation is 92%, and the patient reports pain at a level 8 (on a scale of 0 to 10). Which action prescribed by the health care provider will the nurse implement **first**?
   1. Administer morphine sulfate 4 to 8 mg IV.
   2. Give oxygen at 4 L/min per nasal cannula.
   3. Start an infusion of normal saline at 200 mL/hr.
   4. Apply warm packs to painful joints.

10. These activities are included in the care plan for a 78-year-old patient admitted to the hospital with anemia caused by possible gastrointestinal bleeding. Which activity can the nurse delegate to an experienced assistive personnel (AP)?
    1. Obtaining stool specimens for the fecal occult blood test (FOBT)
    2. Having the patient sign a colonoscopy consent form
    3. Giving the prescribed polyethylene glycol electrolyte solution
    4. Checking for allergies to contrast dye or shellfish

11. The charge nurse is making the daily assignments on the medical-surgical unit. Which patient is **best** assigned to a float RN who has come from the post-anesthesia care unit (PACU)?
    1. A 30-year-old patient with thalassemia major who has an order for subcutaneous infusion of deferoxamine
    2. A 43-year-old patient with multiple myeloma who requires discharge teaching
    3. A 52-year-old patient with chronic gastrointestinal bleeding who has returned to the unit after a colonoscopy
    4. A 65-year-old patient with pernicious anemia who has just been admitted to the unit

12. The nurse is making a room assignment for a newly arrived patient whose laboratory test results indicate pancytopenia. Which patient will be the **best** roommate for the new patient?
    1. Patient with digoxin toxicity
    2. Patient with viral pneumonia
    3. Patient with shingles
    4. Patient with cellulitis

13. A 67-year-old patient who is receiving chemotherapy for lung cancer is admitted to the hospital with thrombocytopenia. Which statement made by the patient when the nurse is obtaining the admission history is of **most** concern?
    1. "I've noticed that I bruise more easily since the chemotherapy started."
    2. "My bowel movements are soft and dark brown."
    3. "I take ibuprofen every day because of my history of osteoarthritis."
    4. "My appetite has decreased since the chemotherapy started."

14. After a car accident, a patient with a medical alert bracelet indicating hemophilia A is admitted to the emergency department. Which action prescribed by the health care provider will the nurse implement **first**?
    1. Transport the patient to the radiology department for cervical spine radiography.
    2. Transfuse factor VII concentrate.
    3. Type and cross-match for 4 units of packed red blood cells.
    4. Infuse normal saline at 250 mL/hr.

15. The home health nurse is obtaining a history for a patient who has deep vein thrombosis and is taking warfarin 2 mg/day. Which statement by the patient is the **best** indicator that additional teaching about warfarin may be needed?
    1. "I have started to eat more healthy foods like green salads and fruit."
    2. "The doctor said that it is important to avoid becoming constipated."
    3. "Warfarin makes me feel a little nauseated unless I take it with food."
    4. "I will need to have some blood testing done once or twice a week."

16. A patient is admitted to the intensive care unit with disseminated intravascular coagulation associated with a gram-negative infection. Which assessment information has the **most** immediate implications for the patient's care?
    1. There is no palpable radial or pedal pulse.
    2. The patient reports chest pain.
    3. The patient's oxygen saturation is 87%.
    4. There is mottling of the hands and feet.

 Answer Key for this chapter begins on p. 89

17. A patient with iron deficiency anemia who is taking oral iron supplements is evaluated by the nurse in the outpatient clinic. Which finding by the nurse is of **most** concern?
    1. The patient reports that stools are black.
    2. The patient complains of occasional constipation.
    3. The patient takes a multivitamin tablet every day.
    4. The patient takes an antacid with the iron to avoid nausea.

18. When the nurse is assessing a patient with chronic kidney disease who is receiving epoetin alfa (erythropoietin) injections, which finding **most** indicates a need to talk with the health care provider (HCP) before giving the medication?
    1. Hemoglobin level is 8.9 g/dL (89 g/L).
    2. Blood pressure is 198/92 mm Hg.
    3. The patient does not like subcutaneous injections.
    4. The patient has a history of myocardial infarction.

19. A 22-year-old patient with stage I Hodgkin disease is admitted to the oncology unit for radiation therapy. During the initial assessment, the patient tells the nurse, "Sometimes I'm afraid of dying." Which response is **most** appropriate at this time?
    1. "Many individuals with this diagnosis have some fears."
    2. "Perhaps you should ask the doctor about medication."
    3. "Tell me a little bit more about your fear of dying."
    4. "Most people with stage I Hodgkin disease survive."

20. After the nurse receives a change-of-shift report, which patient should be seen **first**?
    1. A 26-year-old patient with thalassemia who has a hemoglobin level of 8 g/dL (80 g/L) and orders for a blood transfusion
    2. A 44-year-old patient admitted 3 days previously for sickle cell crisis who is scheduled for a computed tomographic scan
    3. A 50-year-old patient with stage IV non-Hodgkin lymphoma who is crying and saying, "I'm not ready to die"
    4. A 69-year-old patient with chemotherapy-induced neutropenia who has an oral temperature of 100.1°F (37.8°C)

21. A patient in a long-term care facility who has anemia reports chronic fatigue and dizziness with minimal activity. Which nursing activity will the nurse delegate to the assistive personnel (AP)?
    1. Evaluating the patient's response to normal activities of daily living
    2. Obtaining the patient's blood pressure and pulse with position changes
    3. Determining which self-care activities the patient can do independently
    4. Assisting the patient in choosing a diet that will improve strength

22. A transfusion of packed red blood cells has been infusing for 5 minutes when the patient becomes flushed and tachypneic and says, "I'm having chills. Please get me a blanket." Which action should the nurse take **first**?
    1. Obtain a warm blanket for the patient.
    2. Check the patient's oral temperature.
    3. Stop the transfusion.
    4. Administer oxygen.

23. A group of patients is assigned to an RN-LPN/LVN team. The LPN/LVN should be assigned to provide patient care and administer medications to which patient?
    1. A 36-year-old patient with chronic kidney failure who will need a subcutaneous injection of epoetin alfa
    2. A 39-year-old patient with hemophilia B who has been admitted to receive a blood transfusion
    3. A 50-year-old patient with newly diagnosed polycythemia vera who will require a phlebotomy
    4. A 55-year-old patient with a history of stem cell transplantation who has a bone marrow aspiration scheduled

24. The nurse obtains the following data about a patient admitted with multiple myeloma. Which information requires the **most** rapid action by the nurse?
    1. The patient reports chronic bone pain.
    2. The blood uric acid level is very elevated.
    3. The 24-hour urine test shows Bence Jones proteins.
    4. The patient reports new-onset leg numbness.

25. The nurse in the outpatient clinic is assessing a 22-year-old patient who needs a physical exam before starting a new job. The patient reports a history of a splenectomy several years previously after an accident but has otherwise been healthy. Which information obtained during the assessment will be of **most** immediate concern to the nurse?
    1. The patient engages in unprotected sex.
    2. The patient's oral temperature is 100°F (37.8°C).
    3. The patient's blood pressure is 148/76 mm Hg.
    4. The patient admits to daily marijuana use.

26. A patient with graft-versus-host disease after bone marrow transplantation is being cared for on the medical unit. Which nursing activity is **best** assigned to a traveling RN?
    1. Administering oral cyclosporine
    2. Assessing the patient for signs of infection
    3. Infusing 5% dextrose in 0.45% saline at 125 mL/hr
    4. Educating the patient about ways to prevent infection

27. The nurse is caring for a patient who takes warfarin daily for a diagnosis of atrial fibrillation. Which information about the patient is **most** important to report to the health care provider (HCP)?
    1. The international normalized ratio (INR) is 5.2.
    2. Bruising is noted at sites where blood has been drawn.
    3. The patient reports eating a green salad for lunch every day.
    4. The patient has questions about whether a different anticoagulant can be used.

28. A patient with an absolute neutrophil count of 300/μL $(0.3 \times 10^9/L)$ is admitted to the oncology unit. Which staff member should the charge nurse assign to provide care for this patient, under the supervision of an experienced oncology RN?
    1. LPN/LVN who has floated from the same-day surgery unit
    2. RN from a staffing agency who is being oriented to the oncology unit
    3. LPN/LVN with 2 years of experience on the oncology unit
    4. RN who recently transferred to the oncology unit from the emergency department

29. The nurse is transferring a patient with newly diagnosed chronic myeloid leukemia to a long-term care facility. Which information is **most** important to communicate to the nurse at the long-term care facility before transferring the patient?
    1. Philadelphia chromosome is present in the patient's blood smear.
    2. The patient's glucose level is elevated as a result of prednisone therapy.
    3. There has been a 20-lb (9.1-kg) weight loss over the last year.
    4. The patient's chemotherapy has resulted in neutropenia.

30. A patient with acute myelogenous leukemia is receiving induction-phase chemotherapy. Which assessment finding requires the **most** rapid action?
    1. Serum potassium level of 7.8 mEq/L (7.8 mmol/L)
    2. Urine output less than intake by 400 mL
    3. Inflammation and redness of the oral mucosa
    4. Ecchymoses present on the anterior trunk

31. A patient who has been receiving cyclosporine after an organ transplantation is experiencing these symptoms. Which one is of **most** concern?
    1. Bleeding of the gums while brushing the teeth
    2. Nontender lump in the right groin
    3. Occasional nausea after taking the medication
    4. Numbness and tingling of the feet

32. A patient with Hodgkin lymphoma who is receiving radiation therapy to the groin area has skin redness and tenderness in the area being irradiated. Which nursing activity should the nurse delegate to the assistive personnel (AP) caring for the patient?
    1. Checking the skin for signs of redness or peeling
    2. Assisting the patient in choosing appropriate clothing
    3. Explaining good skin care to the patient and family
    4. Cleaning the skin over the area daily with a mild soap

33. After the nurse receives the change-of-shift report, which patient should be assessed **first**?
    1. A 20-year-old patient with possible acute myelogenous leukemia who has just arrived on the medical unit
    2. A 38-year-old patient with aplastic anemia who needs teaching about decreasing infection risk before discharge
    3. A 40-year-old patient with lymphedema who requests help in putting on compression stockings before getting out of bed
    4. A 60-year-old patient with non-Hodgkin lymphoma who is refusing the prescribed chemotherapy regimen

34. A patient with severe iron deficiency anemia is to receive iron dextran complex 25 mg IV. The medication is diluted in 250 mL of normal saline and is to be infused over 6 hours. The nurse will infuse _____ mL/hr. (Round to two decimal points.)

PART 2 Common Health Scenarios

Answer Key for this chapter begins on p. 89

35. Enhanced Hot Spot _____

Case Study

The nurse is providing care for a 65-year-old patient who is being seen for a yearly physical exam. She is 65 inches tall and weighs 81kg. Her fasting blood sugar is 134 and her total cholesterol level is 250. Family history includes an aunt who died of breast cancer at age 55. Her parents are alive and in good health. She does not smoke and drinks a couple of glasses of wine on the Jewish Sabbat every week. Her mammograms indicate she has dense breast tissue. She is married and has one adult child who is 30 years old.

Instructions: Underline or highlight information that increases the patient's risk for developing breast cancer.

Vital signs:
Temperature 97.8°F (36.5°C)
Pulse 100 beats/min
Respirations 18 breaths/min
Blood Pressure (BP) 150/90 mmHg
Oxygen Saturation 98%

36. Cloze _____

Scenario: The RN is caring for a patient with thrombocytopenia and leukopenia after receiving 3 days of chemotherapy. Her skin turgor is poor with dry mucous membranes. The patient has no allergies. The patient's white blood cell count (WBC) is 2,000 /mm^3, platelet count is 150,000/mm^3, red blood cell count (RBC) 5.0 million cells/mcL.

Instructions: Complete the sentences below by choosing the most probable option for the missing information that corresponds with the same numbered list of options provided.

Vital signs:
Temperature 99°F (37.2°C)
Pulse 96 beats/min
Respirations 16 breaths/min
Blood Pressure 100/72 mmHg
Oxygen Saturation 90% on room air

The RN ___1___ and admits the patient to a ___2___. The RN anticipates the healthcare provider will prescribe ___3___ to prevent infection.

Option 1	Option 2	Option 3
Inserts a #18 gauge IV and administers normal saline to keep vein open	Semi-private room	1 unit of platelets
Establishes a #22-gauge saline lock	Negative pressure room	Pegfilgrastin 6mg subcutaneous injection
Administers oxygen at 2 Liters by nasal cannula	Private room	Vancomycin 500mg IV every 6 hours
Applies a 100% oxygen non-rebreather mask	Positive pressure room	Fresh frozen plasma

Common Health Scenarios PART 2

Answers

1. **Ans: 2** The most important assessment to carry out before the procedure is to review the platelet count to ensure that the platelets are within normal limits. A complication of a bone marrow aspiration is bleeding and platelets are necessary for normal clotting to take place. The RN should also review the prothrombin time, partial thromboplastin time, and international normalized ratio for the same reason. A patient's DNR status should be reviewed in case of an emergency on all ill patients as a general rule. The leukocyte count in leukemia is expected to be altered and is not important when considering the bleeding complication. Usually it is not necessary for a patient to be NPO before the procedure. **Focus:** Prioritization.

2. **Ans: 2** Guidelines for the management of vaso-occlusive crisis suggest the rapid use of parenteral opioids for patients who have moderate to severe pain. The other medications may also be appropriate for the patient as the crisis resolves but are not the best choice for rapid treatment of severe pain. **Focus:** Prioritization.

3. **Ans: 3** Because the patient is severely hypotensive, correction of hypovolemia caused by the splenic sequestration is the most urgent action. Nevertheless, the other actions are appropriate because a complete assessment will be needed to plan care, a transfusion is likely to be needed, and vaccination history is pertinent for patients with sickle cell disease. Infusion of saline, however, is the priority need. **Focus:** Prioritization. **Test-Taking Tip:** Although a thorough assessment of a newly admitted patient is always needed, when the primary assessment (focused on airway, breathing, circulation, and disability) indicates a need for rapid treatment, the treatment should be initiated before proceeding with the rest of the assessment.

4. **Ans: 1** AP education and role includes obtaining vital signs, which will be reported to the RN before the initiation of the transfusion. Monitoring for transfusion reactions, adjusting the transfusion rate, and ensuring that the blood type and number are correct require critical thinking and should be done by the RN. **Focus:** Delegation.

5. **Ans: 2** Thigh swelling after an injury in a patient with hemophilia likely indicates acute bleeding, which can compromise blood flow and nerve function in the leg and should be treated immediately with the administration of factor replacement. The other patients also need assessment, treatment, or both, but the data do not indicate any immediate threat to life or function. **Focus:** Prioritization.

6. **Ans: 3** Leukocytosis is an adverse effect of filgrastim and indicates a need to stop the medication or decrease dosage. Bone pain is a common adverse effect as the bone marrow starts to produce more neutrophils; the patient should receive analgesics, but the medication will be continued. Stinging with injection may occur; the nurse should administer the medication more slowly. The patient's platelet count is low and should be reported, but the level of 110,000 mm^3 (110 × 10^9/L) does not increase risk for spontaneous bleeding. **Focus:** Prioritization.

7. **Ans: 4** Centers for Disease Control and Prevention guidelines for the prevention of surgical site infections indicate that surgery should be postponed when there is evidence of a preexisting infection such as an elevation in white blood cell count. The other values are slightly abnormal but would not be likely to cause postoperative problems for knee arthroscopy. **Focus:** Prioritization.

8. **Ans: 3** Normal saline, an isotonic solution, should be used when priming the IV line to avoid causing hemolysis of red blood cells (RBCs). Ideally, blood products should be infused as soon as possible after they are obtained; however, a 20-minute delay would not be unsafe. Large-bore IV catheters are preferable for blood administration; if a smaller catheter must be used, normal saline may be used to dilute the RBCs. Although the new RN should avoid increasing patient anxiety by indicating that a serious transfusion reaction may occur, this action is not as high a concern as using an inappropriate fluid for priming the IV tubing. **Focus:** Prioritization.

9. **Ans: 2** National guidelines for sickle cell crisis indicate that oxygen should be administered if the oxygen saturation is less than 95%. Hypoxia and deoxygenation of the blood cells are the most common cause of sickling, so administration of oxygen is the priority intervention here. Pain control (including the administration of morphine and application of warm packs to joints) and hydration are also important interventions for this patient and should be accomplished rapidly. **Focus:** Prioritization.

10. **Ans: 1** An experienced AP will have been taught how to obtain a stool specimen for the FOBT because this is a common screening test for hospitalized patients. Having the patient sign an informed consent form should be done by the health care provider who will be performing the colonoscopy. Administering medications and checking for allergies are within the scope of practice of licensed nursing staff. **Focus:** Delegation.

11. **Ans: 3** A nurse who works in the post anesthesia care unit will be familiar with the monitoring needed for a patient who has just returned from a procedure such as a colonoscopy, which requires moderate sedation or monitored anesthesia care (conscious sedation). Care of the other patients requires staff with more experience

with various types of hematologic disorders and would be better to assign to nursing personnel who regularly work on the medical-surgical unit. **Focus:** Assignment.

12. **Ans: 1** Patients with pancytopenia are at higher risk for infection. The patient with digoxin toxicity presents the least risk of infecting the new patient. Viral pneumonia, shingles, and cellulitis are infectious processes. **Focus:** Prioritization.

13. **Ans: 3** Because nonsteroidal antiinflammatory drugs will decrease platelet aggregation, patients with thrombocytopenia should not use ibuprofen routinely. Patient teaching about this should be included in the care plan. Bruising is consistent with the patient's admission problem of thrombocytopenia. Soft, dark brown stools indicate that there is no frank or occult blood in the bowel movements. Although the patient's decreased appetite requires further assessment by the nurse, this is a common complication of chemotherapy. **Focus:** Prioritization.

14. **Ans: 2** When a hemophiliac patient is at high risk for bleeding, the priority intervention is to maximize the availability of clotting factors. The other prescribed actions should also be implemented rapidly but do not have as high a priority as administering clotting factors. **Focus:** Prioritization.

15. **Ans: 1** Patients taking warfarin are advised to avoid making sudden dietary changes because changing the oral intake of foods high in vitamin K (e.g., green leafy vegetables and some fruits) will have an impact on the effectiveness of the medication. The other statements suggest that further teaching may be indicated, but more assessment for teaching needs is required first. **Focus:** Prioritization.

16. **Ans: 3** Because the decrease in oxygen saturation will have the greatest immediate effect on all body systems, improvement in oxygenation should be the priority goal of care. The other data also indicate the need for rapid intervention, but improvement of oxygenation is the most urgent need. **Focus:** Prioritization.

17. **Ans: 4** Concurrent use of antacids with iron supplements will decrease absorption of the iron and decrease the efficacy in resolving the patient's anemia. Black stools are expected when taking oral iron. The patient's occasional constipation may indicate a need for information about prevention of constipation while taking iron. Use of a multivitamin tablet is safe when taking iron supplements (although the patient may need to avoid taking combined vitamin and mineral supplements). **Focus:** Prioritization.

18. **Ans: 2** Epoetin alfa can cause hypertension, and blood pressure should be controlled before administering the medication. Because patients with chronic kidney disease have chronic anemia, a hemoglobin level of 8.9 g/dL (89 g/L) is not unusual. Although the nurse could ask the HCP about IV administration of the medication, subcutaneous administration requires a lower dose of the medication and is preferred. Epoetin

alfa can cause angina or myocardial infarction, but the risk is highest when hemoglobin levels are greater than 11 g/dL (110 g/L). **Focus:** Prioritization.

19. **Ans: 3** More assessment about what the patient means is needed before any interventions can be planned or implemented. All of the other statements indicate an assumption that the patient is afraid of dying of Hodgkin disease, which may not be the case. **Focus:** Prioritization. **Test-Taking Tip:** When determining how to respond to a patient concern or comment, always consider whether further assessment or clarification is needed before appropriate actions can be planned and implemented.

20. **Ans: 4** Any temperature elevation in a neutropenic patient may indicate the presence of a life-threatening infection, so actions such as drawing blood for culture and administering antibiotics should be initiated quickly. The other patients need to be assessed as soon as possible but are not critically ill. **Focus:** Prioritization.

21. **Ans: 2** AP education covers routine nursing skills such as assessment of vital signs. Evaluation, baseline assessment of patient abilities, and nutrition planning are activities appropriate to RN practice. **Focus:** Delegation.

22. **Ans: 3** The patient's symptoms indicate that a transfusion reaction may be occurring, so the first action should be to stop the transfusion. Chills are an indication of a febrile reaction, so warming the patient may not be appropriate. Checking the patient's temperature and administering oxygen are also appropriate actions if a transfusion reaction is suspected; however, stopping the transfusion is the first priority. **Focus:** Prioritization.

23. **Ans: 1** LPNs/LVNs should be assigned to care for stable patients. Subcutaneous administration of epoetin is within the LPN/LVN scope of practice. Blood transfusions should be administered by RNs because evaluation for and management of transfusion reactions require an RN-level education and scope of practice. The other patients will require teaching about phlebotomy and bone marrow aspiration, which should be implemented by the RN. **Focus:** Assignment **Test-Taking Tip:** When assigning patients or nursing actions to an LPN/LVN, remember that the LPN/LVN education and scope of practice is focused on the care of more stable patients.

24. **Ans: 4** The leg numbness may indicate spinal cord compression, which should be evaluated and treated immediately by the health care provider to prevent further loss of function. Chronic bone pain, hyperuricemia, and the presence of Bence Jones proteins in the urine all are typical of multiple myeloma and do require assessment or treatment; however, the loss of motor or sensory function is an emergency. **Focus:** Prioritization.

25. **Ans: 2** Because the spleen has an important role in the phagocytosis of microorganisms, the patient is at higher risk for severe infection after a splenectomy. Antibiotic administration is usually indicated for any symptoms of infection. The other information also indicates the need for more assessment and

intervention, but prevention and treatment of infection are the highest priorities for this patient. **Focus:** Prioritization.

26. **Ans: 3** The infusion of IV fluids is a common intervention that can be implemented by RNs who do not have experience in caring for patients who are severely immunosuppressed. Administering cyclosporine, assessing for subtle indications of infection, and patient teaching are more complex tasks that should be done by RN staff members who have experience caring for immunosuppressed patients. **Focus:** Assignment.

27. **Ans: 1** An INR of 2 to 3 is the goal for patients who are taking warfarin for atrial fibrillation; an INR of 5.2 will require that the medication dose be adjusted. Because bleeding times are prolonged when patients receive anticoagulants, bruising is a common adverse effect. Green leafy vegetables contain vitamin K and have an impact on the effectiveness of warfarin, but if patients eat these vegetables consistently, then warfarin dosing will also be consistent. The HCP may need to discuss use of the newer oral anticoagulants (which do not require blood testing) with the patient, but the highest concern is the very prolonged INR. **Focus:** Prioritization.

28. **Ans: 3** Because many aspects of nursing care need to be modified to prevent infection when a patient has a low absolute neutrophil count, care should be provided by the staff member with the most experience with neutropenic patients. The other staff members have the education required to care for this patient but are not as clinically experienced. When LPN/LVN staff members are given acute care patient assignments, they must work under the supervision of an RN. The LPN/LVN in this case would report to the RN assigned to the patient. **Focus:** Assignment.

29. **Ans: 4** A patient with neutropenia is at increased risk for infection, and the nurse who will be receiving the patient needs to know about the neutropenia to make decisions about the patient's room assignment and to plan care. The other information will also impact planning for patient care, but the charge nurse needs the information about neutropenia before the patient is transferred. **Focus:** Prioritization.

30. **Ans: 1** Fatal hyperkalemia may be caused by tumor lysis syndrome, a potentially serious consequence of chemotherapy in acute leukemia. The other symptoms also indicate a need for further assessment or interventions but are not as critical as the elevated potassium level, which requires immediate treatment. **Focus:** Prioritization.

31. **Ans: 2** A nontender lump in this area (or near any lymph node) may indicate that the patient has developed lymphoma, a possible adverse effect of

immunosuppressive therapy. The patient should receive further evaluation immediately. The other symptoms may also indicate side effects of cyclosporine (gingival hyperplasia, nausea, and paresthesia, respectively) but do not indicate the need for immediate action. **Focus:** Prioritization.

32. **Ans: 4** Skin care is included in the AP's education and job description. Assessment and patient teaching are more complex tasks that should be delegated to RNs. Because the patient's clothes need to be carefully chosen to prevent irritation or damage to the skin, the RN should assist the patient with this. **Focus:** Delegation.

33. **Ans: 1** The newly admitted patient should be assessed first because the baseline assessment and plan of care need to be completed. The other patients also need assessments or interventions but do not need immediate nursing care. **Focus:** Prioritization.

34. **Ans: 41.67 mL/hr.** To infuse 250 mL of solution over 6 hours, the nurse will need to infuse 41.67 mL/hr. **Focus:** Prioritization.

35. **Ans:** The nurse is providing care for a **65-year-old patient** who is being seen for a yearly physical exam. Vital signs include: T 97.8°F (36.5°C), HR 100/min, RR 18, BP 150/90mm Hg. O$_2$ Sat 98%. She is **65 inches tall and weighs 81kg.** Her fasting **blood sugar is 134** and her total cholesterol level is 250. Family history includes an aunt who died of breast cancer at age 55. Her parents are alive, and in good health. She does not smoke and drinks a couple of glasses of wine on the **Jewish Sabbat every week.** Her mammograms indicate she has **dense breast tissue.** She is married and has **one adult child who is 30 years old.**

36. **Ans: Option 1, Oxygen at 2 Liters by nasal cannula; Option 2, Positive pressure room; Option 3, Pegfilgrastin 6mg subcutaneous injection.** Oxygen should be administered to keep the oxygen saturation levels above 90%. Two liters of oxygen increases the percentage of oxygen by approximately 6% so 100% is not necessary. The patient with leukopenia is susceptible to infection and should be admitted to a positive pressure room to protect them from pathogens. A negative pressure room is used to protect others from the patient's pathogens. Platelets should be transfused if the platelet count is below 100,000/mm^3. Fresh frozen plasma contains clotting factors but not white blood cells to prevent infection.

Pegfilgrastin stimulates the bone marrow to increases white blood cells to prevent infection. There is no evidence of infection so Vancomycin would not be anticipated. **Focus:** Priority.

CHAPTER 9

Neurologic Problems

Questions

1. The nurse in the ER assesses a 21-year-old new admission who was in a motor vehicle crash. On assessment, the nurse discovers the patient has the pictured manifestation. Which injury does this finding indicate to the nurse?

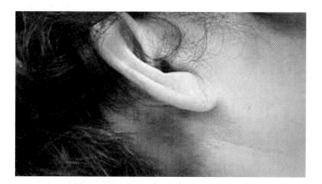

   1. Frontal skull fracture
   2. Basilar skull fracture
   3. Orbital fracture
   4. Temporal fracture

2. The nurse is assessing a patient with a neurologic health problem and discovers a change in level of consciousness from alert to lethargic. What is the nurse's **best** action?
   1. Perform a complete neurologic assessment.
   2. Assess the cranial nerve functions.
   3. Contact the rapid response team.
   4. Reassess the patient in 30 minutes.

3. The nurse on the neurologic acute care unit is assessing the orientation of a patient with severe headaches. Which questions would the nurse use to determine orientation? **Select all that apply.**
   1. When did you first experience the headache symptoms?
   2. Did the mayor of Cleveland run as a Democrat or Republican?
   3. What is your health care provider's name?
   4. What year and month is it?

5. What is the color of your parents' house?
6. What is the name of this health care facility?

4. What is the **priority** nursing concern for a patient experiencing a migraine headache?
   1. Pain
   2. Anxiety
   3. Hopelessness
   4. Risk for brain injury

5. The nurse is creating a teaching plan for a patient with newly diagnosed migraine headaches. Which key items will be included in the teaching plan? **Select all that apply.**
   1. Foods that contain tyramine, such as alcohol and aged cheese, should be avoided.
   2. Drugs such as nitroglycerin and nifedipine should be avoided.
   3. Abortive therapy is aimed at eliminating the pain during the aura.
   4. A potential side effect of medications is rebound headache.
   5. Complementary therapies such as biofeedback and relaxation may be helpful.
   6. Estrogen therapy should be continued as prescribed by the patient's health care provider.

6. After a patient has a seizure, which action can the nurse delegate to the assistive personnel (AP)?
   1. Documenting the seizure
   2. Performing neurologic checks
   3. Checking the patient's vital signs
   4. Restraining the patient for protection

7. The nurse is preparing to admit a patient with a seizure disorder. Which action can be assigned to an LPN/LVN?
   1. Completing the admission assessment
   2. Setting up oxygen and suction equipment
   3. Placing a padded tongue blade at the bedside
   4. Padding the side rails before the patient arrives

8. A nursing student is teaching a patient and family about epilepsy before the patient's discharge. For which statement should the nurse intervene?
   1. "You should avoid consumption of all forms of alcohol."
   2. "Wear your medical alert bracelet at all times."
   3. "Protect your loved one's airway during a seizure."
   4. "It's OK to take over-the-counter medications."

9. A patient with Parkinson disease has a problem with decreased mobility related to neuromuscular impairment. The nurse observes the assistive personnel (AP) performing all of these actions. For which action must the nurse intervene?
   1. Helping the patient ambulate to the bathroom and back to bed
   2. Reminding the patient not to look at his feet when he is walking
   3. Performing the patient's complete bathing and oral care
   4. Setting up the patient's tray and encouraging the patient to feed himself

10. The nurse is preparing to discharge a patient with chronic low back pain. Which statement by the patient indicates the need for additional teaching?
    1. "I will avoid exercise because the pain gets worse."
    2. "I will use heat or ice to help control the pain."
    3. "I will not wear high-heeled shoes at home or work."
    4. "I will purchase a firm mattress to replace my old one."

11. A patient with a spinal cord injury reports a sudden severe throbbing headache that started a short time ago. Assessment of the patient reveals increased blood pressure (168/94 mm Hg) and decreased heart rate (48 beats/min), diaphoresis, and flushing of the face and neck. What action should the nurse take **first**?
    1. Administer the ordered acetaminophen.
    2. Check the indwelling catheter tubing for kinks or obstruction.
    3. Adjust the temperature in the patient's room.
    4. Notify the health care provider (HCP) about the change in status.

12. Which patient should the charge nurse assign to a newly graduated RN who is orienting to the neurologic care unit?
    1. A 28-year-old newly admitted patient with a spinal cord injury
    2. A 67-year-old patient who had a stroke 3 days ago and has left-sided weakness
    3. An 85-year-old patient with dementia who is to be transferred to long-term care today
    4. A 54-year-old patient with Parkinson disease who needs assistance with bathing

13. A patient with a spinal cord injury at level C3 to C4 is being cared for by the nurse in the emergency department. What is the **priority** nursing assessment?
    1. Determine the level at which the patient has intact sensation.
    2. Assess the level at which the patient has retained mobility.
    3. Check blood pressure and pulse for signs of spinal shock.
    4. Monitor respiratory effort and oxygen saturation level.

14. The nurse is floated from the emergency department to the neurologic floor. Which action should the nurse delegate to the assistive personnel (AP) when providing nursing care for a patient with a spinal cord injury?
    1. Assessing the patient's respiratory status every 4 hours
    2. Checking and recording the patient's vital signs every 4 hours
    3. Monitoring the patient's nutritional status, including calorie counts
    4. Instructing the patient how to turn, cough, and breathe deeply every 2 hours

15. The nurse is helping a patient with a spinal cord injury (SCI) to establish a bladder retraining program. Which strategies may stimulate the patient to void? **Select all that apply.**
    1. Stroking the patient's inner thigh
    2. Pulling on the patient's pubic hair
    3. Initiating intermittent straight catheterization
    4. Pouring warm water over the patient's perineum
    5. Tapping the bladder to stimulate the detrusor muscle
    6. Reminding the patient to void in a urinal every hour while awake

16. A patient with a cervical spinal cord injury has been placed in fixed skeletal traction with a halo fixation device. When caring for this patient, the nurse may assign which actions to the LPN/LVN? **Select all that apply.**
    1. Checking the patient's skin for pressure from the device
    2. Assessing the patient's neurologic status for changes
    3. Observing the halo insertion sites for signs of infection
    4. Cleaning the halo insertion sites with hydrogen peroxide
    5. Developing the nursing plan of care for the patient
    6. Administering oral medications as prescribed

Answer Key for this chapter begins on p. 98

17. The nurse is preparing a nursing care plan for a patient with a spinal cord injury (SCI) for whom problems of decreased mobility and inability to perform activities of daily living (ADLs) have been identified. The patient tells the nurse, "I don't know why we're doing all this. My life's over." Based on this statement, which additional nursing concern takes **priority**?
    1. Risk for injury
    2. Decreased nutrition
    3. Difficulty with coping
    4. Impairment of body image

18. Which patient should the charge nurse assign to the traveling nurse, new to neurologic nursing care, who has been on the neurologic unit for 1 week?
    1. A 34-year-old patient with newly diagnosed multiple sclerosis (MS)
    2. A 68-year-old patient with chronic amyotrophic lateral sclerosis (ALS)
    3. A 56-year-old patient with Guillain-Barré syndrome (GBS) in respiratory distress
    4. A 25-year-old patient admitted with a C4-level spinal cord injury (SCI)

19. The critical care nurse is assessing a patient whose baseline Glasgow Coma Scale (GCS) score in the emergency department was 5. The current GCS score is 3. What is the nurse's **best** interpretation of this finding?
    1. The patient's condition is improving.
    2. The patient's condition is deteriorating.
    3. The patient will need intubation and mechanical ventilation.
    4. The patient's medication regime will need adjustments.

20. A patient with multiple sclerosis tells the assistive personnel after physical therapy that she is too tired to take a bath. What is the **priority** nursing concern at this time?
    1. Fatigue
    2. Impaired safety
    3. Decreased mobility
    4. Muscular weakness

21. An LPN/LVN, under the RN's supervision, is assigned to provide nursing care for a patient with Guillain-Barré syndrome (GBS). What observation should the LPN/LVN be instructed to report **immediately**?
    1. Reports of numbness and tingling
    2. Facial weakness and difficulty speaking
    3. Rapid heart rate of 102 beats/min
    4. Shallow respirations and decreased breath sounds

22. The RN notes that a patient with myasthenia gravis has an elevated temperature (102.2°F [39°C]), an increased heart rate (120 beats/min), and a rise in blood pressure (158/94 mm Hg) and is incontinent of urine and stool. What is the nurse's **best** action at this time?
    1. Administer an acetaminophen suppository.
    2. Notify the health care provider (HCP) immediately.
    3. Recheck vital signs in 1 hour.
    4. Reschedule the patient's physical therapy.

23. The nurse is providing care for a patient with an acute hemorrhagic stroke. The patient's spouse tells the nurse that he has been reading a lot about strokes and asks why his wife has not received alteplase. What is the nurse's **best** response?
    1. "Your wife was not admitted within the time frame that alteplase is usually given."
    2. "This drug is used primarily for patients who experience an acute heart attack."
    3. "Alteplase dissolves clots and may cause more bleeding into your wife's brain."
    4. "Your wife just had gallbladder surgery 6 months ago, so we can't use alteplase."

24. The RN is supervising a senior nursing student who is caring for a patient with a right hemisphere stroke. Which action by the student nurse requires that the RN intervene?
    1. Instructing the patient to sit up straight and the patient responds with a puzzled expression
    2. Moving the patient's food tray to the right side of his over-bed table
    3. Assisting the patient with passive range-of-motion exercises
    4. Combing the hair on the left side of the patient's head when the patient always combs his hair on the right side

25. Which actions should the nurse delegate to an experienced assistive personnel (AP) when caring for a patient with a thrombotic stroke who has residual left-sided weakness? **Select all that apply.**
    1. Assisting the patient to reposition every 2 hours
    2. Reapplying pneumatic compression boots
    3. Reminding the patient to perform active range-of-motion exercises
    4. Assessing the extremities for redness and edema
    5. Setting up meal trays and assisting with feeding
    6. Using a lift to assist the patient up to a bedside chair

Answer Key for this chapter begins on p. 98

26. A patient who had a stroke needs to be fed. What instruction should the nurse give to the assistive personnel (AP) who will feed the patient?
    1. Position the patient sitting up in bed before he or she is fed.
    2. Check the patient's gag and swallowing reflexes.
    3. Feed the patient quickly because there are three more patients to feed.
    4. Suction the patient's secretions between bites of food.

27. The nurse has just admitted a patient with bacterial meningitis who reports a severe headache with photophobia (sensitivity to light) and has a temperature of 102.6°F (39.2°C) orally. Which prescribed intervention should be implemented **first**?
    1. Administer codeine 15 mg orally for the patient's headache.
    2. Infuse ceftriaxone 2000 mg IV to treat the infection.
    3. Give acetaminophen 650 mg orally to reduce the fever.
    4. Give furosemide 40 mg IV to decrease intracranial pressure.

28. The nurse is mentoring a student nurse in the intensive care unit while caring for a patient with meningococcal meningitis. Which action by the student requires that the nurse intervene **most** rapidly?
    1. Entering the room without putting on a protective mask and gown
    2. Instructing the family that visits are restricted to 10 minutes
    3. Giving the patient a warm blanket when he says he feels cold
    4. Checking the patient's pupil response to light every 30 minutes

29. A 23-year-old patient with a recent history of encephalitis is admitted to the medical unit with new-onset generalized tonic-clonic seizures. Which nursing activities included in the patient's care would be **best** to assign to an LPN/LVN under the nurse's supervision? **Select all that apply.**
    1. Observing and documenting the onset and duration of any seizure activity
    2. Administering phenytoin 200 mg PO three times a day
    3. Teaching the patient about the need for frequent tooth brushing and flossing
    4. Developing a discharge plan that includes referral to the Epilepsy Foundation
    5. Assessing for adverse effects caused by new antiseizure medications
    6. Turning the patient to his or her side to avoid aspiration

30. Which nursing action will be implemented **first** if a patient has a generalized tonic-clonic seizure?
    1. Turn the patient to one side.
    2. Give lorazepam 2 mg IV.
    3. Administer oxygen via a nonrebreather mask.
    4. Assess the patient's level of consciousness.

31. A patient who recently started taking phenytoin to control simple partial seizures is seen in the outpatient clinic. Which information obtained during the nurse's chart review and assessment will be of **greatest** concern?
    1. The gums appear enlarged and inflamed.
    2. The white blood cell count is 2300/mm^3 (2.3 x 10^9/L).
    3. The patient sometimes forgets to take the phenytoin until the afternoon.
    4. The patient wants to renew her driver's license in the next month.

32. After the nurse receives the change-of-shift report at 7:00 AM, which patient must the nurse assess **first**?
    1. A 23-year-old patient with a migraine headache who reports severe nausea associated with retching
    2. A 45-year-old patient who is scheduled for a craniotomy in 30 minutes and needs preoperative teaching
    3. A 59-year-old patient with Parkinson disease who will need a swallowing assessment before breakfast
    4. A 63-year-old patient with multiple sclerosis (MS) who has an oral temperature of 101.8°F (38.8°C) and flank pain

33. All of the following nursing care activities are included in the care plan for a 78-year-old man with Parkinson disease who has been referred to the home health agency. Which activities will the nurse delegate to the assistive personnel (AP)? **Select all that apply.**
    1. Checking for orthostatic changes in pulse and blood pressure
    2. Assessing for improvement in tremor after levodopa is given
    3. Reminding the patient to allow adequate time for meals
    4. Monitoring for signs of toxic reactions to anti-Parkinson medications
    5. Assisting the patient with prescribed strengthening exercises
    6. Adapting the patient's preferred activities to his level of function

     Answer Key for this chapter begins on p. 98

34. The nurse is in charge of developing a standard plan of care for an Alzheimer disease care facility and is responsible for assigning and supervising resident care given by LPNs/LVNs and delegating and supervising care given by assistive personnel (AP). Which activity is **best** to assign to the LPN/LVN team leaders?
    1. Checking for improvement in resident memory after medication therapy is initiated
    2. Using the Mini-Mental State Examination to assess residents every 6 months
    3. Assisting residents in using the toilet every 2 hours to decrease risk for urinary incontinence
    4. Developing individualized activity plans after consulting with residents and family

35. A patient who has Alzheimer disease is hospitalized with new-onset angina. Her spouse tells the nurse that he does not sleep well because he needs to be sure the patient does not wander during the night. He insists on checking each of the medications the nurse gives the patient to be sure they are "the same pills she takes at home." Based on this information, which nursing problem is **most** appropriate for this patient?
    1. Acute patient confusion
    2. Care provider role stress
    3. Increased risk for falls
    4. Noncompliance with therapeutic plan

36. The nurse is caring for a patient with a glioblastoma who is receiving dexamethasone 4 mg IV push every 6 hours to relieve symptoms of right arm weakness and headache. Which assessment information concerns the nurse the **most**?
    1. The patient no longer recognizes family members.
    2. The blood glucose level is 234 mg/dL (13 mmol/L).
    3. The patient reports a continuing headache.
    4. The daily weight has increased 2.2 lb (1 kg).

37. A 70-year-old patient with alcoholism who has become lethargic, confused, and incontinent during the last week is admitted to the emergency department. His wife tells the nurse that he fell down the stairs about a month ago but that "he didn't have a scratch afterward." Which collaborative interventions will the nurse implement **first**?
    1. Place the patient on the hospital alcohol withdrawal protocol.
    2. Transport the patient to the radiology department for a computed tomography scan.
    3. Make a referral to the social services department.
    4. Give the patient phenytoin 100 mg PO.

38. Which patient in the neurologic intensive care unit should the charge nurse assign to an RN who has been floated from the medical unit?
    1. A 26-year-old patient with a basilar skull fracture who has clear drainage coming out of the nose
    2. A 42-year-old patient admitted several hours ago with a headache and a diagnosis of a ruptured berry aneurysm
    3. A 46-year-old patient who was admitted 48 hours ago with bacterial meningitis and has an intravenous antibiotic dose due
    4. A 65-year-old patient with an astrocytoma who has just returned to the unit after undergoing a craniotomy

39. The nurse is providing care for a patient newly diagnosed with early Alzheimer disease (AD). On assessment, which finding would the nurse expect to discover?
    1. Short-term memory impairment
    2. Rapid mood swings
    3. Physical aggressiveness
    4. Increased confusion at night

40. For which patient with severe migraine headaches would the nurse question a prescription for sumatriptan?
    1. A 58-year-old patient with gastroesophageal reflux disease
    2. A 48-year-old patient with hypertension
    3. A 65-year-old patient with mild emphysema
    4. A 72-year-old patient with hyperthyroidism

41. A patient with Guillain-Barré syndrome is to undergo plasmapheresis to remove circulating antibodies thought to be responsible for the disease. Which patient care action should the nurse delegate to the experienced assistive personnel (AP)?
    1. Observe the access site for ecchymosis or bleeding.
    2. Instruct the patient that there will be three or four treatments.
    3. Weigh the patient before and after the procedure.
    4. Assess the access site for bruit and thrill every 2 to 4 hours.

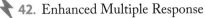

42. Enhanced Multiple Response

Case Study and Question

The nurse is supervising a senior nursing student who will provide nursing care for a 63-year-old man diagnosed with amyotrophic lateral sclerosis (ALS).

Which statements by the student indicate accurate understanding of the disease process, assessment findings, and nursing care needed for this patient?

Instructions: Read the case study on the left and circle the numbers that best answer the question. **Select all that apply.**

1. Patients usually die within 10 to 15 years of diagnosis.
2. Early symptoms include tripping, dropping things, and fatigue of extremities
3. ALS always leads to changes in consciousness and confusion.
4. Nursing care for a patient with ALS includes decreasing risk for aspiration and falls
5. There are no drugs and there is no cure for ALS.
6. The patient is likely to exhibit signs of depression.
7. The most common cause of death is respiratory tract infection.
8. Riluzole is a drug that can slow the progression of ALS.

Answer Key for this chapter begins on p. 98

PART 2 Common Health Scenarios

Answers

Common Health Scenarios

PART 2

1. **Ans: 2**   The location of a fracture determines the signs and symptoms that develop over several hours. This figure shows Battle sign (postauricular ecchymosis), which is a common clinical sign for a basilar skull fracture (a type of linear fracture involving the base of the skull). Another sign of this type of fracture is raccoon eyes (periorbital ecchymosis). It is usually accompanied by a tear in the dura with leaking of cerebrospinal fluid so rhinorrhea (nose) or otorrhea (ears) are also present. The other three types of fracture have different signs depending on the location. **Focus:** Prioritization.

2. **Ans: 3**   A change in level of consciousness and orientation is the earliest and most reliable indication that central neurologic function has declined. If a decline occurs, the nurse should contact the rapid response team or health care provider immediately. The nurse should also perform a focused assessment to determine if there are any other changes. **Focus:** Prioritization.

3. **Ans: 1, 3, 4, 6**   After determining alertness in a patient, the next step is to evaluate orientation. When the patient's attention is engaged, ask him or her questions to determine orientation. Varying the sequence of questioning on repeated assessments prevents the patient from memorizing the answers. Responses that indicate orientation include the ability to answer questions about person, place, and time, so the nurse should ask for information relating to the onset of the patient's symptoms, the name of his or her health care provider or nurse, the year and month, his or her address, and the name of the referring physician or health care agency. Asking about the mayor's affiliation or for his or her parents' address may be inappropriate to assess orientation. **Focus:** Prioritization. **Test-Taking Tip:** Remember that the type of questions the nurse would ask a patient with acute onset of headache are different than would be appropriate for a patient with brain injury or delirium.

4. **Ans: 1**   The priority for interdisciplinary care for the patient experiencing a migraine headache is pain management. All of the other problems are accurate, but none of them is as urgent as the issue of pain, which is often incapacitating. **Focus:** Prioritization.

5. **Ans: 1, 2, 3, 4, 5**   Medications such as estrogen supplements may actually trigger a migraine headache attack and should be avoided. All of the other statements are accurate and should be included in the teaching plan. **Focus:** Prioritization.

6. **Ans: 3**   Measurement of vital signs is within the education and scope of practice of APs. The nurse should perform neurologic checks and document the seizure.

Patients with seizures should not be restrained; however, the nurse may guide the patient's movements if necessary to prevent injury. **Focus:** Delegation, Supervision.

7. **Ans: 2**   The LPN/LVN scope of practice includes setting up the equipment for oxygen and suctioning. The RN should perform the complete initial assessment. Controversy exists as to whether padded side rails actually provide safety, and their use may embarrass the patient and family. Tongue blades should never be at the bedside and should never be inserted into the patient's mouth after a seizure begins. **Focus:** Assignment, Supervision.

8. **Ans: 4**   A patient with a seizure disorder should not take over-the-counter medications without consulting with the health care provider first. The other three statements are appropriate teaching points for patients with seizure disorders and their families. **Focus:** Delegation, Supervision. **Test-Taking Tip:** Remember that there are many drug interactions. For this reason, patients should consult with their health care provider before taking over-the-counter drugs.

9. **Ans: 3**   Although all of these actions fall within the scope of practice for an AP, the AP should help the patient with morning care as needed, but the goal is to keep the patient as independent and mobile as possible. The patient should be encouraged to perform as much morning care as possible. Assisting the patient in ambulating, reminding the patient not to look at his feet (to prevent falls), and encouraging the patient to feed himself are all appropriate to the goal of maintaining independence. **Focus:** Delegation, Supervision.

10. **Ans: 1**   Exercises are used to strengthen the back, relieve pressure on compressed nerves, and protect the back from reinjury. Ice, heat, and firm mattresses are appropriate interventions for back pain. People with chronic back pain should avoid wearing high-heeled shoes at all times. **Focus:** Prioritization.

11. **Ans: 2**   The patient's signs and symptoms are characteristic of autonomic dysreflexia, a neurologic emergency that must be promptly treated to prevent a hypertensive stroke. The cause of this syndrome is noxious stimuli, most often a distended bladder or constipation, so checking for poor catheter drainage, bladder distention, and fecal impaction is the first action that should be taken. Adjusting the room temperature may be helpful because too cool a temperature in the room may contribute to the problem. Acetaminophen will not decrease the autonomic dysreflexia that is causing the patient's headache. Notifying the HCP may be

necessary if nursing actions do not resolve symptoms. **Focus:** Prioritization.

12. **Ans: 2** The newly graduated RN who is on orientation to the unit should be assigned to care for patients with stable, noncomplex conditions, such as the patient with stroke. The task of helping the patient with Parkinson disease to bathe is best delegated to the assistive personnel. The patient being transferred to the nursing home and the newly admitted patient with a spinal cord injury should be assigned to nurses with experience in neurological nursing care. **Focus:** Assignment.

13. **Ans: 4** The first priority for the patient with a spinal cord injury is assessing respiratory patterns and ensuring an adequate airway. A patient with a high cervical injury is at risk for respiratory compromise because spinal nerves C3 through C5 innervate the phrenic nerve, which controls the diaphragm. The other assessments are also necessary but are not as high a priority. **Focus:** Prioritization.

14. **Ans: 2** The AP's training and education covers measuring and recording vital signs. The AP may help with turning and repositioning the patient and may remind the patient to cough and deep breathe, but he or she does not teach the patient how to perform these actions. Assessing and monitoring patients require additional education and are appropriate to the scope of practice of professional nurses. **Focus:** Delegation, Supervision.

15. **Ans: 1, 2, 4, 5** All of the strategies except straight catheterization may stimulate voiding in patients with an SCI. Intermittent bladder catheterization can be used to empty the patient's bladder, but it will not stimulate voiding. To use a urinal, the patient must have bladder control, which is often absent after an SCI. In addition, every hour while awake would be too often and would ignore the bladder filling at night. **Focus:** Prioritization.

16. **Ans: 1, 3, 4, 6** Checking and observing for signs of pressure or infection is within the scope of practice of the LPN/LVN. The LPN/LVN also has the appropriate skills for cleaning the halo insertion sites with hydrogen peroxide. Administering oral drugs is within the scope of practice for an LPN/LVN. Neurologic examination and care plan development require additional education and skill appropriate to the professional RN. **Focus:** Assignment, Supervision. **Test-Taking Tip:** The RN must be aware of the scope of practice for an LPN/LVN. This may vary from state to state and may depend on whether the LPN/LVN has additional education. Generally, in-depth assessment, care plan development, and in-depth patient education remain within the scope of practice of the professional RN.

17. **Ans: 3** The patient's statement indicates difficulty with coping in adjusting to the limitations of the injury and the need for additional counseling, teaching,

and support. The other three nursing problems may be appropriate for a patient with an SCI but are not related to the patient's statement. **Focus:** Prioritization.

18. **Ans: 2** The traveling nurse is relatively new to neurologic nursing and should be assigned patients whose condition is stable and not complex, such as the patient with chronic ALS. The newly diagnosed patient with MS will need a lot of teaching and support. The patient with GBS in respiratory distress will need frequent assessments and may need to be transferred to the intensive care unit. The patient with a C4-level SCI is at risk for respiratory arrest. All three of these patients should be assigned to nurses experienced in neurologic nursing care. **Focus:** Assignment.

19. **Ans: 2** The GCS is used in many acute care settings to establish baseline data in these areas: eye opening, motor response, and verbal response. The patient is assigned a numeric score for each of these areas. The lower the score, the lower the patient's neurologic function. A decrease of two or more points in the Glasgow Coma Scale score total is clinically significant and should be communicated to the health care provider immediately. **Focus:** Prioritization.

20. **Ans: 1** At this time, based on the patient's statement, the priority is inability to perform ADLs most likely related to being tired (fatigue) after physical therapy. The other three nursing concerns are appropriate to a patient with MS but are not related to the patient's statement. **Focus:** Prioritization.

21. **Ans: 4** The priority intervention for a patient with GBS is maintaining adequate respiratory function. Patients with GBS are at risk for respiratory failure, which requires urgent intervention. The other findings are important and should be reported to the nurse, but they are not life threatening. **Focus:** Prioritization.

22. **Ans: 2** The changes that the RN notes are characteristic of myasthenic crisis, which often follows some type of infection. The patient is at risk for inadequate respiratory function. In addition to notifying the HCP or rapid response team, the nurse should carefully monitor the patient's respiratory status. The patient may need intubation and mechanical ventilation. **Focus:** Prioritization.

23. **Ans: 3** Alteplase is a clot buster. In a patient who has experienced hemorrhagic stroke, there is already bleeding into the brain. A drug, such as alteplase, dissolves the clot and can cause more bleeding in the brain. The other statements about the use of alteplase are accurate but are not pertinent to this patient's diagnosis and do not answer the spouse's question. **Focus:** Prioritization.

24. **Ans: 1** Patients with right cerebral hemisphere stroke often manifest neglect syndrome. They lean to the left and, when asked, respond that they believe they are sitting up straight. They often neglect the left side of their bodies and ignore food on the left side of their food trays. The nurse needs to remind the

student of this phenomenon and discuss the appropriate interventions. **Focus:** Delegation, Supervision.

25. **Ans: 1, 2, 3, 5, 6**   An experienced AP would know how to reposition the patient, reapply compression boots, and feed a patient and would remind the patient to perform activities the patient has been taught to perform. APs are also trained to use a patient lift to get patients into or out of bed. Assessing for redness and swelling (signs of deep vein thrombosis) requires additional education and skill, appropriate to the professional nurse. **Focus:** Delegation, Supervision.

26. **Ans: 1**   Positioning the patient in a sitting position decreases the risk of aspiration. The AP is not trained to assess gag or swallowing reflexes. The patient should not be rushed during feeding. A patient who needs suctioning performed between bites of food is not handling secretions and is at risk for aspiration. Such a patient should be assessed further before feeding. **Focus:** Delegation, Supervision.

27. **Ans: 2**   Bacterial meningitis is a medical emergency, and antibiotics are administered even before the diagnosis is confirmed (after specimens have been collected for culture). The other interventions will also help to reduce central nervous system stimulation and irritation and should be implemented as soon as possible but are not as important as starting antibiotic therapy. **Focus:** Prioritization.

28. **Ans: 1**   Meningococcal meningitis is spread through contact with respiratory secretions, so use of a mask and gown is required to prevent transmission of the infection to staff members or other patients. The other actions may or may not be appropriate. The presence of a family member at the bedside may decrease patient confusion and agitation. Patients with hyperthermia frequently report feeling chilled, but warming the patient is not an appropriate intervention. Checking the pupils' response to light is appropriate but is not needed every 30 minutes and is uncomfortable for a patient with photophobia. **Focus:** Prioritization.

29. **Ans: 1, 2, 6**   Any nursing staff member who is involved in caring for the patient should observe for the onset and duration of seizures (although a more detailed assessment of seizure activity should be done by the RN). Administration of oral medications is included in LPN/LVN education and scope of practice. Turning the patient on his or her side to avoid aspiration is certainly within the scope of practice for an LPN/LVN. Teaching, discharge planning, and assessment for adverse effects of new medications are complex activities that require RN-level education and scope of practice. **Focus:** Assignment.

30. **Ans: 1**   The priority action during a generalized tonic-clonic seizure is to protect the airway by turning the patient to one side to prevent aspiration. Administering lorazepam should be the next action because it will act rapidly to control the seizure. Although oxygen may be useful during the postictal phase, the hypoxemia during tonic-clonic seizures is caused by apnea, which cannot be corrected by oxygen administration. Checking the level of consciousness is not appropriate during the seizure because generalized tonic-clonic seizures are associated with a loss of consciousness. **Focus:** Prioritization.

31. **Ans: 2**   Leukopenia is a serious adverse effect of phenytoin therapy and would require discontinuation of the medication. The other data indicate a need for further assessment or patient teaching but will not require a change in medical treatment for the seizures. **Focus:** Prioritization.

32. **Ans: 4**   Urinary tract infections (UTIs) are a frequent complication in patients with MS because of the effect of the disease on bladder function, and UTIs may lead to sepsis in these patients. The elevated temperature and flank pain suggest that this patient may have pyelonephritis. The health care provider should be notified immediately so that IV antibiotic therapy can be started quickly. The other patients should be assessed as soon as possible, but their needs are not as urgent as those of this patient. **Focus:** Prioritization.

33. **Ans: 1, 3, 5**   AP education and scope of practice include checking pulse and blood pressure measurements. The nurse would be sure to instruct the AP to report heart rate and blood pressure findings. In addition, APs can reinforce previous teaching or skills taught by the RN or personnel in other disciplines, such as speech or physical therapists. Evaluating patient response to medications and developing and individualizing the plan of care require RN-level education and scope of practice. **Focus:** Delegation.

34. **Ans: 1**   LPN/LVN education and team leader responsibilities include checking for the therapeutic and adverse effects of medications. Changes in the residents' memory would be communicated to the RN supervisor, who is responsible for overseeing the plan of care for each resident. Assessing for changes in score on the Mini-Mental State Examination and developing the plan of care are RN responsibilities. Assisting residents with personal care and hygiene would be delegated to APs working at the long-term care facility. **Focus:** Assignment.

35. **Ans: 2**   The husband's statement about lack of sleep and concern about whether his wife is receiving the correct medications are behaviors that support the problem of care provider role stress. The husband's statements about how he monitors the patient and his concern with medication administration do not indicate difficulty complying with the therapeutic plan. The patient may be confused, but the nurse would need to gather more data, and this is not the main focus of the husband's concerns. Falls are not an immediate concern at this time. **Focus:** Prioritization.

36. **Ans: 1**   The inability to recognize family members is a new neurologic deficit for this patient and indicates a possible increase in intracranial pressure (ICP). This

change should be communicated to the health care provider immediately so that treatment can be initiated. The continuing headache also indicates that the ICP may be elevated but is not a new problem. The glucose elevation and weight gain are common adverse effects of dexamethasone that may require treatment but are not emergencies. **Focus:** Prioritization.

37. **Ans: 2** The patient's history and assessment data indicate that he may have a chronic subdural hematoma. The priority goal is to obtain a rapid diagnosis and send the patient to surgery to have the hematoma evacuated. The other interventions also should be implemented as soon as possible, but the initial nursing activities should be directed toward diagnosis and treatment of any intracranial lesion. **Focus:** Prioritization.

38. **Ans: 3** Of the patients listed, the patient with bacterial meningitis is in the most stable condition and likely the least complex. An RN from the medical unit would be familiar with administering IV antibiotics. The other patients require assessments and care from RNs more experienced in caring for patients with neurologic diagnoses. **Focus:** Assignment.

39. **Ans: 1** One of the first symptoms of AD is short-term memory impairment. Behavioral changes that occur late in the disease progression include rapid mood swings, tendency toward physical and verbal aggressiveness, and increased confusion at night (when light is inadequate) or when the patient is excessively fatigued. **Focus:** Prioritization.

40. **Ans: 2** Sumatriptan is a triptan preparation developed to treat migraine headaches. Most are contraindicated in patients with actual or suspected ischemic heart disease, cerebrovascular ischemia, hypertension, and peripheral vascular disease and in those with Prinzmetal angina because of the potential for coronary vasospasm. **Focus:** Prioritization.

41. **Ans: 3** The scope of practice for an experienced AP would include weighing patients. Observing, assessing, and providing instructions all require additional educational preparation and are appropriate to the scope of practice for a professional nurse. **Focus:** Delegation.

42. **Ans: 2, 4, 6, 7** Early symptoms include tripping, dropping things, extremity fatigue, slurred speech, and muscle cramps or twitching. Nursing care focuses on facilitating communication, decreasing risk for aspiration and falls, early identification of respiratory problems, decreasing pain related to muscle weakness, and providing diversion activities. With ALS, patients are usually cognitively intact while their bodies waste away. This can lead to depression. Death most commonly occurs 2 to 5 years after diagnosis. Riluzole (Rilutek) is a drug that can be used to slow the progression of ALS; however, there is no cure. **Focus:** Supervision.

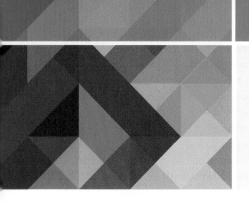

CHAPTER 10

Visual and Auditory Problems

Questions

1. According to evidence-based guidelines from the American Optometric Association, which modifiable risk factor is the **most** important to emphasize during patient teaching to reduce the risk for age-related macular degeneration?
   1. Initiate smoking cessation.
   2. Take vitamin D and E supplements.
   3. Eat dark green, leafy vegetables.
   4. Wear protective eyewear as needed.

2. The nurse is reviewing prescriptions for several patients who have disorders of the eye. Which medication prescription is the **most** important to discuss with the health care provider?
   1. Timolol for open-angle glaucoma
   2. Cromolyn sodium for allergic conjunctivitis
   3. Atropine for acute angle-closure glaucoma
   4. Ranibizumab for wet age-related macular degeneration

3. A patient calls the clinic and reports redness of the sclera, itching of the eyes, and increased lacrimation for several hours. What should the nurse direct the caller to do **first**?
   1. "Please call your health care provider" (i.e., decline to advise).
   2. "Apply a cool compress to your eyes."
   3. "If you are wearing contact lenses, remove them."
   4. "Take an over-the-counter antihistamine."

4. The nurse is teaching a community group about the prevention of accidental eye injuries. Which advice is the **most** important to stress?
   1. Workplace policies for handling chemicals should be followed.
   2. Children and parents should be cautious about aggressive play.
   3. Protective eyewear should be worn during sports or hazardous work.
   4. Emergency eyewash stations should be established in the workplace.

5. Which finding should be **immediately** reported to the health care provider?
   1. A change in color vision
   2. Crusty yellow drainage on the eyelashes
   3. Increased lacrimation
   4. A curtainlike shadow across the visual field

6. A patient has a hordeolum (sty) on the right upper eyelid. Which intervention would the nurse recommend **first**?
   1. Apply warm compresses four times per day.
   2. Gently perform hygienic eyelid scrubs.
   3. Obtain a prescription for antibiotic drops.
   4. Contact the ophthalmologist.

7. After cataract surgery, which symptom needs to be **immediately** reported to the health care provider?
   1. A scratchy sensation in the operative eye
   2. Loss of depth perception with the patch in place
   3. Poor vision 6 to 8 hours after patch removal
   4. Pain not relieved by prescribed medication

8. For a patient who has multiple risk factors for primary open-angle glaucoma (POAG), which sign or symptom should be investigated as an **early** sign of POAG?
   1. Loss of central visual field
   2. Seeing halos around lights
   3. Mild eye aching
   4. Loss of peripheral vision

9. According to evidence-based guidelines from the American Optometric Association, which patient needs to have an annual (or sooner, as recommended) eye examination?
   1. 18-year-old who is asymptomatic and has low risk
   2. 40-year-old who is asymptomatic and has low risk
   3. 55-year-old who is asymptomatic and has low risk
   4. 67-year-old who is asymptomatic and has low risk

10. Which tasks are appropriate to assign to an LPN/LVN who is functioning under the supervision of an RN? **Select all that apply.**

1. Administering sulfacetamide sodium 10% to a child with conjunctivitis
2. Reviewing hand-washing and hygiene practices with patients who have eye infections
3. Showing patients how to gently cleanse the eyelid margins to remove crusting
4. Assessing nutritional factors for a patient with age-related macular degeneration
5. Reviewing the health history of a patient to identify risk for ocular manifestations
6. Performing a routine check of a patient's visual acuity using the Snellen eye chart

11. The nurse is on a camping trip. A man who is chopping wood gets struck in the eye with a piece of debris. On examination, a wood splinter is protruding from his eyeball. What should the nurse do **first**?
    1. Have the man lie in the back seat of the car and drive him to the emergency department.
    2. Gently remove the piece of wood and place a sterile dressing over the eye.
    3. Carefully rest a plastic cup on the orbital rim and tape it in place.
    4. Flush the eye with copious amounts of clean tepid water; then check visual acuity.

12. The home health nurse discovers that an older patient has been taking her glaucoma eyedrops by mouth for the past week. What should the nurse do **first**?
    1. Obtain a prescription for tonometry so that her intraocular pressure can be checked.
    2. Try to determine the frequency and the amount that she has been ingesting.
    3. Ask her how she decided to take the drops orally instead of instilling them as eyedrops.
    4. Call the Poison Control Center and be prepared to describe untoward side effects.

13. A nursing student is assisting an older patient who has decreased vision related to macular degeneration. The patient is alert, conversant, and cognitively intact. When would the supervising nurse intervene?
    1. Student puts the call bell and personal items within reach and locates each item by guiding the patient's hand.
    2. Student closes the curtains and turns off all of the lights at the end of the shift to encourage rest and sleep.
    3. Student talks to the patient about family and asks, "So, when was the last time that you saw your uncle?"
    4. Student assists during mealtime by opening packages and describing location of foods by using clock coordinates.

14. In the care of a patient who recently sustained blindness, which tasks would be delegated to assistive personnel (AP)? **Select all that apply.**
    1. Counseling the patient to express grief or loss
    2. Assisting the patient with ambulating in the hall
    3. Orienting the patient to the surroundings
    4. Encouraging independence
    5. Obtaining supplies for hygienic care
    6. Storing personal items to reduce clutter

15. Which patients would be **best** to assign to the most experienced nurse in an ambulatory care center that specializes in vision problems and eye surgery? **Select all that apply.**
    1. Patient who requires postoperative instructions after cataract surgery
    2. Patient who needs an eye pad and a metal shield applied
    3. Patient who requests a home health referral for dressing changes and eyedrop instillation
    4. Patient who needs teaching about self-administration of eyedrops
    5. Patient who requires an assessment for recent and sudden loss of sight
    6. Patient who requires preoperative teaching for laser trabeculoplasty

16. The nurse is preparing to administer a beta-adrenergic blocking glaucoma agent. Which statement made by the patient warrants additional assessment and a notification to the health care provider?
    1. "My blood pressure runs a little high if I gain too much weight."
    2. "Occasionally, I have palpitations, but they pass very quickly."
    3. "My joints feel stiff today, but that's just my arthritis."
    4. "My pulse rate is a little low today because I take digoxin."

17. The nurse is supervising a new nurse who has just finished assessing a patient for redness and discomfort to the right eye. The new nurse documents "visual acuity N/A." Which action would the supervising nurse take?
    1. Do nothing; the documentation is minimal but acceptable.
    2. Ask her to explain the rationale for the documentation.
    3. Reassess the patient's eye and vision to validate findings.
    4. Suggest contacting the clinical educator for documentation tips.

Answer Key for this chapter begins on p. 108

PART 2 Common Health Scenarios

18. Phenylephrine, an adrenergic agonist, has been prescribed as a topical application for a patient who had intraocular surgery. Although systemic toxicity is unlikely, which adverse physiologic response is the concern?
    1. Cardiovascular response, such as hypertension or ventricular dysrhythmias
    2. Renal response, such as urinary retention or urinary incontinence
    3. Respiratory response, such as bronchospasm or mucus plugs
    4. Musculoskeletal response, such as bone pain or joint stiffness

19. An older patient had ranibizumab injected into his eye for treatment of wet age-related macular degeneration several days ago. He is now experiencing redness, light sensitivity, and pain. Which advice would the nurse give to the patient?
    1. These are common side effects that should pass after a few more days.
    2. Contact the health care provider (HCP) immediately for possible eye infection.
    3. Rest eyes as much as possible and wear sunglasses if lights are too bright.
    4. Inform the HCP before the next treatment so that the dosage can be adjusted.

20. The nurse is aware that many eyedrops that are prescribed for glaucoma could cause potentially serious systemic effects. On the figure below identify the area where the nurse will teach the patient to apply punctal occlusion to prevent systemic absorption.

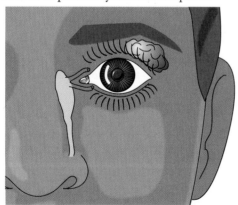

21. Which tasks are appropriate to assign to an LPN/LVN who is functioning under the supervision of a team leader or RN? **Select all that apply.**
    1. Irrigating the ear canal to loosen impacted cerumen
    2. Administering amoxicillin to a child with otitis media
    3. Reminding the patient not to blow the nose after tympanoplasty

    4. Counseling a patient with Ménière disease
    5. Developing communication techniques for the family of a hearing-impaired older adult
    6. Assessing a patient with labyrinthitis for headache and level of consciousness

22. The nurse is interviewing an older adult patient who reports that "lately there has been a roaring sound in my ears." What additional assessments should the nurse include? **Select all that apply.**
    1. Obtain a medication history.
    2. Ask about exposure to loud noises.
    3. Observe the canal for earwax or foreign body.
    4. Assess for signs and symptoms of ear infection.
    5. Ask about method of ear hygiene.
    6. Ask about diet and nutrition.

23. A cheerful older widow comes to the community clinic for her annual checkup. She is in reasonably good health, but she has a hearing loss of 40 dB. She confides, "I don't get out much. I used to be really active, but the older I get, the more trouble I have hearing. It can be really embarrassing." What is the **priority** nursing concept to consider in planning care for this patient?
    1. Safety
    2. Sensory perception
    3. Mood and affect
    4. Functional ability

24. Which combination of drugs is cause for **greatest** concern if the patient reports tinnitus or other problems with hearing?
    1. Gentamycin and ethacrynic acid
    2. Furosemide and metoprolol
    3. Vancomycin and nitroglycerin patch
    4. Aspirin and calcium supplement

25. Which physical assessment findings should be reported to the health care provider?
    1. Pearly gray or pink tympanic membrane
    2. Dense whitish ring at the circumference of the tympanum
    3. Bulging red or blue tympanic membrane
    4. Cone of light at the innermost part of the tympanum

26. Which description by a patient reporting vertigo is cause for **greatest** concern?
    1. Dizziness with hearing loss
    2. Episodic vertigo
    3. Vertigo without hearing loss
    4. "Merry-go-round" vertigo

Answer Key for this chapter begins on p. 108

27. The nurse is caring for several patients who are having problems with their ears. Which patient condition is cause for **greatest** concern?
    1. Has discomfort of the ear preceded by a viral infection; the tympanic membrane is erythematous
    2. Has been treated with antibiotics for recurrent acute otitis media four times within the past 6 months
    3. Reports rapid onset ear pain with pruritus and a sensation of fullness that started after cleaning the ear canal with a finger
    4. Reports progressive severe otic pain with purulent discharge and is positive for human immunodeficiency virus

28. The nurse performed postoperative stapedectomy teaching several days ago for a patient. Which comment by the patient is cause for **greatest** concern?
    1. "I'm going to take swimming lessons in a couple of months."
    2. "I have to take a long overseas flight in several weeks."
    3. "I can't wait to get back to my regular weightlifting class."
    4. "I have been coughing a lot with my mouth open."

29. The nurse is working in a clinic that specializes in the care of patients with ear disorders. A patient tells the nurse that he has been taking meclizine. Which question is the nurse **most** likely to ask to evaluate the effectiveness of the medication?
    1. Has the medication helped to relieve the pain in the ear canal?
    2. Are you still experiencing the whirling and turning sensations?
    3. Have you been able to hear better since you started the medication?
    4. Are you still having itching and discomfort in the outer ear?

30. Which information is **most** important to convey to the health care provider before he/she prescribes amoxicillin, which is the first-line antibiotic for acute otitis media in children?
    1. Child took amoxicillin several months ago for a similar problem
    2. Child has a personal and family history of penicillin allergies
    3. Child has concurrent allergic rhinitis with sneezing and congestion
    4. Child is 18 months old and goes to day care and his parents smoke

31. Drag and Drop

Scenario: After examining the patient's ear canal with an otoscope, the health care provider (HCP) instructs the nurse to irrigate the ear canal.

Instructions: Steps for ear irrigation are listed in the left-hand column. In the right-hand column, indicate the order in which the nurse will perform each step.

Steps for ear irrigation	Correct order for steps
1. Place the tip of the syringe at an angle in the external canal.	
2. Watch for fluid return and signs of cerumen	
3. If cerumen does not appear, wait 10 minutes and repeat the irrigation.	
4. Fill a syringe with warm irrigating solution.	
5. After completion of the irrigation, have the patient turn the head to the side to facilitate drainage.	
6. Apply gentle but continuous pressure to the syringe plunger.	
7. Document how the patient tolerated procedure and appearance of drainage	
8. Place patient in sitting position; drape the shoulder with a waterproof pad and towel	
9. Instruct the patient to hold the basin against the neck to catch drainage.	
10. Straighten the ear canal by pulling upward and backward	

 Answer Key for this chapter begins on p. 108

32. Extended Multiple Response

Case Study and Question

A first semester nursing student is preparing the equipment to irrigate a patient's ear canal. The student has practiced setting up the equipment in the skills lab, but the nursing instructor recognizes that the student may lack experience regarding the contraindications for this procedure.

In which circumstances would the nursing instructor intervene before the student starts the irrigation?

Instructions: Read the case study on the left and circle or highlight each circumstance where the nursing instructor would intervene before the student starts the procedure. **Select all that apply.**

1. Patient has a probable perforated eardrum.
2. Patient has a foreign body, probably a bean, in the ear canal.
3. Patient has a foreign body, probably an insect, in the ear canal.
4. Patient has hearing loss related to cerumen accumulation.
5. Patient is currently being treated for acute otitis media.
6. Patient has used ear candles in the past to remove ear wax.
7. Patient reports tinnitus and transient vertigo.
8. Patient has an impaction that did not resolve with over-the-counter earwax softeners or irrigation at home with a bulb syringe.

33. Cloze

Scenario: A 73-year-old woman comes to the clinic for an annual wellness visit. The patient is alert, oriented and conversant. She has mild heart failure, rheumatoid arthritis hypercholesterolemia and occasional anxiety. Medications include lisinopril 2.5 mg/day, acetaminophen 500 mg every 12 hours, aspirin 1000 mg every 4 to 6 hours, pravastatin 40 mg/day, and lorazepam 1 mg PRN.

Instructions: Complete the sentences below by choosing the most probable option for the missing information that corresponds with the same numbered list of options provided.

As the nurse is interviewing, assessing, and administering standardized tests, the nurse suspects a hearing problem when the patient ____**1**____. A ____**2**____ supports the nurse's suspicion of hearing loss. The nurse collects further information about ____**3**____ and ____**4**____ because of the potential for ototoxicity, as a medication side effect. To facilitate two-way communication with the patient, the nurse would first try ____**5**____.

Option 1	Option 2	Options 3 and 4	Option 5
tilts her head toward the nurse	Mini-Mental State Exam score of 30	lisinopril 2.5 mg/day	speaking very loudly
watches the nurse's hands	Rinne Test-negative	acetaminophen 500 mg every 12 hours	clearly enunciating unfamiliar terms
appears distracted and disinterested	Get up and Go Test of 30 seconds	aspirin 1000 mg every 4 to 6 hours	writing messages on a white board
tells long rambling stories	Mini-Cog test score of 5	pravastatin 40 mg/day	facing patient with eye contact
asks to go to the bathroom	Snellen score of 20/40	lorazepam 1 mg PRN	using simple, brief commands

Common Health Scenarios

PART 2

34. Extended Multiple Response

Case Study and Question

A 67-year-old African American patient reports a sudden excruciating pain in the left eye with the visual change of colored halos around lights and blurred vision. The health care provider makes the medical diagnosis of angle-closure glaucoma.

Which interventions should the nurse expect and perform for this emergency condition?

Instructions: Read the case study on the left and circle or highlight each intervention that nurse would expect to perform for this patient. **Select all that apply.**

1. Prepare the patient for photodynamic therapy.
2. Instill a mydriatic agent, such as phenylephrine.
3. Instill a miotic agent, such as pilocarpine.
4. Instill a cycloplegic agent, such as tropicamide.
5. Administer an oral hyperosmotic agent, such as isosorbide.
6. Apply a cool compress to the forehead.
7. Provide a darkened, quiet, and private space for the patient.
8. Inform patient that decreased visual acuity in dim light is an expected side effect of the medications.
9. Prepare teaching materials about laser peripheral iridotomy or surgical iridectomy as needed for long-term management.
10. Prepare the patient for cataract extraction.

PART 2 · Common Health Scenarios

Answer Key for this chapter begins on p. 108

Answers

1. **Ans: 1**   According to the American Optometric Association, smoking cessation is the most important modifiable factor for decreasing risk for age-related macular degeneration. Consumption of dark green vegetables and use of vitamin supplements are recommended, but the evidence is less compelling. Use of protective eyewear is recommended to prevent eye injuries during active sports or hazardous occupations, but this preventative measure is not related to age-related macular degeneration. **Focus:** Prioritization.

2. **Ans: 3**   Atropine should not be used for acute angle-closure glaucoma. Atropine causes dilation of the pupil, which impedes outflow of aqueous humor and increases intraocular pressure. This action could precipitate or worsen the condition. **Focus:** Prioritization.

3. **Ans: 3**   If the patient is wearing contact lenses, the lenses may be causing the symptoms, and removing them will prevent further eye irritation or damage. Policies on giving telephone advice vary among institutions, and knowledge of the facility policy is essential. The other options may be appropriate, but additional information is needed before suggesting anything else. **Focus:** Prioritization.

4. **Ans: 3**   Most accidental eye injuries (90%) could be prevented by wearing protective eyewear for sports and hazardous work. The other options should be considered in the overall prevention of injuries. **Focus:** Prioritization.

5. **Ans: 4**   A curtainlike shadow is a symptom of retinal detachment, which is an emergency situation. A change in color vision is a symptom of a cataract. Crusty drainage is associated with conjunctivitis. Increased lacrimation is associated with many eye irritants, such as allergies, contact lenses, or foreign bodies. **Focus:** Prioritization. **Test-Taking Tip:** NCLEX® Examination questions frequently test the ability to identify life-threatening conditions, or in this case, the risk for permanent disability. In preparing to take the NCLEX® Examination, pay attention to signs and symptoms that signal life-threatening conditions and those that could lead to permanent injury.

6. **Ans: 1**   Warm compresses usually provide relief. If the problem persists, eyelid scrubs and antibiotic drops would be appropriate. The ophthalmologist could be consulted, but other providers such as the family physician or the nurse practitioner could give a prescription for antibiotics. **Focus:** Prioritization.

7. **Ans: 4**   Pain may signal hemorrhage, infection, or increased ocular pressure. A scratchy sensation and loss of depth perception with the patch in place are common. Adequate vision may not return for 24 hours. **Focus:** Prioritization.

8. **Ans: 3**   POAG develops slowly, and irreversible damage to the optic nerve can occur before any signs or symptoms are manifested; however, mild eye aching or headaches should be investigated as possible early signs of POAG. Loss of peripheral vision, seeing halos, and loss of central vision are late signs. **Focus:** Prioritization.

9. **Ans: 4**   People 65 years or older are advised to have eye examinations annually or even more frequently, even if they have low risk. People who are 18 to 64 years old with low risk are advised to have eye examinations at least every 2 years. Examples of risk factors include: family history for eye disease; systemic health conditions that affect the eyes, such as diabetes; racial or ethnic backgrounds with increased risk, such as African-Americans; occupations that are eye hazardous; prescription or nonprescription drugs with ocular side effects; contact lenses; previous eye surgery or eye injury; and having functional vision in only one eye. **Focus:** Prioritization.

10. **Ans: 1, 2, 3, 6**   Administering medications, reviewing and demonstrating standard procedures, and performing standardized assessments with predictable outcomes in noncomplex cases are within the scope of practice for the LPN/LVN. Assessing for systemic manifestations and behaviors, risk factors, and nutritional factors is the responsibility of the RN. **Focus:** Assignment.

11. **Ans: 3**   Penetrating objects should not be removed or disturbed by anyone except an eye specialist because the object may be creating a tamponade effect. Removing or disrupting the object could result in additional damage to the eye. The man needs to have emergency care, and 911 should be called, but if there are no emergency services available, the man should sit in the back seat of the car with a seat belt in place for transport to the nearest facility. After a penetrating eye injury has been assessed and treated by an ophthalmologist, there is a possibility that based on the ophthalmologist's recommendations, foreign body removal, flushing, and dressing application could be accomplished in the emergency department; however, penetrating objects frequently require surgical removal. Antibiotics and a tetanus immunization are administered before the patient is transferred to the operating room. **Focus:** Prioritization.

12. **Ans: 2**   Try to find out the amount and frequency that she has been taking the drops by mouth. This information will be needed when calling the ophthalmologist or Poison Control. A good follow-up question is to try to find out why she is taking the drops by mouth. She may be very confused, or there may

have been an error of omission in patient education by all health care team members who were involved in the initial prescription. **Focus:** Prioritization. **Test-Taking Tip:** Remember that the first step of the nursing process is assessment and gathering sufficient data. Always assess first unless taking the time to assess would be life threatening.

13. **Ans: 2** For patients who retain some vision, the room should be well-lit; even at night, there should be a night light. Other options are correct actions. Words such as "see," "look," or "view" are parts of normal speech, and it's acceptable and natural to use these terms (e.g., "Well, it looks like you had a quiet day today"). **Focus:** Supervision.

14. **Ans: 2, 5** Assisting the patient with ambulating in the hall and obtaining supplies are within the scope of practice of the AP. Counseling for emotional problems, orienting the patient to the room, and encouraging independence require formative evaluation to gauge readiness, and these activities should be the responsibility of the RN. Storing items and rearranging furniture are inappropriate actions because the patient needs be able to consistently locate objects in the immediate environment. **Focus:** Delegation. **Test-Taking Tip:** Remember to differentiate whether the question is about an acute or chronic condition. The nurse could delegate more tasks to the AP if the patient's condition is chronic. For example, a patient who has been blind for a long time is less likely to need the nurse to prompt or assess independence. For a patient with a severely depressed respiratory rate, however, the nurse would not delegate the vital signs to the AP.

15. **Ans: 1, 3, 5, 6** Providing postoperative and preoperative instructions, making home health referrals, and assessing for needs related to loss of vision should be done by an experienced nurse who can give specific details and specialized information about follow-up eye care and adjustment to loss. The principles of applying an eye pad and shield and teaching the administration of eyedrops are basic procedures that should be familiar to all nurses. **Focus:** Assignment.

16. **Ans: 4** All beta-adrenergic blockers are contraindicated in bradycardia. Alpha-adrenergic agents can cause tachycardia and hypertension. Carbonic anhydrase inhibitors should not be given to patients with rheumatoid arthritis who are taking high dosages of aspirin. **Focus:** Prioritization. **Test-Taking Tip:** Beta-adrenergic blockers "block" the receptor sites for epinephrine and norepinephrine, which are responsible for the "fight-or-flight" response; thus these medications will slow the pulse rate.

17. **Ans: 2** Asking the nurse to explain the documentation is a way of assessing her knowledge of documentation, her understanding of how the patient's report guides the focused assessment, and her understanding of the use of abbreviations. The nurse may have a good reason for charting "N/A," but a reader could misunderstand. For example, "visual acuity N/A" could be interpreted as the nurse making a clinical judgment that assessing vision was not applicable (important) for this patient. The documentation is not acceptable because the patient's report indicates that vision should be tested if at all possible. Redoing the assessment does not help the nurse to correct mistakes. Contacting the educator for assistance is an option that is based on assessment of her rationale. **Focus:** Supervision, Prioritization.

18. **Ans: 1** Topical phenylephrine usually does not cause systemic reactions because the amount of absorption is very small. Cardiac responses (hypertension, dysrhythmias, or cardiac arrest) are the concern. Other possible reactions may include sweating, tremors, agitation, or confusion. **Focus:** Prioritization.

19. **Ans: 2** Ranibizumab is an angiogenesis inhibitor that is directly injected into the vitreous humor of the eye. The purpose of the medication injection is to inhibit the growth of new blood vessels in patients who have neovascular age-related macular degeneration. The biggest concern about adverse effects of the treatment is endophthalmitis. This can be caused by bacteria, virus, or fungus. Redness, light sensitivity, or pain are signs of possible endophthalmitis that should be immediately reported to the provider. **Focus:** Prioritization.

20. **Ans:**
Punctal occlusion decreases systemic absorption of eyedrops. The nurse teaches the patient to place pressure on the corner of the eye near the nose immediately after eyedrop instillation. **Focus:** Prioritization.

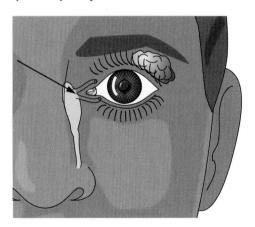

21. **Ans: 1, 2, 3** Irrigating the ear, giving medication, and reminding the patient about postoperative instructions that were given by an RN are within the scope of practice of the LPN/LVN. Counseling patients and families and assessing for meningitis signs in a patient with labyrinthitis are the responsibilities of the RN. **Focus:** Assignment.

22. **Ans: 1, 2, 3, 4, 5**   Medications such as aspirin or diuretics (and many others) can cause tinnitus (ringing in the ears). Loud noises, impacted earwax or foreign bodies in the ear canal, or ear infections can also cause tinnitus. Ask about method of hygiene; insertion of cotton-tipped swabs may be contributing to the impaction of earwax. Diet and nutrition should always be assessed for older adult patients, but in this case, there is no direct relationship to the patient's report of roaring sound. **Focus:** Prioritization.

23. **Ans: 2**   This patient has a hearing loss, and it seems likely that a referral for a hearing aid or rehabilitation program will allow her to participate in her baseline social habits. **Focus:** Prioritization.

24. **Ans: 1**   The combination of gentamycin and ethacrynic acid can have additive effects because both are considered ototoxic. Furosemide, vancomycin, and aspirin are also considered ototoxic drugs. There could be a few patients who report tinnitus with metoprolol, nitroglycerin, and calcium supplements, but these drugs are generally not known to have ototoxic effects. **Focus:** Prioritization.

25. **Ans: 3**   A bulging red or blue tympanic membrane is a possible sign of otitis media or perforation. The other signs are considered normal anatomy. **Focus:** Prioritization.

26. **Ans: 3**   The patient reporting vertigo without hearing loss should be further assessed for nonvestibular causes, such as cardiovascular or metabolic causes. The other descriptions are more commonly associated with inner ear or labyrinthine causes. **Focus:** Prioritization.

27. **Ans: 4**   Progressive severe otic pain with purulent discharge and granulation tissue of the external auditory canal are signs or symptoms of necrotizing otitis externa. This is a rare but potentially fatal condition because bacteria can spread from the ear to the brain and cause meningitis. Immunocompromised patients, such as those who are positive for human immunodeficiency virus and older patients with diabetes, have an increased risk for this condition. Option 1 describes acute otitis media, which is treated with antibiotics. Option 2, recurrent acute otitis media, can be treated with short-term antibiotic therapy, prophylactic antibiotic therapy, or tympanostomy tubes. Option 3 is describing swimmer's ear; this condition readily responds to antibiotic and antifungal eardrops. **Focus:** Prioritization. **Test-Taking Tip:** Recall that any immunocompromised person has an increased risk for infection. Signs and symptoms that signal infection should be immediately reported to the health care provider because even minor infections can become life threatening.

28. **Ans: 3**   Heavy lifting should be strictly avoided for at least 3 weeks after stapedectomy. Water in the ear and air travel should be avoided for at least 1 week. Coughing and sneezing should be performed with the mouth open to prevent increased pressure in the ear. **Focus:** Prioritization.

29. **Ans: 2**   Meclizine can be helpful for patients who have vertigo (sensation of whirling or turning in space). Meclizine is also prescribed for the symptoms of motion sickness. **Focus:** Prioritization.

30. **Ans: 2**   According to the American Academy of Pediatrics, amoxicillin is the antibiotic of choice unless the child is allergic to penicillin. It would not be prescribed if the child had received it within the previous 30 days or has concurrent purulent conjunctivitis. Allergy symptoms, such as sneezing or rhinorrhea, are not a contraindication. Secondhand smoke, day care attendance, and ages 6 to 18 months are factors associated with an increased incidence of acute otitis media. **Focus:** Prioritization.

31. **Ans: 8, 9, 4, 10, 1, 6, 2, 3, 5, 7**   First, the HCP or the nurse should use an otoscope to assess the ear (perforation, acute infection, or organic foreign bodies are contraindications for irrigation). The patient sits and the shoulder on the affected side is draped. The patient is instructed on how to hold the basin to catch the drainage. The syringe is filled with warm fluid and angled in the ear canal to allow the fluid to flow along the side of the canal, not directly at the eardrum. Continuous gentle pressure is applied rather than a pumping action. Fluid should return with cerumen. If not, the nurse waits at least 10 minutes and repeats the irrigation. Tipping the head allows gravity drainage of fluid from the ear canal. Documentation includes patient response and appearance of drainage. **Focus:** Prioritization.

32. **Ans: 1, 2, 3, 5, 8**   Ear canal irrigation is not performed if the patient has a perforated eardrum or otitis media because of potential to spread the infection to the inner ear. Vegetable matter or other organic matter can swell if it gets wet, so this would worsen the impaction. For insects, attempts should be made to coax the insect out with a flashlight if they are alive or smothering with oil before attempting removal. If there is an impaction that did not resolved with softeners and irrigation, the health care provider should perform the procedure with concurrent evaluation of pain and possible complications. Tinnitus and vertigo are common symptoms caused by excessive cerumen in the ear canal. Hearing loss related to cerumen is alleviated with earwax softeners and irrigation. Patients should be advised not to use ear candles or to insert other foreign objects into the ear canal. **Focus:** Supervision.

33. **Ans: Option 1, tilts her head toward the nurse; Option 2, Rinne Test- negative; Option 3, lisinopril 2.5 mg/day; Option 4, aspirin 1000 mg every 4 to 6 hours; Option 5, facing patient with eye contact.** Tilting the head or ear towards the speaker, straining to hear, physically leaning in and watching the speaker's lips are behaviors that people use to compensate for hearing loss. In a Rinne test, a tuning fork

is struck and placed on the mastoid bone, if the sound is louder through bone conduction then through the air, the result is negative and consider abnormal. Lisinopril (commonly prescribed for heart failure) and aspirin (commonly prescribed for pain associated with rheumatoid arthritis) have the potential for ototoxicity. In addition, the aspirin dosage that the patient is taking is in the higher range. Facing the patient and making eye contact is the first intervention that the nurse would try, because people with hearing impairment will watch the lips and look for nonverbal cues, such as facial expression or gesturing. Facing the patient also directs sound towards the patient's pinna, which is designed to catch and amplify sounds. **Focus:** Prioritization.

34. **Ans: 3, 5, 6, 7, 8, 9** For angle-closure glaucoma, immediate inventions include instillation of miotics, which open the trabecular network and facilitate aqueous outflow, and intravenous or oral administration of hyperosmotic agents to move fluid from the intracellular space to the extracellular space. Deceased visual acuity after the instillation of a miotic agent is an expected side effect. Applying cool compresses and providing a dark, quiet space are appropriate comfort measures. Either laser peripheral iridotomy or surgical iridectomy may be performed for long-term management and to prevent recurrent episodes. Photodynamic therapy is a treatment for age-related macular degeneration. Use of mydriatic and cycloplegic agents are contraindicated because dilation of the pupil will further block the outflow. Cataract extraction is not related to the treatment of acute angle-closure glaucoma. **Focus:** Prioritization.

PART 2 Common Health Scenarios

CHAPTER 11

Musculoskeletal Problems

Questions

1. The nurse is assisting with a student assessment screening of 6th graders at the local grade school. A student presents with a back and spine as in the following illustration. What is the nurse's best interpretation of this finding?
   1. Dupuytren contracture
   2. Colles fracture
   3. Scoliosis
   4. Lordosis

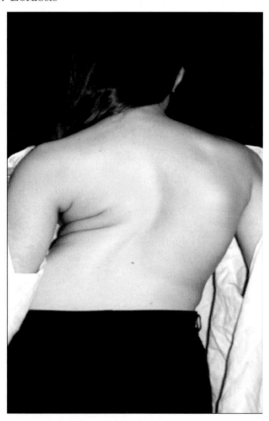

2. The nurse is caring for a patient who had a dual-energy x-ray absorptiometry scan and is now prescribed calcium with vitamin D twice a day. The patient asks the nurse the purpose of this drug. What is the nurse's **best** response? **Select all that apply.**
   1. "When your calcium and vitamin D levels are low, your risk for osteoporosis and osteomalacia increases."
   2. "When your vitamin D level is high, your bones release calcium to keep your blood calcium level in the normal range."
   3. "When your blood calcium is low, calcium is released from your bones increasing your risk for fractures."
   4. "When blood calcium is normal, long bones are formed, increasing a person's height."
   5. "The extra calcium and vitamin D will help protect your bones from damage such as fractures."
   6. "You can also get extra vitamin D by increasing your intake of beef and pork sources."

3. The nurse is preparing a discussion of musculoskeletal health maintenance for a group of older adults. Which key points would the nurse be sure to include? **Select all that apply.**
   1. Be aware of and consume foods rich in calcium and vitamin D.
   2. Wear hats and long sleeves to avoid sun exposure at all times.
   3. Consider exercise with low impact to avoid risk for injury.
   4. If you smoke, consider a smoking cessation program.
   5. Excessive alcohol intake can interfere with vitamins and nutrients for bone growth.
   6. Weight-bearing activities decrease the risk for osteoporosis.

4. The nurse is caring for a patient with osteoporosis who is at an increased risk for falls. Which intervention should the nurse delegate to the assistive personnel (AP)?
   1. Identifying environmental factors that increase the risk for falls
   2. Monitoring gait, balance, and fatigue level with ambulation
   3. Collaborating with the physical therapist to provide the patient with a walker
   4. Assisting the patient with ambulation to the bathroom and in the halls

5. The nurse is preparing to teach a patient with a new diagnosis of osteoporosis about strategies to prevent falls. Which teaching points should the nurse be sure to include? **Select all that apply.**
   1. Wear a hip protector when ambulating.
   2. Remove throw rugs and other obstacles at home.
   3. Exercise to help build your strength.
   4. Expect a few bumps and bruises when you go home.
   5. Rest when you are tired.
   6. Avoid consuming three or more alcoholic drinks per day.

6. The nurse's assessment reveals all of these data when a patient with Paget disease is admitted to the acute care unit. Which finding should the nurse notify the health care provider about **first**?
   1. There is a bowing of both legs, and the knees are asymmetrical.
   2. The base of the skull is invaginated (platybasia).
   3. The patient is only 5 feet tall and weighs 120 lb.
   4. The skull is soft, thick, and larger than normal.

7. The charge nurse observes an LPN/LVN assigned to provide all of these interventions for a patient with Paget disease. Which action requires that the charge nurse intervene?
   1. Administering 600 mg of ibuprofen to the patient
   2. Encouraging the patient to perform exercises recommended by a physical therapist
   3. Applying ice and gentle massage to the patient's lower extremities
   4. Reminding the patient to drink milk and eat cottage cheese

8. The charge nurse is making assignments for the day shift. Which patient should be assigned to the nurse who was floated from the postanesthesia care unit (PACU) for the day?
   1. A 35-year-old patient with osteomyelitis who needs teaching before hyperbaric oxygen therapy
   2. A 62-year-old patient with osteomalacia who is being discharged to a long-term care facility
   3. A 68-year-old patient with osteoporosis given a new orthotic device whose knowledge of its use must be assessed
   4. A 72-year-old patient with Paget disease who has just returned from surgery for total knee replacement

9. The nurse delegates the measurement of vital signs to an experienced assistive personnel (AP). Osteomyelitis has been diagnosed in a patient. Which vital sign value would the nurse instruct the AP to report immediately for this patient?
   1. Temperature of 101°F (38.3°C)
   2. Blood pressure of 136/80 mm Hg
   3. Heart rate of 96 beats/min
   4. Respiratory rate of 24 breaths/min

10. The nurse is working with an assistive personnel (AP) to provide care for six patients. At the beginning of the shift, the nurse carefully tells the AP what patient interventions and tasks he or she is expected to perform. Which "Four Cs" guide the nurse's communication with the AP? **Select all that apply.**
    1. Clear
    2. Comprehensive
    3. Concise
    4. Credible
    5. Correct
    6. Complete

11. The nurse is caring for a patient with carpal tunnel syndrome (CTS) who has been admitted for surgery. Which intervention should be delegated to the assistive personnel (AP)?
    1. Initiating placement of a splint for immobilization during the day
    2. Assessing the patient's wrist and hand for discoloration and brittle nails
    3. Assisting the patient with daily self-care measures such as bathing and eating
    4. Testing the patient for painful tingling in the five digits of the hand

12. The nurse observes the assistive personnel (AP) performing all of these interventions for a patient with carpal tunnel syndrome (CTS). Which action requires that the nurse intervene immediately?
    1. Arranging the patient's lunch tray and cutting his meat
    2. Providing warm water and assisting the patient with his bath
    3. Replacing the patient's splint in hyperextension position
    4. Reminding the patient not to lift very heavy objects

13. A patient is scheduled for endoscopic carpal tunnel release surgery in the morning. What would the nurse be sure to teach the patient?
    1. Pain and numbness are expected to be experienced for several days to weeks.
    2. Immediately after surgery, the patient will no longer need assistance.
    3. After surgery, the dressing will be large, and there will be lots of drainage.
    4. The patient's pain and paresthesia will no longer be present.

 Answer Key for this chapter begins on p. 117

14. The charge nurse assigns the nursing care of a patient who has just returned from open carpal tunnel release surgery to an experienced LPN/LVN, who will perform under the supervision of an RN. Which instructions would the RN provide for the LPN/LVN? **Select all that apply.**
    1. Check the patient's vital signs every 15 minutes in the first hour.
    2. Check the dressing for drainage and tightness.
    3. Elevate the patient's hand above the heart.
    4. The patient will no longer need pain medication.
    5. Check the neurovascular status of the fingers every hour.
    6. Instruct the patient to perform range of motion on the affected wrist.

15. The nurse is preparing a patient who had carpal tunnel release surgery for discharge. Which information is important to provide for this patient?
    1. The surgical procedure is a cure for carpal tunnel syndrome (CTS).
    2. Do not lift any heavy objects.
    3. Frequent doses of pain medication will no longer be necessary.
    4. The health care provider should be notified immediately if there is any pain or discomfort.

16. The nurse is providing care for a patient with a rotator cuff tear. What treatment does the nurse expect the health care provider (HCP) will prescribe **first** for this patient?
    1. Arthroscopic repair of the rotator cuff tear
    2. Elimination of movements in the affected shoulder
    3. Conservative therapies such as nonsteroidal anti-inflammatory drugs (NSAIDs) and physical therapy
    4. Pendulum exercises that start slow and progress over 2 weeks

17. The emergency department nurse receives a call about a patient with a traumatic finger amputation. What instructions will the nurse provide to the patient's wife? **Select all that apply.**
    1. Wrap the completely severed finger in dry sterile gauze (if available) or a clean cloth.
    2. Put the finger in a watertight, sealed plastic bag.
    3. Place the bag directly on ice.
    4. Elevate the affected extremity above the patient's heart.
    5. Examine the amputation site and apply direct pressure with layers of dry gauze.
    6. After performing these steps, call 911 and check the patient for breathing.

18. When receiving discharge instructions, a patient with osteoporosis makes all of these statements. Which statement indicates to the nurse that the patient needs additional teaching?
    1. "I take my ibuprofen every morning as soon as I get up."
    2. "My daughter removed all of the throw rugs in my home."
    3. "My husband helps me every afternoon with range-of-motion exercises."
    4. "I rest in my reclining chair every day for at least an hour."

19. A patient has a fractured femur. Which finding would the nurse instruct the assistive personnel to report immediately?
    1. The patient reports pain.
    2. The patient appears confused.
    3. The patient's blood pressure is 136/88 mm Hg.
    4. The patient voided using the bedpan.

20. After the nurse receives the change-of-shift report, which patient should be assessed **first**?
    1. A 42-year-old patient with carpal tunnel syndrome who reports pain
    2. A 64-year-old patient with osteoporosis awaiting discharge
    3. A 28-year-old patient with a fracture who reports that the cast is tight
    4. A 56-year-old patient with a left leg amputation who reports phantom pain

21. A patient with a fractured fibula is receiving skeletal traction and has skeletal pins in place. What would the nurse instruct the assistive personnel to report immediately?
    1. The patient wants to change position in bed.
    2. There is a small amount of clear fluid at the pin sites.
    3. The traction weights are resting on the floor.
    4. The patient reports pain and muscle spasm.

22. The nurse is supervising a newly graduated RN caring for a patient with a fracture of the right ankle who is at risk for complications of immobility. For which action should the supervising nurse intervene?
    1. Encouraging the patient to go from a lying to a standing position
    2. Administering pain medication before the patient begins exercises
    3. Explaining to the patient and family the purpose of the exercise program
    4. Reminding the patient about the correct use of crutches

23. The charge nurse is assigning the nursing care of a patient who had a left below-the-knee amputation 1 day ago to an experienced LPN/LVN, who will function under an RN's supervision. What will the RN tell the LPN/LVN is the **major** focus for the patient's care today?
    1. To attain pain control over phantom pain
    2. To monitor for signs of sufficient tissue perfusion
    3. To assist the patient to ambulate as soon as possible
    4. To elevate the residual limb when the patient is supine

24. A patient with a right above-the-knee amputation asks the nurse why he has phantom limb pain. What is the nurse's **best** response?
    1. "Phantom limb pain is not explained or predicted by any one theory."
    2. "Phantom limb pain occurs because your body thinks your leg is still present."
    3. "Phantom limb pain will not interfere with your activities of daily living."
    4. "Phantom limb pain is not real pain but is remembered pain."

25. During morning care, a patient with a below-the-knee amputation asks the assistive personnel (AP) about prostheses. How will the nurse instruct the AP to respond?
    1. "You should get a prosthesis so that you can walk again."
    2. "Wait and ask your health care provider (HCP) that question the next time he comes in."
    3. "It's too soon to be worrying about getting a prosthesis."
    4. "I'll ask the nurse to come in and discuss this with you."

26. During the assessment of a patient with fractures of the medial ulna and radius, the nurse finds all of these data. Which assessment finding should the nurse report to the health care provider immediately?
    1. The patient reports pressure and pain.
    2. The cast is in place and is dry and intact.
    3. The skin is pink and warm to the touch.
    4. The patient can move all the fingers and the thumb.

27. A patient who underwent a right above-the-knee amputation 4 days ago also has a diagnosis of depression. Which prescription would the nurse clarify with the health care provider?
    1. Give fluoxetine 40 mg once a day.
    2. Administer acetaminophen with codeine 1 or 2 tablets every 4 hours as needed.
    3. Assist the patient to the bedside chair every shift.
    4. Reinforce the dressing to the right residual limb as needed.

28. The nurse is caring for a postoperative patient with a hip replacement. Which patient care actions can be delegated to the experienced assistive personnel (AP)? **Select all that apply.**
    1. Inspect heels and other bony prominences every 8 hours.
    2. Turn and reposition the patient every 2 hours.
    3. Ensure that the patient's heels are elevated off the bed.
    4. Assess the patient's calf regions for redness and swelling.
    5. Check vital signs and oxygen saturation via pulse oximetry.
    6. Assess for pain and administer pain medication.

29. The emergency department (ED) nurse should question which health care provider prescription when providing care for an older adult with a fracture of the left ulna?
    1. Get x-rays of the left forearm.
    2. Give meperidine IM for pain.
    3. Monitor vital signs every hour.
    4. Elevate left arm on pillows.

30. The RN is mentoring a student nurse who is caring for a patient with carpal tunnel syndrome of the right hand with a neurovascular check ordered every 2 hours. For which action by the student nurse must the RN intervene?
    1. Student nurse checks the patient's radial pulse every 2 hours.
    2. Student nurse checks for sensation in the patient's right hand.
    3. Student nurse assesses color, temperature, and pain in right wrist and hand.
    4. Student nurse instructs the patient to avoid movement because of the pain.

31. The nurse is preparing a patient for magnetic resonance imaging. Which action can the nurse delegate to the experienced assistive personnel (AP)?
    1. Teach the patient what to expect during the test.
    2. Instruct the patient to remove metal objects including zippers.
    3. Witness that the patient has signed the consent form.
    4. Check and record preprocedure vital signs.

32. The nurse is teaching an older patient about risks for fractures and osteoporosis. Which diagnostic test should the nurse teach about when the goal is to establish the patient's bone strength and determine if osteoporosis is present?
    1. Computed tomography scan
    2. Magnetic resonance imaging scan
    3. Dual-energy x-ray absorptiometry (DXA or DEXA) scan
    4. Joint x-rays

Answer Key for this chapter begins on p. 117

33. The RN is receiving a patient with peripheral vascular disease from the postanesthesia care unit after a Syme amputation of the right lower extremity. At which level on this diagram would the RN expect to find the amputation?
    1. A
    2. B
    3. C
    4. D

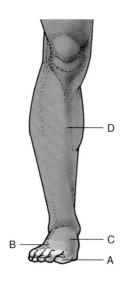

34. The nurse is providing care for a patient with a connective tissue disorder exacerbation for whom the health care provider has prescribed an IV dose of methylprednisolone 20 mg in 50 mL normal saline to be infused over 30 minutes. At what rate will the nurse set the IV infusion pump to administer this drug correctly?

_____

 35. Enhanced Drag and Drop _____

Scenario: The patient has rheumatoid arthritis. Which health care team member listed in the right column would be best to assign to each care task listed below.

Instructions: Place the correct letter in the space in front of each task listed in the left column.

1. _____ Reinforce medication teaching and disease management strategies.
2. _____ Assess need related to obtaining necessary medical equipment.
3. _____ Establish exercise regimen for patient.
4. _____ Assist patient with self-care needs.
5. _____ Assess disease impact on quality of life and joint function.
6. _____ Assess impact of patient's condition on ability to perform activities of daily living.
7. _____ Administer oral ibuprofen for pain.
8. _____ Provide patient with specialized equipment for self-feeding.

a. RN
b. LPN/LVN
c. Assistive personnel (AP)
d. Physical therapist
e. Occupational therapist
f. Social worker

Answers

1. **Ans: 3** Scoliosis occurs when the vertebrae rotate and begin to compress; the spinal column moves into a lateral curve. On assessment, findings include asymmetry of hip and shoulder height with prominent thoracic ribs and scapula on one side. Dupuytren contracture is a hand deformity with slow progressive thickening of the palmar fascia leading to flexion contracture of the 4th and 5th fingers. Colles fracture occurs in the distal radius. Lordosis is a loss of lumbar curvature sometimes called "flat back," which may also be present with scoliosis. **Focus:** Prioritization.

2. **Ans: 1, 3, 5** Vitamin D and its metabolites are produced in the body and transported in the blood to promote the absorption of calcium and phosphorus from the small intestine. There is a relationship between calcium and phosphorus so that if a patient's phosphorus level is higher than normal, the calcium level will drop, and vice versa. A decrease in the body's vitamin D level can result in osteomalacia (softening of bone) in an adult. When serum calcium levels are lowered, parathyroid hormone (PTH, or parathormone) secretion increases and stimulates bone to promote osteoclastic activity and release calcium to the blood. PTH reduces the renal excretion of calcium and facilitates its absorption from the intestine. Sources of vitamin D include sunlight, fatty fish, and vitamin D–enriched foods. **Focus:** Prioritization.

3. **Ans: 1, 3, 4, 5, 6** Many health problems of the musculoskeletal system can be prevented through health promotion strategies and avoidance of risky lifestyle behaviors. Weight-bearing activities such as walking can reduce risk factors for osteoporosis and maintain muscle strength. Young men are at the greatest risk for trauma related to motor vehicle crashes. Older adults are at the greatest risk for falls that result in fractures and soft tissue injury. High-impact sports, such as excessive jogging or running, can cause musculoskeletal injury to soft tissues and bone. Tobacco use slows the healing of musculoskeletal injuries. Excessive alcohol intake can decrease vitamins and nutrients a person needs for bone and muscle tissue growth. Hats and long sleeves are recommended to prevent sunburn, but the nurse would recommend 20 minutes of sun exposure several times a week for vitamin D, which contributes to bone health. **Focus:** Prioritization.

4. **Ans: 4** Assisting with activities of daily living, including assisting with ambulation to the bathroom and in the halls, is within the scope of the AP's practice. The other three interventions require additional educational preparation and are within the scope of practice of licensed nurses. **Focus:** Delegation, Supervision.

5. **Ans: 1, 2, 3, 5** The purpose of this teaching is to help the patient prevent falls. The hip protector can prevent hip fractures if the patient falls. Throw rugs and obstacles in the home increase the risk of falls. Patients who are tired are also more likely to fall. Exercise helps to strengthen muscles and improve coordination. Women should not consume more than one drink per day, and men should not consume more than two drinks per day. **Focus:** Prioritization. **Test-Taking Tip:** A question like this is asking which actions should be taken to prevent injury and keep the patient safe. Think about patient safety when choosing the best answers.

6. **Ans: 2** Platybasia (basilar skull invagination) causes brainstem manifestations that threaten life. Patients with Paget disease are usually short and often have bowing of the long bones that results in asymmetrical knees or elbow deformities. The skull is typically soft, thick, and enlarged. **Focus:** Prioritization.

7. **Ans: 3** Applying heat, not ice, is the appropriate measure to help reduce the patient's pain. Ibuprofen is useful to manage mild to moderate pain. Exercise prescribed by a physical therapist would be nonimpact in nature and provide strengthening for the patient. A diet rich in calcium promotes bone health. **Focus:** Assignment, Supervision. **Test-Taking Tip:** The charge nurse would be familiar with the usual care of a patient with Paget disease. Supervise the LPN/LVN so that he or she will stop the ice treatment and explain to the LPN/LVN that the use of heat is preferable to reduce the patient's pain.

8. **Ans: 4** The PACU nurse is very familiar with the assessment skills necessary to monitor a patient who just underwent surgery. For the other patients, nurses familiar with musculoskeletal system–related nursing care are needed to provide teaching and assessment and prepare a report to the long-term care facility. **Focus:** Assignment.

9. **Ans: 1** An elevated temperature indicates infection and inflammation. This patient needs IV antibiotic therapy. The other vital sign values are normal or high normal. **Focus:** Delegation, Supervision.

10. **Ans: 1, 3, 5, 6** Clear, concise, correct, and complete are the "Four Cs" of communication. Implementing the four Cs of communication helps the nurse ensure that the AP understands what is being said; that the AP does not confuse the nurse's directions; that the directions comply with policies, procedures, job descriptions, and the law; and that the AP has all the information necessary to complete the tasks assigned. **Focus:** Delegation, Supervision. **Test-Taking Tip:** When an NCLEX question involves the nurse giving

PART 2 Common Health Scenarios

instructions to an AP, examine the options. The option that is clear, concise, correct, and complete is likely to be the correct answer.

11. **Ans: 3** Helping with activities of daily living (e.g., bathing, feeding) is within the scope of practice of APs. Placing a splint for the first time is appropriate to the scope of practice of physical therapists. Assessing and testing for paresthesia are not within the scope of practice of APs and are appropriate for professional nurses. **Focus:** Delegation, Supervision.

12. **Ans: 3** When a patient with CTS has a splint to immobilize the wrist, the wrist is placed either in the neutral position or in slight extension, not hyperextension. The other interventions are correct and are within the scope of practice of an AP. APs may remind patients about elements of their care plans that have already been taught, such as avoiding heavy lifting. **Focus:** Delegation, Supervision.

13. **Ans: 1** Postoperative pain and numbness occur for a longer period of time with endoscopic carpal tunnel release than with an open procedure. Patients often need assistance postoperatively, even after they are discharged. The dressing from the endoscopic procedure is usually very small, and there should not be a lot of drainage. **Focus:** Prioritization.

14. **Ans: 1, 2, 3, 5** Postoperatively, patients undergoing open carpal tunnel release surgery experience pain and numbness, and their discomfort may last for weeks to months. Hand movements may be restricted for 4 to 6 weeks after surgery. All of the other directions are appropriate for the postoperative care of this patient. It is important to monitor for drainage, tightness, and neurovascular changes. Raising the hand and wrist above the heart reduces the swelling from surgery, and this is often done for several days. **Focus:** Assignment, Supervision.

15. **Ans: 2** Hand movements, including heavy lifting, may be restricted for 4 to 6 weeks after surgery. Patients experience discomfort for weeks to months after surgery. The surgery is not always a cure; in some cases, CTS may recur months to years after surgery. **Focus:** Prioritization.

16. **Ans: 3** For the patient with a torn rotator cuff, the HCP usually treats the patient conservatively with NSAIDs, intermittent steroid injections, physical therapy, and activity limitations while the tear heals. Physical therapy treatments may include ultrasound, electrical stimulation, ice, and heat. **Focus:** Prioritization.

17. **Ans: 1, 2, 4, 5** For a person who has a traumatic amputation in the community, first call 911 and then assess the patient for airway or breathing problems. Examine the amputation site and apply direct pressure with layers of dry gauze or cloth. Elevate the extremity above the patient's heart to decrease the bleeding. Do not remove the dressing to prevent dislodging the clot. Wrap the completely severed finger in dry sterile

gauze (if available) or a clean cloth. Put the finger in a watertight, sealed plastic bag. Place the bag in ice water, never directly on ice, with 1 part ice and 3 parts water. Avoid contact between the finger and the water to prevent tissue damage. Do not remove any semidetached parts of the digit. Be sure that the part goes with the patient to the hospital. **Focus:** Prioritization.

18. **Ans: 1** Ibuprofen can cause abdominal discomfort or pain and ulceration of the gastrointestinal tract. In such cases, it should be taken with meals or milk. Removal of throw rugs helps prevent falls. Range-of-motion exercises and rest are important strategies for coping with osteoporosis. **Focus:** Prioritization.

19. **Ans: 2** Fat embolism syndrome is a serious complication that often results from fractures of long bones. Its earliest manifestation is altered mental status caused by a low arterial oxygen level. The nurse would want to know about and treat the pain, but it is not life threatening. The nurse would also want to know about the blood pressure and the patient's voiding; however, this information is not urgent to report. **Focus:** Prioritization, Delegation, Supervision.

20. **Ans: 3** The patient with the tight cast is at risk for circulation impairment and peripheral nerve damage. Although all of the other patients' concerns are important and the nurse will want to see them as soon as possible, none of their complaints is urgent. The patient with the tight cast may have risk for injury to a limb, which is more urgent. **Focus:** Prioritization.

21. **Ans: 3** When the weights are resting on the floor, they are not exerting pulling force to provide reduction and alignment or to prevent muscle spasm. The weights should always hang freely. Attending to the weights may reduce the patient's pain and spasms. With skeletal pins, a small amount of clear fluid drainage is expected. It is important to inspect the traction system after a patient changes position because position changes may alter the traction. **Focus:** Delegation, Supervision, Prioritization.

22. **Ans: 1** Moving directly from a lying to a standing position does not allow the patient to establish balance. The supervising nurse should instruct the newly graduated RN about moving the patient from a lying position first, then to a sitting position, and finally to a standing position, which will allow the patient to establish balance before standing. Administering pain medication before the patient begins exercising decreases pain with exercise. Explanations about the purpose of the exercise program and proper use of crutches are appropriate interventions for this patient. **Focus:** Delegation, Supervision.

23. **Ans: 2** Monitoring for sufficient tissue perfusion is the priority at this time. Phantom pain is a concern but is more common in patients with above-the-knee amputations. Early ambulation is a goal, but at this time, the patient is more likely to be engaged in muscle-strengthening exercises. Elevating the residual limb on a

pillow is controversial because it may promote knee flexion contracture. **Focus:** Delegation, Supervision.

24. **Ans: 1** Three theories are being researched with regard to phantom limb pain. The peripheral nervous system theory suggests that sensations remain as a result of the severing of peripheral nerves during the amputation. The central nervous system theory states that phantom limb pain results from a loss of inhibitory signals that were generated through afferent impulses from the amputated limb. The psychological theory helps predict and explain phantom limb pain because stress, anxiety, and depression often trigger or worsen a pain episode. **Focus:** Prioritization.

25. **Ans: 4** The patient is indicating an interest in learning about prostheses. The experienced nurse can initiate discussion and begin educating the patient. Certainly, the HCP can also discuss prostheses with the patient, but the patient's wish to learn should receive a quick response. The nurse can then notify the HCP about the patient's request. **Focus:** Delegation, Supervision.

26. **Ans: 1** Pressure and pain may be caused by increased compartment pressure and can indicate the serious complication of acute compartment syndrome. This situation is urgent. If it is not treated, cyanosis, tingling, numbness, paresis, and severe pain can occur. The other findings are normal and should be documented in the patient's chart. **Focus:** Prioritization.

27. **Ans: 1** Doses of fluoxetine, a drug used to treat depression, that are greater than 20 mg should be given in two divided doses, not once a day. The other three prescriptions are appropriate for a patient who underwent amputation 4 days earlier. **Focus:** Prioritization.

28. **Ans: 2, 3, 5** The AP's scope of practice includes repositioning patients and checking vital signs, and an experienced AP would know how to check pulse oximetry and elevate the patient's heels off the bed. Assessing and inspecting patients is more appropriate to the educational level of the professional nurse. **Focus:** Delegation.

29. **Ans: 2** Meperidine should not be used because of its toxic metabolites that can cause seizures and other adverse drug events, especially in the older adult population. X-rays are used to confirm the diagnosis. Vital signs and elevation are common actions for a patient in the ED, and elevation can decrease the swelling in the affected extremity. **Focus:** Prioritization. **Test-Taking Tip:** Questions often focus on actions

or findings specific to older adults because there are many differences as adults age. Meperidine is seldom used for pain relief in any patient now because of its negative effects.

30. **Ans: 4** Performing complete neurovascular assessment (also called a "circ check") includes palpation of pulses in the extremities below the level of injury and assessment of sensation, movement, color, temperature, and pain in the injured part. If pulses are not palpable, use of a Doppler helps find pulses in the extremities. After surgery, the patient should be given pain medication and encouraged to move the fingers frequently. Some hand movements such as lifting heavy objects may be restricted for 4 to 6 weeks after surgery. **Focus:** Prioritization.

31. **Ans: 4** The AP's scope of practice includes checking and recording patient vital signs. Teaching and instructing, as well as witnessing consent forms, is appropriate to the professional RN's scope of practice. The AP could remind the patient about the removal of metal objects after the patient receives that instruction. **Focus:** Delegation.

32. **Ans: 3** Testing bone density (how strong the bones are) is the only way to know for sure whether or not a patient has osteoporosis. A diagnostic test commonly prescribed by health care providers is DXA or DEXA. This type of scan focuses on two main areas, the hip and the spine. The forearm can be tested, however, if the hip or spine cannot be tested. The other tests may be prescribed but are not as commonly used to test bone strength. **Focus:** Prioritization.

33. **Ans: 3** When a patient has a Syme amputation, most of the foot is removed but the ankle remains. Advantages of this surgery over below the knee include that the patient can still be weight bearing (with a prosthesis) and that there is less pain. **Focus:** Prioritization.

34. **Ans: 100 mL/hr.** To infuse 50 mL over 30 minutes (0.5 hr), the nurse would have to set the infusion rate at 100 mL/hr. **Focus:** Prioritization.

35. **Ans: 1b, 2f, 3d, 4c, 5a, 6e, 7b, 8e** Care for a patient with rheumatoid arthritis requires a thorough program of education and drug therapy. In addition to the health care provider, team members include the RN, LPN/ LVN, AP, physical therapist, occupational therapist, and social worker. All of these roles contribute to patient care including teaching, assessment, and assistance. **Focus:** Prioritization.

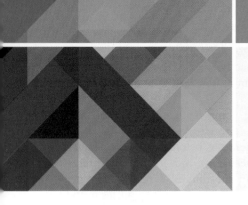

CHAPTER 12

Gastrointestinal and Nutritional Problems

Questions

1. Which question will the RN ask the LPN/LVN who is assigned to do an enteral feeding for a patient with a small-bore feeding tube?
   1. Have you evaluated the nutritional status of the patient?
   2. Is the patient tolerating the supine position after feedings?
   3. Have you had any problems checking the residual?
   4. Is the patient developing any problems related to the feedings?

2. When a patient is being prepared for a colonoscopy procedure, which task is **most** suitable to delegate to assistive personnel (AP)?
   1. Explaining how to assume the side-lying position
   2. Reinforcing the need for a clear liquid diet
   3. Administering laxatives as needed
   4. Administering an enema to prepare the bowel

3. Which laboratory results would the nurse check to determine if there are untoward effects associated with vomiting, nasogastric suction, or lavage?
   1. White blood cell (WBC) counts
   2. Hematocrit and hemoglobin
   3. Serum electrolytes
   4. Blood urea nitrogen (BUN) and serum creatinine

4. The nurse would be **most** concerned about a prescription for a total parenteral nutrition (TPN) fat emulsion for a patient with which condition?
   1. Gastrointestinal (GI) obstruction
   2. Severe anorexia nervosa
   3. Chronic diarrhea and vomiting
   4. Fractured femur

5. For a patient with short bowel syndrome, the nurse would question the prescription of which enteral formula?
   1. High sodium content
   2. High fat content
   3. High protein content
   4. Modified carbohydrate content

6. The nurse is caring for a patient with peptic ulcer disease (PUD). Which assessment finding is the **most** serious?
   1. Projectile vomiting
   2. Burning sensation 2 hours after eating
   3. Coffee-ground emesis
   4. Board-like abdomen with shoulder pain

7. The nurse is taking an initial history for a patient seeking surgical treatment for obesity. Which finding should be called to the attention of the surgeon?
   1. Obesity for approximately 5 years
   2. History of counseling for body dysmorphic disorder
   3. Failure to reduce weight with other forms of therapy
   4. Body weight 100% above the ideal for age, gender, and height

8. The nurse is taking a report on an older patient who was admitted with abdominal pain, nausea, vomiting, and diarrhea. The patient also has a history of chronic dementia. Which comment by the night shift nurse is **most** concerning?
   1. The patient has a flat affect and rambling and repetitive speech.
   2. The patient has memory impairments and thinks the year is 1948.
   3. The patient lacks motivation and demonstrates early morning awakening.
   4. The patient has a fluctuating level of consciousness and mood swings.

9. In the care of a patient with gastroesophageal reflux disease, which task would be appropriate to delegate to assistive personnel (AP)?
   1. Sharing successful strategies for weight reduction
   2. Encouraging the patient to express concerns about lifestyle modification
   3. Reminding the patient not to lie down for 2 to 3 hours after eating
   4. Explaining the rationale for eating small frequent meals

120

PART 2 Common Health Scenarios

10. The patient needs diagnostic testing to confirm symptoms of peptic ulcer disease (PUD), and the health care provider tells the nurse that the patient prefers noninvasive methods. Which brochure is the nurse **most** likely to prepare for the patient?
    1. "Three Simple Ways to Detect *H. pylori* Using Your Blood, Breath, or Stool."
    2. "How Your Doctor Uses a Barium Contrast Study to Detect PUD."
    3. "Esophagogastroduodenoscopy: The Major Diagnostic Test for PUD."
    4. "Common Questions and Answers About Nuclear Medicine Scans."

11. The nurse is providing the immediate postoperative care for a patient who had fundoplication to reinforce the lower esophageal sphincter for the purpose of a hiatal hernia repair. What is the **priority** action in the care of this patient?
    1. Elevate the head of the bed at least 30 degrees.
    2. Assess the nasogastric tube for yellowish-green drainage.
    3. Assist the patient to start taking a clear liquid diet.
    4. Assess the patient for gas bloat syndrome.

12. A patient with chronic hepatitis C has been taking a daily dose of the antiviral medication ledipasvir–sofosbuvir for the past month. Which information is the **most** important for the nurse to communicate to the health care provider?
    1. The patient reports mild headaches that come and go.
    2. The patient complains of feeling chronically tired.
    3. The patient has missed a period and is having unprotected sex.
    4. The patient reports nausea and occasional diarrhea.

13. Which patient is the **most** appropriate to assign to an LPN/LVN under the supervision of an RN?
    1. A patient with oral cancer who is scheduled for a glossectomy in the morning
    2. An obese patient who has returned from surgery after a vertical banded gastroplasty
    3. A patient with anorexia nervosa who has muscle weakness and decreased urine output
    4. A patient with intermittent nausea and vomiting after chemotherapy

14. For patients with peptic ulcer disease (PUD), what is the **most** important lifestyle modification?
    1. Avoiding caffeine
    2. Decreasing alcohol intake
    3. Smoking cessation
    4. Controlling stress

15. For the postoperative care of a morbidly obese patient, which task **best** utilizes the expertise of the LPN/LVN, under the supervision of the RN team leader?
    1. Obtaining an oversized blood pressure cuff and a large-size bed
    2. Setting up a reinforced trapeze bar
    3. Assisting in the planning of toileting, turning, and ambulation
    4. Assigning tasks to assistive personnel (AP) and other ancillary staff

16. A patient with proctitis needs a rectal suppository. A senior nursing student assigned to care for this patient tells the nurse that she is afraid to insert a suppository because she has never done it before. What is the **most** appropriate action in supervising this student?
    1. Give the medication and tell the student to talk to the instructor.
    2. Ask the student to leave the clinical area because she is unprepared.
    3. Reassign the patient to an LPN/LVN and send the student to observe.
    4. Show the student how to insert the suppository and talk to the instructor.

17. A nursing student is performing a colostomy irrigation. When would the nurse intervene?
    1. Student hangs the prepared irrigation container on the bed rail.
    2. Student puts 500 to 1000 mL of lukewarm water in the container.
    3. Student cleans, rinses, and dries the skin and applies a new drainage pouch.
    4. Student encourages the patient to walk for 30 to 45 minutes for secondary evacuation.

18. Which task, related to a nasogastric (NG) tube, can be delegated to an experienced assistive personnel (AP)?
    1. Removing the NG tube at the prescribed time
    2. Securing the tape if the patient accidentally dislodges the tube
    3. Disconnecting the suction to allow ambulation to the toilet
    4. Checking the suction after the patient has ambulated

19. The nurse is planning a treatment and prevention program for chronic bowel incontinence for an older patient. Which intervention should the nurse try **first**?
    1. Administer a glycerin suppository 15 minutes before evacuation time.
    2. Insert a rectal tube at specified intervals each day.
    3. Assist the patient to the commode or toilet 30 minutes after meals.
    4. Use incontinence briefs or adult-sized diapers.

Answer Key for this chapter begins on p. 128

PART 2 Common Health Scenarios

20. In which case would fecal microbiota transplantation (FMT) be considered for a patient with *Clostridium difficile* infection (CDI)?
    1. Patient has had multiple recurrences of CDI treated with vancomycin or fidaxomicin.
    2. Patient has CDI and a healthy donor who meets the criteria for donation is available.
    3. Patient has had a recurrence of CDI after receiving a full course of metronidazole.
    4. Patient has many risk factors for CDI and has poor nutritional and fluid reserves.

21. The charge nurse is reviewing the medication administration records for several patients. Which situation needs to be brought to the attention of the prescribing health care provider?
    1. A patient with gastroesophageal reflux disease is receiving omeprazole.
    2. An older adult patient with constipation is getting psyllium three times a day.
    3. A patient who needs a bowel prep is getting polyethylene glycol-electrolyte solution.
    4. A patient with abdominal pain secondary to diverticulitis is receiving bisacodyl.

22. What question is the home health nurse **most** likely to ask the patient to evaluate the efficacy of cimetidine?
    1. "Are you still having problems with constipation?"
    2. "Has the medication helped to relieve the acid indigestion?"
    3. "Did the medication relieve the nausea and vomiting?"
    4. "Do you feel like your appetite has improved?"

23. The nurse is caring for an obese postoperative patient who underwent surgery for bowel resection. As the patient is moving in bed, he comments, "Something popped open." Upon examination, the nurse notes wound evisceration. Place the steps in order for handling this complication.
    1. Cover the intestine with sterile moistened gauze.
    2. Stay calm and stay with the patient.
    3. Check the vital signs, especially blood pressure and pulse.
    4. Ask assistive personnel (AP) to get sterile supplies.
    5. Put the patient into semi-Fowler position with knees slightly flexed.
    6. Prepare the patient for surgery as ordered.
    7. Ask charge nurse to call the surgeon.
    _____, _____, _____, _____, _____, _____, _____

24. The nurse is providing postoperative care for a patient who underwent laparoscopic cholecystectomy. What should be reported **immediately** to the health care provider?
    1. The patient cannot void 5 hours postoperatively.
    2. The patient reports shoulder pain.
    3. The patient reports right upper quadrant pain.
    4. Output does not equal input for the first few hours.

25. An older adult patient tells the home health nurse that he puts 17 g of polyethylene glycol in a large cup of coffee every morning. Which assessment will the nurse perform **first**?
    1. Assess for signs and symptoms of dehydration or electrolyte imbalances.
    2. Assess for signs and symptoms of malnutrition and nutritional deficiencies.
    3. Ask the patient to describe frequency and consistency of bowel movements.
    4. Ask the patient what he understands about the purpose of the medication.

26. In the care of a patient with acute viral hepatitis, which task would be delegated to assistive personnel (AP)?
    1. Emptying the bedpan while wearing gloves
    2. Engaging the patient in diversional activities
    3. Monitoring dietary preferences
    4. Reporting signs and symptoms of jaundice

27. The nurse is caring for a patient with cirrhosis and portal hypertension. Which statement by the patient is cause for **greatest** concern?
    1. "I'm very constipated and have been straining during bowel movements."
    2. "I can't button my pants anymore because my belly is so swollen."
    3. "I have a tight sensation in my lower legs when I forget to put my feet up."
    4. "When I sleep, I have to sit in a recliner so that I can breathe more easily."

28. For patients coming to the ambulatory care gastrointestinal clinic, which task would be **most** appropriate to assign to an LPN/LVN?
    1. Teaching a patient self-care measures for an ulcer
    2. Assisting the health care provider to incise and drain a pilonidal cyst
    3. Evaluating a patient's response to sitz baths for an anorectal abscess
    4. Describing the basic pathophysiology of an anal fistula to a patient

29. A patient underwent an exploratory laparotomy 2 days ago. The health care provider (HCP) should be called **immediately** for which assessment finding?
    1. Abdominal distention and rigidity
    2. Absent or hypoactive bowel sounds
    3. Nausea and occasional vomiting
    4. Displacement of the nasogastric (NG) tube

30. Which instruction will the RN give to the LPN/LVN to determine if the prescribed dronabinol is having the desired therapeutic effect?
    1. Monitor and report bouts of nausea and vomiting.
    2. Monitor the frequency and amount of diarrheal episodes.
    3. Ask the patient if heartburn has decreased or resolved.
    4. Assess for abdominal pain in the upper right quadrant.

31. The nurse is caring for a patient who was recently admitted for severe diverticulitis. Which task is appropriate to delegate or assign for the care of this patient?
    1. Tell the unit secretary to call radiology and schedule a barium enema.
    2. Ask the LPN/LVN to give as needed (PRN) laxatives for constipation.
    3. Instruct the nursing student to help the patient ambulate up and down the hall.
    4. Tell assistive personnel to save a stool specimen to test for occult blood.

32. A patient is admitted to the medical-surgical unit for observation after being evaluated in the emergency department for blunt trauma to the abdomen. Which instructions would the RN give to assistive personnel (AP)?
    1. Check the patient's skin temperature and report if the skin feels cool.
    2. Check the urometer every hour and observe for red- or pink-tinged urine.
    3. Check vital signs every hour and report all of the values.
    4. Check the patient's pain and report worsening of pain or discomfort.

33. After a nasogastric tube is inserted, which assessment finding is cause for **greatest** concern?
    1. The patient reports that the tube is irritating nose and throat feels sore.
    2. Gastric contents have a coffee-ground appearance.
    3. The patient demonstrates coughing and cannot speak clearly.
    4. Gastric fluid is bright red and has small clots.

34. Patients who are undernourished or starved for prolonged periods are at risk for refeeding syndrome when nourishment is first given. What is the **priority** nursing assessment to prevent complications associated with this syndrome?
    1. Monitor for peripheral edema, crackles in the lungs, and jugular vein distention.
    2. Monitor for decreased bowel sounds, nausea, bloating, and abdominal distention.
    3. Observe for signs of secret purging and ingestion of water to increase weight.
    4. Assess for alternating constipation and diarrhea and pale clay-colored stools.

35. The patient with advanced cirrhosis has: massive ascites, peripheral-dependent edema in the lower extremities, nausea and vomiting, and dyspnea related to pressure on the diaphragm. Which indicator is the **most** reliable for tracking fluid retention?
    1. Auscultating the lung fields for crackles every day
    2. Measuring the abdominal girth every morning
    3. Performing daily weights with the same amount of clothing
    4. Checking the extremities for pitting edema and comparing with baseline

36. The nurse hears in the hand-off report that, 1 hour ago, the health care provider requested that the patient be given the maximum dose of magnesium hydroxide. Which instruction is the nurse **most** likely to give to assistive personnel?
    1. Patient will frequently need assistance to the bathroom for bowel evacuation.
    2. Patient may experience some dizziness when ambulating or changing position.
    3. Patient is frequently vomiting and may need linen and gown changes.
    4. Patient needs to be encouraged and assisted to eat and drink as much as possible.

37. A patient with end-stage liver disease is talking to the nurse about being on the transplant list. Which statement by the patient is cause for **greatest** concern?
    1. "I have a family history of diabetes."
    2. "I had symptoms of asthma when I was a kid."
    3. "I guess I should cut back on my alcohol consumption."
    4. "I am not very good about taking prescribed medication."

38. The nurse is supervising a nursing student who is caring for a patient who had a cholecystectomy. There is a T-tube in place. The nurse would intervene if the student performed which action?
    1. Maintained the patient in a semi-Fowler position
    2. Checked the amount, color, and consistency of the drainage
    3. Gently aspirated the drainage from the tube
    4. Inspected the skin around the tube for redness or irritation

Answer Key for this chapter begins on p. 128

39. An older adult patient tells the home health nurse that she is taking methylcellulose for chronic constipation. Which behavior is cause for **greatest** concern?
    1. Patient primarily eats white bread and drinks low-fat milk.
    2. Patient takes the methylcellulose three or four times a day.
    3. Patient takes the medication with a few sips of water.
    4. Patient does not promptly act on the urge to defecate.

40. A male nurse tells an older male patient that he needs to perform a digital examination of the rectum to check for possible fecal impaction. The patient responds, "I'm not letting any homosexual get near me." What should the nurse do **first**?
    1. Explain that the procedure is a nursing action, not a sexual advance.
    2. Ask the charge nurse to reassign that patient to a different nurse.
    3. Document that the patient refused to allow the examination.
    4. Ask the patient if the presence of a female staff member would be acceptable.

41. The patient has portal hypertension and hepatic encephalopathy secondary to liver disease and is being treated with lactulose. Which laboratory result will the nurse check **first** to see if the medication is having the desired effect?
    1. White blood cell count
    2. Ammonia level
    3. Potassium level
    4. Platelet count

42. The nurse is reviewing medication lists for patients who are being treated for peptic ulcer disease (PUD). The nurse is **most** likely to question the use of which medication?
    1. Ibuprofen
    2. Omeprazole
    3. Amoxicillin
    4. Clarithromycin

43. The patient has a medical diagnosis of acute appendicitis. On the figure below, mark the area of the abdomen where the patient is **most** likely to report abdominal pain and tenderness.

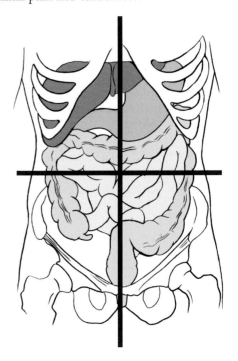

44. Drag and Drop

Case Study and Question

The charge nurse must review the conditions and status of patients to determine who could be placed in the same room as roommates.

Based on current condition and status, which **two** patients could be roomed together?

Instructions: Patients are listed in the left-hand column. In the right-hand column, use an X to indicate which two patients could be cohorted.

Patients on the unit	Two Patients for cohorting
1. 35-year-old woman with copious intractable nausea and vomiting	
2. 43-year-old woman who underwent cholecystectomy 2 days ago	
3. 53-year-old woman with pain related to alcohol-associated pancreatitis	
4. 70-year-old woman with stool culture results that show *Clostridium difficile*	
5. 55-year-old woman who is having symptoms after an exposure to norovirus	
6. 62-year-old woman with colon cancer who is receiving chemotherapy and radiation	
7. 59-year-old woman who has a wound infection; methicillin-resistant *Staphylococcus aureus* is suspected.	

45. Enhanced Multiple Response

Case Study and Question

The nurse is selecting personal protective equipment (PPE) to don before inserting a nasogastric (NG) tube.

Which factors will the nurse consider before selecting PPE?

Instructions: Read the case study on the left and circle or highlight the numbers that best answer the question.
1. Facility policies for procedures
2. Likelihood of exposure to blood and body fluids
3. Patient's ability and willingness to cooperate
4. PPE causes awkwardness when handling equipment
5. Own skill level and proficiency at procedure
6. Patient's health history and medical conditions
7. Availability of PPE at the bedside or on the unit
8. The type of tube that is ordered
9. The purpose of the tube (e.g., decompression of the stomach or enteral feedings)
10. Recent episodes of nausea and vomiting

Answer Key for this chapter begins on p. 128

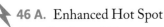

46 A. Enhanced Hot Spot
Case Study and Question

A 72-year old man living alone in poor conditions had prolonged hospitalization for a respiratory infection that was treated with ciprofloxacin. He was then transferred to a long-term care center. He uses over-the-counter (OTC) esomeprazole for heartburn. He has "heart problems" but can't afford to go to the doctor. The resident had two episodes of watery diarrhea in the past hour.

Vital signs:
Temperature 100.3° F (37.9°C)
Pulse 120 beats/min
Respirations 24 breaths /min
Blood Pressure 98/68 mmHg
Oxygen Saturation 93% on room air

Assessment findings: Admission weight: 120 lbs. (54 kg), Admission height 5′ 8″ (172.7 cm). Alert and oriented. Breath sounds clear and equal bilaterally. Respirations even and unlabored. Skin is warm and turgor is poor. Mucous membranes dry. Reports abdominal pain and cramping that is partially relieved after a diarrheal stool. Hyperactive bowel sounds and mild tenderness x 4 quadrants. Reports nausea and loss of appetite. To bathroom during assessment for a large watery bloody diarrheal stool. Specimen obtained. Has mild dizziness but is able to ambulate with assistance.

Which information from the history, vital signs and assessment findings support the nurse's suspicion of *Clostridium difficile* (CDI)?

Instructions: Underline or highlight history, vital signs and assessment findings that support the nurse's suspicion for CDI.

46 B. Expanded Multiple Response
Case Study and Question

For a suspicion of CDI, the nurse initiates nursing interventions to protect the environment and the other residents. The health care provider (HCP) must be notified to order diagnostic testing to confirm CDI and to prescribe additional therapies.

Which nursing interventions can be delegated to the AP?

Instructions: Read the case study on the left and circle or highlight each intervention that the nurse can delegate to the AP. **Select all that apply.**
1. Measure intake and output
2. Assess abdominal pain
3. Encourage sips of oral fluids as tolerated
4. Assist patient to ambulate to the bathroom
5. Take vital signs q 2 hours; report all values
6. Use fall precautions as directed
7. Gather supplies for contact precautions
8. Call SBAR report to HCP
9. Assist with perineal hygiene after diarrheal episodes
10. Assess condition of skin; perineal area and buttocks
11. Hold PRN laxatives, stool softeners and antidiarrheal agents

Common Health Scenarios   PART 2

47. Enhanced Multiple Response

Scenario: While transferring a dirty laundry bag, an assistive personnel (AP) sustains a puncture wound to the finger from a contaminated needle. The unit has several patients with hepatitis and acquired immunodeficiency syndrome; the needle source is unknown.

Which of the following instructions will the charge nurse give to the AP?

1. Have blood test(s) performed per protocol.
2. Interview the patients who are potential source of infection.
3. Attend a mandatory in-service for the prevention of needlesticks.
4. Follow up for laboratory results and counseling.
5. Perform a thorough aseptic hand washing.
6. Wear a mask, gown and gloves while giving patient care.
7. Take unpaid leave until laboratory results are definitive.
8. Expect that the incident will be reported to the board of nursing.
9. Begin prophylactic drug therapy as prescribed.
10. Report to the occupational health nurse.
11. Fill out an incident report.

Instructions: Read the scenario on the left then circle or highlight each instruction that the charge nurse will give to the AP. **Select all that apply.**

PART 2

Common Health Scenarios

Answer Key for this chapter begins on p. 128

Answers

Common Health Scenarios

PART 2

1. **Ans: 3** Checking for residual is within the scope of practice for the LPN/LVN. A disadvantage of small-bore feeding tubes is that they are prone to clogging, and checking for residual can be difficult. If the tube gets clogged, it may have to be removed and reinserted. Evaluating nutritional status and monitoring for complications are the responsibility of the RN. Placing the patient in a supine position is incorrect. The head of the bed needs to be elevated 30° to 45° during feedings and for 30 to 60 minutes after the feeding to reduce the risk of aspiration. **Focus:** Supervision.

2. **Ans: 2** The AP can reinforce dietary and fluid restrictions after the RN has explained the information to the patient. Teaching the patient about what to expect is the RN's duty. An enema is not typically part of the bowel prep but might be ordered if the bowel is not empty or well visualized. The AP may administer enemas with special training and under certain circumstances, such as home care, but in this situation it is unlikely that this task would be delegated to the AP. Medication administration should be performed by the RN or LPN/LVN. **Focus:** Delegation.

3. **Ans: 3** The nurse monitors all laboratory results, but vomiting, nasogastric suction, and lavage (if it is ordered) can cause fluid and electrolyte imbalances. Fluid loss can cause hemoconcentration and artificially elevated levels for hematocrit, hemoglobin, and BUN. BUN is generally more affected by fluid loss than serum creatinine. The WBC count could be elevated because of stress, inflammation, or infection. **Focus:** Prioritization. **Test-Taking Tip:** Use concept-based learning to recognize that vomiting, suctioning, and lavage share a common effect: altering fluid and electrolyte balance.

4. **Ans: 4** A patient with a fractured femur is at risk for fat embolism, so a fat emulsion should be used with caution. TPN is commonly used for patients with GI obstruction, severe anorexia nervosa, and chronic diarrhea or vomiting. **Focus:** Prioritization.

5. **Ans: 2** Patients with short bowel syndrome have impaired fat absorption as a result of limited surface area. Formulas with high sodium content would not be prescribed for heart failure. High-protein formulas can contribute to dehydration if adequate water is not given. Modified carbohydrate content is prescribed for patients with chronic obstructive pulmonary disease when they require nutritional support. **Focus:** Prioritization.

6. **Ans: 4** A board-like abdomen with shoulder pain is a symptom of a perforation, which is the most lethal complication of PUD. A burning sensation is a typical report and can be controlled with medications. Projectile vomiting can signal an obstruction.

Coffee-ground emesis is typical of slower bleeding, and the patient will require diagnostic testing. **Focus:** Prioritization.

7. **Ans: 2** Body dysmorphic disorder is a preoccupation with an imagined physical defect. Corrective surgery can exacerbate this disorder when the patient continues to feel dissatisfied with the results. The other findings are criterion indicators for this treatment. **Focus:** Prioritization.

8. **Ans: 4** A fluctuating level of consciousness and mood swings are associated more with acute delirium, which could be caused by many things, such as electrolyte imbalances, sepsis, or medications. Information about the patient's baseline behavior is essential; however, based on knowledge of pathophysiology, the nurse knows that flat affect and rambling and repetitive speech, memory impairments, and disorientation to time are behaviors typically associated with chronic dementia. Lack of motivation and early morning awakening are associated with depression. **Focus:** Prioritization. **Test-Taking Tip:** A sudden change in the level of consciousness and mental status of a patient signals a need to conduct further assessment for an acute process. This question requires the ability to differentiate between acute and chronic disease processes and accompanying symptoms.

9. **Ans: 3** Reminding the patient to follow through on advice given by the nurse is an appropriate task for the AP. The RN should take responsibility for teaching rationale, discussing strategies for the treatment plan, and assessing patient concerns. **Focus:** Delegation.

10. **Ans: 1** *H. pylori* is frequently associated with PUD, and the organism can be detected through breath, blood, or stool. Esophagogastroduodenoscopy is the best test for PUD; however, it is considered an invasive procedure. A barium contrast study may be ordered for a patient who cannot undergo an endoscopy. A nuclear medicine scan may be ordered if gastrointestinal bleeding is present or to detect gastric emptying disorders. **Focus:** Prioritization.

11. **Ans: 1** The primary concern in the immediate postoperative period is the potential for airway complications. Elevating the head at least 30 degrees decreases the chance for aspiration and facilitates respiratory effort. The other options are also correct but will occur later in the postoperative period. **Focus:** Prioritization. **Test-Taking Tip:** The ABCs (airway, breathing, and circulation) underlie the priorities of care when the patient has an invasive procedure. You can use the concept of gas exchange to answer this question, even if you are not familiar with the specific details of the procedure.

12. **Ans: 3** During pregnancy, this medication is prescribed with caution and only if clearly needed. The health care provider must discuss the risk versus benefits with the patient and then decide to continue or discontinue the medication. Headache, fatigue, nausea, and diarrhea are common adverse effects of ledipasvir–sofosbuvir and should be reported if persistent or recurrent. **Focus:** Prioritization.

13. **Ans: 4** Nausea and vomiting are common after chemotherapy. Administration of antiemetics and fluid monitoring can be done by an LPN/LVN. The RN should perform the preoperative teaching for the glossectomy patient. Patients returning from surgery need extensive assessment. The patient with anorexia is showing signs of hypokalemia and is at risk for cardiac dysrhythmias. **Focus:** Assignment.

14. **Ans: 3** Smoking is associated with PUD. The other lifestyle modifications may be desirable, but the current evidence does not show strong linkage to the development of or recovery from PUD. **Focus:** Prioritization.

15. **Ans: 3** The LPN/LVN can offer valuable assistance in planning the interventions, but the RN has ultimate responsibility for the care plan. The LPN/LVN can delegate and assign tasks to APs; however, if the RN is the team leader, it is better if APs are not receiving instructions from multiple people. Obtaining equipment should be delegated to an AP. A physical therapist should set up specialized equipment. **Focus:** Assignment.

16. **Ans: 4** Showing the student how to insert the suppository meets both the immediate patient need and the student's learning need. The instructor can address the student's fears and long-term learning needs after he or she is aware of the incident. It is preferable that students express fears and learning needs. The other options will discourage the student's future disclosure of clinical limitations and need for additional training. **Focus:** Supervision, Assignment.

17. **Ans: 1** The nurse would remind the student that the container has to be hung at shoulder level. If the container is too low, the flow will be sluggish. If the container is below the entry site, the solution will flow retrograde. If the container is too high, the solution will flow too quickly and cause cramping. The other actions are correct. **Focus:** Supervision.

18. **Ans: 3** Disconnecting the tube from suction is an appropriate task to delegate, but the nurse must give specific instructions or verify that the AP knows how to do this task. Suction should be reconnected by the nurse so that correct pressure is checked. If the AP is permitted to reconnect the tube, the RN is still responsible for checking that the pressure setting is correct. During removal of the tube, there is a potential for aspiration, so the nurse should perform this task. If the tube is dislodged, the nurse should recheck placement before it is secured. **Focus:** Delegation.

19. **Ans: 3** The goal of bowel training is to establish a pattern that mimics normal defecation, and many people have the urge to defecate after a meal. If this is not successful, a suppository can be used to stimulate the urge. The use of incontinence briefs is embarrassing for the patient, and they must be changed frequently to prevent skin breakdown. Routine use of rectal tubes is not recommended because of the potential for damage to the mucosa and sphincter tone. **Focus:** Prioritization.

20. **Ans: 1** FMT is considered after the failure of medication therapy and after multiple reoccurrences. Vancomycin or fidaxomicin is the first-line therapy. Rifaximin is an adjunctive postvancomycin treatment regimen for patients with recurrent CDI. Previously, metronidazole was considered a first-line treatment; however, it is now used only when vancomycin or fidaxomicin are not an option for the patient. **Focus:** Prioritization.

21. **Ans: 4** Bisacodyl is a laxative and laxatives should not be administered to patients with undiagnosed abdominal pain, cramps, or nausea. Appendicitis, diverticulitis, ulcerative colitis, acute surgical abdomens, and bowel obstruction are also contraindications for laxative use. The other patients are receiving medications that are appropriate for their conditions. Omeprazole is a proton pump inhibitor that reduces stomach acid and relieves heartburn. Psyllium is a bulk-forming laxative that is used to treat constipation; the medication needs to be taken with a full glass of water. Polyethylene glycol-electrolyte solution is a laxative solution that is prescribed to prepare the colon for procedures, such as a colonoscopy. **Focus:** Prioritization.

22. **Ans: 2** Cimetidine is available over the counter and is used to relieve heartburn, acid indigestion, and sour stomach. **Focus:** Prioritization.

23. **Ans: 2, 5, 3, 7, 4, 1, 6** Stay calm and stay with the patient. Any increase in intra-abdominal pressure will worsen the evisceration; placement of the patient in a semi-Fowler position with knees flexed will decrease the strain on the wound site. (Note: If shock develops, the patient's head should be lowered.) Continuously monitor vital signs (particularly for a decrease in blood pressure or increase in pulse rate) while the charge nurse notifies the surgeon. An AP can obtain sterile supplies. Covering the site protects the tissue. Ultimately, the patient will need emergency surgery. **Focus:** Prioritization.

24. **Ans: 3** Right upper quadrant pain is a sign of hemorrhage or bile leakage. The ability to void should return within 6 hours postoperatively. Right shoulder pain is related to unabsorbed carbon dioxide and will be resolved by placing the patient in a Sims position. For the first several hours after surgery, output is not expected to equal input. **Focus:** Prioritization.

PART 2 Common Health Scenarios

25. **Ans: 3** The patient is taking the recommended dose of polyethylene glycol. Polyethylene glycol is used for the treatment of chronic constipation, so the nurse would assess the effect that the medication is having on bowel movements. Older adult patients generally have a greater risk for dehydration, fluid and electrolyte imbalances, and nutritional deficiencies so these would be included in routine assessment. Reviewing understanding of medications is always a good idea if the nurse has time. **Focus:** Prioritization.

26. **Ans: 1** The AP should use infection control precautions for the protection of self, employees, and other patients. Monitoring is an RN responsibility. APs can report valuable information; however, they are not responsible for detecting signs and symptoms that can be subtle or hard to detect, such as skin changes. Engaging patients in diversional activities is the ideal; however, it is rarely possible on a busy medical-surgical unit. **Focus:** Delegation.

27. **Ans: 1** Portal hypertension increases pressure in the venous system and contributes to the development of esophageal varices, which are very fragile. Straining increases thoracic or abdominal pressure, which can cause a sudden rupture of fragile blood vessels with massive hemorrhage. The patient could have fluid accumulation in the abdomen (ascites) that may be mild and hard to detect or severe enough to cause orthopnea. Patients will compensate for orthopnea by assuming a more upright position. This symptom warrants additional investigation. Dependent peripheral edema can also be observed but is less urgent. **Focus:** Prioritization. **Test-Taking Tip:** Generally respiratory issues are the priority; however, this question calls for knowledge of pathophysiology of cirrhosis and portal hypertension. Rupture with hemorrhage is the most serious complication.

28. **Ans: 2** Assisting with procedures for patients in stable condition with predictable outcomes is within the educational preparation of the LPN/LVN. Teaching the patient about self-care or pathophysiology and evaluating the outcome of interventions are responsibilities of the RN. **Focus:** Assignment.

29. **Ans: 1** Distention and rigidity can signal hemorrhage or peritonitis. The HCP may also decide that these symptoms require a medication to stimulate peristalsis. Absence of bowel sounds is expected within the first 24 to 48 hours. Nausea and vomiting are not uncommon and are usually self-limiting, and an as needed prescription for an antiemetic is usually part of the routine postoperative care. The NG tube should be assessed for displacement, and the correct position of the tube must be confirmed. The nurse then secures the tube as necessary. **Focus:** Prioritization.

30. **Ans: 1** Dronabinol (medical marijuana) is prescribed to treat nausea and vomiting. **Focus:** Supervision.

31. **Ans: 4** Diverticulitis can cause chronic or severe bleeding, so if there is no obvious blood in the stool, the stool may be tested for occult blood. A barium enema is not usually ordered because of the danger of perforation. Laxatives and ambulation increase intestinal motility and are to be avoided in the initial phase of treatment. If a barium enema, PRN laxative, or ambulation is prescribed, the nurse should check with the health care provider before delegating or assigning the intervention. **Focus:** Delegation.

32. **Ans: 3** The AP can take vital signs and report all of the values to the RN. In this case, all of the values are needed to detect trends. In other cases, the nurse may decide to give parameters for reporting. The RN should assess skin temperature and pain. The RN must also closely monitor the urine output, which is an indicator of perfusion and fluid status. In addition, red or pink urine can signal damage to the urinary system, transfusion reaction, or rhabdomyolysis. **Focus:** Delegation.

33. **Ans: 3** Coughing and an inability to speak or difficulty in speaking clearly suggests that the tube has been inserted into the trachea. The tube should be removed immediately. Bright red blood with clots indicates active bleeding; this should be immediately reported to the health care provider. Coffee-ground appearance of gastric contents indicates old blood; this finding should also be reported but is less urgent. Irritation of the throat and around the nares is commonly reported. Perform hygiene around the nares as needed; irritation of the throat usually subsides, but an anesthetic throat spray may offer some temporary relief. **Focus:** Prioritization.

34. **Ans: 1** Refeeding syndrome occurs when aggressive and rapid feeding results in fluid retention and heart failure. Electrolytes, especially phosphorus, should be monitored, and the patient should be observed for signs of fluid overload. Changes in bowel sounds, nausea, and distention may occur but are also appropriate for any patient with nutritional issues or for patients receiving enteral feedings. Observing for purging and water ingestion would be appropriate for a patient with an eating disorder. Changes in stool patterns may occur but are not related to refeeding syndrome. **Focus:** Prioritization.

35. **Ans: 3** All of these measures should be performed for total care of the patient; however, weighing the patient every day is considered the single best indicator of fluid volume. **Focus:** Prioritization. **Test-Taking Tip:** In studying for the NCLEX® Examination, don't neglect your fundamentals textbook. This question is based on fundamental knowledge of fluids and fluid management.

36. **Ans: 1** The maximum dose of magnesium hydroxide is given for bowel evacuation and cleansing. It is expected that the medication should take effect within 2 to 6 hours. **Focus:** Supervision.

37. **Ans: 3** If alcohol abuse has contributed to liver failure, a person's intent to continue alcohol consumption might be an exclusion for a liver transplant, so the

nurse should conduct an additional assessment about this comment. The comment about the difficulty in taking prescription medications should also be investigated because a true inability to follow the treatment regimen could exclude a patient from being on a transplant list (for any organ). **Focus:** Prioritization.

38. **Ans: 3** T-tubes should not be irrigated, aspirated, or clamped without specific directions from the health care provider. All of the other actions are appropriate in the care of this patient. **Focus:** Supervision.

39. **Ans: 3** Methylcellulose can cause esophageal obstruction if taken with insufficient amounts of fluid. Intestinal obstruction is also a possibility if the passage is slowed or impeded. The patient should be reminded that three times a day is the acceptable dose range. High fiber and a prompt response to urge to defecate should be encouraged to restore natural and normal bowel movements. **Focus:** Prioritization.

40. **Ans: 4** The nurse is likely to feel upset, even angry; however, ideally, the nurse focuses on the patient and tries to find a solution that allows the care to continue. Having a female witness in the room may reassure the patient that nothing untoward will happen. If the patient continues to express hostility and rejection, then the nurse could ask the charge nurse to reassign the patient. In cases of emergency, the nurse would acknowledge the patient's feelings but politely and firmly explain that the intervention can't be delayed. (e.g., "I see you are displeased, but this _____ is an emergency procedure.") All attempts and interventions should be documented. **Test-Taking Tip:** Stay current with trends in healthcare for patients who are LGBTQIA (lesbian, gay, bisexual, transgender, queer/questioning, intersex, asexual/allied.). Issues, interventions, and support for these patients also applies to colleagues and coworkers who are LGBTQIA. **Focus:** Prioritization.

41. **Ans: 2** The healthy liver breaks down ammonia, but in liver disease, the ammonia accumulates, and serum levels increase. Lactulose helps by enhancing intestinal excretion of ammonia. **Focus:** Prioritization.

42. **Ans: 1** Ibuprofen is a nonsteroidal anti-inflammatory drug (NSAID), and NSAIDs are thought to be one of the aggravating factors of PUD. Omeprazole, amoxicillin, and clarithromycin are used as a triple combination therapy for the treatment of PUD. **Focus:** Prioritization. **Test-Taking Tip:** NSAIDs are commonly prescribed and self-selected as over-the-counter medications; thus knowing the pharmacology, drug–drug interactions, and side effects are worthwhile for test taking purposes and clinical practice.

43. The patient is likely to report pain and tenderness over the right lower quadrant. Deep palpation should not be performed because of the possibility of rupture. If the medical diagnosis has been confirmed, palpation may be deferred because even light and gentle palpation may be very painful. **Focus:** Prioritization.

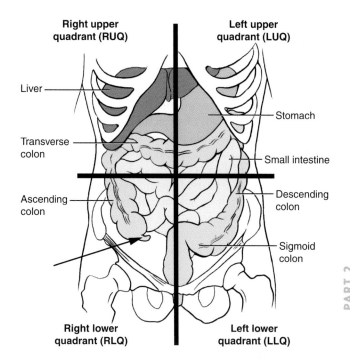

44. **Ans: 2, 3** The patient who had a cholecystectomy and the patient with pancreatitis will need frequent pain assessments and medications. Patients with copious diarrhea or vomiting may need contact isolation. *Clostridium difficile* is frequently identified in health care–acquired infections; contact isolation is usually ordered. Norovirus is highly contagious, and symptoms include abdominal pain, vomiting, and diarrhea. Patients with cancer receiving chemotherapy are at risk for immunosuppression and are likely to need protective isolation. If *methicillin-resistant Staphylococcus aureus* is suspected, the patient would be placed on contact precaution. **Focus:** Assignment.

45. **Ans: 1, 2, 3, 5, 6, 8, 9, 10** Facility policies will vary. For example, gloves, a gown, and an eye shield might be part of the protocol. (Note to student: You may see nurses only wearing gloves for NG tube insertion; this may or may not be a violation of facility policy.) The likelihood of exposure to blood or body fluids is increased by patient behaviors, such as pulling the tube out or thrashing movements, and by the nurse's skill level (e.g., unskilled attempts increase gagging, vomiting, coughing, and sneezing; repeated attempts increase saliva, tears, and mucus production). The patient's health history (e.g., tuberculosis or other respiratory disorders) may prompt the nurse to don a filter mask. The nurse may opt to wear shoe covers if the person has copious or projectile vomiting. The type of tube makes a difference because the larger bore tubes are more likely to trigger gagging, vomiting, and secretions. The purpose of the tube

is also a consideration. For example, if the person has been actively vomiting or very nauseated, the chance of vomiting during the insertion is higher than if the person has not been eating or drinking and needs the tube for feeding and hydration. If the PPE causes awkward movements, the user needs to practice the skill. Disregarding or removing gloves or the eye shield is not the solution. Lack of PPE is not a deciding factor; the supervisor is notified if adequate PPE is not available. **Focus:** Prioritization.

46 A. Ans: A **72-year-old** man living alone in **poor conditions** had **prolonged hospitalization** for a respiratory infection that was treated with **ciprofloxacin**. He was then transferred to a long-term care center. He uses over-the-counter (OTC) esomeprazole for heartburn. He has **"heart problems" but can't afford to go to the doctor**. The resident had **two episodes of watery diarrhea in the past hour**. Vital signs: **Temperature 100.3° F (37.9°C), Pulse 120 beats/min**, Respirations 24 breaths/min, **Blood Pressure 98/68 mmHg**, Oxygen Saturation 93% on room air. Assessment findings: Admission weight: 120 lbs. (54 kg), Admission height 5' 8" (172.7 cm). Alert and oriented. Breath sounds clear and equal bilaterally. Respirations even and unlabored. Skin is warm and **turgor is poor. Mucous membranes dry. Reports abdominal pain and cramping** that is partially relieved after a **diarrheal stool. Hyperactive bowel sounds and mild tenderness** x 4 quadrants. Reports **nausea and loss of appetite**. To bathroom during assessment for a **large watery bloody diarrheal stool**. Specimen obtained. Has **mild dizziness** but is able to ambulate with assistance.

The resident has several risk factors for CDI, which is the most common health-care related gastrointestinal (GI) illness in the United States. Older people have a higher risk because of changes in the GI system. Prolonged hospitalization, broad-spectrum antibiotics such as cephalosporins or fluoroquinolones (destroys normal GI flora) and weak immune system (underweight, living in poor conditions, unknown and untreated chronic health conditions) are risk factors. In addition, medications such as esomeprazole decrease the amount of acid produced in the stomach (stomach acid kills pathogens) so the risk is increased. The signs and symptoms of CDI include: large watery diarrheal stools which may have pus or blood, dehydration (poor skin turgor, dry mucous membranes, low blood pressure, mild dizziness), nausea, anorexia, abdominal pain and cramping, fever, and tachycardia. Focus: Prioritization.

46 B. Ans: 1, 3, 4, 5, 6, 7, 9 The nurse can instruct the AP to: measure intake and output, encourage sips of oral fluid, assist with ambulation, take and report vital signs, use fall precautions as directed, gather supplies and assist with hygiene. Assessment, calling the HCP and decision-making related to PRN medications cannot be delegated. The nurse would hold laxatives, stool softeners and antidiarrheal agents, because these medications may worsen CDI. **Focus:** Delegation.

47. Ans: 1, 4, 5, 9, 10, 11 The nurse supports the AP through the process of getting immediate and follow-up care. Immediate decontamination is appropriate because exposure time can affect the viral load. The occupational health nurse will direct the AP to get the appropriate laboratory tests, obtain prophylaxis within 72 hours (the sooner the better), file the correct forms, and follow up on results. The AP might be tempted to talk to patients who are potential sources of infection, but this is not appropriate, and any follow-up investigation is performed by the infection control nurse. A mandatory in-service might be warranted if an employee has repeated incidents of careless behavior. Using additional personal protective equipment is not necessary. Standard precautions are adequate. The AP would not need to take unpaid leave. The incident will not be reported to the board of nursing unless there are additional circumstances that impact the patient's well-being. **Focus:** Prioritization, Supervision.

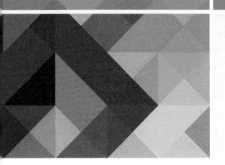

CHAPTER 13
Diabetes Mellitus

Questions

1. A patient with type 1 diabetes asks the nurse if he will ever be able to stop taking insulin. What is the nurse's best response?
   1. "When your sugar is controlled by use of exercise and diet, you may no longer need insulin."
   2. "Yes, because in time your pancreas will develop the ability to make insulin again."
   3. "No, your pancreas no longer makes insulin so you have to take insulin on a daily basis."
   4. "It may be possible that you can take oral antiglycemics most days and insulin only on sick days."

2. The nurse is caring for an older patient with type 1 diabetes and diabetic retinopathy. What is the nurse's **priority** concern for assessing this patient?
   1. Assess ability to measure and inject insulin and to monitor blood glucose levels.
   2. Assess for damage to motor fibers, which can result in muscle weakness.
   3. Assess which modifiable risk factors can be reduced.
   4. Assess for albuminuria, which may indicate kidney disease.

3. An older patient with type 2 diabetes has cardiovascular autonomic neuropathy (CAN). Which instruction would the nurse provide for the assistive personnel (AP) assisting the patient with morning care?
   1. Provide a complete bed bath for this patient.
   2. Sit the patient up slowly on the side of the bed before standing.
   3. Only let the patient wash his or her face and brush his or her teeth.
   4. Be sure to provide rest periods between activities.

4. The nurse is preparing to review a teaching plan for a patient with type 2 diabetes mellitus. To determine the patient's level of compliance with his prescribed diabetic regimen, which value would the nurse be sure to review?
   1. Fasting glucose level
   2. Oral glucose tolerance test results
   3. Glycosylated hemoglobin (HgbA$_{1c}$) level
   4. Fingerstick glucose findings for 24 hours

5. A patient has newly diagnosed type 2 diabetes. Which task should the RN delegate to an experienced assistive personnel (AP)?
   1. Arranging a consult with the dietitian
   2. Assessing the patient's insulin injection technique
   3. Teaching the patient to use a glucometer to monitor glucose at home
   4. Checking the patient's glucose level before each meal

6. A patient with newly diagnosed diabetes has peripheral neuropathy. Which key points should the nurse include in the teaching plan for this patient? **Select all that apply.**
   1. "Clean and inspect your feet every day."
   2. "Be sure that your shoes fit properly."
   3. "Nylon socks are best to prevent friction on your toes from shoes."
   4. "Only a podiatrist should trim your toenails."
   5. "Report any nonhealing skin breaks to your health care provider (HCP)."
   6. "Use a thermometer to check the temperature of water before taking a bath."

7. An LPN/LVN is assigned to perform assessments on two patients with diabetes. Assessments reveal all of these findings. Which finding would the RN instruct the LPN/LVN to report immediately?
   1. Fingerstick glucose reading of 185 mg/dL (10.3 mmol/L)
   2. Numbness and tingling in both feet
   3. Profuse perspiration
   4. Bunion on the left great toe

8. The plan of care for a patient with diabetes includes all of these interventions. Which intervention should the nurse delegate to assistive personnel (AP)?
   1. Reminding the patient to put on well-fitting shoes before ambulating
   2. Discussing community resources for diabetic outpatient care
   3. Teaching the patient to perform daily foot inspections
   4. Assessing the patient's technique for drawing insulin into a syringe

9. A 58-year-old patient with type 2 diabetes was admitted to the acute care unit with a diagnosis of chronic obstructive pulmonary disease (COPD) exacerbation. When the RN prepares a care plan for this patient, what would he or she be sure to include? **Select all that apply.**
   1. Fingerstick blood glucose checks before meals and at bedtime
   2. Sliding-scale insulin dosing as prescribed
   3. Bed rest until the COPD exacerbation is resolved
   4. Teaching about the Atkins diet for weight loss
   5. Demonstration of the components of foot care
   6. Discussing the relationship between illness and glucose levels

10. An assistive personnel (AP) tells the nurse that while assisting with the morning care of a postoperative patient with type 2 diabetes who has been given insulin, the patient asked if she will always need to take insulin now. What is the RN's **priority** for teaching the patient?
    1. Explain to the patient that she is now considered to have type 1 diabetes.
    2. Tell the patient to monitor fingerstick glucose level every 4 hours after discharge.
    3. Teach the patient that a person with type 2 diabetes does not always need insulin.
    4. Discuss the relationship between illness and increased glucose levels.

11. An LPN/LVN is assigned to administer a rapid-acting insulin (lispro) to a patient with type 1 diabetes. What essential information would the RN be sure to tell the LPN/LVN?
    1. Give this insulin when the food tray has been delivered and the patient is ready to eat.
    2. Only give this insulin when the fingerstick glucose reading is above 200 mg/dL (11.1 mmol/L).
    3. This insulin mimics the basal glucose control of the pancreas.
    4. Lispro insulin should be given subcutaneously at least 20 to 30 minutes before eating.

12. In the care of a patient with type 2 diabetes, which actions should the nurse delegate to an assistive personnel (AP)? **Select all that apply.**
    1. Providing the patient with extra packets of artificial sweetener for coffee
    2. Assessing how well the patient's shoes fit
    3. Recording the liquid intake from the patient's breakfast tray
    4. Teaching the patient what to do if dizziness or lightheadedness occurs
    5. Checking and recording the patient's blood pressure
    6. Assisting the patient to ambulate to the bathroom

13. In the emergency department, during the initial assessment of a newly admitted patient with diabetes, the nurse discovers all of these findings. Which finding should be reported to the health care provider immediately?
    1. Hammer toe of the left second metatarsophalangeal joint
    2. Rapid respiratory rate with deep inspirations
    3. Numbness and tingling bilaterally in the feet and hands
    4. Decreased sensitivity and swelling of the abdomen

14. The nurse is caring for a patient with diabetes who is developing diabetic ketoacidosis (DKA). Which task delegation or assignment is **most** appropriate?
    1. Ask the unit clerk to page the health care provider (HCP) to come to the unit.
    2. Ask the LPN/LVN to administer IV push insulin according to a sliding scale.
    3. Ask the assistive personnel (AP) to hang a new bag of normal saline.
    4. Ask the AP to get the patient a cup (236 mL) of orange juice.

15. The RN is serving as preceptor to a newly graduated nurse who has recently passed the RN licensure (NCLEX®) examination. The new nurse has only been on the unit for 2 days. Which patient should be assigned to the newly graduated nurse?
    1. A 68-year-old patient with diabetes who is showing signs of hyperglycemia
    2. A 58-year-old patient with diabetes who has cellulitis of the left ankle
    3. A 49-year-old patient with diabetes who just returned from the postanesthesia care unit after a below-knee amputation
    4. A 72-year-old patient with diabetes who has diabetic ketoacidosis and is receiving IV insulin

16. A patient with diabetes has hot, dry skin; rapid and deep respirations; and a fruity odor to his breath. The charge nurse observes a newly graduated RN performing all of the following patient tasks. Which action requires that the charge nurse intervene immediately?
    1. Checking the patient's fingerstick glucose level
    2. Encouraging the patient to drink orange juice
    3. Checking the patient's order for sliding-scale insulin dosing
    4. Assessing the patient's vital signs every 15 minutes

17. A patient has newly diagnosed type 2 diabetes. Which action should the RN assign to an LPN/LVN rather than an experienced assistive personnel (AP)?
    1. Measuring the patient's vital signs every shift
    2. Checking the patient's glucose level before each meal
    3. Administering subcutaneous insulin on a sliding scale as needed
    4. Assisting the patient with morning care

18. A patient with type 1 diabetes reports feeling dizzy. What should the nurse do **first**?
    1. Check the patient's blood pressure.
    2. Give the patient some orange juice.
    3. Give the patient's morning dose of insulin.
    4. Use a glucometer to check the patient's glucose level.

19. The nurse is responsible for the care of a patient with diabetes who is unable to swallow, is unconscious and seizing, and has a blood glucose level of less than 20 mg/dL (1.1 mmol/L). Which actions are the **most** appropriate responses for this patient at this time? **Select all that apply.**
    1. Check the chart for the patient's most recent A_{1c} level.
    2. Give glucagon 1 mg subcutaneously or intramuscularly (IM).
    3. Repeat the dose of glucagon in 10 minutes if the patient remains unconscious.
    4. Apply aspiration precautions because glucagon can cause vomiting.
    5. Give the patient an oral simple sugar or snack.
    6. Notify the health care provider (HCP) immediately.

20. While working in the diabetes clinic, the RN obtains the following information about an 8-year-old patient with type 1 diabetes. Which finding is **most** important to address when planning child and parent education?
    1. Most recent hemoglobin A_{1c} level of 7.8%
    2. Many questions about diet choices from the parents
    3. Child's participation in soccer practice after school 2 days a week
    4. Morning preprandial glucose range of 55 to 70 mg/dL (3.1 to 3.9 mmol/L)

21. Which actions can the school nurse delegate to an experienced assistive personnel (AP) who is working with a 7-year-old child with type 1 diabetes in an elementary school? **Select all that apply.**
    1. Obtaining information about the child's usual insulin use from the parents
    2. Administering oral glucose tablets when the blood glucose level falls below 60 mg/dL (3.3 mmol/L)
    3. Teaching the child about what foods have high carbohydrate levels
    4. Obtaining blood glucose readings using the child's blood glucose monitor
    5. Reminding the child to have a snack after the physical education class
    6. Assessing the child's knowledge level about his or her type 1 diabetes

22. While the RN is performing an admission assessment on a patient with type 2 diabetes, the patient states that he routinely drinks three beers a day. What is the nurse's **priority** follow-up question at this time?
    1. "Do you have any days when you do not drink?"
    2. "When during the day do you drink your beers?"
    3. "Do you drink any other forms of alcohol?"
    4. "Have you ever had a lipid profile completed?"

23. The assistive personnel reports to the RN that a patient with type 1 diabetes has a question about exercise. What important points would the RN be sure to teach this patient? **Select all that apply.**
    1. Exercise guidelines are based on blood glucose and urine ketone levels.
    2. Be sure to test your blood glucose only after exercising.
    3. You can exercise vigorously if your blood glucose is between 100 and 250 mg/dL (5.6 and 13.9 mmol/L).
    4. Exercise will help resolve the presence of ketones in your urine.
    5. A 5- to 10-minute warm-up and cool-down period should be included in your exercise.
    6. For unplanned exercise, increased intake of carbohydrates is usually needed.

24. The experienced assistive personnel (AP) has been delegated to take vital signs and check fingerstick glucose on a postoperative patient with diabetes. Which vital sign change would the RN instruct the AP to report immediately?
    1. Blood pressure increase from 132/80 to 138/84 mm Hg
    2. Temperature increase from 98.4°F to 99°F (36.9°C to 37.2°C)
    3. Respiratory rate increase from 18 to 22 breaths/min
    4. Glucose increase from 190 to 236 mg/dL (10.6 to 13.1 mmol/L)

 Answer Key for this chapter begins on p. 138

25. The RN is the preceptor for a senior nursing student who will teach a patient with diabetes about self-care during sick days. For which statement by the student must the RN intervene?
    1. "When you are sick, be sure to monitor your blood glucose at least every 4 hours."
    2. "Test your urine for ketones whenever your blood glucose level is less than 240 mg/dL (13.3 mmol/L)."
    3. "To prevent dehydration, drink 8 ounces (236 mL) of sugar-free liquid every hour while you are awake."
    4. "Continue to eat your meals and snacks at the usual times."

26. The nurse is caring for an 81-year-old adult with type 2 diabetes, hypertension, and peripheral vascular disease. Which admission assessment findings increase the patient's risk for development of hyperglycemic-hyperosmolar syndrome (HHS)? **Select all that apply.**
    1. Hydrochlorothiazide prescribed to control blood pressure
    2. Weight gain of 6 lb (2.7 kg) over the past month
    3. Avoids consuming liquids in the evening
    4. Blood pressure of 168/94 mm Hg
    5. Urine output of 50 to 75 mL/hr
    6. Glucose greater than 600 mg/dL (33.3 mmol/L)

27. The RN is orienting a newly graduated nurse who is providing diabetes education for a patient about insulin injection. For which teaching statement by the new nurse must the RN intervene?
    1. "To prevent lipohypertrophy, be sure to rotate injection sites from the abdomen to the thighs."
    2. "To correctly inject the insulin, lightly grasp a fold of skin and inject at a 90-degree angle."
    3. "Always draw your regular insulin into the syringe first before your NPH (neutral protamine Hagedorn) insulin."
    4. "Avoid injecting the insulin into scarred sites because those areas slow the absorption rate of insulin."

28. The patient with type 2 diabetes has a health care provider prescription of NPO status for a cardiac catheterization. An LPN/LVN who is assigned to administer medications to this patient asks the supervising RN whether the patient should receive his prescribed repaglinide. What is the RN's **best** response?
    1. "Yes, because this drug will increase the patient's insulin secretion and prevent hyperglycemia."
    2. "No, because this drug may cause the patient to experience gastrointestinal symptoms such as nausea."
    3. "No, because this drug should be given 1 to 30 minutes before meals and the patient is NPO."
    4. "Yes, because this drug should be taken three times a day whether the patient eats or not."

29. The RN is caring for a patient with diabetes admitted with hypoglycemia that occurred at home. Which teaching points for treatment of hypoglycemia at home would the nurse include in a teaching plan for the patient and family before discharge? **Select all that apply.**
    1. Signs and symptoms of hypoglycemia include hunger, irritability, weakness, headache, and blood glucose less than 60 mg/dL (3.3 mmol/L).
    2. Treat hypoglycemia with 4 to 8 g of carbohydrates such as glucose tablets or 1/4 cup (60 mL) of fruit juice.
    3. Retest blood glucose in 30 minutes.
    4. Repeat the carbohydrate treatment if the symptoms do not resolve.
    5. Eat a small snack of carbohydrates and protein if the next meal is more than an hour away.
    6. If the patient has severe hypoglycemia, does not respond to treatment, and is unconscious, transport to the emergency department (ED).

30. The nurse is evaluating a patient with diabetes for foot risk category. The patient lacks protective sensation and shows evidence of peripheral vascular disease. According to the American Diabetes Association (ADA), which foot risk category **best** fits this patient?
    1. Risk category 0
    2. Risk category 1
    3. Risk category 2
    4. Risk category 3

31. The nurse is preparing a teaching plan for a patient with type 2 diabetes who has been prescribed albiglutide. Which key points would the nurse include? **Select all that apply.**
    1. The drug works in the intestine in response to food intake and acts with insulin for glucose regulation.
    2. This drug increases the cellular utilization of glucose, which lowers blood glucose levels.
    3. This drug is used with diet and exercise to improve glycemic control in adults with type 2 diabetes.
    4. The drug is an oral insulin that should be given only when the patient has something to eat immediately available.
    5. Albiglutide is administered by the subcutaneous route once a week.
    6. Albiglutide should be given with caution for a patient with a history of pancreatic problems.

32. The nurse is assessing a newly admitted older adult with diabetes. Assessment reveals an abnormal appearance of the feet (see the figure below). The nurse recognizes this as which deformity?

1. Claw toe deformity
2. Hammer toe deformity
3. Charcot foot deformity
4. Hypertrophic ungula labium deformity

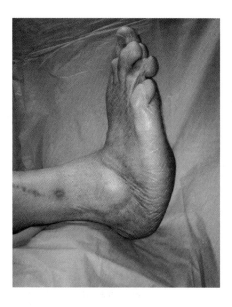

33. The critical care nurse is to start an IV insulin drip on a patient with type 2 diabetes who was admitted with a diagnosis of hyperosmolar hyperglycemic state. The patient weighs 178 lbs. Serum glucose is 600 mg/dL (33.3 mmol/L). The concentration of the drip is 250 units regular insulin in 250 mL normal saline. The health care provider prescribes an initial IV bolus of 0.15 unit per Kg to be followed by a continuous IV drip of 0.1 unit per Kg per hour. How much insulin would the nurse give the patient for the bolus? At what rate in mL/hr would the nurse set the IV pump for the continuous drip?

Bolus_____

Continuous IV _____

34. Extended Multiple Response _____
Case Study and Question

The nurse is providing diabetic teaching for an 18-year-old patient with newly diagnosed type 1 diabetes.

Vital signs:
Temperature 98.7°F (37.06°C)
Pulse 98 beats/min
Respirations 27 breaths/min
Blood Pressure 168/94 mmHg

Which key information would the nurse be sure to include in the teaching plan for this patient?

Instructions: Read the case study on the left and circle or highlight the numbers that best answer the question. **Select all that apply.**
1. Fingerstick glucose monitoring
2. Insulin injection
3. Types of oral hypoglycemic drugs
4. Signs of hypoglycemia and hyperglycemia
5. Avoidance of fast foods and carbohydrates
6. Need for daily foot care
7. Relationship of mealtime and action of insulin
8. Sick day procedures

Answer Key for this chapter begins on p. 138

Answers

1. **Ans: 3** The patient is a type 1 diabetic. These patients no longer make their own insulin and require an external injectable form of insulin. The other three statements are more appropriate to patients with type 2 diabetes. **Focus:** Prioritization.

2. **Ans: 1** The older patient with diabetic retinopathy also has general age-related vision changes, and the ability to perform self-care may be seriously affected. He or she may have blurred vision, distorted central vision, fluctuating vision, loss of color perception, and mobility problems resulting from loss of depth perception. When a patient has visual changes, it is especially important to assess his or her ability to measure and inject insulin and to monitor blood glucose levels to determine if adaptive devices are needed to assist in self-management. The other options are important but are not specific to diabetic retinopathy. **Focus:** Prioritization.

3. **Ans: 2** CAN affects sympathetic and parasympathetic nerves of the heart and blood vessels. It may lead to orthostatic (postural) hypotension and syncope (brief loss of consciousness on standing) caused by failure of the heart and arteries to respond to position changes by increasing heart rate and vascular tone. The nurse should be sure to instruct the AP to have the patient change positions slowly when moving from lying to sitting and standing. **Focus:** Supervision, Delegation.

4. **Ans: 3** The higher the blood glucose level is over time, the more glycosylated the hemoglobin becomes. The HgbA$_{1c}$ level is a good indicator of the average blood glucose level over the previous 120 days. Fasting glucose and oral glucose tolerance tests are important diagnostic tools. Fingerstick blood glucose monitoring provides information that allows for the adjustment of the patient's therapeutic regimen. **Focus:** Prioritization.

5. **Ans: 4** The experienced AP would have been taught to perform tasks such as checking pulse oximetry and glucose checks, and these actions would be part of his or her scope of practice. The RN would be responsible for ensuring that the AP had mastered this skill. Arranging for a consult with the dietitian is appropriate for the unit clerk. Teaching and assessing require additional education and should be carried out by licensed nurses. **Focus:** Delegation, Supervision, Assignment.

6. **Ans: 1, 2, 5, 6** Sensory alterations are the major cause of foot complications in patients with diabetes, and patients should be taught to examine their feet on a daily basis. Properly fitted shoes protect the patient from foot complications. Broken skin increases the risk of infection. Cotton socks are recommended to absorb moisture. Using a bath thermometer can prevent burn injuries. Patients, family, or HCPs may trim toenails. **Focus:** Prioritization. **Test-Taking Tip:** When caring for patients with diabetes, the nurse must be knowledgeable about safety issues with the potential for injuries to these patients. A key nursing role is patient teaching regarding these concerns so patients can perform protective interventions in the home to prevent injuries.

7. **Ans: 3** Profuse perspiration is a symptom of hypoglycemia, a complication of diabetes that requires urgent treatment. A glucose level of 185 mg/dL (10.3 mmol/L) will need coverage with sliding-scale insulin, but this is not urgent. Numbness and tingling, as well as bunions, are related to the chronic nature of diabetes and are not urgent problems. **Focus:** Prioritization.

8. **Ans: 1** Reminding the patient to put on well-fitting shoes (after the nurse has taught the patient about the importance of this action) is part of assisting with activities of daily living and is within the education and scope of practice of the AP. It is a safety measure that can prevent injury. Discussing community resources, teaching, and assessing require a higher level of education and are appropriate to the scope of practice of licensed nurses. **Focus:** Delegation.

9. **Ans: 1, 2, 5, 6** When a patient with diabetes is ill, glucose levels become elevated and administration of insulin may be necessary. Administration of sliding-scale insulin is guided by fingerstick blood glucose checks. Teaching or reviewing the components of proper foot care is always a good idea with a patient with diabetes. Bed rest is not necessary, and glucose levels may be better controlled when a patient is more active. The Atkins diet recommends decreasing the consumption of carbohydrates and is not a good diet for patient with diabetes. **Focus:** Prioritization.

10. **Ans: 4** When a patient with diabetes is ill or has surgery, glucose levels become elevated and administration of insulin may be necessary. This is a temporary change that usually resolves with recovery from the illness or surgery. Option 3 is correct but does not explain why the patient may currently need insulin. The patient does not have type 1 diabetes, and fingerstick glucose checks are usually prescribed for before meals and at bedtime. **Focus:** Prioritization.

11. **Ans: 1** The onset of action for a rapid-acting insulin such as lispro is within minutes, so it should be given only when the patient has food and is ready to eat. Because of this, rapid-acting insulin is sometimes called "see food" insulin. Options 2, 3, and 4 are incorrect with regard to rapid-acting insulin. Option 2 is

incorrect with regard to all forms of insulin. Long-acting insulins mimic the action of the pancreas. Regular insulin should be given 20 to 30 minutes before a patient eats. **Focus:** Assignment, Supervision.

12. **Ans: 1, 3, 5, 6** Giving the patient extra sweetener, recording oral intake, assisting with ambulation, and checking blood pressure are all within the scope of practice of the AP. Assessing shoe fit and patient teaching are within the professional nurse's scope of practice. **Focus:** Delegation.

13. **Ans: 2** Rapid, deep respirations (Kussmaul respirations) are symptomatic of diabetic ketoacidosis. Hammer toe, as well as numbness and tingling, are chronic complications associated with diabetes. Decreased sensitivity and swelling (lipohypertrophy) occur at a site of repeated insulin injections, and treatment involves teaching the patient to rotate injection sites within one anatomic site. **Focus:** Prioritization.

14. **Ans: 1** The nurse should not leave the patient. The scope of the unit clerk's job includes calling and paging HCPs. LPNs/LVNs generally do not administer IV push medication, although in some states, with additional training, this may be done. (Be sure to check the scope of practice in your specific state.) IV fluid administration is not within the scope of practice of APs. Patients with DKA already have a high glucose level and do not need orange juice. **Focus:** Delegation, Supervision, Assignment.

15. **Ans: 2** The new nurse is very early in orientation to the unit. Appropriate patient assignments at this time include patients whose conditions are stable and not complex. Patients 1, 3, and 4 are more complex and will benefit from care by a nurse experienced in the care of patients with diabetes. **Focus:** Assignment. **Test-Taking Tip:** For nurses new to a unit, always assign patients who are the most stable and least complex.

16. **Ans: 2** The signs and symptoms the patient is exhibiting are consistent with hyperglycemia. The RN should not give the patient additional glucose. All of the other interventions are appropriate for this patient. The RN should also notify the health care provider at this time. **Focus:** Prioritization.

17. **Ans: 3** The AP's scope of practice includes checking vital signs and assisting with morning care. Experienced APs with special training can check the patient's glucose level before meals and at bedtime. It is not within the AP's scope of practice to administer medications, but this is within the scope of practice of the LPN/LVN. **Focus:** Assignment.

18. **Ans: 4** Before orange juice or insulin is given, the patient's blood glucose level should be checked. Checking blood pressure is a good idea but is not the first action the nurse should take. **Focus:** Prioritization.

19. **Ans: 2, 3, 4, 6** This patient's manifestations suggest severe hypoglycemia. Essential actions at this time include notifying the HCP immediately and giving glucagon 1 mg subcutaneously or IM. Glucagon is the main counterregulatory hormone to insulin and is used as first-line therapy for severe hypoglycemia in patients with diabetes. The dose of glucagon is repeated after 10 minutes if the patient remains unconscious. Aspiration precautions are important because this drug can cause vomiting. Checking the patient's A_{1c} level is not important at this time. Offering oral glucose or a snack when a patient is unable to swallow or unconscious is inappropriate. **Focus:** Prioritization.

20. **Ans: 4** The low morning fasting blood glucose level indicates possible nocturnal hypoglycemia. Research indicates that it is important to avoid hypoglycemic episodes in pediatric patients because of the risk for permanent neurologic damage and adverse developmental outcomes. Although a lower hemoglobin A_{1c} might be desirable, the upper limit for hemoglobin A_{1c} levels ranges from 7.5% to 8.5% in pediatric patients. The parents' questions about diet and the child's activity level should also be addressed, but the most urgent consideration is education about the need to avoid hypoglycemia. **Focus:** Prioritization.

21. **Ans: 2, 4, 5** National guidelines published by the American Diabetes Association indicate that administering emergency treatment for hypoglycemia (e.g., glucose tablets), obtaining blood glucose readings, and reminding children about content they have already been taught by licensed caregivers are appropriate tasks for non–health care professional personnel such as teachers, paraprofessionals, and APs. Assessments and education require more specialized education and scope of practice and should be done by the school nurse. **Focus:** Delegation.

22. **Ans: 2** Alcohol has the potential for causing alcohol-induced hypoglycemia. It is important to know when the patient drinks alcohol and to teach the patient to ingest it shortly after meals to prevent this complication. The other questions are important but not urgent. The lipid profile question is important because alcohol can raise plasma triglycerides but is not as urgent as the potential for hypoglycemia. **Focus:** Prioritization.

23. **Ans: 1, 3, 5, 6** Guidelines for exercise are based on blood glucose and urine ketone levels. Patients should test blood glucose before, during, and after exercise to be sure that it is safe to exercise. When ketones are present in urine, the patient should not exercise because ketones indicate that current insulin levels are not adequate. Vigorous exercise is permitted in patients with type 1 diabetes if glucose levels are between 100 and 250 mg/dL (5.6 and 13.9 mmol/L). Warm-up and cool-down should be included in exercise to gradually increase and decrease the heart rate. For planned exercise, reduction in insulin dosage is used for hypoglycemia prevention. For unplanned exercise, intake of additional carbohydrates is usually needed. **Focus:** Prioritization.

24. **Ans: 4** An unexpected rise in blood glucose is associated with increased mortality and morbidity after surgical procedures. American Diabetes Association guidelines recommend insulin protocols to maintain blood glucose levels between 140 and 180 mg/dL (7.8 and 10 mmol/L). Also, unexpected rises in blood glucose values may indicate wound infection. Options 1, 2, and 3 reflect small changes and should be monitored but are not as urgent as the increase in glucose. **Focus:** Delegation, Supervision, Prioritization.

25. **Ans: 2** Urine ketone testing should be done whenever a patient's blood glucose is greater than 240 mg/dL (13.3 mmol/L). All of the other teaching points are appropriate "sick day rules." For dehydration, teaching should also include that if the patient's blood glucose is lower than the target range, he or she should drink fluids containing sugar. **Focus:** Supervision, Delegation.

26. **Ans: 1, 3, 6** HHS often occurs in older adults with type 2 diabetes. Risk factors include taking diuretics and inadequate fluid intake. Serum glucose is greater than 600 mg/dL (33.3 mmol/L). Weight loss (not weight gain) would be a symptom. Although the patient's blood pressure is high, this is not a risk factor. A urine output of 50 to 75 mL/hr is adequate. **Focus:** Prioritization.

27. **Ans: 1** Although it is important to rotate injection sites for insulin, it is preferred that the injection sites be rotated within one anatomic site (e.g., the abdomen) to prevent day-to-day changes in the absorption rate of the insulin. All of the other teaching points are appropriate. **Focus:** Supervision, Prioritization.

28. **Ans: 3** Repaglinide is a meglitinide analog drug and should not be given. It is a short-acting agent used to prevent postmeal blood glucose elevation. It should be given within 1 to 30 minutes before meals and can cause hypoglycemia shortly after dosing if a meal is delayed or omitted. **Focus:** Supervision, Assignment, Prioritization.

29. **Ans: 1, 4, 5, 6** The manifestations listed in option 1 are correct. The symptoms should be treated with carbohydrates, but 10 to 15 g (not 4 to 8 g). Glucose should be retested at 15 minutes; 30 minutes is too long to wait. Options 4 and 5 are correct. When a patient has severe hypoglycemia, does not respond to administration of glucagon, and remains unconscious, he or she should be transported to the ED and the health care provider should be notified. **Focus:** Prioritization.

30. **Ans: 3** The ADA's foot risk categories are category 0 (has protective sensation, has no evidence of peripheral vascular disease, has no evidence of foot deformity), category 1 (does not have protective sensation and may have evidence of foot deformity), category 2 (does not have protective sensation and has evidence of peripheral vascular disease), and category 3 (has history of ulcer or amputation). **Focus:** Prioritization.

31. **Ans: 1, 3, 5** Albiglutide is an incretin mimetic. These drugs work like the natural "gut" hormones, glucagon-like peptide-1 (GLP-1) and glucose-dependent insulinotropic polypeptide, that are released by the intestine in response to food intake and act with insulin for glucose regulation. They are used in addition to diet and exercise to improve glycemic control in adults with type 2 diabetes. Albiglutide is administered subcutaneously once a week. **Focus:** Prioritization.

32. **Ans: 3** Charcot foot is a diabetic foot deformity. The foot is warm, swollen, and painful. Walking collapses the arch, shortens the foot, and gives the sole of the foot a "rocker bottom" shape. **Focus:** Prioritization.

33. **Ans: 12.1 units; 8 mL/hr.** Bolus 12.1 units -178 lb equals 80.7 Kg. 80.7 Kg X 0.15 units equals 12.1 units. Continuous IV drip 8 mL/hr - 0.1 unit X 80.7 Kg equals 8.07 mL/hr (round down to 8 mL/hr). **Focus:** Prioritization.

34. **Ans: 1, 2, 4, 6, 7, 8** The patient is type 1 diabetic and insulin dependent. Carbohydrates should not be avoided; however, teaching should include which type of carbohydrates and how much should be consumed. The other focus areas are appropriate to patient teaching for type 1 diabetes. Remember that there are additional important teaching points that should also be covered (e.g., exercise, complications, and pathophysiology). **Focus:** Prioritization.

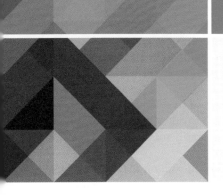

CHAPTER 14

Other Endocrine Problems

Questions

1. The RN is serving as preceptor for a senior nursing student who is assessing an endocrine patient. For which action must the nurse intervene immediately?
   1. Student nurse observes patient skin for areas of pigment loss or excess.
   2. Student nurse asks patient about slower than normal healing processes.
   3. Student nurse auscultates patient's chest to assess heart rate and rhythm.
   4. Student nurse vigorously palpates patient's thyroid while standing behind him.

2. The nurse is caring for a 25-year-old patient admitted to the acute care unit with an intense thirst and dilute, excessive straw-colored urine output (up to 15 L/day). What does the nurse suspect?
   1. Type 2 diabetes
   2. Diabetes insipidus (DI)
   3. Cushing disease
   4. Addison disease

3. The nurse is providing care for a male patient with hypogonadotropin who is receiving sex steroid replacement therapy with testosterone. Which changes indicate to the nurse that therapy is successful? **Select all that apply.**
   1. Decreased facial hair
   2. Increased libido
   3. Decreased bone size
   4. Increased muscle mass
   5. Increased axillary hair growth
   6. Increased breast tissue

4. A patient is admitted to the medical unit with possible Graves disease (hyperthyroidism). Which assessment finding by the nurse supports this diagnosis?
   1. Periorbital edema
   2. Bradycardia
   3. Exophthalmos
   4. Hoarse voice

5. Which change in vital signs for a patient with hyperthyroidism would the nurse instruct the assistive personnel (AP) to report immediately?
   1. Rapid heart rate
   2. Decreased systolic blood pressure
   3. Increased respiratory rate
   4. Decreased oral temperature

6. For a patient with hyperthyroidism, which task should the nurse delegate to an experienced assistive personnel (AP)?
   1. Instructing the patient to report any occurrence of palpitations, dyspnea, vertigo, or chest pain
   2. Monitoring the apical pulse, blood pressure, and temperature every 4 hours
   3. Drawing blood to measure levels of thyroid-stimulating hormone, triiodothyronine, and thyroxine
   4. Teaching the patient about side effects of the drug propylthiouracil

7. As the shift begins, the nurse is assigned to care for the following patients. Which patient should the nurse assess **first**?
   1. A 38-year-old patient with Graves disease and a heart rate of 94 beats/min
   2. A 63-year-old patient with type 2 diabetes and a fingerstick glucose level of 137 mg/dL (7.6 mmol/L)
   3. A 58-year-old patient with hypothyroidism and a heart rate of 48 beats/min
   4. A 49-year-old patient with Cushing disease and dependent edema rated as + 1

8. A patient is hospitalized with adrenocortical insufficiency. Which nursing activity should the nurse delegate to assistive personnel (AP)?
   1. Reminding the patient to change positions slowly
   2. Assessing the patient for muscle weakness
   3. Teaching the patient how to collect a 24-hour urine sample
   4. Revising the patient's nursing plan of care

9. Assessment findings for a patient with Cushing disease include all of the following. For which finding would the nurse notify the health care provider immediately?
   1. Purple striae present on the abdomen and thighs
   2. Weight gain of 1 lb (0.5 kg) since the previous day
   3. Dependent edema rated as + 1 in the ankles and calves
   4. Crackles bilaterally in the lower lobes of the lungs

10. The nurse is preparing to discharge a patient with hyperpituitarism caused by a benign pituitary tumor. The patient has been prescribed the drug bromocriptine. Which key points would the nurse teach the patient about this drug? **Select all that apply.**
    1. Take this drug with a meal or snack to avoid gastrointestinal (GI) symptoms.
    2. Side effects of bromocriptine include severe fatigue and reflux after meals.
    3. Seek medical care if you experience chest pain or dizziness while taking this drug.
    4. If the drug causes headaches, you can take over-the-counter acetaminophen.
    5. Treatment starts with a high dose, which is gradually lowered.
    6. The purpose of bromocriptine is to shrink your pituitary gland to normal size.

11. A patient with pheochromocytoma underwent surgery to remove his adrenal glands. Which nursing intervention should the nurse delegate to an assistive personnel (AP)?
    1. Revising the nursing care plan to include strategies to provide a calm and restful environment postoperatively
    2. Instructing the patient to avoid smoking and drinking caffeine-containing beverages
    3. Assessing the patient's skin and mucous membranes for signs of adequate hydration
    4. Checking lying and standing blood pressure every 4 hours with a cuff placed on the same arm

12. The LPN/LVN is assigned to provide care for a patient with pheochromocytoma. Which physical assessment technique would the RN instruct the LPN/LVN to avoid?
    1. Listening for abdominal bowel sounds in all four quadrants
    2. Palpating the abdomen in all four quadrants
    3. Checking the blood pressure every hour
    4. Assessing the mucous membranes for hydration status

13. A patient with adrenal insufficiency is to be discharged and will take prednisone 10 mg orally each day. Which instruction would the nurse be sure to teach the patient?
    1. Excessive weight gain or swelling should be reported to the health care provider.
    2. Changing positions rapidly may cause hypotension and dizziness.
    3. A diet with foods low in sodium may be beneficial to prevent side effects.
    4. Signs of hypoglycemia may occur while taking this drug.

14. The nurse is caring for a patient who has just undergone a hypophysectomy for hyperpituitarism. Which postoperative finding requires immediate intervention?
    1. Presence of glucose in the nasal drainage
    2. Presence of nasal packing in the nares
    3. Urine output of 40 to 50 mL/hr
    4. Patient reports of thirst

15. Which patient should the charge nurse assign to the care of an LPN/LVN under the supervision of the RN team leader?
    1. A 51-year-old patient who has just undergone a bilateral adrenalectomy
    2. An 83-year-old patient with type 2 diabetes and chronic obstructive pulmonary disease
    3. A 38-year-old patient with myocardial infarction preparing for discharge
    4. A 72-year-old patient with mental status changes admitted from a long-term care facility

16. The nurse is providing care for a patient who underwent a thyroidectomy 2 days ago. Which laboratory value requires close monitoring by the nurse?
    1. Calcium level
    2. Sodium level
    3. Potassium level
    4. White blood cell count

17. A 24-year-old patient with diabetes insipidus (DI) makes all of these statements when the nurse is preparing the patient for discharge from the hospital. Which statement indicates to the nurse that the patient needs additional teaching?
    1. "I will drink fluids equal to the amount of my urine output."
    2. "I will weigh myself every day using the same scale."
    3. "I will wear my medical alert bracelet at all times."
    4. "I will gradually wean myself off the vasopressin."

18. The RN is supervising a senior student nurse who is caring for a fresh postoperative patient who had a hypophysectomy. The RN observes the student nurse perform all of these actions. For which action must the RN intervene?
    1. Assess for changes in vision or mental status.
    2. Keep the head of the bed elevated.
    3. Remind the patient to perform deep breathing every hour while awake.
    4. Encourage the patient to cough vigorously.

19. The nurse is caring for a patient with syndrome of inappropriate antidiuretic hormone secretion. Which patient care actions should the nurse delegate to the experienced assistive personnel? **Select all that apply.**
    1. Monitor and record strict intake and output.
    2. Provide the patient with ice chips when requested.
    3. Remind the patient about his or her fluid restriction.
    4. Weigh the patient every morning using the same scale.
    5. Report a weight gain of 2.2 lb (1 kg) to the nurse.
    6. Provide mouth care and allow the patient to swallow the rinses.

20. The nurse is preparing a care plan for a patient with Cushing disease. Which abnormal laboratory values would the nurse expect? **Select all that apply.**
    1. Increased serum calcium level
    2. Increased salivary cortisol level
    3. Increased urinary cortisol level
    4. Decreased serum glucose level
    5. Decreased sodium level
    6. Increased serum cortisol level

21. When providing care for a patient with Addison disease, the nurse should be alert for which laboratory value change?
    1. Decreased hematocrit
    2. Increased sodium level
    3. Decreased potassium level
    4. Decreased calcium level

22. A female patient is admitted with a diagnosis of primary hypofunction of the adrenal glands. Which nursing assessment finding supports this diagnosis?
    1. Patchy areas of pigment loss over the face
    2. Decreased muscle strength
    3. Greatly increased urine output
    4. Scalp alopecia

23. The nurse is instructing a senior nursing student on the techniques for palpation of the thyroid gland. What instruction would the nurse be sure to include when instructing the student about thyroid palpation?
    1. Always stand to the side of the patient.
    2. Instruct the patient not to swallow.
    3. Palpate using one hand and then the other.
    4. Palpate the thyroid gland for size, symmetry, shape, and presence of nodules.

24. Two assistive personnel (AP) are assisting a patient with Cushing disease to move up in bed. Which action by the APs requires the nurse's immediate intervention?
    1. Positioning themselves on opposite sides of the patient's bed
    2. Grasping under the patient's arms to pull him up in bed
    3. Lowering the side rails of the patient's bed before moving him
    4. Removing the pillow before moving the patient up in bed

25. The nurse is caring for the following patients with endocrine disorders. Which patient must the nurse assess **first**?
    1. A 21-year-old patient with diabetes insipidus whose urine output overnight was 2000 mL
    2. A 55-year-old patient with syndrome of inappropriate antidiuretic hormone secretion who is demanding that the assistive personnel refill his water pitcher
    3. A 65-year-old patient with Addison disease whose morning potassium level is 6.2 mEq/L (6.2 mmol/L)
    4. A 48-year-old patient with Cushing disease with a weight gain of 1.5 lb (0.7 kg) over the past 4 days

26. Which actions prescribed by the health care provider for the patient with Addison disease should the nurse delegate to the experienced assistive personnel (AP)? **Select all that apply.**
    1. Weigh the patient every morning.
    2. Obtain fingerstick glucose before each meal and at bedtime.
    3. Check vital signs every 2 hours.
    4. Monitor for cardiac dysrhythmias.
    5. Administer oral prednisone 10 mg every morning.
    6. Record intake and output.

Answer Key for this chapter begins on p. 146

27. The LPN/LVN who is assigned to care for a patient with Cushing disease asks the RN why the patient has bruising and petechiae across her abdomen. What is the RN's **best** response?
    1. "Patients with Cushing disease often have bleeding disorders."
    2. "Patients with Cushing disease have very fragile capillaries."
    3. "Please ask the patient if she slipped or fell during the night."
    4. "Thin and delicate skin can result in development of bruising."

28. The patient with hyperparathyroidism who is not a candidate for surgery asks the nurse why she is receiving IV normal saline and IV furosemide. What is the nurse's **best** response?
    1. "This therapy is to protect your kidney function."
    2. "You are receiving these therapies to prevent edema formation."
    3. "Diuretic and hydration therapies are used to reduce your serum calcium."
    4. "These therapies may help to improve your candidacy for surgery."

29. Which actions should the nurse assign to the experienced LPN/LVN for the care of a patient with hypothyroidism? **Select all that apply.**
    1. Assessing and recording the rate and depth of respirations
    2. Auscultating lung sounds every 4 hours
    3. Creating an individualized nursing care plan for the patient
    4. Administering sedation medications every 6 hours
    5. Checking blood pressure, heart rate, and respirations every 4 hours
    6. Reminding the patient to report any episodes of chest pain or discomfort

30. The nurse is caring for a patient with hyperthyroidism who had a partial thyroidectomy yesterday. Which change in assessment would the nurse report to the health care provider **immediately**?
    1. Temperature elevation to 100.2°F (37.9°C)
    2. Heart rate increase from 64 to 76 beats/min
    3. Respiratory rate decrease from 26 to 16 breaths/min
    4. Pulse oximetry reading of 92%

31. The nurse admits a patient whose assessment reveals prominent brow ridge, large hands and feet, and large lips and nose. Which pituitary hormone does the nurse suspect is elevated?
    1. Thyroid-stimulating hormone
    2. Growth hormone
    3. Adrenocorticotropic hormone
    4. Vasopressin antidiuretic hormone

32. The nurse is orienting a newly graduated RN who is providing care for a postoperative patient after a thyroidectomy. The new RN assesses the patient and notes laryngeal stridor with a pulse oximetry measure of 89%. What is the **priority** action for the nurse and new RN?
    1. Immediately notify the rapid response team (RRT).
    2. Apply oxygen by face mask.
    3. Prepare to suction the patient.
    4. Assess for numbness and tingling around the mouth.

33. Which prescribed order for a patient with diabetes insipidus (DI) would the nurse be sure to question?
    1. Monitor and record accurate intake and output.
    2. Check urine specific gravity.
    3. Restrict fluids for 6 hours.
    4. Weigh the patient every morning.

34. The nurse assesses a newly admitted patient with a diagnosis of hyperthyroidism (see the figure). How would the nurse **best** document the finding in this patient?

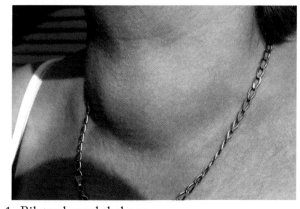

    1. Bilateral exophthalmos
    2. Large visible goiter
    3. Myxedema
    4. Moon face

35. Enhanced Drag and Drop _____

Which clinical findings in the right column are the result of the age-related changes listed in the left column?

Instructions: Write the correct number in the space in the right column.

Endocrine Changes Related to Aging	Clinical Findings
1. Decreased antidiuretic hormone (ADH) production 2. Decreased ovarian production of estrogen 3. Decreased glucose tolerance 4. Decreased general metabolism	a. _____ Decreased appetite b. _____ Urine is more dilute c. _____ Decreased bone density d. _____ Slow wound healing e. _____ Thinner, drier skin f. _____ Decreased heart rate g. _____ Weight gain h. _____ Decreased cold tolerance

36. The nurse is to administer an initial dose of propylthiouracil (PTU) 150 mg orally every 8 hours to a patient. The drug comes in 50 mg tablets.

1. How many tablets will the nurse give with each dose?

Answer: _____

2. For which endocrine disorder is PTU prescribed?

Answer: _____

PART 2 · Common Health Scenarios

Answer Key for this chapter begins on p. 146

Answers

1. **Ans: 4** When assessing the thyroid gland, always palpate gently because vigorous palpation can lead to thyroid storm if a patient is suspected of having hyperthyroidism. During thyroid storm the patient's heart rate, blood pressure, and body temperature can rise to dangerously high levels, and if not treated rapidly, death can occur. The other three techniques are appropriate for endocrine assessment. **Focus:** Prioritization.

2. **Ans: 2** DI is a disorder of the posterior pituitary gland in which water loss is caused by either an antidiuretic hormone (ADH) deficiency or an inability of the kidneys to respond to ADH. The result of DI is the excretion of large volumes of dilute urine because the distal kidney tubules and collecting ducts do not reabsorb water; this leads to polyuria. Dehydration from massive water loss increases plasma osmolarity, which stimulates the sensation of thirst. Thirst promotes increased fluid intake and aids in maintaining hydration. **Focus:** Prioritization.

3. **Ans: 2, 4, 5** Therapy for gonadotropin deficiency begins with high-dose testosterone and is continued until virilization (presence of male secondary sex characteristics) is achieved, with responses that include increases in penis size, libido, muscle mass, bone size, and bone strength. Chest, facial, pubic, and axillary hair growth also increase. Patients usually report improved body image after therapy is initiated. Side effects of therapy include gynecomastia (male breast tissue development), acne, baldness, and prostate enlargement. **Focus:** Prioritization.

4. **Ans: 3** Exophthalmos (abnormal protrusion of the eyes) is characteristic of patients with hyperthyroidism caused by Graves disease. Periorbital edema, bradycardia, and a hoarse voice are all characteristics of patients with hypothyroidism. **Focus:** Prioritization.

5. **Ans: 1** The cardiac problems associated with hyperthyroidism include tachycardia, increased systolic blood pressure, and decreased diastolic blood pressure. Patients with hyperthyroidism may also have increased body temperature related to increased metabolic rate. Respiratory changes are usually not symptomatic of this condition. **Focus:** Delegation, Supervision.

6. **Ans: 2** Monitoring vital signs and recording their values are within the education and scope of practice of APs. An experienced AP should have been taught how to monitor the apical pulse. Nevertheless, a nurse should observe the AP to be sure that the AP has mastered this skill. Instructing and teaching patients, as well as performing venipuncture to obtain laboratory samples, are more suited to the education and scope of practice of licensed nurses. In some facilities, an experienced AP may perform venipuncture but only after special training. **Focus:** Delegation, Supervision, Assignment.

7. **Ans: 3** Although patients with hypothyroidism often have cardiac problems that include bradycardia, a heart rate of 48 beats/min may have significant implications for cardiac output and hemodynamic stability. Patients with Graves disease usually have a rapid heart rate, but 94 beats/min is within normal limits. The patient with diabetes may need sliding-scale insulin dosing. This is important but not urgent. Patients with Cushing disease frequently have dependent edema. **Focus:** Prioritization.

8. **Ans: 1** Patients with hypofunction of the adrenal gland often have hypotension and should be instructed to change positions slowly. After a patient has been so instructed, it is appropriate for the AP to remind the patient of the instructions. Assessing, teaching, and planning nursing care require more education and should be done by licensed nurses. **Focus:** Delegation, Supervision.

9. **Ans: 4** The presence of crackles in the patient's lungs indicates excess fluid volume caused by excess water and sodium reabsorption and may be a symptom of pulmonary edema, which must be treated rapidly. Striae (stretch marks), weight gain, and dependent edema are common findings in patients with Cushing disease. These findings should be monitored but do not require urgent action. **Focus:** Prioritization. **Test-Taking Tip:** Findings that the nurse should immediately report to the HCP are those that can indicate a worsening of the patient's condition that must be treated to prevent further worsening or threat to life.

10. **Ans: 1, 3, 4, 6** Bromocriptine is a dopamine agonist drug that stimulates dopamine receptors in the brain and inhibits the release of growth hormone and prolactin. In most cases, small tumors decrease until the pituitary gland is of normal size. Side effects of bromocriptine include orthostatic (postural) hypotension, headaches, nausea, abdominal cramps, and constipation. Give bromocriptine with a meal or a snack to reduce GI side effects. Treatment starts with a low dose and is gradually increased until the desired level is reached. Patients taking bromocriptine should be taught to seek medical care immediately if chest pain, dizziness, or watery nasal discharge occurs because of the possibility of serious side effects, including cardiac dysrhythmias, coronary artery spasms, and cerebrospinal fluid leakage. Also, if the patient is a female of childbearing age who becomes pregnant, the drug should be stopped. **Focus:** Prioritization.

11. **Ans: 4** Monitoring vital signs is within the education and scope of practice for APs. The nurse must ensure

that the AP knows how to perform orthostatic BP measurements and should be sure to instruct the AP that blood pressure measurements are to be taken with the cuff on the same arm each time. The AP should be instructed to record the blood pressures and inform the nurse of the results. Revising the care plan and instructing and assessing patients are beyond the scope of practice for APs and fall within the purview of licensed nurses. **Focus:** Delegation, Supervision.

12. **Ans: 2**   Palpating the abdomen can cause the sudden release of catecholamines and severe hypertension. All of the other assessments are appropriate for the LPN/LVN assigned to care for this patient. **Focus:** Assignment, Supervision. **Test-Taking Tip:** Students should be aware of assessment techniques that may cause injury or death to a patient and must be avoided. Another example is vigorous palpation of the thyroid.

13. **Ans: 1**   Rapid weight gain and edema are signs of excessive drug therapy, and the dosage of the drug would need to be adjusted. Hypertension, hyponatremia, hyperkalemia, and hyperglycemia are common in patients with adrenal hypofunction. **Focus:** Prioritization.

14. **Ans: 1**   The presence of glucose in nasal drainage indicates that the fluid is cerebrospinal fluid (CSF) and suggests a CSF leak. Packing is normally inserted in the nares after the surgical incision is closed. A urine output of 40 to 50 mL/hr is adequate, and patients may experience thirst postoperatively. When patients are thirsty, nursing staff should encourage fluid intake. **Focus:** Prioritization.

15. **Ans: 2**   The 83-year-old has no complicating factors at the moment. Providing care for patients in stable and uncomplicated condition falls within the LPN/LVN's educational preparation and scope of practice, with the care always being provided under the supervision and direction of an RN. The RN should assess the patient who has just undergone surgery and the newly admitted patient. The patient who is preparing for discharge after myocardial infarction may need some complex teaching. **Focus:** Assignment, Supervision.

16. **Ans: 1**   The parathyroid glands are located on the back of the thyroid gland. The parathyroids are important in maintaining the calcium and phosphorus balance. The nurse should be attentive to all patient laboratory values, but calcium and phosphorus levels are especially important to monitor after thyroidectomy because abnormal values could be the result of removal of the parathyroid glands during the procedure. **Focus:** Prioritization.

17. **Ans: 4**   A patient with permanent DI requires lifelong vasopressin therapy. All of the other statements are appropriate to the home care of this patient. **Focus:** Prioritization.

18. **Ans: 4**   After a hypophysectomy, the nurse should monitor the patient's neurologic response and document any changes in vision or mental status, altered level of consciousness, or decreased strength of the extremities. The head of the bed should be kept elevated. Patients should be reminded to perform deep-breathing exercises hourly while awake to prevent pulmonary problems. The patient should be taught to avoid coughing early after surgery because it increases pressure in the incision area and may lead to a cerebrospinal fluid (CSF) leak. **Focus:** Delegation, Supervision.

19. **Ans: 1, 3, 4, 5**   Fluid restriction is essential because fluid intake further dilutes plasma sodium levels. In some cases, fluid intake may be kept as low as 500 to 1000 mL over 24 hours. All oral fluids count, including ice chips and mouth rinses, and strict intake and output is required. Measure intake, output, and daily weights to assess the degree of fluid restriction needed. A weight gain of 2.2 lb (1 kg) or more per day or a gradual increase over several days is cause for concern. A 2.2-lb (1-kg) weight increase is equal to a 1000-mL fluid retention (1 kg = 1 L). Keep the mouth moist by offering frequent oral rinsing (warn patients not to swallow the rinses). **Focus:** Delegation, Supervision.

20. **Ans: 2, 3, 6**   A patient with Cushing disease experiences increased levels of serum, urinary, and salivary cortisol. Other laboratory findings may include increased blood glucose level, decreased lymphocyte count, increased sodium level, and decreased serum calcium level. **Focus:** Prioritization.

21. **Ans: 1**   A patient with Addison disease is at risk for anemia. The nurse should expect this patient's sodium level to decrease and potassium and calcium levels to increase. **Focus:** Prioritization.

22. **Ans: 1**   Vitiligo, or patchy areas of pigment loss with increased pigmentation at the edges, is seen with primary hypofunction of the adrenal glands and is caused by autoimmune destruction of melanocytes in the skin. The other findings are signs of pituitary hypofunction. **Focus:** Prioritization.

23. **Ans: 4**   The thyroid gland should always be palpated for size, symmetry, shape, and presence of nodules or other irregularities. The student nurse should stand either behind or in front of the patient and use both hands to palpate the thyroid. Having the patient swallow can help with locating the thyroid gland. **Focus:** Supervision, Delegation.

24. **Ans: 2**   Patients with Cushing disease usually have paper-thin skin that is easily injured. The APs should use a lift or a draw sheet to carefully move the patient and prevent injury to the skin. All of the other actions are appropriate when moving this patient up in bed. **Focus:** Delegation, Supervision.

25. **Ans: 3**   This patient's potassium level is very high, placing him or her at risk for cardiac dysrhythmias that could be life threatening. The other patients also need to be seen but are not as urgent. **Focus:** Prioritization.

26. **Ans: 1, 2, 3, 6** Weighing patients, recording intake and output, and checking vital signs are all within the scope of practice for a AP. An experienced AP would have been trained to perform fingerstick glucose monitoring. The nurse should make sure that the AP has mastered this skill and then instruct the AP to record and inform him or her about the results. Administering medications and monitoring for cardiac dysrhythmias are within the scope of practice of licensed nurses. **Focus:** Delegation.

27. **Ans: 2** A key cardiovascular feature seen in patients with Cushing disease is capillary fragility, which results in bruising and petechiae. Bleeding disorders are not a sign of Cushing disease, and although these patients have delicate skin, this is not the cause of the bruising. The nurse may want to investigate whether the patient fell, but these patients can have bruising and petechiae without falls. **Focus:** Assignment, Supervision, Prioritization.

28. **Ans: 3** Diuretics and hydration help reduce serum calcium for patients with hyperparathyroidism who are not surgery candidates. Furosemide increases kidney excretion of calcium when combined with IV saline in large volumes. **Focus:** Prioritization.

29. **Ans: 1, 2, 5, 6** Assessment, auscultation, and reminding patients about information that has been taught to them are within the scope of practice of the LPN/LVN. The LPN/LVN could be assigned to check the patient's vital signs, and this is certainly within the scope of practice. Checking vital signs could also be delegated to the assistive personnel. Creating nursing care plans falls within the scope of practice of the RN. The use of sedation is discouraged for patients with hypothyroidism because it may make respiratory problems more difficult. If sedation is used, the dosage is reduced, and it is not given around the clock. **Focus:** Assignment, Supervision.

30. **Ans: 1** When caring for a patient with hyperthyroidism, even after a partial thyroidectomy, a temperature elevation of 1°F must be reported immediately because it may indicate an impending thyroid crisis. The other changes should be monitored but are not urgent. **Focus:** Prioritization.

31. **Ans: 2** These assessment findings are classic initial manifestations of growth hormone excess. **Focus:** Prioritization.

32. **Ans: 1** The first priority is to monitor the patient after surgery to identify symptoms of obstruction (stridor, dyspnea, falling oxygen saturation, inability to swallow, drooling) after thyroid surgery. If any are present, respond by immediately notifying the RRT. If the airway is obstructed, oxygen therapy will not be helpful, and the patient may need airway management such as intubation. For this reason, the RRT needs to be activated first. Emergency tracheostomy equipment, oxygen, and suctioning equipment should already be in the patient's room and have been checked to be sure that they are in working order. **Focus:** Prioritization. **Test-Taking Tip:** This is a life-threatening situation, so the nurse's priority is to notify the RRT and health care provider immediately to safeguard the patient's life.

33. **Ans: 3** Ensure that no patient suspected of having DI is deprived of fluids for more than 4 hours, because reduced urine output and severe dehydration can result. Interventions for DI include accurately measuring fluid intake and output, checking urine specific gravity, and recording the patient's weight daily. **Focus:** Prioritization.

34. **Ans: 2** A patient with hyperthyroidism may have an enlarged thyroid gland (goiter) that can be four times the size of a normal gland. Exophthalmos refers to the wide-eyed, startled look resulting from edema in the extraocular muscled and increased fatty tissue behind the eye that pushes the eye forward. Myxedema occurs often in patients with hypothyroidism, and moon face is a common characteristic of Cushing disease. **Focus:** Prioritization.

35. **Ans: a4, b1, c2, d3, e2, f4, g3, h4** As a patient ages and ADH decreases, urine becomes more dilute and less able to be concentrated. A decreased production of estrogen leads to decreased bone density, thin and dry skin (with risk of injury), and drier perineal and vaginal tissues. Decreased glucose tolerance results in weight gain greater than ideal, along with changes in glucose levels (fasting and random), slow wound healing, yeast infections, polydipsia, and polyuria. Decreased general tolerance manifests as less tolerance for cold and decreased appetite, as well as decreased heart rate and blood pressure. **Focus:** Prioritization.

36. **Ans: 1. 3 tablets; 2. Hyperthyroidism** 50 mg/1 tablet: 150 mg/X tablets = 3 tablets. PTU is prescribed for hyperthyroidism. **Focus:** Prioritization.

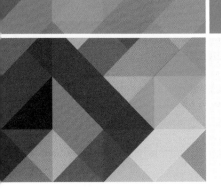

CHAPTER 15

Integumentary Problems

Questions

1. The nurse assigns a dressing change to the LPN/LVN on a stage III pressure injury that is draining large amounts of purulent serosanguinous fluid. Which type of dressing should the nurse instruct the LPN/LVN to utilize?
   1. A hydrophobic dressing
   2. Wet to damp saline moistened gauze
   3. A hydrophilic dressing
   4. A transparent dressing

2. Which actions will the nurse use when treating a patient with a venous ulcer on the right lower leg? **Select all that apply.**
   1. Position the right leg lower than the heart.
   2. Use compression wraps consistently.
   3. Administer analgesics before wound care.
   4. Maintain a dry wound environment.
   5. Encourage right ankle flexion exercises.
   6. Clean wound with a nonirritating solution.

3. After the nurse has performed a skin assessment on a recently admitted 19-year-old patient, which finding is the **highest** priority to report to the health care provider?
   1. Mole 2 mm in diameter on the chest
   2. Tenting of the skin on the forearms
   3. Patches of vitiligo around both eyes
   4. Scattered brown macules on the face

4. The home health nurse is caring for a patient with a fungal infection of the toenails who has a new prescription for oral itraconazole. Which patient information is **most** important to discuss with the health care provider (HCP) before administration of the itraconazole?
   1. The patient's toenails are thick and yellow.
   2. The patient is embarrassed by the infection.
   3. The patient is also taking simvastatin daily.
   4. The patient is allergic to iodine and shellfish.

5. The health care provider (HCP) prescribes permethrin application for all family members of a patient who has scabies. Which patient information will be **most** important for the nurse to discuss with the HCP before teaching the patient about the medication?
   1. The patient has a newborn infant.
   2. Burrows are noted on the wrists.
   3. The patient and family live in a homeless shelter.
   4. Family members are asymptomatic.

6. The nurse is caring for a patient who has just had a squamous cell carcinoma removed from the face. Which action can be assigned to an experienced LPN/LVN?
   1. Teaching the patient about risk factors for squamous cell carcinoma
   2. Showing the patient how to care for the surgical site at home
   3. Monitoring the surgical site for swelling, bleeding, or pain
   4. Discussing the reasons for avoiding aspirin use for 1 week after surgery

7. The charge nurse in a long-term care (LTC) facility that employs RNs, LPNs/LVNs, and assistive personnel (AP) is planning care for a resident with a stage III sacral pressure injury. Which nursing intervention is **best** to assign to an LPN/LVN?
   1. Choosing the type of dressing to be used on the injury
   2. Using the Braden scale to assess for pressure injury risk factors
   3. Assisting the patient in changing position at frequent intervals
   4. Cleaning and changing the dressing on the injury every morning

8. The nurse has just received a change-of-shift report for the burn unit. Which patient should be assessed **first**?
   1. Patient with deep partial-thickness burns on both legs who reports severe and continuous leg pain
   2. Patient who has just arrived from the emergency department with facial burns sustained in a house fire
   3. Patient who has just been transferred from the postanesthesia care unit after having skin grafts applied to the anterior chest
   4. Patient admitted 3 weeks ago with full-thickness leg and buttock burns who has been waiting for 3 hours to receive discharge teaching

9. The nurse is performing a sterile dressing change for a patient with infected deep partial-thickness burns of the chest and abdomen. List the steps in the order in which each should be accomplished.
   1. Apply silver sulfadiazine ointment.
   2. Obtain specimens for aerobic and anaerobic wound cultures.
   3. Administer morphine sulfate 10 mg IV.
   4. Debride the wound of eschar using gauze sponges.
   5. Cover the wound with a sterile gauze dressing.

   _____, _____, _____, _____, _____

10. Which patient is **best** for the nurse manager on the burn unit to assign to an RN who has floated from the oncology unit?
    1. A 23-year-old patient who has just been admitted with burns over 30% of the body after a warehouse fire
    2. A 36-year-old patient who requires discharge teaching about nutrition and wound care after having skin grafts
    3. A 45-year-old patient with infected partial-thickness back and chest burns who has a dressing change scheduled
    4. A 57-year-old patient with full-thickness burns on both arms who needs assistance in positioning hand splints

11. After the nurse performs a skin assessment on a 70-year-old new resident in a long-term care facility, which finding is of **most** concern?
    1. Numerous striae are noted across the abdomen and buttocks.
    2. All the toenails are thickened and yellow.
    3. Silver scaling is present on the elbows and knees.
    4. An irregular border is seen on a black mole on the scalp.

12. Which assessment finding calls for the **most** immediate action by the nurse?
    1. Bluish color around the lips and earlobes
    2. Yellow color of the skin and sclera
    3. Bilateral erythema of the face and neck
    4. Dark brown spotting on the chest and back

13. The nurse obtains this information about a 60-year-old patient who has a shingles infection. Which finding is of **most** concern?
    1. The patient has had symptoms for about 2 days.
    2. The patient has severe burning-type discomfort.
    3. The patient has not had the herpes zoster vaccination.
    4. The patient's spouse is currently receiving cancer chemotherapy.

14. Which of these actions will the nurse take **first** for a patient who has arrived in the emergency department with sudden-onset urticaria and intense itching?
    1. Ask the patient about any new medications.
    2. Administer the prescribed cetirizine.
    3. Apply topical corticosteroid cream.
    4. Auscultate the patient's breath sounds.

15. A 22-year-old woman who has been taking isotretinoin to treat severe cystic acne makes all these statements while being seen for a follow-up examination. Which statement is of **most** concern?
    1. "My husband and I are thinking of starting a family soon."
    2. "I don't think there has been much improvement in my skin."
    3. "Sometimes I get nauseated after taking the medication."
    4. "I have been experiencing a lot of muscle aches and pains."

16. A patient is scheduled for patch testing to determine allergies to several substances. Which action associated with this test should the nurse delegate to assistive personnel (AP) working in the allergy clinic?
    1. Explaining the purpose of the testing to the patient
    2. Examining the patch area for evidence of a reaction
    3. Scheduling a follow-up appointment for the patient in 2 days
    4. Monitoring the patient for anaphylactic reactions to the testing

17. The nurse is planning hospital discharge teaching for four patients. For which patient is it **most** important to instruct about the need to use sunscreen?
    1. A 32-year-old patient with pneumonia who has a new prescription for doxycycline
    2. A fair-skinned 55-year-old patient with psoriasis who works outside for 8 hours daily
    3. A dark-skinned 62-year-old patient who has had keloids injected with hydrocortisone
    4. A 78-year-old patient with a red, pruritic rash caused by an allergic reaction to penicillin

18. The home health nurse is caring for a 72-year-old patient who has a stage II pressure injury, with risk factors of poor nutrition, bladder incontinence, and immobility. Which nursing action should be delegated to the assistive personnel (AP)?
    1. Telling the patient and family to apply the skin barrier cream in a smooth, even layer
    2. Completing a diet assessment and suggesting changes in diet to improve the patient's nutrition
    3. Reminding the family to help the patient to the commode every 2 hours during the day
    4. Evaluating the patient for improvement in documented areas of skin breakdown or damage

19. The charge nurse in a long-term care facility that employs RNs, LPNs/LVNs, and assistive personnel (AP) as staff members is planning the care for an 80-year-old patient who has candidiasis in the skinfolds of the abdomen and groin. Which intervention is **best** to assign to an LPN/LVN?
    1. Applying nystatin powder to the area three times daily
    2. Cleaning the skinfolds every 8 hours and drying thoroughly
    3. Evaluating the need for further antifungal treatment at least weekly
    4. Assessing for ongoing risk factors for skin breakdown and infection

20. After reviewing the medical record for a patient who has an oral herpes simplex infection after being treated with chemotherapy, which intervention has the **highest** priority?

Physical Assessment	Nutritional Assessment	Social and Emotional Assessment
• Vesicular lesions throughout mouth and lips	• Taking only a few bites of each meal	• States, "I feel like a monster with these herpes sores all over my mouth!"
• Reports level 9 oral pain (on a scale of 0 to 10)	• 2-lb (1-kg) weight loss in past 3 days	• Refuses to see visitors

1. Offer reassurance that herpes can be treated with antiviral medication.
2. Administer prescribed analgesics before meals.
3. Offer the patient frequent small meals and snacks.
4. Encourage the patient to maintain contact with some family members.

21. A patient admitted to the emergency department reports new-onset itching of the trunk and groin. The nurse notes multiple reddened wheals on the chest, back, and groin. Which question should the nurse ask **next**?
    1. "Do you have a family history of eczema?"
    2. "Have you been using sunscreen regularly?"
    3. "How do you usually manage stress?"
    4. "Are you taking any new medications?"

22. A patient who has extensive blister injuries to the back and both legs caused by exposure to toxic chemicals at work is transferred to the emergency department. Which prescribed intervention will the nurse implement **first**?
    1. Infuse lactated Ringer's solution at 250 mL/hr.
    2. Rinse the back and legs with 4 L of sterile normal saline.
    3. Obtain blood for a complete blood count and electrolyte levels.
    4. Document the percentage of total body surface area burned.

23. The nurse has just received the change-of-shift report in the burn unit. Which patient requires the **most** immediate assessment or intervention?
    1. A 22-year-old patient admitted 4 days previously with facial burns due to a house fire who has been crying since recent visitors left
    2. A 34-year-old patient who returned from skin-graft surgery 3 hours ago and is reporting level 8 pain (on a scale of 0 to 10)
    3. A 45-year-old patient with partial-thickness leg burns who has a temperature of 102.6°F (39.2°C) and a blood pressure of 98/46 mm Hg
    4. A 57-year-old patient who was admitted with electrical burns 24 hours ago and has a blood potassium level of 5.1 mEq/L (5.1 mmol/L)

24. A patient with cellulitis is to receive linezolid 600 mg IV over 2 hours. Based on the medication label, the nurse will set the infusion pump for _____ mL/hr.

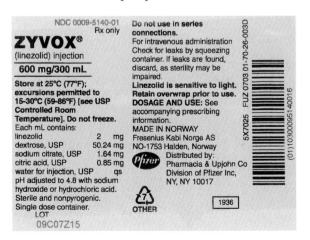

PART 2

Common Health Scenarios

Answer Key for this chapter begins on p. 154

25. In which order will the nurse take these actions that are needed for a patient seen in the family medicine clinic and diagnosed with impetigo?
    1. Obtain specimen for culture.
    2. Apply topical antibiotic ointment.
    3. Give the patient a hand hygiene handout.
    4. Clean off the crust from the lesion.
    5. Apply a sterile dressing to the wound.

    _____, _____, _____, _____, _____

26. Which personal protective equipment will the nurse need when planning a dressing change for a patient with a methicillin-resistant *Staphylococcus aureus*–infected skin wound? **Select all that apply.**
    1. Gown
    2. Gloves
    3. Goggles
    4. Surgical mask
    5. Booties
    6. Sterile gloves

27. The nurse takes the health history of a patient who has been admitted to the same-day surgery unit for elective facial dermabrasion. Which information is **most** important to convey to the plastic surgeon?
    1. The patient does not routinely use sunscreen.
    2. The patient has a family history of melanoma.
    3. The patient has not eaten anything for 8 hours.
    4. The patient takes 325 mg of aspirin daily.

28. The charge nurse on a medical-surgical unit is working with a newly graduated RN who has been on orientation to the unit for 3 weeks. Which patient is **best** to assign to the new graduate?
    1. A 34-year-old patient who was just admitted to the unit with periorbital cellulitis
    2. A 40-year-old patient who needs discharge instructions after having skin grafts to the thigh
    3. A 67-year-old patient who requires a dressing change after hydrotherapy for a pressure injury
    4. A 78-year-old patient who needs teaching before a punch biopsy of a facial lesion

29. When the nurse is evaluating a patient who has been taking prednisone 30 mg/day to treat contact dermatitis, which finding is **most** important to report to the health care provider?
    1. The glucose level is 136 mg/dL (7.6 mmol/L).
    2. The patient states, "I am eating all the time."
    3. The patient reports frequent epigastric pain.
    4. The blood pressure is 148/84 mm Hg.

30. The charge nurse is supervising a newly hired RN. Which action by the new RN requires the **most** immediate action by the charge nurse?
    1. Obtaining an anaerobic culture specimen from a superficial burn wound
    2. Giving doxycycline with a glass of milk to a patient with cellulitis
    3. Discussing the use of herpes zoster vaccine with a 25-year-old patient
    4. Teaching a newly admitted burn patient about the use of pressure garments

31. Which finding about a patient who has been taking adalimumab to treat psoriasis is **most** indicative of a need for a change in therapy?
    1. Temperature 100.9°F (38.3°C)
    2. Patches of scaly skin on chest
    3. Erythema on sun-exposed areas of skin
    4. Patient report of worsening depression

32. At the beginning of the shift, an assistive personnel (AP) tells the nurse, "I have several patients today who have wound infections. I will do my best, but if I put on a gown and gloves every time I go into their rooms, I will never get all the care done!" Which response by the nurse is **best**?
    1. "I know you are busy, but please try to comply with the standard infection control measures because these patients have serious infections."
    2. "Let's look at the patient assignments for today and make changes so that you can give the needed care and maintain good infection control."
    3. "If you are unable to follow infection control standards, perhaps you need a review class in correct use of personal protective equipment."
    4. "Tell me what you think are the most important times to use personal protective equipment to prevent infections from spreading."

33. Cloze _____

Scenario: A 50-year-old patient with no known allergies has sustained 30% partial and full thickness burns. The patient's blood pressure has dropped significantly since admission 18 hours ago. The significant decrease in blood pressure after major burns is due to __1__. His arterial blood gases indicate a metabolic acidosis. Metabolic acidosis in burn victims and is caused by __2__. First line treatment of metabolic acidosis includes administration of __3__. __4__ will be administered to prevent infection with *Clostridium tetani*. To prevent hypertrophic scars and contractures, compression dressings or garments are applied. The patient must wear the compression garments for at least 23 hours a day for __5__ in order to be effective.

Instructions: Complete the sentences below by choosing the most probable option for the missing information that corresponds with the same numbered list of options provided.

Option 1	Option 2	Option 3	Option 4	Option 5
Patient controlled analgesia with Morphine	High bicarbonate levels	Sodium Bicarbonate	Vancomycin	6 months to a year
Insufficient fluid replacement	Hypoventilation	Intravenous fluids	Piperacillin-tazobactam	3 months to 6 months
Septicemia	Decreased tissue perfusion	High flow oxygen	Tetanus toxoid	1 to 2 years
Capillary leak syndrome	Hypoxia	Antibiotics	Amphotericin B	3 to 4 years

Answer Key for this chapter begins on p. 154

Answers

1. **Ans: 3** A hydrophilic dressing will draw the fluid material away from the surface of the wound, preventing the skin surrounding the wound from breaking down. A hydrophobic dressing is used for dry wounds or those with little drainage. In the past when wet to dry dressings were removed, new tissue growth was disrupted. The current practice is to remove dressings while they are damp. This spares the new growth but mechanically removes necrotic tissue. A transparent dressing is used to easily monitor a dry healing wound. **Focus:** Assignment.

2. **Ans: 2, 3, 5, 6** Current guidelines for promotion of venous ulcer healing suggest the use of compression, appropriate analgesia, exercises to improve venous return, and wound cleansing with a nonirritating solution such as normal saline. The extremity should be elevated to promote venous return and decrease swelling. A moist environment encourages wound healing. **Focus:** Prioritization.

3. **Ans: 2** Tenting of the skin on younger patients may indicate dehydration and the need for oral or IV fluid administration. The other data will be recorded but do not require any rapid interventions. **Focus:** Prioritization.

4. **Ans: 3** The "azole" antifungal medications inhibit drug-metabolizing enzymes (when used orally or intravenously) and can lead to toxic levels of many other medications, including some commonly prescribed statins. Thick and yellow toenails are typical with fungal infections in this area, and patients may be embarrassed by the appearance of the nails, but antifungal treatment will improve the appearance of the nails. The patient's iodine allergy will be reported to the HCP but will not impact the use of itraconazole. **Focus:** Prioritization. **Test-Taking Tip:** Be aware that the "azole" medications affect cytochrome P450, an enzyme system that is responsible for the metabolism of many medications. When a patient is taking an azole, plan to check any newly prescribed medications for possible drug interactions that might lead to toxicity.

5. **Ans: 1** Although all family members (symptomatic or not) should be treated for scabies, permethrin is contraindicated in patients who are younger than 2 months of age because of concerns that the medication may be absorbed systemically. Burrows on the wrist are commonly seen with scabies. The patient's homelessness may affect teaching about how to launder clothes and linens but will not affect the use of permethrin for treating the scabies infestation. **Focus:** Prioritization.

6. **Ans: 3** An LPN/LVN who is experienced in working with postoperative patients will know how to monitor for pain, bleeding, or swelling and will notify the supervising RN. Patient teaching requires more education and a broader scope of practice and is appropriate for RN staff members. **Focus:** Assignment.

7. **Ans: 4** LPN/LVN education and scope of practice includes sterile and nonsterile wound care. LPNs/LVNs do function as wound care nurses in some LTC facilities, but the choice of dressing type and assessment for risk factors are more complex skills that are appropriate to the RN level of practice. Assisting the patient to change position is a task included in AP education and would be more appropriate to delegate to the AP. **Focus:** Assignment.

8. **Ans: 2** Facial burns are frequently associated with airway inflammation and swelling, so this patient requires the most immediate assessment. The other patients also require rapid assessment or interventions, but their situations are not as urgent as that of the patient with facial burns. **Focus:** Prioritization.

9. **Ans: 3, 4, 2, 1, 5** Pain medication should be administered before changing the dressing because changing dressings for partial-thickness burns is painful, especially if the dressing change involves removal of eschar. The wound should be debrided before obtaining wound specimens for culture to avoid including bacteria that are skin contaminants rather than causes of the wound infection. Culture specimens should be obtained before the application of antibacterial creams. The antibacterial cream should then be applied to the area after debridement to gain the maximum effect. Finally, the wound should be covered with a sterile dressing. **Focus:** Prioritization.

10. **Ans: 3** A nurse from the oncology unit would be familiar with dressing changes and the sterile technique. The charge RN in the burn unit would work closely with the float RN to assist in providing care and to answer any questions. Admission assessment and development of the initial care plan, discharge teaching, and splint positioning in burn patients all require expertise in caring for patients with burns. These patients should be assigned to RNs who regularly work on the burn unit. **Focus:** Assignment.

11. **Ans: 4** Irregular borders and a black or variegated color are characteristics associated with malignant skin lesions. Striae and toenail thickening or yellowing are common in older adults. Silver scaling is associated with chronic conditions such as psoriasis and eczema, which may need treatment but are not as urgent a concern as the appearance of the mole. **Focus:** Prioritization.

12. **Ans: 1** A blue color or cyanosis may indicate that the patient has significant problems with circulation or ventilation. Further assessment of respiratory and circulatory status is needed immediately to determine if actions such as administration of oxygen or medications are appropriate. The other data may also indicate health problems in major body systems, but potential respiratory or circulatory abnormalities are the priority. **Focus:** Prioritization.

13. **Ans: 4** Because exposure to patients with shingles may cause herpes zoster infection (including systemic infection) in individuals who are immune suppressed, teaching about how to prevent transmission and possible evaluation and treatment of the patient's spouse is needed. Antiviral treatment is most effective when started within 72 hours of symptom development. The patient will need analgesics to treat the pain associated with shingles and may receive vaccination, but the biggest concern is possible infection of the patient's spouse. **Focus:** Prioritization.

14. **Ans: 4** Because urticaria can be associated with anaphylaxis, assessment for clinical manifestations of anaphylaxis (e.g., respiratory distress, wheezes, or hypotension) should be done immediately. The other actions are also appropriate, but therapy will change if an anaphylactic reaction is occurring. **Focus:** Prioritization.

15. **Ans: 1** Because isotretinoin is associated with a high incidence of birth defects, it is important that the patient stop using the medication at least 1 month before attempting to become pregnant. Nausea and muscle aches are possible adverse effects of isotretinoin that would require further assessment but are not as urgent as discussing the fetal risks associated with this medication. The patient's concern about whether treatment is effective should be addressed, but this is a lower priority intervention. **Focus:** Prioritization.

16. **Ans: 3** Scheduling a follow-up appointment for the patient is within the legal scope of practice and training for the AP role. Patient teaching, assessment for positive skin reactions to the test, and monitoring for serious allergic reactions are appropriate to the education and practice role of licensed nursing staff. **Focus:** Delegation.

17. **Ans: 1** Systemic use of tetracyclines such as doxycycline is associated with severe photosensitivity reactions to ultraviolet (UV) light. All individuals should be taught about the potential risks of overexposure to sunlight or other UV light, but the patient taking doxycycline is at the most immediate risk for severe adverse effects. **Focus:** Prioritization.

18. **Ans: 3** Although it is not appropriate for APs to plan or implement initial patient or family teaching, reinforcement of previous teaching is an important function of APs (who are likely to be in the home on a daily basis). Teaching about medication use, nutritional assessment and planning, and evaluation for improvement are included in the RN scope of practice. **Focus:** Delegation.

19. **Ans: 1** Medication administration is included in LPN/LVN education and scope of practice. Bathing and cleaning patients require the least education and would be better delegated to an AP. Assessment and evaluation of outcomes of care are more complex skills best performed by RNs. **Focus:** Assignment. **Test-Taking Tip:** When deciding what nursing actions should be done by staff with various levels of education, remember to consider effective use of resources and use staff to the level of their education. Although LPN/LVN staff members can provide more basic care, it's best to assign them to interventions that take advantage of their education and scope of practice.

20. **Ans: 2** The highest priority problems for this patient are pain and inadequate nutrition. Administration of analgesics is the most important action because the patient's acute oral pain will need to be controlled to increase the ability to eat and to improve nutrition. The patient's concern about appearance and refusal to see visitors are also concerns but are not as high priority as the need for pain control and improved nutrition. **Focus:** Prioritization.

21. **Ans: 4** Wheals are frequently associated with allergic reactions, so asking about exposure to new medications is the most appropriate question for this patient. The other questions would be useful in assessing the skin health history but do not directly relate to the patient's symptoms. **Focus:** Prioritization.

22. **Ans: 2** With chemical injuries, it is important to remove the chemical from contact with the skin to prevent ongoing damage. The other actions also should be accomplished rapidly; however, rinsing the chemical off is the priority for this patient. **Focus:** Prioritization.

23. **Ans: 3** This patient's vital signs indicate that the life-threatening complications of sepsis and septic shock may be developing. The other patients also need rapid assessment or nursing interventions, but their symptoms do not indicate that they need care as urgently as the febrile and hypotensive patient. **Focus:** Prioritization. **Test-Taking Tip:** Remember that when skin integrity is affected due to large burn injuries, patients are at high risk for complications such as sepsis and hypovolemia. You should monitor for changes in vital signs that might indicate these complications are occurring.

24. **Ans: 150** The label indicates 600 mg of medication in 300 mL. To infuse 300 mL in 2 hours, the nurse will need to give 150 mL/hr. **Focus:** Prioritization.

25. **Ans: 4, 1, 2, 5, 3** Culture of the wound will be needed before any antibiotic therapy, but the crust should be removed before wound culture to obtain a specimen that is not contaminated by normal skin bacteria. Application of topical antibiotic will be most effective with the crust removed and should be followed by covering the wound with a sterile

dressing. The nurse will provide written teaching materials when the patient is not distracted by the culture and dressing activities. **Focus:** Prioritization.

26. **Ans: 1, 2**   Contact precautions include gown and gloves when doing dressing changes for a patient with an infected wound. Booties are not needed for contact precautions. Goggles and a surgical mask may be needed if splashes or sprays are anticipated (e.g., with wound irrigation). Sterile gloves may be needed to change a sterile dressing but are not used as a contact precaution. **Focus:** Prioritization.

27. **Ans: 4**   Because aspirin affects platelet aggregation, the patient is at an increased risk for postprocedural bleeding, and the surgeon may need to reschedule the procedure. The other information is also pertinent but will not affect the scheduling of the procedure. **Focus:** Prioritization.

28. **Ans: 3**   A new graduate would be familiar with the procedure for a sterile dressing change, especially after working for 3 weeks on the unit. Patients whose care requires more complex skills such as admission assessments, preprocedure teaching, and discharge teaching should be assigned to more experienced RN staff members. **Focus:** Assignment.

29. **Ans: 3**   Epigastric pain may indicate that the patient is developing peptic ulcers, which require collaborative interventions such as the use of antacids, histamine$_2$ receptor blockers, and proton pump inhibitors. The elevation in blood glucose level, increased appetite, and slight elevation in blood pressure may be related to prednisone use but are not clinically significant when steroids are used for limited periods and do not require treatment. **Focus:** Prioritization.

30. **Ans: 2**   Dairy products inhibit the absorption of doxycycline, so this action would decrease the effectiveness of the antibiotic. The other activities are not appropriate but would not cause as much potential harm as the administration of doxycycline with milk. Anaerobic bacteria would not be likely to grow in a superficial wound. The herpes zoster vaccine is recommended for patients who are 60 years or older. Pressure garments may be used after graft wounds heal and during the rehabilitation period after a burn injury, but this should be discussed when the patient is ready for rehabilitation, not when the patient is admitted. **Focus:** Prioritization.

31. **Ans: 1**   Biologic immunomodulating agents such as adalimumab (which are frequently used in autoimmune disorders) increase infection risk and should be discontinued in patients with manifestations of infection. Scaly patches, erythema after sun exposure, and depression need further investigation and may require changes in therapy, but the highest concern is risk for worsening infection if the medication is continued. **Focus:** Prioritization.

32. **Ans: 2**   Seeking the AP's input into changes is respectful and helps with team dynamics. This response also most directly addresses the AP's concern about difficulties with time management. Asking the AP to try to comply suggests that noncompliance with needed infection control actions is an option. The suggestion that the AP will have to attend a class is disrespectful because it sounds like a threat, and there is no indication that the AP needs more training on infection control. Asking the AP to clarify when personal protective equipment is needed may lead to useful discussion about infection control but should be done when more time is available for discussion. **Focus:** Delegation.

33. **Ans: Option 1, Capillary leak syndrome; Option 2, Decreased tissue perfusion; Option 3, Intravenous fluids; Option 4, Tetanus Toxoid; Option 5, 1-2 years.**   After a major burn blood pressure initially increases due to vasoconstriction; however, within 12 hours, the BP will decrease due to capillary leak syndrome (third spacing), caused by dilation of the blood vessels that are near the burns. Morphine, insufficient fluid and septicemia can also lower blood pressure but are not unique to the physiology of major burns. Metabolic acidosis occurs as fluid, protein and electrolytes leak out of the vascular space. This action leads to decreased tissue perfusion which releases acids. Hyperkalemia worsens the acidosis as potassium from inside the destroyed cells is lost. In order to treat the metabolic acidosis intravenous fluids are given according to burn protocols in order to maintain urine output at 0.5mg/kg. Fluid resuscitation is necessary to maintain tissue perfusion in order to lessen the acidosis. Adequate renal function is necessary to excrete excess acid. Usually, sodium bicarbonate is administered only if the pH is less than 7.0 and is controversial. Fluids are first line therapy. *Clostridium tetani* is the bacteria that causes tetanus. The correct treatment for tetanus is tetanus toxoid. Vancomycin and Piperacillin-tazobactam are broad spectrum antibiotics that may be given to cover for septicemia, but they do not treat tetanus and Amphotericin B is an antifungal. Compression garments must be worn for 1-2 years for the full benefit to be realized. **Focus:** Priority.

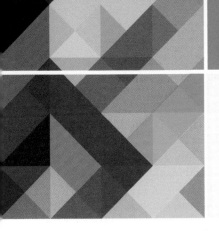

CHAPTER 16

Renal and Urinary Problems

Questions

1. The RN is supervising an LPN/LVN who is providing care for a patient with type 2 diabetes who is to have a renal computer tomography (CT) scan with contrast tomorrow morning. Which instruction would the RN be sure to provide to the LPN/LVN?
   1. "Remind the patient that the purpose of this scan is to measure kidney function."
   2. "Tell the assistive personnel to remove the patient's water pitcher from the bedside at 10 PM."
   3. "The patient's metformin should be discontinued 24 hours before the procedure."
   4. "Keep the patient on bedrest for at least 8 hours after returning to the unit."

2. The nurse is reviewing the lab values for a patient with risk for urinary problems. Which finding is of **most** concern to the nurse?
   1. Blood urea nitrogen of 10 mg/mL (3.6 mmol/L)
   2. Presence of glucose and protein in urine
   3. Serum creatinine of 0.6 mg/mL (53 mcmol/L)
   4. Urinary pH of 8

3. For which patient is the nurse **most** concerned about the risk for developing kidney disease?
   1. A 25-year-old patient who developed a urinary tract infection during pregnancy
   2. A 55-year-old patient with a history of kidney stones
   3. A 63-year-old patient with type 2 diabetes
   4. A 79-year-old patient with stress urinary incontinence

4. The nurse is caring for a patient at risk for kidney disease for whom a urinalysis has been ordered. What time would the nurse instruct the assistive personnel is **best** to collect this sample?
   1. With first morning void
   2. Before any meal
   3. At bedtime
   4. Immediately

5. The nurse has delegated collection of a urinalysis specimen to an experienced assistive personnel (AP). For which action must the nurse intervene?
   1. The AP provides the patient with a specimen cup.
   2. The AP reminds the patient of the need for the specimen.
   3. The AP assists the patient to the bathroom.
   4. The AP allows the specimen to sit for more than 1 hour.

6. The nurse is caring for a patient with risk for incomplete bladder emptying. Which noninvasive finding **best** supports this problem?
   1. Patient is able to void additional 100 mL after nurse massages over the bladder.
   2. Patient voids additional 350 mL with insertion of an intermittent catheter.
   3. Patient has postvoid residual of 275 mL documented by bedside bladder scanner.
   4. Patient has constant dribbling between voidings.

7. The nurse is providing care for a patient after a kidney biopsy. Which actions should the nurse delegate to an experienced assistive personnel (AP)? **Select all that apply.**
   1. Check vital signs every 4 hours for 24 hours.
   2. Remind the patient about strict bed rest for 2 to 6 hours.
   3. Reposition the patient by log-rolling with supporting backroll.
   4. Measure and record urine output.
   5. Assess the dressing site for bleeding and check complete blood count results.
   6. Teach the patient to resume normal activities after 24 hours if there is no bleeding.

8. The nurse is providing nursing care for a 24-year-old female patient admitted to the acute care unit with a diagnosis of cystitis. Which intervention should the nurse delegate to the assistive personnel (AP)?
   1. Teaching the patient how to secure a clean-catch urine sample
   2. Assessing the patient's urine for color, odor, and sediment
   3. Reviewing the nursing care plan and adding nursing interventions
   4. Providing the patient with a clean-catch urine sample container

9. Which laboratory result is of **most** concern to the nurse for an adult patient with cystitis?
   1. Serum white blood cell (WBC) count of 9000/mm^3 (9 × 109/L)
   2. Urinalysis results showing 1 or 2 WBCs present
   3. Urine bacteria count of 100,000 colonies per milliliter
   4. Serum hematocrit of 36%

10. The charge nurse would assign the nursing care of which patient to an LPN/LVN, working under the supervision of an RN?
    1. A 48-year-old patient with cystitis who is taking oral antibiotics
    2. A 64-year-old patient with kidney stones who has a new order for lithotripsy
    3. A 72-year-old patient with urinary incontinence who needs bladder training
    4. A 52-year-old patient with pyelonephritis who has severe acute flank pain

11. The nurse is admitting a 66-year-old male patient suspected of having a urinary tract infection (UTI). Which part of the patient's medical history supports this diagnosis?
    1. Patient's wife had a UTI 1 month ago
    2. Followed for prostate disease for 2 years
    3. Intermittent catheterization 6 months ago
    4. Kidney stone removal 1 year ago

12. A patient is being admitted to rule out interstitial cystitis. What should the nurse's plan of care for this patient include that is specific to this diagnosis?
    1. Take daily urine samples for urinalysis.
    2. Maintain accurate intake and output records.
    3. Obtain an admission urine sample to determine electrolyte levels.
    4. Teach the patient about the cystoscopy procedure.

13. The RN is supervising a new graduate nurse who is orientating to the unit. The new nurse asks why the patient with uncomplicated cystitis is being discharged with a prescription for ciprofloxacin 250 mg twice a day for only 3 days. What is the RN's **best** response?
    1. "We should check with the health care provider because the patient should take this drug for 10 to 14 days."
    2. "A 3-day course of ciprofloxacin is not the appropriate treatment for a patient with uncomplicated cystitis."
    3. "Research has shown that a 3-day course of ciprofloxacin is effective for uncomplicated cystitis and there is increased patient adherence to the plan of care."
    4. "Longer courses of antibiotic therapy are required for hospitalized patients to prevent nosocomial infections."

14. A 28-year-old married female patient with cystitis requires instruction about how to prevent future urinary tract infections (UTIs). The supervising RN has assigned this teaching to a newly graduated nurse. Which statement by the new graduate requires that the supervising RN intervene?
    1. "You should always drink 2 to 3 L of fluid every day."
    2. "Empty your bladder regularly even if you do not feel the urge to urinate."
    3. "Drinking cranberry juice daily will decrease the number of bacteria in your bladder."
    4. "It's okay to soak in the tub with bubble bath because it will keep you clean."

15. The nurse is creating a care plan for older adult patients with incontinence. For which patient will a bladder-training program be an appropriate intervention?
    1. Patient with functional incontinence caused by mental status changes
    2. Patient with stress incontinence due to weakened bladder neck support
    3. Patient with urge incontinence and abnormal detrusor muscle contractions
    4. Patient with transient incontinence related to loss of cognitive function

16. A patient with incontinence will be taking oxybutynin chloride 5 mg by mouth three times a day after discharge. Which information would the nurse be sure to teach this patient before discharge?
    1. "Drink fluids or use hard candy when you experience a dry mouth."
    2. "Be sure to notify your health care provider (HCP) if you experience a dry mouth."
    3. "If necessary, your HCP can increase your dose up to 40 mg/day."
    4. "You should take this medication with meals to avoid stomach ulcers."

17. The nurse is providing care for a patient with reflex urinary incontinence. Which action could be appropriately assigned to a new LPN/LVN?
    1. Teaching the patient bladder emptying by the Credé method
    2. Demonstrating how to perform intermittent self-catheterization
    3. Discussing when to report the side effects of bethanechol chloride to the health care provider (HCP)
    4. Reinforcing the importance of proper hand washing to prevent infection

18. A patient has urolithiasis and is passing the stones into the lower urinary tract. What is the **priority** nursing concern for the patient at this time?
    1. Pain
    2. Infection
    3. Injury
    4. Anxiety

19. The RN is supervising a nurse orientating to the acute care unit who is discharging a patient admitted with kidney stones and who underwent lithotripsy. Which statement by the orienting nurse to the patient requires that the supervising RN intervene?
    1. "You should finish all of your antibiotics to make sure that you don't get a urinary tract infection."
    2. "Remember to drink at least 3 L of fluids every day to prevent another stone from forming."
    3. "Report any signs of bruising to your health care provider (HCP) immediately because this indicates bleeding."
    4. "You can return to work in 2 days to 6 weeks, depending on what your HCP prescribes."

20. The RN is teaching a patient how to perform intermittent self-catheterization for a long-term problem with incomplete bladder emptying. Which are the **most** important points for teaching this technique? **Select all that apply.**
    1. Always use sterile techniques.
    2. Proper hand washing and cleaning of the catheter reduce the risk for infection.
    3. A small lumen and good lubrication of the catheter prevent urethral trauma.
    4. A regular schedule for bladder emptying prevents distention and mucosal trauma.
    5. The social work department can help you with the purchase of sterile supplies.
    6. If you are uncomfortable with this procedure, a home health nurse can do it.

21. The charge nurse must rearrange room assignments to admit a new patient. Which two patients would be **best** suited to be roommates?
    1. A 58-year-old patient with urothelial cancer receiving multiagent chemotherapy
    2. A 63-year-old patient with kidney stones who has just undergone open ureterolithotomy
    3. A 24-year-old patient with acute pyelonephritis and severe flank pain
    4. A 76-year-old patient with urge incontinence and a urinary tract infection

22. The problem of constipation related to compression of the intestinal tract has been identified in a patient with polycystic kidney disease. Which care action should the nurse assign to a newly-trained LPN/LVN?
    1. Instructing the patient about foods that are high in fiber
    2. Teaching the patient about foods that assist in promoting bowel regularity
    3. Assessing the patient for previous bowel problems and bowel routine
    4. Administering docusate sodium 100 mg by mouth twice a day

 Answer Key for this chapter begins on p. 163

23. Drag and Drop

Case Study

Scenario: A male patient must undergo intermittent catheterization. The nurse is preparing to ina catheter to assess the patient for postvoid residual.

Instructions: In the left column are the steps for intermittent catheter insertion. In the right column write the number to indicate the correct order of the steps, 1 being the first step and 8 being the last step.

Steps for intermittent catheter insertion	Order of steps
A. Assist the patient to the bathroom and ask the patient to attempt to void.	
B. Retract the foreskin and hold the penis at a 60-to 90-degree angle.	
C. Open the catheterization kit and put on sterile gloves.	
D. Lubricate the catheter and insert it through the meatus of the penis.	
E. Position the patient supine in bed or with the head slightly elevated.	
F. Drain all the urine present in the bladder into a container.	
G. Cleanse the glans penis starting at the meatus and working outward.	
H. Remove the catheter, clean the penis, and measure the amount of urine returned.	

24. The nurse is admitting a patient with nephrotic syndrome. Which assessment finding supports this diagnosis?
1. Edema formation
2. Hypotension
3. Increased urine output
4. Flank pain

25. When the nurse must apply containment strategies for a patient with incontinence, what is the **major** risk?
1. Incontinence-associated dermatitis
2. Skin breakdown
3. Infection
4. Fluid imbalance

26. The nurse is caring for a patient with renal cell carcinoma (adenocarcinoma of the kidney). While serving as preceptor for a new nurse orienting to the unit, the nurse is asked why this patient is not receiving chemotherapy. What is the **best** response?
1. "The prognosis for this form of cancer is very poor, and we will be providing only comfort measures."
2. "Nephrectomy is the preferred treatment because chemotherapy has been shown to have only limited effectiveness against this type of cancer."
3. "Research has shown that the most effective means of treating this form of cancer is with radiation therapy."
4. "Radiofrequency ablation is a minimally invasive procedure that is the best way to treat renal cell carcinoma."

27. The nurse is teaching a patient how to prevent renal trauma after an injury that required a left nephrectomy. Which points would the nurse include in the teaching plan? **Select all that apply.**
1. Always wear a seat belt.
2. Avoid contact sports.
3. Practice safe walking habits.
4. Wear protective clothing if you participate in contact sports.
5. Use caution when riding a bicycle.
6. Always avoid use of drugs that may damage the kidney.

28. The nurse is providing nursing care for a patient with acute kidney failure for whom volume overload has been identified. Which actions should the nurse delegate to an experienced assistive personnel? **Select all that apply.**
1. Measuring and recording vital sign values every 4 hours
2. Weighing the patient every morning using a standing scale
3. Administering furosemide 40 mg orally twice a day
4. Reminding the patient to save all urine for intake and output measurement
5. Assessing breath sounds every 4 hours
6. Ensuring that the patient's urinal is within reach

29. An assistive personnel (AP) reports to the RN that a patient with acute kidney failure had a urine output of 350 mL over the past 24 hours after receiving furosemide 40 mg IV push. The AP asks the nurse how this can happen. What is the nurse's **best** response?
    1. "During the oliguric phase of acute kidney failure, patients often do not respond well to either fluid challenges or diuretics."
    2. "There must be some sort of error. Someone must have failed to record the urine output."
    3. "A patient with acute kidney failure retains sodium and water, which counteracts the action of the furosemide."
    4. "The gradual accumulation of nitrogenous waste products results in the retention of water and sodium."

30. Which patient will the charge nurse assign to an RN floated to the acute care unit from the surgical intensive care unit (SICU)?
    1. A patient with kidney stones scheduled for lithotripsy this morning
    2. A patient who has just undergone surgery for renal stent placement
    3. A newly admitted patient with an acute urinary tract infection
    4. A patient with chronic kidney failure who needs teaching on peritoneal dialysis

31. The patient is receiving IV piggyback doses of gentamicin every 12 hours. Which would be the nurse's **priority** for monitoring during the period that the patient is receiving this drug?
    1. Serum creatinine and blood urea nitrogen (BUN) levels
    2. Patient weight every morning
    3. Intake and output every shift
    4. Temperature every 4 hours

32. A patient diagnosed with acute kidney failure had a urine output of 1560 mL for the past 8 hours. The LPN/LVN who is caring for this patient under the RN's supervision asks how a patient with kidney failure can have such a large urine output. What is the RN's **best** response?
    1. "The patient's kidney failure was caused by hypovolemia, and we have given him IV fluids to correct the problem."
    2. "Acute kidney failure patients go through a diuretic phase when their kidneys begin to recover and may put out as much as 10 L of urine per day."
    3. "With that much urine output, there must have been a mistake in the patient's diagnosis."
    4. "An increase in urine output like this is an indicator that the patient is entering the recovery phase of acute kidney failure."

33. A patient on the medical-surgical unit with acute kidney failure is to begin continuous arteriovenous hemofiltration (CAVH) as soon as possible. What is the **priority** collaborative action at this time?
    1. Call the charge nurse and arrange to transfer the patient to the intensive care unit.
    2. Develop a teaching plan for the patient that focuses on CAVH.
    3. Assist the patient with morning bath and mouth care before transfer.
    4. Notify the health care provider (HCP) that the patient's mean arterial pressure is 68 mm Hg.

34. The nurse is caring for a patient admitted with dehydration secondary to deficient antidiuretic hormone (ADH). Which specific gravity value supports this diagnosis?
    1. 1.010
    2. 1.035
    3. 1.020
    4. 1.002

35. The RN is supervising a senior nursing student who is caring for a 78-year-old patient scheduled for an intravenous pyelography test. What information would the RN be sure to stress about this procedure to the nursing student?
    1. "After the procedure, monitor urine output because contrast dye increases the risk for kidney failure in older adults."
    2. "The purpose of this procedure is to measure kidney size."
    3. "Because this procedure assesses kidney function, there is no need for a bowel prep."
    4. "Keep the patient NPO after the procedure because during the procedure the patient will receive drugs that may affect the gag reflex."

36. The RN supervising a senior nursing student is discussing methods for preventing acute kidney injury (AKI). Which points would the RN be sure to include in this discussion? **Select all that apply.**
    1. Encourage patients to avoid dehydration by drinking adequate fluids.
    2. Instruct patients to drink extra fluids during periods of strenuous exercise.
    3. Immediately report a urine output of less than 2 mL/kg/hr.
    4. Record intake and output and weigh patients daily.
    5. Question any prescriptions for potentially nephrotoxic drugs.
    6. Monitor laboratory values that reflect kidney function.

Answer Key for this chapter begins on p. 163

37. The nurse is caring for a patient with chronic kidney disease after hemodialysis. Which patient care action should the nurse delegate to the experienced assistive personnel (AP)?
    1. Assess the patient's access site for a thrill and bruit.
    2. Monitor for signs and symptoms of postdialysis bleeding.
    3. Check the patient's postdialysis blood pressure and weight.
    4. Instruct the patient to report signs of dialysis disequilibrium syndrome immediately.

38. The RN is to administer a subcutaneous injection of epoetin alfa 100 units/kg three times a week for a patient on dialysis. The patient weight 156 lb. Epoetin alfa comes from the pharmacy in a vial 10,000 units /1 mL.
    1. How many units will the RN give with each injection? _____
    2. How many mL will the RN give the patient? **(Round to two digits.)** _____
    3. What type of syringe would the nurse use to administer the medication? _____

39. Enhanced Multiple Response _____
Case Study and Question

The nurse is providing care for a patient with end stage kidney disease who is receiving hemodialysis 3 days a week. On return from dialysis, the RN notes a positive bruit and thrill at the dialysis site on the left arm. Bruising is noted distal and medial to the access. The patient states that she has no pain or discomfort.

Which tasks could be appropriately delegated to an experienced assistive personnel (AP)?

1. Check the patient's blood pressure in both arms.
2. Weigh the patient on return from dialysis treatment.
3. Reassess the patient's dialysis site for a bruit and thrill.
4. Assist the patient up to the chair for meals.
5. Record accurate intake and output.
6. Report any patient bleeding to the RN immediately.
7. Assess the patient for signs of hypotension after dialysis.
8. Administer evening medications as ordered.
9. Place a sign over the bed stating "No blood pressures, IV, or venipunctures in left arm."

Instructions: Read the case study on the left and circle the numbers that best answer the question.

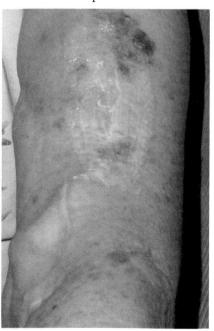

Answers

PART 2

Common Health Scenarios

1. **Ans: 3**   Patients receiving metformin are at risk for lactic acidosis when given iodinated contrast media. The drug should be discontinued for at least 24 hours before and 48 hours after the procedure and kidney function should be re-evaluated before the patient resumes taking metformin. The purpose of the scan is get three-dimensional information about the kidneys. A patient having this scan is not kept NPO and is not kept on bedrest. **Focus:** Supervision, Assignment.

2. **Ans: 2**   When blood glucose levels are greater than 220 mg/dL (12.2 mmol/L), some glucose stays in the filtrate and is present in the urine. Normally, almost all glucose and most proteins are reabsorbed and are not present in the urine. Report the presence of glucose or proteins in the urine of a patient undergoing a screening examination to the health care provider because this is an abnormal finding and requires further assessment. **Focus:** Prioritization.

3. **Ans: 3**   A history of chronic health problems, especially diabetes and hypertension, increases the risk for development of kidney disease. **Focus:** Prioritization.

4. **Ans: 1**   Urinalysis is a part of any complete physical examination and is especially useful for patients with suspected kidney or urologic disorders. Ideally, the urine specimen is collected at the morning's first voiding. Specimens obtained at other times may be too dilute. **Focus:** Delegation, Supervision.

5. **Ans: 4**   Urine specimens become more alkaline when left standing unrefrigerated for more than 1 hour, when bacteria are present, or when a specimen is left uncovered. Alkaline urine increases cell breakdown; thus the presence of red blood cells may be missed on analysis. Ensure that urine specimens are covered and delivered to the laboratory promptly or refrigerated. Actions 1, 2, and 3 are appropriate for urinalysis specimen collection. **Focus:** Delegation, Supervision.

6. **Ans: 3**   The use of portable ultrasound scanners in the hospital and rehabilitation setting by nurses is a noninvasive method of estimating bladder volume. Bladder scanners are used to screen for postvoid residual volumes and to determine the need for intermittent catheterization based on the amount of urine in the bladder rather than the time between catheterizations. There is no discomfort with the scan, and no patient preparation beyond an explanation of what to expect is required. Use of bladder massage or presence of urinary dribbling is inexact, and intermittent catheterization is invasive. **Focus:** Prioritization.

7. **Ans: 1, 2, 3, 4**   Checking vital signs, repositioning patients, reminding patients what has already been taught, and recording intake and output are within the scope of practice for an AP. Assessing and teaching are more within the scope of practice for professional nurses. If no bleeding occurs, the patient can resume general activities after 24 hours. Nevertheless, instruct him or her to avoid lifting heavy objects, exercising, and performing other strenuous activities for 1 to 2 weeks after the biopsy procedure. Driving may also be restricted. **Focus:** Delegation, Supervision.

8. **Ans: 4**   Providing the equipment that the patient needs to collect the urine sample is within the scope of practice of a AP. Teaching, planning, and assessing all require additional education and skill, which is appropriate to the scope of practice of professional nurses. **Focus:** Delegation, Supervision.

9. **Ans: 3**   The presence of 100,000 bacterial colonies per milliliter of urine or the presence of many WBCs and red blood cells indicates a urinary tract infection. This WBC count is within normal limits, and the hematocrit is a little low, which may require follow-up. Neither of these results indicates infection. **Focus:** Prioritization. **Test-Taking Tip:** It is essential that the nurse be alert to any signs or symptoms of infection for a patient. In this case, the presence of so many bacterial colonies indicates the presence of an infection in the bladder, which needs to be treated with antibiotics.

10. **Ans: 1**   The patient with cystitis who is taking oral antibiotics is in stable condition with predictable outcomes, and caring for this patient is therefore appropriate to the scope of practice of an LPN/LVN under the supervision of an RN. The patient with a new order for lithotripsy will need teaching about the procedure, which should be accomplished by the RN. The patient in need of bladder training will need the RN to plan this intervention. The patient with flank pain needs a careful and skilled assessment by the RN. **Focus:** Assignment.

11. **Ans: 2**   Prostate disease increases the risk of UTIs in men because of urinary retention. The wife's UTI should not affect the patient. The times of the catheter usage and kidney stone removal are too distant to cause this UTI. **Focus:** Prioritization.

12. **Ans: 4**   A cystoscopy is needed to accurately diagnose interstitial cystitis. A urinalysis may show white blood cells and red blood cells but no bacteria. The patient will probably need a urinalysis upon admission, but daily samples do not need to be obtained. Intake and output may be assessed, but results will not contribute to the diagnosis. Cystitis does not usually affect urine electrolyte levels. **Focus:** Prioritization.

13. **Ans: 3**   For uncomplicated cystitis, a 3-day course of antibiotics is an effective treatment, and research has shown that patients are more likely to adhere to shorter antibiotic courses. Seven-day courses of antibiotics are appropriate for complicated cystitis, and 10- to 14-day courses are prescribed for uncomplicated pyelonephritis. This patient is being discharged and should not be at risk for a nosocomial infection. **Focus:** Prioritization.

14. **Ans: 4**   Women should avoid irritating substances such as bubble baths, nylon underwear, and scented toilet tissue to prevent UTIs. Adequate fluid intake, consumption of cranberry juice, and regular voiding are all good strategies for preventing UTIs. **Focus:** Assignment, Supervision, Prioritization.

15. **Ans: 3**   A patient with urge incontinence can be taught to control the bladder as long as the patient is alert, aware, and able to resist the urge to urinate by starting a schedule for voiding, then increasing the intervals between voids. Patients with functional incontinence related to mental status changes or loss of cognitive function are not able to follow a bladder-training program. A better treatment for a patient with stress incontinence involves exercises such as pelvic floor (Kegel) exercises to strengthen the pelvic floor muscles. **Focus:** Prioritization.

16. **Ans: 1**   Oxybutynin is an anticholinergic agent, and these drugs often cause an extremely dry mouth. The maximum dosage is 20 mg/day. Oxybutynin should be taken between meals because food interferes with absorption of the drug. **Focus:** Prioritization.

17. **Ans: 4**   Teaching about bladder emptying, self-catheterization, and when to notify the HCP about medication side effects requires additional knowledge and training and is appropriate to the scope of practice of the RN. The LPN/LVN can reinforce information that has already been taught to the patient. **Focus:** Assignment, Supervision.

18. **Ans: 1**   When patients with urolithiasis pass stones, they can be in excruciating pain for as much as 24 to 36 hours. All of the other nursing concerns for this patient are accurate; however, at this time, pain is the most urgent concern for the patient. **Focus:** Prioritization.

19. **Ans: 3**   Bruising is to be expected after lithotripsy. It may be quite extensive and take several weeks to resolve. All of the other statements are accurate for a patient after lithotripsy. **Focus:** Assignment, Supervision, Prioritization.

20. **Ans: 2, 3, 4**   Intermittent self-catheterization is often used to help patients with long-term problems of incomplete bladder emptying. It is not a sterile procedure and does not require sterile equipment. It is a clean procedure. Important teaching points include responses 2, 3, and 4 of this question. **Focus:** Prioritization.

21. **Ans: 3, 4**   Both of these patients will need frequent assessments and medications. The patient receiving chemotherapy and the patient who has just undergone surgery should not be exposed to any patient with infection. **Focus:** Assignment, Prioritization.

22. **Ans: 4**   Administering oral medications appropriately is covered in the educational program for LPNs/LVNs and is within their scope of practice. Teaching and assessing the patient require additional education and skill and are appropriate to the scope of practice of RNs. **Focus:** Assignment, Supervision.

23. **Ans: 1, 5, 3, 2, 7, 4, 6, 8**   Before checking postvoid residual, the RN should ask the patient to void and then position him. Next the nurse should open the catheterization kit and put on sterile gloves, position the patient's penis, clean the meatus, and then lubricate and insert the catheter. All urine must be drained from the bladder to assess the amount of postvoid residual the patient has. Finally, the catheter is removed, the penis cleaned, and the urine measured. **Focus:** Prioritization. **Test-Taking Tip:** For this type of question, the nurse must stop and think about the correct steps for performing a nursing action and then place them in the correct order.

24. **Ans: 1**   The underlying pathophysiology of nephrotic syndrome involves increased glomerular permeability, which allows larger molecules to pass through the membrane into the urine and be removed from the blood. This process causes massive loss of protein, edema formation, and decreased serum albumin levels. Key features include hypertension and renal insufficiency (decreased urine output) related to concurrent renal vein thrombosis, which may be a cause or an effect of nephrotic syndrome. Flank pain is seen in patients with acute pyelonephritis. **Focus:** Prioritization.

25. **Ans: 2**   A major concern with the use of wearable protective pads is the risk for skin breakdown. Some patients may develop incontinence-associated dermatitis even when the skin is kept free of contact with urine because wearable pads generate heat and sweat in the area and can cause dermatitis. Infection becomes a risk when skin breakdown occurs. **Focus:** Prioritization.

26. **Ans: 2**   Chemotherapy has limited effectiveness against renal cell carcinoma. This form of cancer is usually treated surgically with nephrectomy. **Focus:** Supervision, Prioritization.

27. **Ans: 1, 2, 3, 5**   A patient with only one kidney should avoid all contact sports and high-risk activities to protect the remaining kidney from injury and preserve kidney function. Protective clothing may not be enough to protect the patient's remaining kidney. Drugs that may cause kidney damage may still be prescribed, especially to save a patient's life. All of the other points are key to preventing renal trauma. **Focus:** Prioritization.

28. **Ans: 1, 2, 4, 6**   Administering oral medications is appropriate to the scope of practice for an LPN/LVN or RN. Assessing breath sounds requires additional education and skill development and is most appropriate within the scope of practice of an RN, but it may be part of the observations of an experienced and competent LPN/LVN. All other actions are within the educational preparation and scope of practice of an experienced AP. **Focus:** Delegation, Supervision.

29. **Ans: 1** During the oliguric phase of acute kidney failure, a patient's urine output is greatly reduced. Fluid boluses and diuretics do not work well. This phase usually lasts from 8 to 15 days. Although there are occasionally omissions in recording intake and output, this is probably not the cause of the patient's decreased urine output. Retention of sodium and water is the rationale for giving furosemide, not the reason that it is ineffective. Nitrogenous wastes build up as a result of the kidneys' inability to perform their elimination function. **Focus:** Prioritization, Supervision.

30. **Ans: 2** A nurse from the SICU will be thoroughly familiar and comfortable with the care of patients who have just undergone surgery. The patient scheduled for lithotripsy may need education about the procedure. The newly admitted patient needs an in-depth admission assessment, and the patient with chronic kidney failure needs teaching about peritoneal dialysis. All of these interventions would best be accomplished by an experienced nurse with expertise in the care of patients with kidney problems. **Focus:** Assignment.

31. **Ans: 1** Gentamicin can be a highly nephrotoxic substance. The nurse would monitor creatinine and BUN levels for elevations indicating possible nephrotoxicity. All of the other measures are important but are not specific to gentamicin therapy. **Focus:** Prioritization.

32. **Ans: 2** Patients with acute kidney failure usually go through a diuretic phase 2 to 6 weeks after the onset of the oliguric phase. The diuresis can result in an output of up to 10 L/day of dilute urine. During this phase, it is important to monitor for electrolyte and fluid imbalances. This is followed by the recovery phase. A patient with acute kidney failure caused by hypovolemia would receive IV fluids to correct the problem; however, this would not necessarily lead to the onset of diuresis. **Focus:** Supervision.

33. **Ans: 1** CAVH is a continuous renal replacement therapy that is prescribed for patients with kidney failure who are critically ill and do not tolerate the rapid shifts in fluids and electrolytes that are associated with hemodialysis. The patient will need careful in-depth monitoring in a critical care setting during this procedure. A teaching plan is not urgent at this time. A patient must have a mean arterial pressure (MAP) of at least 60 mm Hg or more for CAVH to be of use. The HCP should be notified about this patient's MAP; it is a priority but not the highest priority. When a patient urgently needs a procedure, morning care does not take priority and may be deferred until later in the day. **Focus:** Prioritization.

34. **Ans: 4** A patient with dehydration as a result of deficient ADH would have dilute urine with a decreased urine specific gravity. Normal urine specific gravity ranges from 1.003 to 1.030. A specific gravity of 1.035 would indicate urine that is concentrated. **Focus:** Prioritization. **Test-Taking Tip:** A way to remember the difference between Increased ADH

and Decreased ADH is: Increased ADH = Increased specific gravity (Kidneys hold on to the water [antidiuretic]) so the urine is concentrated, while Decreased ADH = Decreased specific gravity (Kidneys can't hold on to water because there is no antidiuretic) so the urine is very dilute.

35. **Ans: 1** The risk for contrast-induced kidney failure is greatest in patients who are older or dehydrated. If possible, arrange for the patient to have this procedure early in the day to prevent dehydration. The purpose of this procedure is to assess kidney function and identify anomalies. The administration of drugs that affect the gag reflex is not done during this procedure. **Focus:** Supervision, Prioritization.

36. **Ans: 1, 2, 4, 6** Dehydration reduces perfusion and can lead to AKI. Patients should be encouraged to take in adequate fluids, and extra fluids should be taken in during strenuous exercise. Intake and output, as well as daily weights, should be documented. Lab values that indicate kidney function should be followed. The health care provider should be notified for a urine output of less than 0.5 mL/kg/hr that persists for more than 2 hours. Many drugs are potentially nephrotoxic but are still administered. Patients are encouraged to take in extra fluids, and nurses must monitor for any nephrotoxic effects when these drugs are prescribed. **Focus:** Prioritization.

37. **Ans: 3** Checking vital signs and weighing patients are within the scope of practice for the AP. Nevertheless, the nurse must be sure to caution the AP to check the blood pressure in the arm opposite to the access site. Assessing, teaching, and monitoring require additional skills that fit within the scope of practice for the professional nurse. **Focus:** Delegation.

38. **Ans: 7090 units; .7090 mL (.71 mL)** 156 lb/2.2 = 70.91 × 100 = 7091 units
10,000 units/1 mL : 7091 units/X mL = .7091 mL (.71 mL)
(To administer such a small volume of fluid, use a very small syringe—e.g., a tuberculin syringe.) **Focus:** Prioritization.

39. **Ans: 2, 4, 5, 6, 9** The AP's scope of practice includes checking vital signs, weighing patients, assisting with ambulation and recording intake/output records. Since the patient's dialysis access in is the left arm, no blood pressures, IVs, or blood draws would be done on the left arm. (If there is no sign stating these limits placed above the patient's bed, the RN should instruct the AP to do this.) The AP would certainly notify the RN if there was any bleeding noted after dialysis; however, the RN would also be carefully assessing for this. The RN would also assess and reassess the access site for a bruit and thrill, as well as any signs or symptoms of hypotension after dialysis. The RN would administer medications (an LPN/LVN could also be assigned this task). **Focus:** Delegation, Assignment.

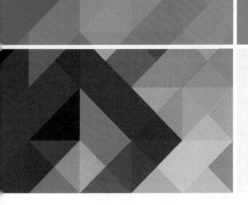

Questions

1. A 59-year-old postmenopausal woman is being interviewed by the nurse. Which statement made by the patient requires the nurse to notify the health care provider **immediately**?
   1. "Every time I cough or sneeze, I spill a little urine."
   2. "My vagina feels so dry and uncomfortable."
   3. "I thought getting my period was finally over but I started bleeding again."
   4. "Having sex is so painful and uncomfortable."

2. The nurse obtains the health history of a 37-year-old woman who is requesting contraceptive therapy. Which information about the patient will have the **most** impact on the choice of contraceptive?
   1. History of uterine fibroids
   2. Blood pressure of 136/80 mm Hg
   3. Cigarette smoking of a pack/day
   4. Planning outpatient oral surgery

3. A postmenopausal woman who is taking raloxifene for osteoporosis calls the clinic nurse with these concerns. Which information indicates a need for **immediate** further evaluation?
   1. Experiences hot flashes several times weekly
   2. Describes family history of coronary artery disease
   3. Reports nasal stuffiness and runny nose
   4. Notices swelling and tenderness in left calf

4. The nurse is assessing a long-term-care patient with a history of benign prostatic hyperplasia. Which information will require the **most** immediate action?
   1. The patient states that he always has trouble starting his urinary stream.
   2. The chart shows an elevated level of prostate-specific antigen.
   3. The bladder is palpable above the symphysis pubis, and the patient is restless.
   4. The patient says he has not voided since having a glass of juice 4 hours ago.

5. While performing a breast examination on a 22-year-old patient, the nurse obtains these data. Which finding is of **most** concern?
   1. Both breasts have many nodules in the upper outer quadrants.
   2. The patient reports bilateral breast tenderness with palpation.
   3. The breast on the right side is slightly larger than the left breast.
   4. An irregularly shaped, nontender lump is palpable in the left breast.

6. After undergoing a modified radical mastectomy, a patient is transferred to the postanesthesia care unit. Which nursing action is **best** to assign to an experienced LPN/LVN?
   1. Monitoring the patient's dressing for any signs of bleeding
   2. Documenting the initial assessment on the patient's chart
   3. Communicating the patient's status report to the charge nurse on the surgical unit
   4. Teaching the patient about the importance of using pain medication as needed

7. The nurse is working with an assistive personnel (AP) to care for a patient who has had a right breast lumpectomy and axillary lymph node dissection. Which nursing action can be delegated to the AP?
   1. Teaching the patient why blood pressure measurements are taken on the left arm
   2. Elevating the patient's arm on two pillows to promote lymphatic drainage
   3. Assessing the patient's right arm for lymphedema
   4. Reinforcing the dressing if it becomes saturated

8. The nurse obtains the following assessment data about a patient who has had a transurethral resection of the prostate (TURP) and has continuous bladder irrigation. Which finding indicates the **most** immediate need for nursing intervention?
   1. The patient states that he feels a continuous urge to void.
   2. The catheter drainage is light pink with occasional clots.
   3. The catheter is taped to the patient's thigh.
   4. The patient reports painful bladder spasms.

9. A patient with benign prostatic hyperplasia has a new prescription for tamsulosin. Which statement about tamsulosin is **most** important to include when teaching this patient?
   1. "This medication will improve your symptoms by shrinking the prostate."
   2. "The force of your urinary stream will probably increase."
   3. "Your blood pressure might decrease as a result of taking this medication."
   4. "You should avoid sitting up or standing up too quickly."

10. The nurse is caring for a patient who has just returned to the surgical unit after a transurethral resection of the prostate (TURP). Which assessment finding will require the **most** immediate action?
    1. Blood pressure reading of 153/88 mm Hg
    2. Catheter that is draining deep red blood
    3. Patient not wearing antiembolism hose
    4. Patient report of abdominal cramping

11. After a radical prostatectomy, a patient is ready to be discharged. Which nursing action included in the discharge plan should be assigned to an experienced LPN/LVN?
    1. Reinforcing the patient's need to check his temperature daily
    2. Teaching the patient how to care for his retention catheter
    3. Documenting a discharge assessment in the patient's chart
    4. Instructing the patient about the prescribed opioid analgesic

12. The day after a radical prostatectomy, a patient has blood clots in the urinary catheter and reports bladder spasms. The patient says that his right calf is sore and that he feels short of breath. Which action will the nurse take **first**?
    1. Irrigate the catheter with 50 mL of sterile saline.
    2. Administer oxybutynin 5 mg orally.
    3. Apply warm packs to the right calf.
    4. Measure oxygen saturation using pulse oximetry.

13. The emergency department nurse receives change-of-shift report about four patients. Which one should be assessed **first**?
    1. A 19-year-old patient with scrotal swelling and severe pain that has not decreased with elevation of the scrotum
    2. A 25-year-old patient who has a painless indurated lesion on the glans penis
    3. A 44-year-old patient with an elevated temperature, chills, and back pain associated with recurrent prostatitis
    4. A 77-year-old patient with abdominal pain and acute bladder distention

14. The nurse obtains this information when taking the health history of a 56-year-old postmenopausal woman. Which information is **most** important to report to the health care provider (HCP)?
    1. Sagging of breasts bilaterally
    2. Vaginal dryness and painful intercourse
    3. Hot flashes occurring during the night
    4. Occasional painless vaginal bleeding

15. The nurse is interviewing a woman who is in the clinic for a well woman examination, and the woman requests a screening test for ovarian cancer. Which response by the nurse is **best**?
    1. "Only a small number of ovarian cancers are diagnosed at an early stage."
    2. "There is no effective screening test for ovarian cancer in low-risk women."
    3. "Benefits of ovarian cancer screening will depend on your medical history."
    4. "Ovarian cancer screening will probably not be covered by your insurance."

16. A patient who has just returned to the surgical unit after a transurethral resection of the prostate (TURP) reports acute bladder spasms. In which order will the nurse perform these prescribed actions?
    1. Administer acetaminophen/oxycodone 325 mg/5 mg.
    2. Irrigate the retention catheter with 30 to 50 mL of sterile normal saline.
    3. Infuse 500 mL of 5% dextrose in lactated Ringer's solution over 2 hours.
    4. Offer the patient oral fluids to at least 2500 to 3000 mL/day.
    _____, _____, _____, _____

17. A 68-year-old patient who is ready for discharge from the emergency department has a new prescription for nitroglycerin 0.4 mg sublingual as needed for angina. Which patient information has the **most** immediate implications for teaching?
    1. The patient has prostatic hyperplasia with some urinary hesitancy.
    2. The patient's father and two brothers all have had myocardial infarctions.
    3. The patient uses sildenafil several times weekly for erectile dysfunction.
    4. The patient is unable to remember when he first experienced chest pain.

18. The nurse is caring for a 21-year-old patient who had a left orchiectomy for testicular cancer on the previous day. Which nursing activity will be **best** to assign to an LPN/LVN?
    1. Educating the patient about postorchiectomy chemotherapy and radiation
    2. Administering the prescribed as needed oxycodone to the patient
    3. Teaching the patient how to do testicular self-examination on the remaining testicle
    4. Assessing the patient's knowledge level about postorchiectomy fertility

19. Which patient is **best** for the oncology unit charge nurse to assign to an RN who has floated from the emergency department?
    1. Patient who needs doxorubicin chemotherapy to treat metastatic breast cancer
    2. Patient who needs discharge teaching after surgery for stage II ovarian cancer
    3. Patient with metastatic prostate cancer who requires frequent assessment and treatment for breakthrough pain
    4. Patient with testicular cancer who requires preoperative teaching about orchiectomy and lymph node resection

20. After receiving the change-of-shift report, in which order will the nurse assess these assigned patients?
    1. A 22-year-old patient who has questions about how to care for the drains placed in her breast reconstruction incision
    2. An anxious 44-year-old patient who is scheduled to be discharged today after undergoing a total vaginal hysterectomy
    3. A 69-year-old patient who reports level 5 pain (on a scale of 0 to 10) after undergoing a perineal prostatectomy 2 days ago
    4. A usually oriented 78-year-old patient who has new-onset confusion after having a bilateral orchiectomy the previous day

    _____, _____, _____, _____

21. A patient has had a needle biopsy of the prostate gland using the transrectal approach. Which statement is **most** important to include in the patient teaching plan?
    1. "The health care provider (HCP) will call you about the test results."
    2. "Serious infections may occur as a complication of this test."
    3. "You will need to call the HCP if you develop a fever or chills."
    4. "It is normal to have a small amount of rectal bleeding after the test."

22. The nurse is working in the postanesthesia care unit caring for a 32-year-old patient who has just arrived after undergoing dilation and curettage to evaluate infertility. Which assessment finding should be **immediately** communicated to the surgeon?
    1. Blood pressure of 162/90 mm Hg
    2. Saturation of the perineal pad after the first 30 minutes
    3. Oxygen saturation of 91% to 95%
    4. Sharp, continuous, level 8 abdominal pain (on a scale of 0 to 10)

23. When the nurse is developing the plan of care for a home health patient who has been discharged after a radical prostatectomy, which activities will be delegated to the home health aide? **Select all that apply.**
    1. Monitoring the patient for symptoms of urinary tract infection
    2. Helping the patient to connect the catheter to the leg bag
    3. Checking the patient's incision for appropriate wound healing
    4. Assisting the patient in ambulating for increasing distances
    5. Helping the patient shower at least every other day
    6. Educating the patient on when he may begin driving

24. The nurse is working in the emergency department when a patient with possible toxic shock syndrome is admitted. Which prescribed intervention will the nurse implement **first**?
    1. Remove the patient's tampon.
    2. Obtain blood specimens for culture.
    3. Give acetaminophen 650 mg.
    4. Infuse nafcillin 1000 mg IV.

25. Which information will the nurse include when teaching a group of 20-year-old women about emergency contraception with levonorgestrel (the morning-after pill)? **Select all that apply.**
    1. Heavier menstrual bleeding is a common side effect of this medication regimen.
    2. Emergency contraception requires a prescription from a licensed health care provider.
    3. Even if pregnancy occurs after using emergency contraception, risk for complications is low.
    4. Because nausea and vomiting may occur, an antiemetic may be used before levonorgestrel.
    5. The medication must be taken within the first 24 hours after unprotected intercourse to be effective.
    6. Levonorgestrel can be used as a regular form of birth control.

26. The clinic nurse reviews information about four patients who are requesting Pap testing. Which patient needs to be scheduled **first**?
    1. A 19-year-old patient who first had intercourse at age 13 years
    2. A 25-year-old patient who has never had a pelvic examination
    3. A 33-year-old patient who had a normal Pap test 2 years previously
    4. A 67-year-old patient who says her previous Pap test results have been normal

27. When assessing a patient with cervical cancer who had a total abdominal hysterectomy yesterday, the nurse obtains the following data. Which information has the **most** immediate implications for planning of the patient's care?
    1. Fine crackles are audible at the lung bases.
    2. The patient's right calf is swollen, and she reports mild calf tenderness.
    3. The patient uses the patient-controlled analgesia device every 30 minutes.
    4. Urine in the collection bag is amber and clear.

28. The nurse is supervising a student nurse who is caring for a patient who has an intracavitary radioactive implant in place to treat cervical cancer. Which action by the student requires that the nurse intervene **immediately**?
    1. Standing next to the patient for 5 minutes while assisting with her bath
    2. Asking the patient how she feels about losing her childbearing ability
    3. Assisting the patient to the bedside commode for a bowel movement
    4. Offering to get the patient whatever she would like to eat or drink

29. A patient who had an abdominal hysterectomy 3 days ago reports burning with urination. Her urine output during the previous shift was 210 mL, and her temperature is 101.3°F (38.5°C). Which of these actions prescribed by the health care provider will the nurse implement **first**?
    1. Insert a straight catheter as needed for output of less than 300 mL/8 hr.
    2. Administer acetaminophen 650 mg now and every 6 hours PRN.
    3. Send a urine specimen to the laboratory for culture and sensitivity testing.
    4. Administer ceftizoxime 1 g IV now and every 12 hours.

30. An 86-year-old woman had an anterior and posterior colporrhaphy (A & P repair) several days ago. Her retention catheter was removed 8 hours ago. Which assessment finding requires that the nurse act **most** rapidly?
    1. Her oral temperature is 100.7°F (38.2°C).
    2. Her abdomen is firm and tender to palpation above the symphysis pubis.
    3. Her breath sounds are decreased, with fine crackles audible at both bases.
    4. Her apical pulse is 86 beats/min and slightly irregular.

31. The nurse is reviewing medication lists for several patients. Which medication is **most** important for the nurse to question?
    1. Testosterone transdermal gel for a patient who has prostate cancer
    2. Metformin for a patient whose only diagnosis is polycystic ovary syndrome
    3. Sildenafil for a patient who is also taking hydrochlorothiazide for hypertension
    4. Methoprogesterone for a patient who has infertility associated with endometriosis

32. The nurse is providing orientation for a new RN on the medical-surgical unit who is caring for a patient with severe pelvic inflammatory disease (PID). Which action by the new RN is **most** important to correct quickly?
    1. Telling the patient that she should avoid using tampons in the future
    2. Offering the patient an ice pack to decrease her abdominal pain
    3. Positioning the patient flat in bed while helping her take a bath
    4. Teaching the patient that she should not have intercourse for 2 months

  Answer Key for this chapter begins on p. 172

33. Which information obtained when taking a patient's health history will be **most** important in determining whether the patient should receive the human papillomavirus (HPV) immunization?
    1. The patient is 19 years old.
    2. The patient is sexually active.
    3. The patient has a positive pregnancy test result.
    4. The patient has tested positive for HPV previously.

34. Three days after undergoing a pelvic exenteration procedure, a patient reports dizziness after experiencing a sudden "giving" sensation along her abdominal incision. The nurse finds that the wound edges are open, and loops of intestine are protruding. Which action should the nurse take **first**?
    1. Notify the surgeon that wound evisceration has occurred.
    2. Cover the wound with saline-soaked dressings.
    3. Use swabs to obtain aerobic and anaerobic wound cultures.
    4. Call for assistance from the rapid response team (RRT).

35. The nurse is working on a medical unit staffed with LPNs/LVNs and assistive personnel (AP) when a patient with stage IV ovarian cancer and recurrent ascites is admitted for paracentesis. Which activity is **best** to assign to an experienced LPN/LVN?
    1. Obtaining a paracentesis tray from the central supply area
    2. Completing the short-stay patient admission form
    3. Measuring vital signs every 15 minutes after the procedure
    4. Providing discharge instructions after the procedure

36. A new nurse who is assigned to care for a transgender patient who has been admitted with pneumonia tells the charge nurse, "I do not feel comfortable caring for this patient." Which action should the charge nurse take **first**?
    1. Teach the new nurse that culturally sensitive care for all patients is an expectation for staff members.
    2. Change the new nurse's assignment for the day and arrange for more training about transgender health.
    3. Ask the new nurse to clarify the specific concerns about providing treatment for a transgender patient.
    4. Explain to the new nurse that the treatment for pneumonia will not be affected by the patient's transgender status.

37. Which action by the nurse will **best** meet the goal of providing culturally competent care for lesbian, gay, bisexual, and transgender patients?
    1. Direct transgender patients to the unisex bathrooms.
    2. Assure patients that they will all be treated the same way.
    3. Ask all patients about sexual orientation and gender identification.
    4. Develop forms that use gender-neutral terms to collect patient information.

38. While the nurse is working in the clinic, a healthy 32-year-old woman whose sister is a carrier of the *BRCA* gene asks which form of breast cancer screening is the most effective for her. Which response is **best**?
    1. "An annual mammogram is usually sufficient screening for women your age."
    2. "Monthly self-breast examination is recommended because of your higher risk."
    3. "A yearly breast examination by a health care provider should be scheduled."
    4. "Magnetic resonance imaging (MRI) is recommended in addition to annual mammography."

39. A patient with toxic shock syndrome is to receive clindamycin 900 mg IV over 60 minutes. The clindamycin is diluted in 100 mL of normal saline. The nurse will infuse _____ mL/hr.

40. A patient who is being treated as an outpatient for pelvic inflammatory disease (PID) with oral antibiotics returns to the clinic after 3 days of treatment. Which finding by the nurse is of **highest** concern?
    1. Patient reports nausea after taking the antibiotics.
    2. Patient's abdominal rebound pain is unchanged.
    3. Patient says she feels ashamed to have the infection.
    4. Patient's cervical culture report shows gonorrhea.

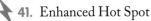

41. Enhanced Hot Spot _____

Case Study

The nurse is assessing a 48-year-old male who is being seen for a yearly physical.

Vital Signs:
Temperature 98.8°F (37.1°C)
Pulse 90 beats/min
Respirations 20 breaths/min
Blood Pressure 150/94 mm Hg
Oxygen Saturation 98% on room air
Body Mass Index 26 kg/m^2

Medications:
Sertraline 25mg QD
Simvastatin 40mg QD
Lisinopril 20mg QD

Social history: Divorced, smokes e-cigarettes and admits to drinking 2 beers a day, employed as construction worker, walks 3 miles a day and lifts weights 3 times a week.

Medical history: Depression, Chronic low back pain, degenerate disk disease L4-L6, hypertension, high cholesterol.

Instructions: Underline or highlight the factors and characteristics that increase the risk for male erectile dysfunction (ED).

PART 2

Common Health Scenarios

 Answer Key for this chapter begins on p. 172

Answers

1. **Ans: 3** Spotting or bleeding after a woman has been in menopause for over a year can be a sign of uterine or ovarian cancer. Vaginal dryness, painful sex, and stress incontinence are common signs and symptoms of menopause and can be treated but are not considered a priority. **Focus:** Prioritization.

2. **Ans: 3** The most commonly prescribed oral contraceptives are combination estrogen-progestin medications, but estrogen-containing oral contraceptives are contraindicated for women who are older than 35 years and who smoke because of the increased risk for thromboembolism. A progestin-only oral contraceptive or an intrauterine device may be prescribed for this patient. Estrogen-containing contraceptives may stimulate fibroid growth and elevate blood pressure, but these are relative contraindications. It is recommended that estrogen-containing contraceptives be discontinued a few weeks before surgeries that might impair mobility and increase venous thromboembolism risk, but oral surgery will not affect mobility. **Focus:** Prioritization.

3. **Ans: 4** Raloxifene increases the risk for deep vein thrombosis and pulmonary embolism, and the patient should be evaluated further with an examination, possible venous ultrasonography, and coagulation studies. Hot flashes and nasal congestion are common side effects of raloxifene but are not reasons to discontinue the medication. Raloxifene lowers myocardial infarction risk in women at high risk. **Focus:** Prioritization.

4. **Ans: 3** A palpable bladder and restlessness are indicators of urinary retention, which would require action (e.g., insertion of a catheter) to empty the bladder. The other data would be consistent with the patient's diagnosis of benign prostatic hyperplasia. More detailed assessment may be indicated, but no immediate action is required. **Focus:** Prioritization.

5. **Ans: 4** Irregularly shaped and nontender lumps are consistent with a diagnosis of breast cancer, so this patient needs immediate referral for diagnostic tests such as mammography or ultrasonography. The other information is not unusual and does not indicate the need for immediate action. **Focus:** Prioritization. **Test-Taking Tip:** Remember to investigate further when a patient has a nontender lump or swelling because lumps that are not painful are a common clinical manifestation of cancer in areas such as the breasts or lymph tissues. Pain is rarely an early manifestation of cancer but occurs as tumors grow and place pressure on other organs or tissues.

6. **Ans: 1** An LPN/LVN working in a postanesthesia care unit would be expected to check dressings for bleeding and alert RN staff members if bleeding occurs. The other tasks are more appropriate for nursing staff with RN-level education and licensure. **Focus:** Assignment.

7. **Ans: 2** Positioning the patient's arm is a task within the scope of practice for the AP working on a surgical unit. Patient teaching and assessment are RN-level skills. The RN should reinforce dressings as necessary because this requires assessment of the surgical site and possible communication with the surgeon. **Focus:** Delegation.

8. **Ans: 4** The bladder spasms may indicate that blood clots are obstructing the catheter, which would indicate the need for irrigation of the catheter with 30 to 50 mL of normal saline using a piston syringe. The other data would all be normal after a TURP, but the patient may need some teaching about the usual post-TURP symptoms and care. **Focus:** Prioritization.

9. **Ans: 4** Because tamsulosin blocks alpha receptors in the peripheral arterial system, the most significant side effects are orthostatic hypotension and dizziness. To avoid falls, it is important that the patient change positions slowly. The other information is also accurate and may be included in patient teaching but is not as important as decreasing the risk for falls. **Focus:** Prioritization. **Test-Taking Tip:** When any medication might lower blood pressure, be aware that safety is a priority. Avoid risk for falls by teaching patients to change position slowly.

10. **Ans: 2** Hemorrhage is a major complication after TURP and should be reported to the surgeon immediately. The other assessment data also indicate a need for nursing action but not as urgently. **Focus:** Prioritization.

11. **Ans: 1** Reinforcement of previous teaching is an expected role of the LPN/LVN. Planning and implementing patient initial teaching and documentation of a patient's discharge assessment should be performed by experienced RN staff members. **Focus:** Assignment.

12. **Ans: 4** It is important to assess oxygenation because the patient's calf tenderness and shortness of breath suggest a possible venous thromboembolism and pulmonary embolus, serious complications of transurethral resection of the prostate. The other activities are appropriate but are not as high a priority as ensuring that oxygenation is adequate. **Focus:** Prioritization. **Test-Taking Tip:** You should rapidly investigate any patient report of shortness of breath because oxygenation is the most basic physiologic need.

13. **Ans: 1** This patient has symptoms of testicular torsion, an emergency that needs immediate assessment and intervention because it can lead to testicular ischemia and necrosis within a few hours. The other patients also have symptoms of acute problems (primary syphilis, acute bacterial prostatitis, and prostatic hyperplasia with urinary retention), which need rapid assessment and intervention, but these are not as urgent as the possible testicular torsion. **Focus:** Prioritization.

14. **Ans: 4** Painless vaginal bleeding in postmenopausal women may indicate endometrial or cervical cancer and will require diagnostic testing such as endometrial biopsy. Breast atrophy, vaginal dryness and painful intercourse, and hot flashes are common after menopause, although these symptoms should also be discussed with the HCP and may need treatment. **Focus:** Prioritization.

15. **Ans: 3** Current guidelines state that there is no effective screening tool for low-risk women, but women who are high risk because of family history or the *BRCA* genes may be screened with transvaginal ultrasonography and serum marker CA-125 levels. The other statements are accurate but do not respond as well to the patient's concern. **Focus:** Prioritization.

16. **Ans: 2, 1, 3, 4** Bladder spasms after a TURP are usually caused by the presence of clots that obstruct the catheter, so irrigation should be the first action taken. Administration of analgesics may help to reduce spasm. Administration of a bolus of IV fluids is commonly used in the immediate postoperative period to help maintain fluid intake and increase urinary flow. Oral fluid intake should be encouraged when the nurse is sure that the patient is not nauseated and has adequate bowel tone. **Focus:** Prioritization.

17. **Ans: 3** Sildenafil is a potent vasodilator and has caused cardiac arrest in patients who were also taking nitrates such as nitroglycerin. The other patient data indicate the need for further assessment or teaching, but it is essential for the patient who uses nitrates to avoid concurrent use of sildenafil. **Focus:** Prioritization.

18. **Ans: 2** Administration of opioids and the associated patient monitoring are included in LPN/LVN education and scope of practice. Assessments and teaching are more complex skills that require RN-level education and are best accomplished by an RN with experience in caring for patients with this diagnosis. **Focus:** Assignment.

19. **Ans: 3** An RN from the emergency department would be experienced in assessment and management of pain. Because of their diagnoses and treatments, the other patients should be assigned to RNs who are experienced in caring for patients with cancer. **Focus:** Assignment. **Test-Taking Tip:** When making assignments for nurses who have floated to a specialty area, it is best to assign the float nurse to patients who require actions that are commonly used in many areas of nursing, such as administration of analgesics, dressing changes, and fluid infusions.

20. **Ans: 4, 3, 2, 1** The bilateral orchiectomy patient needs immediate assessment because confusion may be an indicator of serious postoperative complications such as hemorrhage, infection, or pulmonary embolism. The patient who had a perineal prostatectomy should be assessed next because pain medication may be needed to allow him to perform essential postoperative activities such as deep breathing, coughing, and ambulating. The vaginal hysterectomy patient's anxiety needs further assessment next. Although the breast implant patient has questions about care of the drains at the surgical site, there is nothing in the report indicating that these need to be addressed immediately. **Focus:** Prioritization.

21. **Ans: 3** Although infection occurs only rarely as a complication of transrectal prostate biopsy, it is important that the patient receive teaching about checking his temperature and calling the HCP if there is any fever or other signs of systemic infection. The patient should understand that the test results will not be available immediately but that he will be notified about the results. Transient rectal bleeding may occur after the biopsy, but bleeding that lasts for more than a few hours indicates that there may have been rectal trauma. **Focus:** Prioritization.

22. **Ans: 4** Cramping or aching abdominal pain is common after dilation and curettage; however, sharp, continuous pain may indicate uterine perforation, which would require rapid intervention by the surgeon. The other data indicate a need for ongoing assessment or interventions. Transient blood pressure elevation may occur because of the stress response after surgery. Bleeding after the procedure is expected but should decrease over the first 2 hours. Although the oxygen saturation is not at an unsafe level, interventions to improve the saturation should be carried out. **Focus:** Prioritization.

23. **Ans: 2, 4, 5** Assisting with catheter care, ambulation, and hygiene are included in home health aide education and would be expected activities for this staff member. Patient assessments and education are the responsibility of RN members of the home health care team. **Focus:** Delegation.

24. **Ans: 1** Because the most likely source of the bacteria causing the toxic shock syndrome is the patient's tampon, it is essential to remove it first. The other actions should be implemented in the following order: obtain blood culture samples (best done before initiating antibiotic therapy to ensure accurate culture and sensitivity results), infuse nafcillin (rapid initiation of antibiotic therapy will decrease bacterial release of toxins), and administer acetaminophen (fever reduction may be necessary, but treating the infection has the highest priority). **Focus:** Prioritization.

25. **Ans: 1, 3, 4** Emergency contraception with levonorgestrel (Plan B) may cause heavy menstrual bleeding and nausea with vomiting. Risk for pregnancy complications is not increased. The medication is most effective if taken within 72 hours, but it can be used up to 5 days after unprotected intercourse. Levonorgestrel does not need a prescription when used for emergency contraception by patients age 17 years or older. Levonorgestrel should not be used as a regular form of birth control. **Focus:** Prioritization.

26. **Ans: 2** Current guidelines indicate that Pap testing should be started at age 21 years, regardless of when a woman has become sexually active. The 19-year-old patient should be counseled that there is an increased risk for cervical cancer associated with sexual activity

before age 17 years and encouraged to schedule Pap testing, human papillomavirus testing, or both at age 21 years. The 33-year-old patient will need screening every 3 years, and the 67-year-old will not need further Pap screening if she has had several normal Pap test results within the past 2 to 3 years. **Focus:** Prioritization.

27. **Ans: 2** Right calf swelling and tenderness indicate the possible presence of deep vein thrombosis. This will change the plan of care because the patient may be placed on bed rest and will require diagnostic testing and possible anticoagulant therapy. The other data indicate the need for common postoperative nursing actions such as having the patient cough, assessing her pain, and increasing her fluid intake. **Focus:** Prioritization.

28. **Ans: 3** Patients with intracavitary implants are kept in bed during the treatment to avoid dislodgement of the implant. The other actions may also require the nurse to intervene by providing guidance to the student. Minimal time should be spent close to patients who are receiving internal irradiation. Asking the patient about her reaction to losing childbearing abilities may be inappropriate at this time. Patients are frequently placed on low-residue diets to decrease bowel distention while implants are in place. **Focus:** Prioritization.

29. **Ans: 1** The patient has symptoms of a urinary tract infection. Inserting a straight catheter will enable the nurse to obtain an uncontaminated urine specimen for culture and sensitivity testing before the antibiotic is started. In addition, the patient is probably not emptying her bladder fully because of the painful urination. The antibiotic therapy should be initiated as rapidly as possible after the urine specimen is obtained. Administration of acetaminophen is the lowest priority because the patient's temperature is not dangerously elevated. **Focus:** Prioritization.

30. **Ans: 2** After an A & P repair, it is essential that the bladder be empty to avoid putting pressure on the suture lines. The abdominal firmness and tenderness indicate that the patient's bladder is distended. The health care provider should be notified and an order for catheterization obtained. The other data also indicate a need for further assessment of her cardiac status and actions such as having the patient cough and deep breathe, but these are not such immediate concerns. **Focus:** Prioritization.

31. **Ans: 1** Testosterone is contraindicated in patients who have prostate cancer because it can promote the growth of prostate cancer. Although metformin is most commonly prescribed for type 2 diabetes, it can be helpful in restoring ovulation in patients with polycystic ovary syndrome. Sildenafil lowers blood pressure and should not be used by patients who are taking nitrates or alpha-adrenergic blockers but may be used in patients taking other antihypertensives. Progestin therapy alone will not treat infertility caused by endometriosis but may be used to shrink endometrial tissue. **Focus:** Prioritization.

32. **Ans: 3** The patient should be positioned in a semi-Fowler position to decrease pain and minimize the risk

of abscess development higher in the abdomen. The other actions also require correction but not as rapidly. Tampon use is not contraindicated after an episode of PID, although some sources recommend not using tampons during the acute infection. Heat application to the abdomen and pelvis is used for pain relief. Intercourse is safe a few weeks after effective treatment for PID. **Focus:** Prioritization.

33. **Ans: 3** The Centers for Disease Control and Prevention guidelines indicate that the HPV immunization should not be given during pregnancy. Ideally, the immunization series should start at age 11 or 12 years for girls and boys, but it may be started up through age 26 years. HPV immunization is most effective in preventing HPV infection and cervical cancer when it is started before the individual is sexually active and before any HPV infection, but these are not contraindications for vaccination. **Focus:** Prioritization.

34. **Ans: 2** The initial action should be to ensure that the abdominal contents remain moist by covering the wound and loops of intestine with dressings soaked with sterile normal saline. Because national guidelines addressing the use of RRTs indicate that the role of the RRT is immediate assessment and stabilization of the patient, the nurse's next action should be to activate the RRT. The surgeon should be notified after further assessments of the patient (e.g., pulse and blood pressure) are obtained. Wound cultures may be obtained, but protection of the wound, further assessment of the patient, and then notification of the surgeon so that other actions can be taken are the priority. **Focus:** Prioritization.

35. **Ans: 3** LPN/LVN education includes vital sign monitoring after procedures such as paracentesis; an experienced LPN/LVN would recognize and report significant changes in vital signs to the RN. The paracentesis tray could be obtained by an AP. Patient admission assessment and teaching require RN-level education and experience, although part of the data gathering may be done by an LPN/LVN. **Focus:** Assignment.

36. **Ans: 3** The initial response by the charge nurse should be assessment of the new nurse's concerns about caring for this patient. Acknowledging the new nurse's concerns will be more effective than mandating culturally sensitive care. Changing the assignment and arranging training may be appropriate, but more information about the new nurse's anxieties is needed first. Treatment for pneumonia will not be different for a transgender patient, but it is important that the patient's care is provided in a nonjudgmental manner. **Focus:** Prioritization.

37. **Ans: 4** The Joint Commission suggests that forms should use inclusive and gender-neutral language to allow for patient self-identification. Unisex or single-stall bathrooms should be provided, but transgender patients should also be able to use bathrooms consistent

with their gender identity. Treating all patients the same fails to acknowledge that sexual orientation and gender identity may have an impact on health care needs. The nurse should be receptive of information about patient sexual orientation and gender identity, but self-identification should be at the patient's chosen time. **Focus:** Prioritization.

38. **Ans: 4** The current guidelines, supported by nonrandomized screening trials and observational data, call for first-degree relatives of patients with the *BRCA* gene to be screened with both annual mammography and MRI. Although annual mammography, breast self-examination, and clinical breast examination by a health care provider may help to detect cancer, the best option for this patient is annual mammography and MRI. **Focus:** Prioritization.

39. **Ans: 100** To infuse 100 mL over 60 minutes, the nurse will need to set the infusion pump to give 100 mL/hr. **Focus:** Prioritization.

40. **Ans: 2** Because clinical manifestations of PID should improve with 3 days of effective antibiotic treatment, the patient's ongoing pain indicates a need for actions such as hospitalization for intravenous antibiotic therapy. Nausea is a side effect of many antibiotics, but the patient will be instructed to continue the medications. The patient's feeling of shame should be addressed by the nurse but is not the most important finding. Because *N. gonorrhoeae* is a common cause of PID, all drug regimens that are used will be effective in treating gonorrhea and *C. trachomatis.* **Focus:** Prioritization.

41. **Ans:** The nurse is assessing a 48-year-old male who is being seen for a yearly physical. Vital signs: Temperature 98.8°F (37.1°C), Pulse 90 beats/min, Respirations 20 breaths/min, Oxygen Saturation 98% room air, **Blood Pressure 150/94 mm Hg,** Body Mass Index: 24 kg/m². Medications: Sertraline 25mg QD, Simvastatin 40mg QD, **Hydrochlorothiazide 25mg QD.** Social history: Divorced, **smokes e-cigarettes and admits to drinking 2 beers a day,** employed as construction worker, walks 3 miles a day and lifts weights 3 times a week. Medical history: **Depression, Chronic low back pain, degenerate disk disease L4-L6, hypertension, high cholesterol.** A weakened firmness of the penis and deteriorating ability for the penis to achieve erection signifies ED. ED can be caused by inflammation in the seminal vesicles or urethra, obesity (BMI over 30kg/m²), high cholesterol levels, high blood pressure and some blood pressure medications such as thiazide diuretics. Nicotine (found in E-cigarettes), alcohol, depression, and anxiety also increase the risk for ED. Chronic low back pain as well as lumbosacral injuries can cause ED. Exercise and weights do not cause ED. **Focus:** Prioritization.

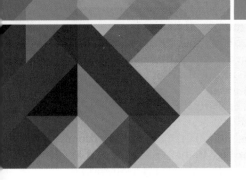

CHAPTER 18

Problems in Pregnancy and Childbearing

Questions

1. A 21-year-old woman at 8 weeks' gestation tells the nurse she has obtained marijuana from the town's marijuana dispensary to help her with the nausea she is experiencing. Which action would be the **priority?**
   1. Inform the patient that there are other treatments for nausea in pregnancy.
   2. Advise the patient that marijuana may have deleterious effects on the neurologic development of the fetus.
   3. Teach the patient that inhaled marijuana will have a more rapid effect than edible marijuana products.
   4. Inform the patient that marijuana is thought to be an effective remedy for nausea.

2. A new RN is working in labor and delivery providing care to a patient who is having an induction of labor with oxytocin. She is gradually increasing the oxytocin according to unit protocol. Which action would the new RN take when she is being ridiculed by the other more experienced RNs on the unit and told that her patient will never deliver if she continues to increase the oxytocin so slowly?
   1. Modify the oxytocin protocol and increase the oxytocin according to her clinical judgment.
   2. Increase the oxytocin as recommended by the more experienced nurses.
   3. Speak with the charge nurse and report her experience.
   4. Page the physician on call for guidance on the oxytocin administration.

3. Which statement by the student nurse to the 21-year-old pregnant woman who smokes would require the supervising RN to intervene?
   1. "Pregnancy is an excellent time to quit smoking."
   2. "Vaping instead of smoking during pregnancy is less risky."
   3. "You should not allow anyone to smoke around you during pregnancy."
   4. "You should not allow anyone to smoke around the baby when she is born."

4. A 30-year-old woman with type 1 diabetes mellitus comes to the clinic for preconception care. Which information would be the **priority** to communicate to her at this time?
   1. Her insulin requirements will likely increase during the second and third trimesters of pregnancy.
   2. Infants of mothers with diabetes can be macrosomic, which can result in a more difficult delivery and a higher likelihood of cesarean section.
   3. Breastfeeding is highly recommended, and insulin use is not a contraindication.
   4. Achievement of optimal glycemic control at this time is of utmost importance in preventing congenital anomalies.

5. Which task could be appropriately delegated to the assistive personnel (AP) working with the nurse at the obstetric clinic?
   1. Checking the blood pressure of a patient who is 36 weeks' pregnant and reports a headache
   2. Removing the adhesive skin closure strips of a patient who had a cesarean section 2 weeks ago
   3. Giving community resource information and emergency numbers to a prenatal patient who may be experiencing domestic violence
   4. Dispensing a breast pump with instruction to a lactating patient having trouble with milk supply 4 weeks postpartum

6. Several patients have just come into the obstetric triage unit. Which patient should the nurse assess **first?**
   1. A 17-year-old gravida 1, para 0 (G1P0) woman at 40 weeks' gestation with contractions every 6 minutes who is crying loudly and is surrounded by anxious family members
   2. A 22-year-old G3P2 woman at 38 weeks' gestation with contractions every 3 minutes who is requesting to go to the bathroom to have a bowel movement
   3. A 32-year-old G4P3 woman at 27 weeks' gestation who noted vaginal bleeding today after intercourse
   4. A 27-year-old G2P1 woman at 37 weeks' gestation who experienced spontaneous rupture of membranes 30 minutes ago but feels no contractions

7. A 19-year-old gravida 1, para 0 patient at 40 weeks' gestation who is in labor is being treated with magnesium sulfate for seizure prophylaxis in preeclampsia. Which are **priority** assessments with this medication? **Select all that apply.**
   1. Check deep tendon reflexes.
   2. Observe for vaginal bleeding.
   3. Check the respiratory rate.
   4. Note the urine output.
   5. Monitor for calf pain.
   6. Watch for early fetal heart rate decelerations.

8. Which action would **best** demonstrate evidence-based nursing practice in the care of a patient who is 1 day postpartum and reporting nipple soreness while breastfeeding?
   1. Inform the mother that a certain amount of soreness is normal.
   2. Assess the mother–baby couplet for nursing position and latch and correct as indicated.
   3. Advise the use of a breast pump until nipple soreness resolves.
   4. Advise alternating breastfeeding and pumping to avoid excess sucking at the nipple.

9. A 24-year-old gravida 2, para 1 woman is being admitted in active labor at 39 weeks' gestation. Which prenatal data would be **most** important for the nurse to address at this time?
   1. Hemoglobin level of 11 g/dL (110 g/L) at 28 weeks' gestation
   2. Positive result on test for group B streptococci at 36 weeks' gestation
   3. Urinary tract infection with *Escherichia coli* treated at 20 weeks' gestation
   4. Elevated level on glucose screening test at 28 weeks' gestation followed by normal 3-hour glucose tolerance test results at 29 weeks' gestation

10. The telephone triage nurse in the prenatal clinic receives the following calls. Which telephone call would require **immediate** notification of the health care provider?
    1. Patient reports leaking vaginal fluid at 34 weeks' gestation.
    2. Patient reports nausea and vomiting at 8 weeks' gestation.
    3. Patient reports pedal edema at 39 weeks' gestation.
    4. Patient reports vaginal itching at 20 weeks' gestation.

11. The nurse identified late fetal heart decelerations and decreased variability in the fetal heart rate of a woman in active labor and notified the health care provider (HCP) on call, who advised the nurse that the pattern is acceptable. What would be the **priority** action at this time?

    1. Advise the patient that a different HCP will be called because the first HCP's response was not adequate.
    2. Discuss the concerns with another labor and delivery nurse.
    3. Document the conversation with the HCP accurately, including the HCP's interpretation and recommendation, and continue close observation of the fetal heart rate.
    4. Go up the chain of command and communicate the assessment of the fetal heart rate findings clearly to the next appropriate person per unit protocol.

12. The nurse is caring for a patient in labor at 39 weeks' gestation and has identified mild variable fetal heart rate decelerations. Which action would the nurse take **first**?
    1. Change the maternal position.
    2. Notify the health care provider.
    3. Prepare for delivery.
    4. Readjust the fetal monitor.

13. A 24-year-old gravida 1, para 0 patient is receiving oxytocin during her labor at 41 weeks' gestation. Which nursing actions are appropriate when late fetal heart rate decelerations are identified? **Select all that apply.**
    1. Discontinue the oxytocin.
    2. Decrease the maintenance IV fluid rate.
    3. Administer oxygen to the mother by mask.
    4. Place the woman in high Fowler position.
    5. Notify the health care provider (HCP).
    6. Discontinue epidural anesthesia.

14. A pregnant woman at 12 weeks' gestation tells the nurse that she is a vegetarian. Which action would the nurse take **first**?
    1. Recommend vitamin B_{12} and iron supplementation.
    2. Recommend consumption of protein drinks daily.
    3. Obtain a 24-hour diet recall history.
    4. Determine the reason for her vegetarian diet.

15. A 26-year-old gravida 1, para 1 patient who underwent a cesarean section 24 hours ago tells the nurse that she is having some trouble breastfeeding. Which tasks could be appropriately delegated to the assistive personnel (AP) on the postpartum floor? **Select all that apply.**
    1. Providing the mother with an ordered abdominal binder
    2. Assisting the mother with breastfeeding
    3. Taking the mother's vital signs
    4. Checking the amount of lochia present
    5. Assisting the mother with ambulation
    6. Checking the incision site

PART 2 Common Health Scenarios

16. Which action by a newly graduated RN during a delivery complicated by shoulder dystocia would require **immediate** correction by the nurse who is orienting her?
    1. Applying fundal pressure
    2. Applying suprapubic pressure
    3. Requesting the immediate presence of the neonatologist
    4. Flexing the maternal legs back across the maternal abdomen

17. Which statements by a new father indicate that additional discharge teaching is needed for this family, who had their first baby 24 hours ago? **Select all that apply.**
    1. "We have a crib ready for our baby with lots of stuffed animals and two quilts that my mother made."
    2. "My wife wants to receive the flu shot before she goes home."
    3. "We will bring our baby to the pediatrician in 3 weeks."
    4. "I will give the baby formula at night so my wife can rest. She will breastfeed in the daytime."
    5. "We will always put our baby to sleep in a face-up position."
    6. "We will watch and be sure that the baby urinates at least 6 times tomorrow."

18. The charge nurse in the labor and delivery unit needs to assign two patients to one of the RNs because of a staffing shortage. Normally the unit has a nurse-patient ratio of 1:1. Which two patients would the charge nurse assign to the RN?
    1. A 30-year-old gravida 1, para 0 (G1P0) woman, 40 weeks, 2 cm/90% effaced/−1 station
    2. A 25-year-old G3P2 woman, 38 weeks, 8 cm/100% effaced/0 station
    3. A 26-year-old G1P1 woman who delivered via normal vaginal delivery 15 minutes ago
    4. A 17-year-old G1P0 woman with premature rupture of membranes, no labor at 35 weeks
    5. A 40-year-old G6P5 woman with contractions at 28 weeks who has not yet been evaluated by the health care provider
    _____, _____

19. While assessing a 29-year-old gravida 2, para 2 patient who had a normal spontaneous vaginal delivery 30 minutes ago, the nurse notes a large amount of red vaginal bleeding. Which nursing action would be the **priority**?
    1. Check vital signs.
    2. Notify the health care provider.
    3. Firmly massage the uterine fundus.
    4. Put the baby to breast.

20. A 30-year-old gravida 1, para 0 woman at 39 weeks' gestation experienced a fetal demise and has just delivered the female infant. Her husband is at the bedside. Which nursing actions are appropriate at this time? **Select all that apply.**
    1. Offer the option of autopsy to the parents.
    2. Stay with the parents and offer supportive care.
    3. Place the infant on the maternal abdomen.
    4. Clean and wrap the baby and offer the infant to the parents to view or hold when desired.
    5. Ask the parents if there are any special rituals in their religion or culture for a baby who has died that they would like to have done.
    6. Tell the parents that they will be able to have more children.

21. A 27-year-old patient underwent a primary cesarean section because of breech presentation 24 hours ago. Which assessment finding would be of the **most** concern?
    1. Small amount of lochia rubra
    2. Temperature of 99°F (37.2°C)
    3. Slight redness and pain of the left calf
    4. Pain rated as 3 of 10 in the incisional area

22. A 22-year-old gravida 1, para 0 woman is being given an epidural anesthetic for pain control during labor and birth. Which are appropriate nursing actions when epidural anesthesia is used during labor? **Select all that apply.**
    1. Request the anesthesiologist to discontinue the epidural anesthetic when the patient's cervix is completely dilated to allow the patient to sense the urge to push.
    2. Insert an indwelling catheter because the woman is likely to be unable to void.
    3. Encourage ambulation to encourage descent of the fetal head.
    4. Encourage the patient to turn from side to side during the course of labor.
    5. Teach the patient that pain relief can be expected to last 1 to 2 hours.
    6. Explain to the patient that she will feel very drowsy after the epidural is given.

23. A 36-year-old gravida 1, para 0 patient has received an epidural anesthetic. Her cervix is 6 cm dilated. Her blood pressure is currently 60/38 mm Hg. Which nursing actions would be the **priority**? **Select all that apply.**
    1. Place the patient in high Fowler position.
    2. Turn the patient to a lateral position.
    3. Notify the anesthesiologist.
    4. Prepare for emergency cesarean section.
    5. Decrease the IV fluid rate.
    6. Observe closely for fetal heart rate decelerations.

24. A 17-year-old gravida 1, para 0 woman at 40 weeks' gestation is in labor. She has chosen natural childbirth with assistance from a doula. Her mother and her boyfriend are at the bedside. Which nursing action can help the patient achieve her goal of an unmedicated labor and birth?
    1. Encourage the patient to stay in bed.
    2. Allow the patient's support people to provide labor support and minimize nursing presence.
    3. Assess the effectiveness of the labor support team and offer suggestions as indicated.
    4. Offer pain medication on a regular basis so the patient knows it is available if desired.

25. A 25-year-old gravida 2, para 1 patient has come to the obstetric triage room at 32 weeks' gestation reporting painless vaginal bleeding. The nurse is providing orientation for a new RN on the unit. Which statement by the new RN to the patient would require the nurse to promptly intervene?
    1. "I'm going to check your vital signs."
    2. "I'm going to apply a fetal monitor to check the baby's heart rate and to see if you are having contractions."
    3. "I'm going to perform a vaginal examination to see if your cervix is dilated."
    4. "I'm going to feel your abdomen to check the position of the baby."

26. A 30-year-old gravida 6, para 5 woman at 12 weeks' gestation has just begun prenatal care, and her initial laboratory work reveals that she has tested positive for human immunodeficiency virus (HIV) infection. Which information would be **priority** evidence-based nursing education for this patient today?
    1. Medication for HIV infection is safe and can greatly reduce transmission of HIV to the infant.
    2. Breastfeeding is still recommended because of the great benefits to the infant.
    3. Pregnancy is known to accelerate the course of HIV disease in the mother.
    4. Cesarean section is not recommended because of the increased risk of HIV transmission with the bleeding at surgery.

27. A 22-year-old woman is 6 weeks postpartum. In the clinic, she admits to crying every day, feeling overwhelmed, and sometimes thinking that she may hurt the baby. Which nursing action would be the **priority** at this time?
    1. Advise the patient of community resources, parent groups, and depression hotlines.
    2. Counsel the mother that the "baby blues" are common at this time and assess her nutrition, rest, and availability of help at home.

3. Contact the health care provider to evaluate the patient before allowing her to leave the clinic.
4. Advise the woman that she cannot use medication for depression because she is breastfeeding.

28. A 23-year-old gravida 1, para 0 patient at 10 weeks' gestation states that she exercises 5 days a week. The nurse has discussed exercise in pregnancy with her. Which statement by the patient indicates that more teaching of evidence-based principles is needed?
    1. "I will continue to exercise 5 days a week."
    2. "I will reduce my exercise at this time in my pregnancy to reduce the risk of miscarriage but will increase it in the second trimester."
    3. "I will drink more fluid before and after exercising."
    4. "I will stop playing football while I am pregnant."

29. A 3-day-old breastfed infant is brought to the clinic by his parents for routine assessment following a normal full-term delivery without complications. Which statement by the parents suggests an abnormal finding on a newborn of this age?
    1. "The baby urinated only three times yesterday."
    2. "The bowel movement of the baby was dark at first, but yesterday it was greenish yellow."
    3. "The baby cried for 2 hours last night."
    4. "The baby ate four times in the past 24 hours."

30. A full-term newborn is at the clinic with his parents. He is 4 days old. His birth weight was 7 lb (3.2 kg). Which assessment made by the RN is **most** significant?
    1. The infant's weight today is 6 lb 9 oz (3 kg).
    2. The infant's skin is peeling.
    3. The infant's breast tissue is swollen.
    4. There is a yellow discharge from the infant's right eye.

31. The nurse has received orders to initiate phototherapy on a 36-hour-old newborn with an elevated bilirubin level. The nurse asks the student nurse to explain how she plans to administer this treatment. Which actions would be expected from the student nurse? **Select all that apply.**
    1. Cover the infant's eyes with a mask.
    2. Monitor the infant's temperature closely.
    3. Keep the infant NPO during the treatment.
    4. Apply ointment to the infant's skin before light exposure.
    5. Offer the infant sterile water feedings during the treatment.
    6. Instruct the mother to pump her breasts because the infant will not be nursing during treatment.

Answer Key for this chapter begins on p. 183

32. A patient in the obstetric clinic is at 8 weeks' gestation. She tells the nurse of her plans to travel next month to visit family in a country that is affected by the Zika virus. What is the **priority** counseling by the nurse today?
    1. It is recommended that a patient not travel to a country impacted by Zika. The Zika virus has been linked to a very serious birth defect called microcephaly.
    2. It is recommended that long-sleeved shirts and long pants be always worn while there and that mosquito repellent be applied because mosquitos carry the virus.
    3. It is recommended that mosquito repellent containing DEET be used because it is most effective.
    4. It is recommended that the patient stay indoors at dusk and dawn because mosquitos are most active at this time.

33. A female same-sex couple is being seen in the clinic today. They inform the nurse that they are planning a pregnancy and plan to use donor sperm that will be inseminated into one of the women. What is the **priority** education at this time?
    1. Refer the couple to another health center specializing in same-sex issues and explain that you do not have the expertise to deal with their issues.
    2. Review all preconception education issues, including vaccines, diet, folic acid use, avoidance of alcohol and medications, and the importance of physical and mental health prior to pregnancy.
    3. Ask the couple if they have considered the effects on a child of having same-sex parents.
    4. Inform them that donor sperm carry an increased risk of infection and chromosomal disorders.

34. A same-sex couple are in the delivery room, and a healthy baby boy has just been born to one of the women. She breastfed the baby with a good latch, and now the baby has fallen asleep. She tells the nurse that both she and her partner are planning to breastfeed the baby. What should the nurse do **next**?
    1. Wake the baby and help the baby to latch on to the other woman's breasts. Alternate the baby between the two women for nursing.
    2. Inquire as to what preparation the partner has done for breastfeeding. Let her know you will work with their plan while also assuring adequate intake for the baby.
    3. Explain that the baby must first suck 20 minutes on each of the birth mother's breasts and then can be placed on the other mother's breasts.
    4. Suggest that the birth mother breastfeed the infant and the partner supplement the baby with formula.

35. The nurse on the locked postpartum unit observes as another nurse with more experience opens the door for a middle-aged woman without a visitor badge and then goes to lunch. The nurse notices the woman wandering in the hall. In what order should the following actions be performed?
    1. Find the nurse who let the woman in and question her about why she did that and see if she knows the woman.
    2. Ask the supervisor to clarify the access policies for the postpartum unit to all staff.
    3. Go up to the woman and ask if you can help her. Confirm with her which patient she is visiting and request that she get a visitor pass.
    4. Ask the unit desk secretary to closely monitor the infant security system.

    _____, _____, _____, _____

36. A patient in labor had a positive QuantiFERON-TB gold tuberculosis (TB) test during pregnancy. A chest x-ray examination was done and showed no active TB in the lungs. The charge nurse has told the RN to isolate the newborn from the mother to reduce the risk of infection. Which action should be taken by the RN?
    1. Isolate the mother, initiate droplet precautions, separate the mother and baby, and do not allow breastfeeding at this time.
    2. Inform the patient that the charge nurse's instructions are incorrect and that the mother will not be isolated from the newborn. Encourage the mother to initiate breastfeeding.
    3. Privately discuss the case with the charge nurse and make sure she understands that the chest x-ray showed no active TB. Offer to consult the infectious disease practitioner and hospital infection control policies to confirm that there is no need for isolation.
    4. Place a face mask on the mother while transporting her outside her room. Isolate her from the baby but encourage her to pump milk, which can be fed to the baby by a healthy family member.

37. The charge nurse is orienting a new nurse on the postpartum floor. Which action by the new nurse would require intervention by the charge nurse?
    1. Telling a patient with active varicella that she may breastfeed her newborn
    2. Telling a patient with active varicella that she should pump her milk to maintain her milk supply, but dump the milk until the varicella has resolved
    3. Telling a patient with active varicella that other family members should be vaccinated against varicella
    4. Telling a patient with active varicella that she must wear a face mask when being transported from her room

PART 2

Common Health Scenarios

38. The health care provider has ordered a flu vaccine for a patient in the prenatal clinic. As the nurse prepares to give it, the patient states she does not want the vaccine because she never gets it and has never had the flu. How can the nurse **best** respond to the patient?
    1. Respect the patient's preference and offer her education on how to avoid getting the flu by good hand washing, good nutrition, and adequate rest. Tell her to notify the clinic if she ever feels like she is getting the flu.
    2. Inform the patient that changes in the heart, lungs, and immune system in pregnancy put her in a higher risk group for complications of flu and that the flu in pregnancy can be associated with pregnancy complications such as premature delivery.
    3. Inform the patient that it is acceptable to defer the vaccine until the postpartum period if she is worried about the vaccine's effects in pregnancy.
    4. Explain that the vaccine is mandatory in pregnancy.

39. The postpartum nurse has just taken the report from the night nurse. Place the following patients in the order in which they should be seen by the oncoming nurse.
    1. A 32-year-old woman gravida 1, para 1 (G1P1) on day 2 after a normal spontaneous vaginal delivery who is tearful because the baby has been up all night crying and not nursing well
    2. A 22-year-old G3P3 6 hours after normal spontaneous vaginal delivery who has expressed a wish to speak with a social worker about giving up her baby for adoption
    3. A 16-year-old G1P1 on day 1 postpartum with a blood pressure reading of 160/90 mm Hg who is complaining of a headache
    4. A 26-year-old G2P2 on day 1 after cesarean section with a temperature of 100.5°F (38.1°C)

    _____, _____, _____, _____

40. Enhanced Multiple Response _____

Scenario: A patient who was recently diagnosed with influenza is in labor. She has been placed on droplet precautions. The student nurse who has been assigned to work with her has given the following information to the patient and her family.

Which of the following instructions would require the nurse to intervene with further explanation?

Instructions: Place an X in the space provided or highlight instructions and information from the student nurse that would require the RN to intervene with further explanation. **Select all that apply.**
1. _____ "I will be wearing gowns and gloves and masks as we care for you today."
2. _____ "I will be putting on a mask as I care for you today."
3. _____ "Any visitors to the room will be offered a mask to wear."
4. _____ "I will be moving you to a negative pressure room to prevent the spread of influenza."
5. _____ "You must wear a mask when you are outside of your room."
6. _____ "Droplets of your breast milk will be infectious at this time, so you will need to pump and dump your milk after delivery."

Answer Key for this chapter begins on p. 183

41. The patient is 32 weeks pregnant with a diagnosis of complete placenta previa and is experiencing heavy vaginal bleeding. The plan of care is immediate blood transfusion and emergency cesarean section. The patient tells the nurse that she does not want the blood transfusion because she is concerned about getting hepatitis from it. Her husband shares this concern, and the couple is declining the transfusion. How should the nurse proceed?
    1. Allow the patient to decline the blood transfusion, move her quickly to the operating room to prepare for emergent cesarean section, and inform the obstetrician that the patient has declined.
    2. Quickly inform the patient that the blood transfusion is mandatory because of the amount of bleeding she is experiencing. State that there is virtually no risk of bloodborne infection.
    3. Speak quickly and intently to the couple while moving to the operating room. Collaborate with the obstetrician and anesthesiologist to quickly counsel the couple about the risk-to-benefit ratio she is facing.
    4. Call the blood bank and request that they come to the bedside and outline the risks and benefits of blood transfusion in this case before the surgery is allowed to start.

42. There are four patients on the busy labor and delivery unit undergoing induction of labor with oxytocin. The nurse supervisor for the unit is reviewing the patients. Which patient situation would require the supervising nurse to alert the bedside nurse to take **immediate** action?
    1. A patient with contractions every 10 minutes with a fetal heart rate of 150 beats/min.
    2. A patient with contractions every 1 ½ minutes with a fetal heart rate of 140 beats/min.
    3. A patient with contractions every 5 minutes with a fetal heart rate of 130 beats/min who is moaning and crying.
    4. A patient with contractions every 6 minutes who is leaking clear amniotic fluid with a fetal heart rate of 120 beats/min.

43. A patient on the postpartum unit tells the nurse she is so happy that her 3-year-old son will visit today and get to meet the new baby. She mentions that the toddler has been sick with vomiting and diarrhea that was going around his day-care center. Which response would the nurse provide?
    1. "Your toddler will need extra love and hugs during his visit because he has been sick. He can stay with you throughout the day."
    2. "I am very sorry, but because of the toddler's illness, he cannot visit you due to the risk of spreading the virus to you, the baby, and other vulnerable mothers and babies on the unit. We will set up another way for you to interact with your toddler today."
    3. "Because of your toddler's illness, you should pump your milk and discard it for 24 hours because of the risk of transmission of the virus to the newborn."
    4. "Because of your exposure to the virus, you should wear a mask, gown, and gloves when holding your newborn today."

44. The nurse works in a high-risk antepartum unit where many of the patients are homeless and have other risk factors. The nurse is concerned because she is unable to secure the patients' follow-up appointments at discharge because the receptionists in the high-risk prenatal clinic do not have time to answer the phone and make appointments much of the time. Which actions would the nurse take? **Select all that apply.**
    1. Give the patient the phone number of one of the high-risk prenatal receptionists and tell her to keep trying to get an appointment.
    2. Speak with the charge nurse of the prenatal clinic to discuss the problem and potential solutions.
    3. Make community connections with community health nurses who may be able to follow the high-risk patients to be sure follow-up care is received.
    4. Contact the hospital social worker to see the high-risk patients and assist with a solid discharge plan.
    5. Instruct the patient to be seen at an urgent care center if she is unable to get a prenatal appointment.
    6. Suggest that the patient access care at another clinic and provide her the phone number.

Answers

1. **Ans: 2** There is evidence that marijuana use during pregnancy can be linked to impaired neurologic development in the fetus and learning and behavioral issues in the child exposed to marijuana in the prenatal period. The first priority would be to prevent harm and to begin educating the mother of the potential risks of marijuana use in pregnancy. It would then be appropriate to provide information to her of other potential treatments for her nausea. The goal would be to educate the woman of the risks and to provide an alternative safer treatment. It is true that inhaled marijuana will have a quicker action and that some studies have found marijuana to be effective in the treatment of nausea; however, that is not priority information for her at this time. **Focus:** Prioritization.

2. **Ans: 3** The new RN should report her experience to the immediate nursing manager; this may be the charge nurse or the nurse manager of the unit. Bullying of a new nurse to encourage unsafe practice should never be tolerated. The new RN would not modify the oxytocin protocol nor follow the advice of the experienced RNs in this matter because oxytocin is a high-risk medication capable of causing harm during labor. Paging the physician would not be appropriate in this case because there is not a medical problem, but rather a problem with the behavior of the experienced RNs. **Focus:** Assignment.

3. **Ans: 2** The nurse would need to intervene to correct erroneous information being given to the patient. Vaping is not safer than smoking in pregnancy. Babies born to mothers who vape have levels of nicotine exposure, low birth weight, and shortened gestational age equal to infants born to mothers who smoke. Clear advice about pregnancy being an excellent time to quit and then providing resources to do so is appropriate education. Advising the mother to avoid secondhand smoke during the pregnancy and after delivery is appropriate advice. **Focus:** Assignment.

4. **Ans: 4** The incidence of congenital anomalies is three times higher in the offspring of women with diabetes. Good glycemic control during preconception and early pregnancy significantly reduces this risk and would be the highest-priority message to this patient at this point. The other responses are correct but are not of greatest importance at this time. **Focus:** Prioritization.

5. **Ans: 1** The AP can check the blood pressure of the patient and report it to the RN. The RN would include this information in her full assessment of the patient, who may be showing signs of preeclampsia. The other tasks listed require nursing assessment, analysis, and planning and should be performed by the RN. Provision of accurate and supportive education about breastfeeding and breast pumping supports the Perinatal Core Measure of increasing the percentage of women who exclusively breastfeed. **Focus:** Delegation.

6. **Ans: 2** A multiparous patient in active labor with an urge to have a bowel movement will probably give birth imminently. She needs to be the first assessed. The health care provider must be notified immediately, and the patient must be moved to a safe location for the birth. She should not be allowed to go to the bathroom at this time. The other patients all have needs requiring prompt assessment, but the imminent birth takes priority. Vaginal bleeding after intercourse could be caused by cervical irritation or a vaginal infection or could have a more serious cause such as placenta previa. This patient should be the second one assessed. **Focus:** Prioritization.

7. **Ans: 1, 3, 4** Magnesium sulfate toxicity can cause fatal cardiovascular events or respiratory depression or arrest, so monitoring of the respiratory rate is of utmost importance. The drug is excreted by the kidneys, and therefore monitoring for adequate urine output is essential. Deep tendon reflexes disappear when serum magnesium is reaching a toxic level. Vaginal bleeding is not associated with magnesium sulfate use. Calf pain can be a sign of a deep vein thrombosis but is not associated with magnesium sulfate therapy. Early fetal heart rate decelerations are not associated with use of magnesium sulfate. **Focus:** Prioritization.

8. **Ans: 2** Improper latch and position are the most common causes of nipple soreness and can be corrected with assessment and assistance to the mother. This practice supports the Perinatal Core Measure of increasing the percentage of newborns who are fed breast milk only. Advising the mother that soreness can be normal does not provide any assessment or assistance to the mother with her problem. Using a pump may be appropriate at some times during lactation, but the first priority is to assess and correct the issue that is causing the soreness. **Focus:** Prioritization.

9. **Ans: 2** The positive group B streptococci result requires immediate action. The health care provider must be notified and orders obtained for prompt antibiotic prophylaxis during labor to reduce the risk of mother-to-newborn transmission of group B streptococci. The other data are not as significant in the care of the patient at this moment. Intrapartum-appropriate antibiotic treatment of the mother with group B streptococci supports the Perinatal Core Measure of reducing health care–acquired bloodstream infections in newborns. **Focus:** Prioritization.

10. **Ans: 1** Leaking vaginal fluid at 34 weeks' gestation requires immediate attention because it could indicate

premature rupture of membranes with the risk of premature birth. An RN in a prenatal clinic can safely give telephone advice regarding nausea, vomiting, and pedal edema, which can be considered normal in pregnancy. The RN would assess the complaint, give the patient evidence-based advice, and define the circumstances under which the patient should call back. Vaginal itching at 20 weeks' gestation could indicate a yeast infection. Depending on clinic protocols, the RN could, after phone assessment, safely recommend an over-the-counter medication or arrange an office visit for the patient. **Focus:** Prioritization.

11. **Ans: 4** The RN must follow through on the findings of a nonreassuring fetal heart rate. When patient safety is concerned, the nurse is obligated to pursue an appropriate response. Documenting the conversation with the HCP and discussing it with a colleague are appropriate, but something must be done to address the immediate safety concern and possible need for intervention at this time. The RN must persist until the safety concern has been addressed appropriately. **Focus:** Prioritization.

12. **Ans: 1** The cause of variable fetal heart decelerations is compression of the umbilical cord, which can often be corrected by a change in maternal position. It is usually a benign condition and would not require the nurse to prepare for delivery or to notify the health care provider unless the variable decelerations are severe and persistent. Adjusting the fetal monitor may be needed after the change in maternal position but would not directly address the variable decelerations. **Focus:** Prioritization.

13. **Ans: 1, 3, 5** Late fetal heart rate decelerations can be an ominous sign of fetal hypoxemia, especially if repetitive and accompanied by decreased variability. Notification of the HCP is indicated. Turning off the oxytocin and administering oxygen to the mother are recommended nursing interventions to improve fetal oxygenation. An increase, not a decrease, in the IV rate can improve hydration, correct hypovolemia, and increase blood flow to the uterus. Putting the woman in a lateral position can increase blood flow to the uterus and increase oxygenation to the fetus. The high Fowler position would not be helpful. Discontinuation of epidural anesthesia would not be indicated in the presence of late fetal heart rate decelerations. The anesthesia may be vitally important if the condition continues or worsens and necessitates a cesarean section. Promptly addressing fetal heart rate changes may allow intrauterine resuscitation and may decrease the need for cesarean section if those measures are effective. This supports the Perinatal Core Measure of reducing cesarean section rates. **Focus:** Prioritization.

14. **Ans: 3** The care of a vegetarian woman who is pregnant should begin with an assessment of her diet because vegetarian practices vary widely. The RN must first assess exactly what the woman's diet consists of

and then determine any deficiencies. It is probable that the woman will need a vitamin B_{12} supplement, but the assessment comes first. Vegetarian diets can be completely adequate in protein, and therefore protein supplementation is not routinely recommended. The reason for the diet is less important than what the diet actually contains. **Focus:** Prioritization.

15. **Ans: 1, 3, 5** The AP could provide an abdominal binder, measure the vital signs of the patient, and assist her to ambulate. The RN would be responsible for evaluating the normality of the vital sign values. The AP should be given parameter limits for vital signs and told to report values outside these limits to the RN. Assisting in breastfeeding for a first-time mother is a very important nursing function because the RN needs to give consistent, evidence-based advice to enhance success at breastfeeding. A common complaint of postpartum patients is inconsistent help with and advice on breastfeeding. The RN should also be the one to check the amount of lochia and the surgical incision site because the evaluation requires nursing judgment. The use of the professionally educated RN to provide evidence-based and consistent information and assistance with breastfeeding supports the Perinatal Core Measure of increasing the percentage of newborns who are fed breast milk only. **Focus:** Delegation.

16. **Ans: 1** Fundal pressure should never be applied in a case of shoulder dystocia because it may worsen the problem by impacting the fetal shoulder even more firmly into the symphysis pubis. This issue of patient safety would require the supervising RN to intervene immediately. The other responses are appropriate actions in a case of shoulder dystocia. **Focus:** Assignment.

17. **Ans: 1, 3, 4, 6** It is recommended that a newborn be placed on the back in a crib with a firm mattress with no toys and a minimum of blankets as a safety measure for prevention of sudden infant death syndrome. A newborn discharged before 72 hours of life should be seen by an RN or health care provider within 2 days of discharge. Breastfeeding women should breastfeed at all feedings, especially in the early weeks of establishing breastfeeding. This supports the Perinatal Core Measure of increasing the percentage of newborns who are fed breast milk only. A more appropriate response would be for the father to help with household chores to allow breastfeeding to be established successfully. A newborn would not be expected to void six times on the second day of life. The baby should void at least twice on the second day of life. A flu shot in flu season is a recommended intervention for a new mother. **Focus:** Prioritization.

18. **Ans: 1, 4** Patient 1 is in the latent phase of labor with her first child; she typically will cope well at this point and will have many hours before labor becomes more active. Patient 4 would most likely be managed expectantly at this point and require observation and assessment for labor or signs of infection. Patient 2 can

PART 2 Common Health Scenarios

be expected to deliver soon and so requires intensive nursing care. Patient 3 is in the first hour of recovery and therefore requires frequent assessments, newborn assessments, and help with initiation of breastfeeding if this is her chosen feeding method. Breastfeeding in the first hour of the baby's life supports the Perinatal Core Measure of increasing the percentage of newborns who are fed breast milk only. Patient 5 could be in premature labor and require administration of tocolytic medications to stop contractions or preparation for a preterm delivery if dilation is advanced. **Focus:** Assignment.

19. **Ans: 3** Fundal massage would be the priority nursing action because it helps the uterus to contract firmly and thus reduces bleeding. The first two answer choices are appropriate nursing actions but do nothing to stop the immediate bleeding. Putting the baby to the breast does release oxytocin, which causes uterine contraction, but it will be slower to do so than fundal massage. **Focus:** Prioritization.

20. **Ans: 2, 4, 5** Staying with the parents at this moment and offering physical and emotional support are appropriate. It is also appropriate to prepare the infant in a way that demonstrates care and respect for the baby and to offer the parents the opportunity to view and hold the infant as they desire. The RN must ask the parents if there are cultural or religious rituals they would like for their child to ensure that they feel that their infant has been treated properly with respect to their religion or culture. Autopsy should be discussed but not moments after birth. The infant should not be placed on the maternal abdomen until the nurse assesses the parents' wishes of when and how to view the infant. It would not be appropriate at this time to tell the parents they can have more children. That statement could be seen as minimizing the importance of the child they have just lost. **Focus:** Prioritization.

21. **Ans: 3** Slight redness and pain in the left calf could be suggestive of thrombophlebitis and requires further investigation. The other findings are within normal limits for this point in the postpartum and postoperative course. **Focus:** Prioritization.

22. **Ans: 2, 4** Insertion of an indwelling catheter is indicated because the woman will usually be unable to void because of the effect of the anesthetic in the bladder area. Positioning the patient on her side enhances blood flow and helps to prevent hypotension. Changing maternal position encourages progress in labor. With epidural anesthesia, ambulation is not usually an option due to decreased sensation in the legs. It is not recommended to routinely discontinue an epidural anesthetic at complete dilation. A continuous epidural infusion provides pain relief throughout labor and birth. Drowsiness is not a common side effect with epidural anesthesia. Drowsiness would be more likely with the use of IV narcotics for pain relief in labor. Use of evidence-based practices with a laboring woman

supports the Perinatal Core Measure of reducing the percentage of women who are delivered by cesarean section. **Focus:** Prioritization.

23. **Ans: 2, 3, 6** The patient may be experiencing supine hypotension caused by the pressure of the uterus on the vena cava and the effects of the epidural medication. Maternal hypotension can cause uteroplacental insufficiency, leading to fetal hypoxia. Placing the woman in a lateral position can relieve the pressure on the vena cava. The anesthesiologist should be notified and may need to treat the patient with ephedrine to correct the hypotension. Fetal heart rate decelerations are common if maternal hypotension is not promptly corrected. IV fluids are increased per protocol when supine hypotension occurs. The correction of common problems in labor supports the Perinatal Core Measure of reducing the percentage of women who are delivered by cesarean section. **Focus:** Prioritization.

24. **Ans: 3** The RN remains an important part of the labor and birth in this scenario. Even with a good support team present, the RN needs to observe and assess the patient's comfort and safety as part of essential nursing care during labor. The RN's expertise allows the RN to make helpful suggestions to both the support people and the patient. The patient should be encouraged to use positions and activities that are most comfortable to her. It is appropriate to let the patient and support people know of all pain control options, but it would not be appropriate to continually offer pain medication to a patient who has chosen natural childbirth. Expert nursing care in labor supports the Perinatal Core Measure of reducing the percentage of women who are delivered by cesarean section. **Focus:** Prioritization.

25. **Ans: 3** Painless vaginal bleeding can be a symptom of placenta previa. A digital vaginal examination is contraindicated until ultrasonography can be performed to rule out placenta previa. If a digital examination is performed when placenta previa is present, it can cause increased bleeding. The other statements reflect appropriate assessment of an incoming patient with vaginal bleeding. **Focus:** Assignment. **Test-Taking Tip:** The nurse should consider the possible causes of the symptom described and choose the answer option that assures patient safety until the specific cause of a symptom is known.

26. **Ans: 1** Administration of antiviral medications to the pregnant woman and the newborn, cesarean birth if HIV RNA levels are greater than 1000 copies/mL, and avoidance of breastfeeding have reduced the incidence of perinatal transmission of HIV from approximately 26% to between 1% to 2%. Pregnancy is not known to accelerate HIV disease in the mother. The most important nursing action is to engage the mother in prenatal care and educate her as to the great benefits of medication for HIV during pregnancy. **Focus:** Prioritization.

27. **Ans: 3**   When a patient discloses fear of hurting herself or her baby, the RN must have the woman immediately evaluated before allowing her to leave. Merely informing the patient about community resources is not sufficient. The "baby blues" are typically milder and occur 1 to 2 weeks postpartum. After the woman has been evaluated, the provider can prescribe antidepressants if indicated that can be safely used while breastfeeding. **Focus:** Prioritization. **Test-Taking Tip:** When a situation presents the potential for harm to a patient, choose the option that best protects patient safety.

28. **Ans: 2**   There is no evidence that exercise should be avoided in the first trimester of pregnancy in a healthy woman without medical or obstetric complications. The American College of Obstetricians and Gynecologists recommends 30 minutes or more of exercise on most if not all days of the week for pregnant women. Exercise in which injury is more likely to occur should be avoided. **Focus:** Prioritization.

29. **Ans: 4**   A newborn baby should feed 8 to 12 times in 24 hours. The other findings are normal for an infant of this age. The baby should void six to eight times a day after the fourth day of life. Helpful guidance at this point may help parents understand infant feeding and help support the Perinatal Core Measure of increasing the percentage of infants who are fed breast milk only. **Focus:** Prioritization. **Test-Taking Tip:** Consider the age of the infant as the most important information when choosing an answer option in many questions in pediatrics because infant and child needs and norms change very significantly with age.

30. **Ans: 4**   The yellow eye discharge could be a conjunctivitis related to an infection acquired during birth or afterward. The other findings are normal variants on a newborn of this age. A newborn normally experiences a weight loss of 5% to 10% in the first days of life. **Focus:** Prioritization.

31. **Ans: 1, 2**   During phototherapy, the infant's eyes must be protected and the temperature carefully monitored to avoid both hypothermia and hyperthermia. Breastfeeding should be continued to avoid dehydration and to increase passage of meconium, which helps to excrete bilirubin. Ointments or lotions should not be applied to the skin during phototherapy because they may cause burns. Encouraging continued breastfeeding and teaching the family the benefits of breastfeeding in this scenario supports the Perinatal Core Measure of increasing the percentage of infants who are fed breast milk only. **Focus:** Supervision.

32. **Ans: 1**   The priority is to communicate clearly to the patient the most recent recommendation of the Centers for Disease Control and Prevention (CDC) which at this time advises pregnant women not to travel to areas where Zika is prevalent. The nurse must always check the most recent recommendations online at CDC.gov. With any disease outbreak, the recommendations may change weekly, and it is a vital nursing responsibility to be sure the advice given to patients is consistent with the latest evidence-based information. The other options are correct and are appropriate information for a patient to have if she lives in a Zika-impacted area, or if the patient in this scenario decides to travel despite the risks. Nevertheless, the first priority is to give clear information that travel to these areas is not recommended in pregnancy. **Focus:** Prioritization.

33. **Ans: 2**   Option 2 provides the correct preconception information that should be given to all couples planning pregnancy. Option 1 does not demonstrate the nurse using her or his professional knowledge to offer appropriate information to the couple. Option 3 suggests judgment of the couple for their choice to have a child and would be inappropriate. Although it can be appropriate for the nurse to discuss a woman's motivations for pregnancy in some cases when the pregnancy might seriously adversely affect the woman's health, it would not be appropriate to do so based on the fact that the women are in a same-sex relationship. Option 4 is incorrect information. **Focus:** Prioritization.

34. **Ans: 2**   The priority of nursing care of a newborn being breastfed is to assure adequate transfer of milk from mother to baby. The process of lactation requires hormonal stimulation during pregnancy and after birth. There are protocols for stimulation of lactation in a woman who has not given birth as in this case or in adoption cases. The protocols involve hormonal stimulation of the breasts before birth and mechanical stimulation with pumping. The nurse would need to find out if the partner has been preparing for lactation in this way to know how to best help them achieve their goal. The nurse must clearly communicate the obligation to follow practices that assure the newborn adequate intake. Option 1 without knowledge of how the partner has been preparing for lactation would be inappropriate and might put the infant at risk for inadequate intake. Options 3 and 4 are not appropriate responses for any couple planning to breastfeed their baby. This item supports the Perinatal Core Measurement of increasing breastfeeding. **Focus:** Prioritization.

35. **Ans: 3, 4, 1, 2**   The correct order of action always puts patient safety first. In this case, the nurse should simply ask the unauthorized visitor to identify herself and her purpose on the unit. If any hostility or combativeness is encountered, security should be immediately called. Alerting the desk secretary to maintain close attentiveness to the infant security system would enhance patient safety and allow a security code to be quickly called if an infant went missing. After patient safety is assured, it is then the professional responsibility of the nurse to look at the system issues that caused the breach. The other nurse should be asked why the unauthorized visitor was allowed into the unit and explain the risk this action caused to others on the unit.

PART 2 Common Health Scenarios

A review of policies with the staff by the unit leadership would then further remind all staff of the need for constant vigilance and adherence to the security systems in place to avoid risk to the patients in their care. **Focus:** Prioritization.

36. **Ans: 3** The key information in the question is that the chest x-ray examination showed no evidence of active TB processes in the lungs. The patient is therefore not considered infectious to other patients or to her newborn (not even through her milk). Treatment of latent TB postpartum is appropriate for most patients depending on their medical profile. The nurse needs to engage the charge nurse in clinical consultation regarding the case and use resources such as infectious disease practitioners or hospital policies with the goal of professional interaction to offer the patient the best evidence-based nursing care. A nursing unit should encourage this type of professional interaction among all levels of nurses and other health professionals. **Focus:** Prioritization, Assignment.

37. **Ans: 2** The charge nurse would need to correct the statement that the mother would need to dump her milk. This is not necessary because the varicella infection is not found in the breast milk. The other advice given by the new nurse is correct. The mother with varicella can breastfeed her infant. The newborn should have received varicella-zoster immune globulin and may room with the mother in isolation from other patients. The mother should avoid having the infant's skin come in contact with any varicella lesions and the pediatrician should be notified of maternal varicella. A mother with varicella should have standard, airborne, and contact precautions. The new nurse should be shown the unit policy on varicella and helped to understand why the mother can breastfeed. The information should be corrected by the new nurse so the mother at this difficult time has no misconceptions or guilt. **Focus:** Supervision.

38. **Ans: 2** Option 2 factually explains to the patient the real risks associated with the disease in pregnancy. Research has shown that describing to patients the specific risks a disease may have for them or their children can help them to accept the vaccine. Option 1 does offer useful information for preventing the flu but does not go far enough in factually explaining the vaccine and the special risks of flu in pregnancy. Option 3 is incorrect because giving the vaccine postpartum does not impact the risk of flu during pregnancy. Option 4 is incorrect. Even though an intervention can be highly recommended, a patient may always decline. **Focus:** Prioritization.

39. **Ans: 3, 1, 2, 4** In prioritization, patient safety always takes precedence. In this case, a 16-year-old woman with elevated blood pressure and a headache is showing symptoms of preeclampsia, which can be life threatening. This patient would need prompt assessment and the health care provider should be notified

immediately to evaluate the patient. The patient who is tearful and discouraged about breastfeeding needs timely help from the nurse because she is at a vulnerable time in breastfeeding when many women give up without compassionate skillful interventions by a nurse or lactation consultant. The nurse could delegate to the unit secretary the task of notifying the social worker of the woman who wants to discuss possible adoption with her. The nurse would also assess the patient and explore her situation, but by delegating the call, the process can begin. A temperature of 100.5°F (38.1°C) on day 1 after a cesarean section is not an unusual finding and needs to be monitored via routine assessments for rising temperature or clinical symptoms of infection. **Focus:** Prioritization.

40. **Ans: 1, 4, 6** Droplet precautions dictate health care providers wear a mask while in the room and discard it before leaving the room. In this case, a gown and gloves would be required only if care involved contact with bodily fluids (which may happen frequently in labor and delivery). Use of a negative pressure room is incorrect because it is a feature of airborne precautions. The breast milk itself does not carry influenza and may contain protective antibodies against influenza, which may benefit the newborn. The other options are correct choices in the case of droplet precautions. The nurse should review with the student nurse the types of isolation procedures and clarify the features of each and the need to review information before communicating it to the patient. **Focus:** Assignment.

41. **Ans: 3** This is a situation no nurse would choose to be in. These conversations would have been better held during the prenatal visits when the diagnosis of placenta previa was made and the discussion could have been more lengthy and thorough. At this moment, however, with active bleeding, the lives of the baby and the mother are at risk, so teaching must be accurate and succinct. Option 3 directly addresses the concerns of the couple and gives them information to quickly consider in their decision. It also brings the obstetrician and anesthesiologist rapidly into the conversation to allow the team to collaborate effectively in communicating to the patient. The essential clinical information to communicate quickly is that the risk of hepatitis B is about 1 in 250,000, and the risk of hepatitis C and HIV are 1 in 1 to 2 million from a blood transfusion in the United States. Explain that because of the bleeding she is having, her anemia, and the surgery she is about to have, she is at risk for significant blood loss and resulting severe anemia, which is linked with slower recovery, breastfeeding problems, increased risk of infection, hemorrhagic shock, and death. Option 1 does not show the nurse using her professional knowledge to educate the patient about the risks and benefits, but instead allows the patient to make a consequential decision without being provided adequate information. Option 2 is inaccurate,

and Option 4 is too time consuming for the clinical scenario at hand. **Focus:** Prioritization.

42. **Ans: 2**   Oxytocin is a high-alert medication, and although frequently used in labor and delivery, it requires meticulous monitoring to avoid complications. In Option 2, the contractions are too close together, which is stressful for the fetus because oxygenation is decreased. If this pattern of tachysystole is allowed to continue, fetal hypoxia may occur. Although the fetal heart rate is now normal, the nursing action required at this time would be to stop the oxytocin or decrease the dose and notify the health care provider while keeping a close eye on the fetal heart rate and placing the patient in the optimal position for maternal fetal circulation. This option involves patient safety and so is the priority case. The other options are normal findings during induction of labor and varying stages of labor. This item addresses the Perinatal Core Measurement of reducing the incidence of cesarean sections. **Focus:** Supervision, Prioritization.

43. **Ans: 2**   Family-centered care and open family visitation is the optimal choice in the postpartum unit. Family members and young children can be welcomed into the units. Nevertheless, mothers and newborns are a vulnerable group, and there are times when concerns regarding infectious disease spread must take precedence. The toddler described likely had norovirus, a highly contagious gastrointestinal disease. Excluding the toddler and any other ill family members from visiting the postpartum unit would be recommended. The nurse must realize this may be extremely disappointing to the family and must work hard to find a substitute way for the mother, toddler, and newborn

to interact, possibly through internet connection, photos, or phone calls. It would also be the nurse's responsibility to discuss the illness of the toddler with associated health care providers and infectious disease nurses at the hospital, as well as to consult Centers for Disease Control and Prevention guidelines to offer the patient evidence-based advice regarding measures to take upon discharge to prevent spread of the infection. The other options would not be recommended. **Focus:** Prioritization.

44. **Ans: 2, 3, 4**   The maternal death rate in the United States is unacceptably high and the nurse is an important link to prevention. One the links of prevention is access to high-quality care for at-risk patients. It is not acceptable for a professional nurse to tell a high-risk patient to keep trying to make an appointment within a dysfunctional system. It is often these types of barriers to care that combine to prevent high-risk women from accessing appropriate prenatal care. Taking initiative to correct systemic problems is vitally important. Making linkages with community health nurses and with the hospital social worker are appropriate nursing actions to reduce the number of women who have inadequate prenatal care. It would not be appropriate to tell a high-risk pregnant woman to go to an urgent care center for comprehensive prenatal care because that is not the type of care offered at such a setting. Giving a high-risk pregnant woman the phone number of another clinic without ensuring that appointments can be made and that vital information will be transferred from the hospital to an outpatient setting is not sufficient to ensure good continuity of care. **Focus:** Prioritization.

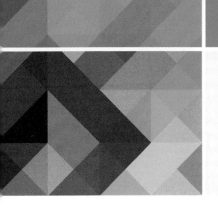

CHAPTER 19
Pediatric Problems

Questions

1. A 3-month-old infant arrives at the health center for a scheduled well-child visit. The parents ask the nurse why the infant extends the arms and legs in response to a loud sound. Which response by the nurse is **best**?
   1. Inform the parents this is a normal reflex that generally disappears by 4 to 6 months of age.
   2. Tell the parents if the behavior does not change by 6 months, the infant will need further evaluation.
   3. Remind the parents this is a normal response that indicates the infant's hearing is intact.
   4. Reassure the parents that the behavior is normal and not an indicator of any problem such as cerebral palsy.

2. Which pediatric pain patient should be assigned to a newly graduated RN?
   1. An adolescent who has sickle cell disease and who was recently weaned from morphine delivered via a patient-controlled analgesia device to an oral analgesic; he has been continually asking for an increased dose.
   2. A child who needs premedication before reduction of a fracture; the child has been crying and is resistant to any touch to the arm or other procedures.
   3. A child who is receiving palliative end-of-life care; the child is receiving opioids around the clock to relieve suffering, but there is a progressive decrease in alertness and responsiveness.
   4. A child who has chronic pain and whose medication and nonpharmacologic regimen has recently been changed; the mother is anxious to see if the new regimen is successful.

3. The nurse caring for a 3-year-old child plans to assess the child's pain using the Wong-Baker FACES® Pain Rating Scale. Which accompanying assessment question would be the **most** useful?
   1. "If number 0 (smiling face) were no pain and number 10 (crying face) were a big pain, what number would your pain be?"
   2. "Can you point to the face picture with one finger and tell me what that pain feels like inside of you?"

   3. "The smiling face has 'no hurting'; the crying face has a 'really big hurting.' Which face is most like your hurting?"
   4. "If you look at these faces and I give you a paper and pencil, can you draw for me the face that looks the most like your pain?"

4. The nurse is caring for several children with cancer who are receiving chemotherapy. The nurse is reviewing the morning laboratory results for each of the patients. Which patient condition combined with the indicated laboratory result would cause the nurse the **greatest** concern?
   1. Nausea and vomiting with a potassium level of 3.3 mEq/L (3.3 mmol/L)
   2. Epistaxis with a platelet count of 100,000/mm^3 (100 × 10^9/L)
   3. Fever with an absolute neutrophil count of 450/mm^3 (450 × 10^9/L)
   4. Fatigue with a hemoglobin level of 8 g/dL (80 g/L)

5. A 7-month-old infant arrives at the health center for a scheduled well-child visit. When the nurse approaches the infant to obtain vital signs, the infant cries vigorously and clings fearfully to the mother. Which of the following phenomena provides the best explanation for the infant's behavior?
   1. Separation anxiety
   2. Disassociation disorder
   3. Stranger anxiety
   4. Autism spectrum

6. A 6-year-old child who received chemotherapy and had anorexia is now cheerfully eating peanut butter, yogurt, and applesauce. When the mother arrives, the child refuses to eat and throws the dish on the floor. What is the nurse's **best** response to this behavior?
   1. Remind the child that foods tasted good today and will help her or his body to get strong.
   2. Allow the mother and child time alone to review and control the behavior.

3. Ask the mother to leave until the child can finish eating and then invite her back.
4. Explain to the mother that the behavior could be a normal expression of anger.

7. An 18-month-old child has oral mucositis secondary to chemotherapy. Which task should the nurse delegate to the assistive personnel (AP)?
1. Reporting evidence of severe mucosal ulceration
2. Assisting the child in swishing and spitting mouthwash
3. Assessing the child's ability and willingness to drink through a straw
4. Feeding the child a bland, moist, soft diet

8. The pediatric unit charge nurse is making patient assignments for the evening shift. Which patient is **most** appropriate to assign to an experienced LPN/LVN?
1. A 1-year-old patient with severe combined immunodeficiency disease who is scheduled to receive chemotherapy in preparation for a stem cell transplant
2. A 2-year-old patient with Wiskott-Aldrich syndrome who has orders for a platelet transfusion
3. A 3-year-old patient who has chronic graft-versus-host disease and is incontinent of loose stools
4. A 6-year-old patient who received chemotherapy 1 week ago and is admitted with increasing lethargy and a temperature of 101°F (38.3°C)

9. The pediatric unit charge nurse is working with a new RN. Which action by the new RN requires the **most** immediate action on the part of the pediatric unit charge nurse?
1. Wearing gloves, gowns, and a mask for a neutropenic child who is receiving chemotherapy
2. Placing a newly admitted child with respiratory syncytial virus (RSV) infection in a room with another child who has RSV
3. Wearing a N95 respirator mask when caring for a child with tuberculosis
4. Performing hand hygiene with soap and water after caring for a child with diarrhea caused by *Clostridium difficile*

10. The nurse is preparing to care for a 6-year-old child who has just undergone allogenic stem cell transplantation. Which nursing tasks should the nurse delegate to the assistive personnel (AP)? **Select all that apply.**
1. Stocking the child's room with standard personal protective equipment items
2. Teaching the child to perform thorough hand washing after using the bathroom
3. Reminding the child to wear a face mask outside of the hospital room

4. Assessing the child's oral cavity for signs and symptoms of infection
5. Talking to the family members about the ways to reduce risk of infection
6. Talk to the parents about local community and health care resources that will support the family after discharge.

11. A 4-month-old infant boy is brought to the emergency department by his parents. He has been vomiting and fussy for the past 24 hours. On examination, there are circular bruises on his back. What **priority** assessment does the nurse anticipate?
1. Chest x-ray examination
2. Ultrasonography of the head
3. Electroencephalography
4. Ophthalmologic examination

12. Which action will the public health nurse take to have the **most** impact on the incidence of infectious diseases in the school?
1. Make soap and water readily available in the classrooms.
2. Ensure that students are immunized according to national recommendations.
3. Provide written information about infection control to all parents.
4. Teach students how to cover their mouths when they cough or sneeze.

13. While working in the pediatric clinic, the nurse receives a telephone call from the parent of a 13-year-old child who is receiving chemotherapy for leukemia. The patient's sibling has chickenpox (varicella). Which action will the nurse anticipate taking **next**?
1. Administer varicella-zoster immune globulin to the patient.
2. Teach the parent about the correct use of acyclovir.
3. Educate the parent about contact and airborne precautions.
4. Prepare to admit the patient to a private room in the hospital.

14. An unimmunized 7-year-old child who attends a local elementary school contracts rubeola (measles). The child has two siblings, ages 9 and 11 years, who also attend the elementary school. Which action by the school nurse is a **priority**?
1. Exclude the child and siblings from attending school for 21 days.
2. Notify all parents of children attending the school of the exposure.
3. Recommend that the siblings receive the measles vaccine.
4. Recommend that the siblings receive measles immunoglobulin.

15. The school nurse is performing developmental screenings for children who will be entering preschool. A 4-year-old girl excitedly tells the nurse about her recent birthday party. As she relates the details of the event, she frequently stutters. Which action by the nurse is **most** appropriate at this time?
    1. Refer the child to an audiologist.
    2. Obtain a detailed birth history from the parents.
    3. Document the findings on the child's school record.
    4. Refer the child to a speech pathologist.

16. An adolescent with cystic fibrosis (CF) is admitted to the pediatric unit with increased shortness of breath and pneumonia. Which nursing activity is **most** important to include in the patient's care?
    1. Allowing the adolescent to decide if aerosolized medications are needed
    2. Scheduling postural drainage and a chest physiotherapy every 4 hours
    3. Placing the adolescent in a room with another adolescent with CF
    4. Encouraging oral fluid intake of 2400 mL/day

17. The nurse has obtained this assessment information about a 3-year-old patient who has just returned to the pediatric unit after having a tonsillectomy. Which finding requires the **most** immediate follow-up?
    1. Frequent swallowing
    2. Hypotonic bowel sounds
    3. Reports of a sore throat
    4. Heart rate of 112 beats/min

18. The nurse is providing nursing care for a newborn infant with respiratory distress syndrome (RDS) who is receiving nasal continuous positive airway pressure ventilation. Which assessment finding is **most** important to report to the health care provider (HCP)?
    1. Apical pulse rate of 156 beats/min
    2. Crackles audible in both lungs
    3. Tracheal deviation to the right
    4. Oxygen saturation of 93%

19. The nurse is assisting with the delivery of a 31-week gestational age premature newborn who requires intubation for respiratory distress syndrome (RDS). Which medication does the nurse anticipate will be needed **first** for this infant?
    1. Theophylline
    2. Surfactant
    3. Dexamethasone
    4. Albuterol

20. The nurse obtains this information when assessing a 3-year-old patient with uncorrected tetralogy of Fallot who is crying. Which finding requires immediate action?
    1. The apical pulse rate is 118 beats/min.

2. A loud systolic murmur is heard in the pulmonic area.
3. There is marked clubbing of the child's nail beds.
4. The lips and oral mucosa are dusky in color.

21. The nurse is observing a preschool classroom of children between the ages of 3 to 4 years of age. When planning actions to ensure that each child meets normal developmental goals, which child will require the **most** immediate intervention?
    1. A 3-year-old boy who needs help dressing
    2. A 4-year-old girl who has an imaginary friend
    3. A 4-year-old girl who engages only in parallel play
    4. A 3-year-old boy who draws stick figures

22. After receiving the change-of-shift report, which patient should the nurse assess **first**?
    1. An 18-month-old patient with coarctation of the aorta who has decreased pedal pulses
    2. A 3-year-old patient with rheumatic fever who reports severe knee pain
    3. A 5-year-old patient with endocarditis who has crackles audible throughout both lungs
    4. An 8-year-old patient with Kawasaki disease who has a temperature of 102.2°F (38.9°C)

23. The pediatric unit charge nurse is working with a newly graduated RN who has been on orientation in the unit for 2 months. Which patient should the charge nurse assign to the new RN?
    1. A 2-year-old patient with a ventricular septal defect for whom digoxin 90 mcg by mouth has been prescribed
    2. A 4-year-old patient who had a pulmonary artery banding and has just been transferred in from the intensive care unit
    3. A 9-year-old patient with mitral valve endocarditis whose parents need teaching about IV antibiotic administration
    4. A 16-year-old patient with a heart transplant who was admitted with a low-grade fever and tachycardia

24. The nurse is obtaining the history and physical information for a child who is recovering from Kawasaki disease and receives aspirin therapy. Which information concerns the nurse the most?
    1. The child attends a day-care center 5 days a week.
    2. The child's fingers have areas of peeling skin.
    3. The child is very irritable and cries frequently.
    4. The child has not received any immunizations.

25. The RN is working with an LPN/LVN to provide care for a 10-year-old patient with severe abdominal, hip, and knee pain caused by a sickle cell crisis. Which action taken by the LPN/LVN requires the RN to intervene immediately?

 Answer Key for this chapter begins on p. 196

1. Administering oral pain medication as needed
2. Positioning cold packs on the child's knees
3. Encouraging increased fluid intake
4. Monitoring vital signs every 2 hours

26. The nurse has just received a change-of-shift report about these pediatric patients. Which patient will the nurse assess **first**?
    1. A 1-year-old patient with hemophilia B who was admitted because of decreased responsiveness
    2. A 3-year-old patient with von Willebrand disease who has a dose of desmopressin scheduled
    3. A 7-year-old patient with acute lymphocytic leukemia who has chemotherapy-induced thrombocytopenia
    4. A 16-year-old patient with sickle cell disease who reports acute right lower quadrant abdominal pain

27. The nurse is reviewing a complete blood count for a 3-year-old patient with idiopathic thrombocytopenic purpura (ITP). Which information should the nurse report immediately to the health care provider (HCP)?
    1. Prothrombin time (PT) of 12 seconds
    2. Hemoglobin level of 6.1 g/dL (61 g/L)
    3. Platelet count of 40,000/mm³ (40 × 10⁹/L)
    4. Leukocyte count of 5600/mm³ (5.6 × 10⁹/L)

28. A 4-year-old patient with acute lymphocytic leukemia has these medications prescribed. Which one is **most** important to double-check with another licensed nurse?
    1. Prednisone 1 mg PO
    2. Amoxicillin 250 mg PO
    3. Methotrexate 10 mg PO
    4. Filgrastim 5 mcg subcutaneously

29. A 6-year-old child arrives in the emergency department with active seizures. Which assessment is the **highest** priority for the nurse to obtain?
    1. Heart rate
    2. Body mass index (BMI)
    3. Blood pressure
    4. Weight

30. The nurse is caring for a 3-year-old patient who has returned to the pediatric intensive care unit after insertion of a ventriculoperitoneal shunt to correct hydrocephalus. Which assessment finding is **most** important to communicate to the surgeon?
    1. The child is crying and says, "It hurts!"
    2. The right pupil is 1 mm larger than the left pupil.
    3. The cardiac monitor shows a heart rate of 130 beats/min.
    4. The head dressing has a 2-cm area of bloody drainage.

31. The nurse is caring for a newborn with a myelomeningocele who is awaiting surgical closure of the defect. Which assessment finding is of **most** concern?
    1. Bulging of the sac when the infant cries
    2. Oozing of stool from the anal sphincter
    3. Flaccid paralysis of both legs
    4. Temperature of 101.8°F (38.8°C)

32. A mother calls the nurse for advice. "My child got cleaning solution in her eyes, and I rinsed her eyes with water for a few minutes. What should I do? She is still screaming!" What does the nurse instruct the caller to do **first**?
    1. Comfort the child and check her vision.
    2. Continue to irrigate the eyes with water.
    3. Call the Poison Control Center.
    4. Call 911 to request an ambulance.

33. The nurse is caring for a child with a foreign body in the ear canal who has not been evaluated by the health care provider (HCP). Which actions should the nurse implement? **Select all that apply.**
    1. Inspect the pinna for trauma.
    2. Irrigate the auditory canal with warm water.
    3. Obtain a history for the type of object.
    4. Attempt to remove the object with forceps.
    5. Use an otoscope to check for perforation.
    6. Use a suction catheter to remove the foreign body.

34. An adolescent who was hospitalized for anorexia nervosa is following the prescribed treatment plan. Her self-esteem and weight have gradually improved, but she continues to refer to herself as "fatty." She is able to verbalize an appropriate diet and exercise plan. At this point, what is the **priority** concern?
    1. Patient needs to continue to gain weight.
    2. Patient has an unrealistic body image.
    3. Patient needs more information about nutrition.
    4. Patient lacks motivation to adhere to therapy.

35. A 6-year-old girl arrives in the emergency department with her parents. She hit her head when she fell from the jungle gym at the school playground. Which questions are appropriate for the nurse to ask to assess the child's neurologic status? **Select all that apply.**
    1. What is your home address?
    2. What time does your family eat dinner?
    3. What grade are you in?
    4. What is your teacher's name?
    5. What time did you fall?
    6. What is the name of your school?

36. A 2-year-old child who has abdominal pain is diagnosed with intussusception. A hydrostatic reduction has been performed. Which finding should be reported immediately before surgery proceeds?

1. Palpable sausage-shaped abdominal mass
2. Passage of normal brown stool
3. Passage of currant jelly–like stools
4. Frequent nausea and vomiting

37. A parent calls the emergency department, saying, "I think my toddler may have swallowed a little toy. He is breathing okay, but I don't know what to do." What is the **most** essential question to ask the caller?
    1. "Has he vomited?"
    2. "Have you been checking his stools?"
    3. "What do you think he swallowed?"
    4. "Has he been coughing?"

38. The nurse is teaching a group of day-care workers about how to avoid transmission of hepatitis A in day-care settings. What is the single **most** effective measure to emphasize?
    1. Hand hygiene should be performed often to prevent and control the spread of infection.
    2. Children in whom hepatitis has been diagnosed should not share toys with others.
    3. Children with episodes of fecal incontinence should be isolated from others.
    4. Immunizations are recommended before children are admitted into day-care settings.

39. These medications have been prescribed for a 9-year-old patient with deep partial- and full-thickness burns. Which medication is **most** important to double-check with another licensed nurse before administration?
    1. Silver sulfadiazine ointment
    2. Famotidine 20 mg IV
    3. Lorazepam 0.5 mg PO
    4. Multivitamin 1 tablet PO

40. The nurse is caring for a 5-year-old whose mother asks why he still wets the bed. What is the **best** response?
    1. "He is old enough that he should no longer be wetting the bed."
    2. "Most children outgrow bed-wetting by the time they start school."
    3. "His bed-wetting may be the result of an immature bladder or deep sleep pattern."
    4. "He will probably stop once he realizes how embarrassing it is to wet the bed."

41. Which intervention for a 5-year-old child who still wets the bed would be **best** assigned to the assistive personnel (AP)?
    1. Reminding the child to use the bathroom before going to bed
    2. Teaching the mother about moisture alarm devices
    3. Administering the prescribed dose of imipramine
    4. Discussing research related to the use of hypnosis with the mother

42. Parents of a 13-year-old adolescent girl expressed concern because she spends "quite a bit of time in her room alone in front of the mirror." The girl's height and weight are in the 50th percentile. In the exam room, the girl is quiet but does answer questions appropriately. What advice should the nurse provide to the parents?
    1. "Further evaluation by a psychologist is needed because your daughter spends a lot of time alone in her room."
    2. "Limit the amount of time that your daughter is allowed to spend alone in her room."
    3. "This behavior is normal. Your daughter is adjusting to the physical changes she is experiencing."
    4. "This behavior may be associated with depression, and further evaluation by a counselor is advised."

43. A 16-year-old female adolescent arrives at the health center. She tells the nurse that she's been sexually active for 6 months "but only with my boyfriend." Her immunizations are up to date. Screening for which sexually transmitted disease (STD) will be **most** important for this patient?
    1. Syphilis
    2. Genital herpes simplex
    3. Human papillomavirus
    4. Chlamydia

44. The health care provider has ordered cooling measures for a child with a fever who is likely to be discharged when the temperature comes down. Which task will the nurse delegate to the assistive personnel (AP)?
    1. Providing explanations of nursing actions to the family
    2. Assisting the child to remove the outer clothing
    3. Advising the parent to use acetaminophen instead of aspirin
    4. Monitoring the child's level of consciousness and orientation level

45. A tearful parent brings a child to the emergency department after the child takes an unknown amount of children's chewable vitamins at an unknown time. The child is currently alert and asymptomatic. What information should be immediately reported to the health care provider?
    1. The ingested children's chewable vitamins contain iron.
    2. The child has been treated previously for ingestion of toxic substances.
    3. The child has been treated several times before for accidental injuries.
    4. The child was nauseated and vomited once at home.

Answer Key for this chapter begins on p. 196

PART 2 Common Health Scenarios

46. The nurse is preparing a child for IV moderate (conscious) sedation before repair of a facial laceration. What information should the nurse immediately report to the health care provider (HCP)?
    1. The parent is unsure about the child's tetanus immunization status.
    2. The child is upset and pulls out the IV.
    3. The parent declines the IV moderate (conscious) sedation.
    4. The parent wants information about the IV moderate (conscious) sedation.

47. A teenager arrives in the triage area alert and ambulatory, but his clothes are covered with blood. His friends are yelling, "We were goofing around, and he got poked in the abdomen with a stick!" Which comment would be of **most** concern?
    1. "There was a lot of blood, and we used three bandages."
    2. "He pulled the stick out, just now, because it was hurting him."
    3. "The stick was really dirty and covered with mud."
    4. "He has diabetes, so he needs attention right away."

48. Enhanced Multiple Response _____

Scenario: The emergency department receives multiple individuals, mostly children, who were injured when the roof of a day-care center collapsed because of a heavy snowfall. The pediatric trauma nurse is aware that there are physiologic differences in children compared with adults.

Based on knowledge of growth and development of children, which injuries and complications does the nurse expect to observe?

Instructions: Place an X in the space provided or highlight each injury or complication that the nurse is most likely to observe among the children. **Select all that apply.**
1. _____ Head injuries
2. _____ Bradycardia or junctional arrhythmias
3. _____ Hypoxemia
4. _____ Liver and spleen contusions
5. _____ Hypothermia
6. _____ Epiphyseal fractures of long bones
7. _____ Lumbar spines injuries

49. A 16-year-old patient arrives at the cystic fibrosis (CF) clinic for a routine 3-month visit. The most recent respiratory culture results are negative. Which action is **best** for the nurse to take?
    1. Place the patient in an exam room immediately upon arrival to the clinic.
    2. Allow the patient to wait in the reception area until the health care provider (HCP) is available to see the patient.
    3. Allow the patient to wait in the reception area with a mask on until the HCP is available to see the patient.
    4. Place the patient in a waiting area with other patients who also have negative respiratory cultures.

50. A child with Hirschsprung disease arrives on the pediatric unit from the operating room with a temporary colostomy. Which task should the nurse delegate to assistive personnel (AP)?
    1. Assess the frequency and consistency of stool.
    2. Instruct the parents on skin care.
    3. Stock the room with ostomy supplies.
    4. Assess the patient for pain.

51. A newborn infant is diagnosed with tracheoesophageal fistula. Which nursing interventions should be implemented in the preoperative period? **Select all that apply.**
    1. Provide small frequent feedings.
    2. Elevate the head of the bed.
    3. Prepare a tracheostomy tray.
    4. Set up suctioning.
    5. Administer IV antibiotics.
    6. Administer Vitamin K.

52. A 2-year-old child arrives at the health center for a routine well-child visit. A complete blood count and lead level are obtained. The lead level is less than 5 mcg/dL (0.483 μmol/L). The hemoglobin is 8 g/dL (80 g/L). The hematocrit is 24% (0.24 volume fraction), and the mean corpuscular volume (MCV) is 65 μm³ (65 fL). What questions should the nurse ask the parent to obtain a more thorough history? **Select all that apply.**
    1. Does your child eat nonfood substances?
    2. Is your child more prone to infections?
    3. Has your child experienced hair loss?
    4. Does your child frequently have nosebleeds?
    5. How much milk does your child drink?
    6. Has your child had any episodes of nausea and vomiting?

53. Liquid supplemental iron is prescribed for a 10-month-old child with iron deficiency anemia. The parents tell the nurse that their child hates the taste of medicine. Which of the following instructions should the nurse provide to the parents? **Select all that apply.**
    1. Give the iron orally with a syringe.
    2. Mix the iron in a little bit of chocolate syrup.
    3. Give the iron with food or milk.
    4. Let the child drink the iron through a straw.
    5. Give the iron with orange juice.
    6. Give the iron with cola.

54. The parents of a 6-month-old girl bring the infant to the emergency department because "she has not held anything down for the entire day." The nurse obtains a fingerstick blood glucose of 94 (5.22 mmol/L). The infant's rectal temperature is 101°F (38.3°C), heart rate is 198 beats/min, respiratory rate is 40 breaths/min, and blood pressure is 60/38 mm Hg in the left arm. Which nursing action is a **priority**?
    1. Administer an antiemetic rectally.
    2. Administer a bolus of D10W.
    3. Administer a bolus of normal saline.
    4. Administer an antipyretic rectally.

55. A 10-year-old girl has completed a course of amoxicillin for a urinary tract infection (UTI). This is the second UTI the child has had this year. The child is in the 95th percentile for weight and has a history of constipation. Her parents ask the nurse for preventive strategies for UTIs. Which of the following preventive strategies is **best** for the nurse to recommend?
    1. Increase whole grains, fruits, and vegetables.
    2. Drink cranberry juice.
    3. Increase vitamin C in her diet.
    4. Limit fluids at bedtime.

56. A 16-year-old boy comes into the office of the school nurse complaining of left hip pain that began when playing basketball in gym class. The boy is in the 85th percentile for height and weight. He complains of increased pain with weight bearing. The nurse observes out-toeing of the left leg with ambulation. Which nursing action is a **priority**?
    1. Administer ibuprofen and instruct the boy to rest.
    2. Apply heat to the hip and elevate the left leg.
    3. Refer the boy to the emergency department.
    4. Apply ice to the hip and immobilize it with a splint.

57. A toddler is brought to the health center for a fever of 102°F (39°C) and a sore throat. As the nurse places the toddler and his parents in the examination room, the child experiences a tonic-clonic seizure. Which nursing action is a **priority**?
    1. Assess the child's level of consciousness.
    2. Obtain an oxygen saturation.
    3. Loosen the child's clothing.
    4. Position the child in a side-lying position.

PART 2   Common Health Scenarios

    Answer Key for this chapter begins on p. 196

Answers

1. **Ans: 1** The infant's behavior is consistent with the Moro and startle reflexes. The Moro reflex usually disappears by 6 months of age. The startle reflex usually disappears by 4 months of age. A hearing test is not based on response to loud sounds alone. Although it is true that further evaluation may be needed if the reflexes do not disappear, there is no need for the nurse to discuss this with the parents at this time. The infant's behavior is not consistent with cerebral palsy. **Focus:** Prioritization. **Test-Taking Tip:** In studying pediatrics, pay attention to the developmental milestones. Moro, startle, and Babinski reflexes are three classic examples of what the nurse observes during physical assessment. Can you name others?

2. **Ans: 2** The set of circumstances is least complicated for the child with the fracture, and this would be the best patient for a new and relatively inexperienced nurse. The child is likely to have a good response to pain medication, and with gentle encouragement and pain management, the anxiety will resolve. The other three children have more complex social and psychological issues related to pain management. **Focus:** Assignment.

3. **Ans: 3** Pain rating scales using faces (depicting smiling, neutral, frowning, crying, and so on) are appropriate for young children who may have difficulty describing pain or understanding the correlation of pain to numerical or verbal descriptors. The other questions require abstract reasoning abilities to make analogies and the use of advanced vocabulary. **Focus:** Prioritization. **Test-Taking Tip:** When caring for children, you must use the principles of growth and development to choose the best assessment tools and to differentiate normal from abnormal findings.

4. **Ans: 3** National guidelines indicate that rapid treatment of infection in neutropenic patients is essential to prevent complications such as overwhelming sepsis and secondary infections; therefore the child with a fever and a low neutrophil count is the priority. A potassium level of 3.3 mEq/L (3.3 mmol/L) is borderline low and should be monitored. Nosebleeds are common, and the patient and parents should be taught to apply direct pressure to the nose, have the child sit upright, and not disturb the clot. Severe spontaneous hemorrhage is not expected until the platelet count drops below 20,000 mm³ (20 × 10⁹/L). Children can withstand low hemoglobin levels. The nurse should help the patient and parents regulate activity to prevent excessive fatigue. **Focus:** Prioritization.

5. **Ans: 3** This infant is displaying stranger anxiety; the child becomes anxious when exposed to unfamiliar people (strangers). Separation anxiety occurs when the child is separated from the primary caregiver; anxiety and crying are also common behaviors. Stranger anxiety and separation anxiety are concurrent and generally begin at 7 to 8 months of age. **Focus:** Prioritization.

6. **Ans: 4** Help the mother to understand that the child may be angry about being left in the hospital or about her inability to prevent the illness and protect the child. Reminding the child about the food and the purpose of the food does not address the strong emotions underlying the outburst. Allowing the mother and child time alone is a possibility, but the assumption would be that the mother understands the child's behavior and is prepared to deal with the behavior in a constructive manner. Asking the mother to leave the child suggests that the mother is a source of stress. **Focus:** Prioritization.

7. **Ans: 4** Helping the child to eat is within the scope of responsibilities for an AP. Assessing ability and willingness to drink and checking for extent of mucosal ulceration are the responsibilities of an RN. An 18-month-old child is not able to swish and spit, which could result in swallowing the mouthwash. Mouthwash is not intended for swallowing because it can contain alcohol and other ingredients not safe for ingestion. **Focus:** Delegation.

8. **Ans: 3** LPN/LVN scope of practice includes the care of patients with chronic and stable health problems, such as the patient with chronic graft-versus-host disease. Chemotherapy medications are considered high-alert medications and should be given by RNs who have received additional education in chemotherapy administration. Platelets and other blood products should be given by RNs. The 6-year-old patient has a history and clinical manifestations consistent with neutropenia and sepsis and should be assessed by an RN as quickly as possible. **Focus:** Assignment.

9. **Ans: 1** Protective isolation (wearing gloves, gowns, and mask) revealed no significant differences in infection rates for children who are neutropenic. General standard precautions are advised with routine patient care. Although private rooms are preferred for patients who need droplet precautions, such as patients with RSV infection, they can be placed in rooms with other patients with exactly the same microorganism. An N95 respirator is recommended for tuberculosis. Washing hands with soap and water after caring for a patient with *C. difficile* is also recommended. **Focus:** Prioritization.

10. **Ans: 1, 3**   Because all patient care staff members should be familiar with standard personal protective equipment, an AP will be able to stock the room. Reminding the child to wear a face mask is also a task that can be done by an AP, although the RN is responsible for the initial teaching. Initially teaching the child a good hand-washing technique, nursing assessments, and family education is within the scope of the registered nurse and not an AP. Talking to the family about local resources post discharge should be done by either the RN or the Social Services department. **Focus:** Delegation.

11. **Ans: 4**   The history and physical examination suggest shaken baby syndrome. An ophthalmologic examination is indicated to determine if the infant has retinal hemorrhages characteristic of shaken baby syndrome. Electroencephalography may be indicated if there is evidence of seizures. Magnetic resonance imaging or computed tomography of the head (not ultrasonography) can detect subdural hematomas. There is no evidence that would support the need for a chest x-ray examination. **Focus:** Prioritization. **Test-Taking Tip:** To answer this type of question, analyze key information: age, symptoms, and injury. Vomiting and fussiness accompany many disorders, but how would a 4-month old infant sustain circular bruises? After you have identified the problem (probable abuse), used knowledge of disorders related to age groups to narrow the field (shaken baby syndrome is common among young infants), and identified common manifestations of the disorder (retinal hemorrhage), then you can select the appropriate assessment technique.

12. **Ans: 2**   The incidence of once-common infectious diseases such as measles, chickenpox, and mumps has been most effectively reduced by the immunization of all school-age children. The other actions are also helpful but will not have as great an impact as immunization. **Focus:** Prioritization.

13. **Ans: 1**   The administration of varicella-zoster immune globulin can prevent the development of varicella in immunosuppressed patients and will typically be prescribed. Acyclovir therapy and hospitalization may be required if the child develops a varicella-zoster virus infection. Contact and airborne precautions will be implemented to prevent the spread of infection to other children if the child is hospitalized with varicella. **Focus:** Prioritization.

14. **Ans: 1**   Rubeola is a highly contagious infectious disease with severe consequences that include death. The Centers for Disease Control and Prevention reports that 9 of 10 susceptible people with close contact to a person with measles will contract the disease. The incubation period is 7 to 21 days. Excluding the infected and exposed children during this period of time is a priority to prevent exposure of healthy children enrolled in the elementary school. Although it is important to notify the parents of the other children in the school of the exposure, limiting exposure of other children is the priority. Mumps, measles, and rubella vaccine administered within 72 hours of initial measles exposure and immunoglobulin administered within 6 days of exposure may provide some protection or modify the clinical course of the disease in unimmunized children; however, the priority is to prevent an epidemic by limiting exposure. **Focus:** Prioritization.

15. **Ans: 3**   Stuttering during the preschool years is a normal variation, particularly when excited or upset. The cause is attributed to preschool children's increased cognitive abilities and imagination such that their speech cannot keep up with their thoughts. Documenting this on the child's record is important for continued observation to determine if it extends beyond the preschool years. **Focus:** Prioritization.

16. **Ans: 2**   National guidelines indicate that airway clearance techniques are critical for patients with CF; thus postural drainage and chest physiotherapy are a priority. National guidelines also indicate that children and adolescents with CF who are hospitalized with respiratory illnesses should be placed on contact precautions. Furthermore, people with CF should be separated from others with CF to reduce droplet transmission of CF pathogens. There is no evidence that increased fluid intake adequately thins respiratory secretions, and chest physiotherapy is the priority. **Focus:** Prioritization.

17. **Ans: 1**   Frequent swallowing after a tonsillectomy may indicate bleeding. The nurse should inspect the back of the throat for evidence of bleeding. The other assessment results are expected in a 3-year-old child after surgery. **Focus:** Prioritization. **Test-Taking Tip:** Be aware of expected findings so that unexpected findings are noticed. In this case, frequent swallowing can indicate bleeding, which should be assessed often and reported to the health care provider if necessary.

18. **Ans: 3**   Tracheal deviation suggests tension pneumothorax, a possible complication of positive-pressure ventilation. The nurse will need to communicate rapidly with the HCP and assist with actions such as chest tube insertion. The heart rate, crackles, and oxygen saturation will be reported to the HCP but are expected in RDS and do not require immediate intervention. **Focus:** Prioritization.

19. **Ans: 2**   Research indicates that the administration of synthetic surfactant improves respiratory status and decreases the incidence of pneumothorax in premature infants with RDS. The other medications may be used if respiratory distress persists, but the first medication administered will be the surfactant. **Focus:** Prioritization.

20. **Ans: 4**   Circumoral cyanosis indicates a drop in the partial pressure of oxygen that may precipitate seizures and loss of consciousness. The nurse should

rapidly place the child in a knee–chest position, administer oxygen, and take steps to calm the child. The other assessment data are expected in a child with congenital heart defects such as tetralogy of Fallot. **Focus:** Prioritization.

21. **Ans: 3** At 4 years of age, children engage in pretend play. Parallel play is seen in younger children between the ages of 2 and 3 years when they play side by side with limited interaction. The other behaviors are developmentally appropriate. The nurse will plan interventions to ensure that all the children meet developmental goals, but the 4-year-old child engaging only in parallel play will require the most immediate intervention. **Focus:** Prioritization. **Test-Taking Tip:** Consider predominant modes of play based on age.

22. **Ans: 3** Crackles throughout both lungs indicate that the child has severe left ventricular failure as a complication of endocarditis. Hypoxemia is likely, so the child needs rapid assessment of oxygen saturation, initiation of supplemental oxygen delivery, and administration of medications such as diuretics. The other children should also be assessed as quickly as possible, but they are not experiencing life-threatening complications of their medical diagnoses. **Focus:** Prioritization.

23. **Ans: 1** This patient requires the least complex assessment and intervention of the four patients. Safe administration of oral medications such as digoxin would have been included in the orientation of the newly graduated RN. The conditions of the other patients are more complex, and they require assessments or interventions (e.g., teaching) that should be carried out by an RN with more experience. **Focus:** Assignment.

24. **Ans: 4** Children who receive aspirin therapy are at risk for the development of Reye syndrome if they contract viral illnesses such as varicella or influenza, so the lack of immunization is the greatest concern for this child. Peeling skin on the fingers and toes and irritability are consistent with Kawasaki disease but do not require any change in therapy. Because Kawasaki disease is not a communicable disease, there is no risk for transmission to other children in the day care (although assuring that immunizations are up to date before returning to day care is important). **Focus:** Prioritization.

25. **Ans: 2** Sickle cell crisis may include vaso-occlusive crisis, splenic sequestration, and aplastic crisis. The symptoms experienced by this child are indicative of both vaso-occlusive crisis and splenic sequestration. Placing cold packs on the knees of a child with vaso-occlusive crisis results in vasoconstriction, placing the child at risk for thrombosis formation. Encouraging increased fluid intake is advised to prevent thrombosis formation. Monitoring vital signs is a method to assess for life-threatening complications associated with both vaso-occlusive crisis and splenic

sequestration. Vaso-occlusive crisis is associated with severe pain and pain medication is recommended. **Focus:** Prioritization.

26. **Ans: 1** Because decreased responsiveness in a 1-year-old patient with a clotting disorder may indicate intracerebral bleeding, this patient should be assessed immediately. The other patients also require assessments or interventions but are not at immediate risk for life-threatening or disabling complications. **Focus:** Prioritization.

27. **Ans: 2** The low hemoglobin count may signify bleeding; therefore alerting the HCP is recommended. ITP is an autoimmune disorder by which circulating platelets are destroyed by autoantibodies. Platelet production from the bone marrow, however, is not affected. Laboratory findings characteristic of ITP include a low platelet count generally less than 20,000/mm^3 (20×10^9/L). Nevertheless, all other indices of the complete blood count are normal. Additionally, the PT and partial thromboplastin time are normal with ITP. In this 3-year-old child, the leukocytes and PT are normal. The platelet count is low but consistent with this disease. **Focus:** Prioritization.

28. **Ans: 3** Methotrexate is a high-alert drug, and extra precautions, such as double-checking with another nurse, should be taken when administering this medication. Although many pediatric units have a policy requiring that all medication administration to children be double-checked, the other medications listed are not on the high-alert list published by the Institute for Safe Medication Practices. **Focus:** Prioritization. **Test-Taking Tip:** For test-taking purposes and for safety in the clinical setting, it is worthwhile to memorize medications that are considered "high-alert" drugs.

29. **Ans: 4** The child will need medication to control the seizures. Medications for children are based on weight in kilograms. Although heart rate and blood pressure may be obtained, the priority is to stop the seizures with medication. There is no clinical indication for BMI for a child with active seizures. **Focus:** Prioritization.

30. **Ans: 2** Pupil dilation may indicate increased intracranial pressure and should be reported immediately to the surgeon. The other data are not unusual in a 3-year-old patient after surgery, although they indicate the need for ongoing assessments or interventions. **Focus:** Prioritization.

31. **Ans: 4** The elevated temperature indicates possible infection and should be reported immediately to the surgeon so that treatment can be started. The other data are typical in an infant with myelomeningocele. **Focus:** Prioritization.

32. **Ans: 2** Even though the child is screaming, the mother must continue to irrigate the eyes for at least 20 minutes. Another adult, if present, should call the Poison Control Center and 911. **Focus:** Prioritization.

33. **Ans: 1, 3** The nurse should assess the pinna for trauma and obtain a history for the type of object as a component of a complete assessment, which could determine the course of action by the HCP. Some foreign bodies may swell when water is used for irrigation, further lodging the object in the auditory canal. Removing the object with forceps could traumatize the tympanic membrane and auditory canal further. Placing an otoscope in the auditory canal could wedge the object further into the canal. **Focus:** Prioritization.

34. **Ans: 2** The patient continues to refer to herself as "fatty" and still has a disturbed body image; however, she has appropriate knowledge, and her self-esteem has improved. The patient has demonstrated an ability to follow the therapeutic plan while in the hospital. Interventions should be designed to help her to continue after discharge. **Focus:** Prioritization.

35. **Ans: 1, 3, 4, 6** This child is in Piaget's stage of concrete operations. Children in this stage can organize experiences and understand some complex information. Children in this age group have difficulty conceptualizing time; therefore asking questions about the time that incidents occur will not be helpful in determining the child's orientation. **Focus:** Prioritization.

36. **Ans: 2** Passage of brown stool indicates resolution of the intussusception, so surgery may not be necessary. The other findings are part of the clinical presentation of this disorder. **Focus:** Prioritization.

37. **Ans: 4** Even though the caller reports that the child is "breathing okay," additional questions about possible airway obstruction are the priority (e.g., coughing, gagging, choking, drooling, refusing to eat or drink). Gastrointestinal symptoms should be assessed but are less urgent. The type of foreign body, in the absence of symptoms, may dictate a wait-and-see approach, in which case the parent would be directed to check the stools for passage of the foreign body. **Focus:** Prioritization. **Test-Taking Tip:** In emergency situations, apply the ABCs (airway, breathing, and circulation) before proceeding to other actions.

38. **Ans: 1** Hand washing is the most important aspect to emphasize. Addressing fecal incontinence and sharing of personal items may be recommended when the disease is in an infectious stage. Immunizations are recommended, but this would be emphasized to parents rather than day-care workers. **Focus:** Prioritization.

39. **Ans: 3** Oral sedation agents such as the benzodiazepines are considered high-alert medications when ordered for children, and extra precautions should be taken before administration. Many facilities require that all medications administered to pediatric patients be double-checked before administration, but the lorazepam is the most important to double-check with another nurse. **Focus:** Prioritization.

40. **Ans: 3** Theories about bed-wetting relate it to immature bladder and deep sleep patterns. Although it is true that most children stop bed-wetting by the time they start school, this does not answer the mother's question. Many boys wet the bed until after the age of 5 years. The fourth response is not accurate because often bed-wetting is not within the control of a 5-year-old child. **Focus:** Prioritization.

41. **Ans: 1** Reminding the child about something that has already been taught is within the scope of practice for an AP. An LPN/LVN could administer the oral medication. Teaching and discussion of other strategies for dealing with bed-wetting require additional education and are more appropriate to the scope of practice of the professional RN. **Focus:** Delegation.

42. **Ans: 3** This is normal behavior in early adolescence. During this time period, adolescents are conscious of their rapid physical changes. As a result, they spend more time in front of the mirror inspecting their bodies. Consider that the height and weight are normal; therefore an eating disorder is not likely. Also, the girl does answer questions appropriately, so mental health issues are not likely. **Focus:** Prioritization. **Test-Taking Tip:** It will be helpful to know what types of physical and mental health disorders are common at various developmental stages because these issues are likely to be on the NCLEX® Examination and will occur commonly in a pediatric nursing practice setting.

43. **Ans: 4** Recommendations by the Centers for Disease Control and Prevention recommend annual screening for chlamydia (and gonorrhea) for all sexually active women younger than the age of 25 years. Chlamydia is the most prevalent STD in the United States. Screening for syphilis and genital herpes simplex is recommended only if other risk factors or evidence of disease are present. The patient is fully immunized, which would include the human papillomavirus vaccine. **Focus:** Prioritization.

44. **Ans: 2** The AP can help with the removal of outer clothing, which allows the heat to dissipate from the child's skin. Assessing, advising, and explaining require an RN-level education and scope of practice. **Focus:** Delegation.

45. **Ans: 1** Iron is a toxic substance that can lead to massive hemorrhage, coma, shock, and hepatic failure. Deferoxamine is an antidote that can be used for severe cases of iron poisoning. The other information needs additional investigation but will not change the immediate diagnostic testing or treatment plan. **Focus:** Prioritization.

46. **Ans: 3** Parental refusal is an absolute contraindication; therefore the HCP must be notified. Tetanus status can be addressed later. The RN can reestablish the IV access and provide information about moderate (conscious) sedation; if the parent is still not satisfied, the provider can give more information. **Focus:** Prioritization.

47. **Ans: 2** An impaled object may be providing a tamponade effect, and removal can precipitate sudden

hemodynamic decompensation. Additional history, including a more definitive description of the blood loss, depth of penetration, and medical history, should be obtained. Other information, such as the dirt on the stick or history of diabetes, is important in the overall treatment plan but can be addressed later. **Focus:** Prioritization.

48. **Ans: 1, 3, 4, 5, 6** Children have proportionately larger heads, which predisposes them to head injuries. Hypoxemia is more likely because of their higher oxygen demand. Liver and spleen injuries are more likely because the thoracic cages of children offer less protection. Hypothermia is more likely because of children's thinner skin and proportionately larger body surface area. They have strong hearts; therefore pulse rate will increase to compensate, but other arrhythmias are less likely to occur. Children have relatively flexible bones compared with those of adults; however they have a greater risk for epiphyseal (growth plate) injuries. The most likely spinal injury in children is injury to the cervical area. **Focus:** Prioritization.

49. **Ans: 1** This is a CF clinic, so this patient may be exposed to others with CF if he or she remains in the reception area. The CF Foundation recommends that all individuals with CF, regardless of respiratory culture results, be separated from others with CF to reduce risk of droplet transmission of CF pathogens. National guidelines indicate that the best solution is that patients with CF not wait in common areas but instead be placed in a private exam room. Nevertheless, when patients must be in common waiting areas, a minimum distance of 3 feet (1 meter) between patients should be maintained if patients have CF. **Focus:** Prioritization.

50. **Ans: 3** Assessment and patient teaching are the responsibilities of the RN. The AP may stock the room with ostomy supplies, but the nurse would give instructions or validate the AP's knowledge of supplies. **Focus:** Delegation.

51. **Ans: 2, 4, 5, 6** A tracheoesophageal fistula is a congenital malformation in which the esophagus ends in a blind pouch and there is a fistula (opening) between the esophagus and the trachea. The infant is at high risk for aspiration of esophageal contents into the trachea; thus the infant is NPO in the preoperative period. IV fluids are administered to maintain hydration. A tracheostomy is not indicated for tracheoesophageal fistula. Surgical interventions for tracheoesophageal fistula include ligation of the fistula and reanastomosis of the esophagus. Suction should be on hand to remove secretions from the blind pouch. IV antibiotics and vitamin K are initiated in the preoperative period. **Focus:** Prioritization.

52. **Ans: 1, 5** Iron deficiency anemia is a microcytic anemia. Laboratory findings consistent with iron deficiency anemia include low hemoglobin, hematocrit, and MCV. Additionally, the patient may have thrombocytosis, which is an increase in the number

of platelets; thus the child will not be more likely to have nosebleeds. The white blood cell count (WBC) and WBC differential are not affected by anemia; therefore the child will not be more prone to infections. Children with iron deficiency anemia experience pica, which is a consumption of nonfood items. Excessive cow's milk intake has been found to cause anemia by irritating the intestine and resulting in microscopic blood loss from the gastrointestinal tract. **Focus:** Prioritization.

53. **Ans: 1, 5** Iron supplementation can stain the teeth and has an unpleasant taste. By administering the iron with a syringe to the back of the throat, it will mask the taste and prevent staining of the teeth. The vitamin C in orange juice increases iron absorption and may mask the unpleasant taste. Chocolate and cola contain caffeine, which interferes with the absorption of iron. Milk and food also interfere with the absorption of iron. Although allowing a child to drink the iron through a straw is feasible for an older child, a 10-month-old child cannot developmentally perform this task. **Focus:** Prioritization.

54. **Ans: 3** This infant is experiencing severe dehydration, which is evidenced by tachycardia and hypotension. The child is at risk for hypovolemic shock, which is a life-threatening event. A bolus of normal saline or lactated Ringer solution of 20 mL/kg is the standard of care to establish hemodynamic stability. The blood glucose is normal. The safety profile for antiemetics have not been established with infants, and the priority for this patient is to establish hemodynamic stability. Fever can cause increased fluid loss; however, the priority in this life-threatening situation is to establish hemodynamic stability. **Focus:** Prioritization.

55. **Ans: 1** Based on the history, this child's constipation is the most likely etiology of the UTI, and increasing whole grains, fruits, and vegetables is the best intervention. Urinary stasis from constipation is the primary cause of UTIs in children. Stool in the intestine prevents complete emptying of the bladder. There is no conclusive evidence to support that cranberry juice and vitamin C prevent UTIs. Limiting fluids at bedtime has not been shown to decrease UTIs. Increasing fluids, however, helps to flush bacteria out of the bladder. **Focus:** Prioritization.

56. **Ans: 3** This boy is presenting with classic symptoms of slipped capital femoral epiphysis (SCFE), which is a slippage of the femoral head at the proximal epiphyseal plate. SCFE is an emergency. A delay in treatment can result in necrosis and death of the femoral head. Although the exact cause of SCFE is unknown, there is an increased incidence in boys. Additionally, obesity is a risk factor for SCFE. **Focus:** Prioritization.

57. **Ans: 4** To ensure safety and prevent aspiration, the first action by the nurse should be to position the child in a side-lying position. Other assessment and actions will follow this initial step. **Focus:** Prioritization.

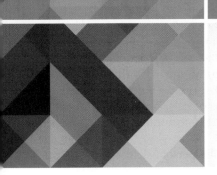

CHAPTER 20
Pharmacology

Questions

1. The patient weighs 80 kg and is about to receive a potassium IV infusion of 10 mEq in 100 mL normal saline. For which finding must the nurse notify the health care provider before completing this prescribed action?
   1. The patient's morning serum sodium level was 136 mEq/L.
   2. The patient's urine output for the past 24 hours was 550 mL.
   3. The patient required placement of a new IV access this morning.
   4. Patient assessment revealed a positive Chvostek sign.

2. The nurse is caring for a patient newly diagnosed with hypertension. Blood pressure readings over the past 8 hours have been: 08:00 164/93 mm Hg, 12:00 158/90 mm Hg, and 16:00 166/94 mm Hg. The health care provider prescribes a no added salt diet and plans to start the patient on hydrochlorothiazide 25 mg. Which action is **most** important for the nurse to take before administering this drug?
   1. Check the patient's serum potassium level.
   2. Review the patient's urine output for the past 24 hours.
   3. Instruct the assistive personnel to check the orthostatic blood pressure.
   4. Check the patient's cardiac monitor for abnormal heart rhythms.

3. A patient is prescribed meloxicam for rheumatoid arthritis. This drug has a long half-life of 51 hours. Which prescription would the nurse be sure to clarify with the health care provider before giving the medication?
   1. Meloxicam 7.5 to 15 mg/day
   2. Meloxicam 15 mg/day before breakfast
   3. Meloxicam 7.5 mg every 4 hours as needed for pain
   4. Meloxicam 7.5 mg/day as needed

4. The RN is a team leader working with an LPN/LVN and two assistive personnel (APs) to provide care for eight medical patients. Which action would be appropriate for the RN to take with regard to nursing care provided by the LPN/LVN?
   1. Delegate the performance of an abdominal dressing change to the LPN/LVN.
   2. Supervise and document the patient assessments completed by the LPN/LVN.
   3. Assign the LPN/LVN the administration of insulin to a patient with type 1 diabetes.
   4. Delegate checking and recording vital signs on all eight patients to the LPN/LVN.

5. A 14-year-old child was recently diagnosed with type 1 diabetes. The patient is prescribed 10 units of regular insulin and 15 units of neutral protamine Hagedorn (NPH) insulin each morning. How should the nurse instruct this patient to give herself the prescribed doses of insulin?
   1. "First draw up and administer the NPH insulin. Wait at least 15 minutes, then draw up and administer the regular insulin."
   2. "First draw up and administer the regular insulin, then draw up and administer the NPH insulin."
   3. "First draw up the NPH insulin, then draw up the regular insulin in the same syringe."
   4. "First draw up the regular insulin, then draw up the NPH insulin in the same syringe."

6. A patient with type 2 diabetes has a prescription for a change in oral antidiabetic agents from glyburide to acarbose. The patient asks the nurse why there is no need to be worried about the new drug causing hypoglycemia. What is the nurse's **best** answer?
   1. "Because your pancreatic function is improving, it does not need as much stimulation, so acarbose is not as powerful as glyburide."
   2. "Glyburide stimulates your pancreas to secrete insulin, increasing your risk for hypoglycemia. Acarbose does not stimulate insulin secretion; rather, it reduces your intestinal uptake of sugar."
   3. "Acarbose increases the cells' uptake of glucose without the need for insulin, so you cannot become hypoglycemic even if you miss a meal on this medication."
   4. "Glyburide is actually an oral form of insulin, and too much could make your blood sugar drop quickly. Acarbose reduces blood sugar by suppressing pancreatic release of glucagon."

7. An adult patient with type 2 diabetes is prescribed miglitol 25 mg three times a day with meals. What specific **priority** instruction about this drug does the RN provide to the LPN/LVN assigned to care for this patient?
   1. "Make certain the patient's meal is actually on the unit before administering the drug and give the drug with the first bite of the meal."
   2. "Check the patient's blood glucose level to determine whether the drug therapy is having an effect on the diabetes."
   3. "Check the patient's daily urine output and current lab work, especially the blood urea nitrogen and serum creatinine levels, because kidney problems increase the effects of the drug."
   4. "Make sure that the patient is able to eat and will do so within 30 minutes of taking the drug."

8. An older adult patient with type 1 diabetes is legally blind and is prescribed daily morning doses of regular and neutral protamine Hagedorn (NPH) insulin. The patient's daughter provides in-home care and will be preparing the insulin syringes on a weekly basis. What does the nurse teach the patient's daughter about storing the prefilled insulin syringes?
   1. "Keep the syringes stored flat and do not attach the needles until you are ready to use a syringe."
   2. "Keep the syringes in the upright position with the needle pointing toward the ceiling."
   3. "Keep the syringes in the upright position with the needle pointing toward the floor."
   4. "Storage position is unimportant as long as the syringes are kept in the refrigerator."

9. A female patient with type 2 diabetes who is breast-feeding her newborn infant has a prescription for glipizide. What is the nurse's **best** action?
   1. Administer the drug as ordered with meals.
   2. Hold the drug and clarify the order with the health care provider.
   3. Assign the LVN/LPN to administer the drug before breakfast.
   4. Instruct the assistive personnel to check the patient's fingerstick glucose, then give the drug.

10. A patient is to receive metoprolol tartrate 5 mg IV to control high blood pressure. IV metoprolol tartrate is administered over 2 minutes. Based on the label for the medication, the nurse will administer? _____ mL/min.

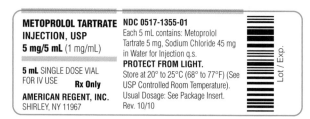

METOPROLOL TARTRATE INJECTION, USP 5 mg/5 mL (1 mg/mL)	NDC 0517-1355-01 Each 5 mL contains: Metoprolol Tartrate 5 mg, Sodium Chloride 45 mg in Water for Injection q.s.
5 mL SINGLE DOSE VIAL FOR IV USE **Rx Only** AMERICAN REGENT, INC. SHIRLEY, NY 11967	**PROTECT FROM LIGHT.** Store at 20° to 25°C (68° to 77°F) (See USP Controlled Room Temperature). Usual Dosage: See Package Insert. Rev. 10/10

11. Which of the following should the nurse be sure to assess before and after giving amlodipine to treat high blood pressure? **Select all that apply.**
    1. Swelling in ankles or feet
    2. Heart rate
    3. Oral temperature
    4. Blood pressure
    5. Lung sounds
    6. Weight
    7. Respiratory rate

12. A patient diagnosed with hypertension has received the first dose of lisinopril. Which interventions will the RN delegate to the assistive personnel (AP)? **Select all that apply.**
    1. Restrict the patient to bed rest for at least 12 hours.
    2. Recheck the patient's vital signs every 4 to 8 hours.
    3. Ensure that the patient's call light is within easy reach.
    4. Keep the patient's bed in a supine position with all side rails up.
    5. Remind the patient to rise slowly from the bed and sit before standing.
    6. Assist the patient to get out of bed and use the bathroom.
    7. Assess the patient for signs of dizziness.

13. An older patient with chronic obstructive pulmonary disease is to be discharged with prescriptions for albuterol, which is a short-acting beta agonist (SABA), and salmeterol, which is a long-acting beta agonist (LABA) bronchodilator. Which statement by the patient indicates to the nurse that the patient requires additional teaching?
    1. "I will insert my inhaler into the spacer and shake the whole unit three or four times before taking my dose of the drug."
    2. "I will use my salmeterol whenever I become suddenly short of breath."
    3. "I will wait at least 1 minute between the first and second puff of my inhaler."
    4. "I will check my pulse before and after using my bronchodilator inhaler."

14. Which patient care action could the nurse delegate to assistive personnel (AP) after administering an inhaled anti-inflammatory drug to a patient with chronic obstructive pulmonary disease?
    1. Assess the patient's mouth for white-colored patches.
    2. Teach the patient how to clean the inhaler and spacer.
    3. Assist the patient to rinse the mouth with water or mouthwash.
    4. Auscultate the patient's lungs for any changes in breath sounds.

15. A patient with familial hypercholesterolemia is prescribed atorvastatin 40 mg once a day. Which finding will the nurse **immediately** report to the health care provider?
    1. Stomach upset
    2. Constipation
    3. Bloating
    4. Muscle soreness

16. What key instruction must the nurse give to the assistive personnel (AP) who is assisting with morning care for an older patient prescribed apixaban, 2.5 mg orally twice a day, for chronic atrial fibrillation?
    1. "Be sure to tell me if you notice any bleeding from the gums when the patient brushes his or her teeth."
    2. "Instruct the patient to avoid using aspirin-containing drugs or nonsteroidal anti-inflammatory drugs."
    3. "Teach the patient to expect some bruising to occur because this is a side effect of the drug."
    4. "Remind the patient that each morning a laboratory technician will stop by early to draw clotting studies."

17. The RN team leader has assigned the LPN/LVN to administer clopidogrel 75 mg orally to a patient with a diagnosis of myocardial infarction. The patient also has an antacid prescribed for a diagnosis of gastric reflux. What must the LPN/LVN remember when administering these drugs? **Select all that apply.**
    1. Clopidogrel can interfere with absorption of the antacid.
    2. The antacid can interfere with absorption of clopidogrel.
    3. Clopidogrel can be given with a meal to prevent nausea or upset stomach.
    4. Clopidogrel should be given 1 hour after giving the antacid.
    5. Clopidogrel and the antacid are compatible and can be given together.
    6. Clopidogrel can be given 1 hour before the antacid.

18. Which drug prescription would the nurse be sure to question for a patient diagnosed with heart failure?
    1. Carvedilol 3.125 mg orally twice a day
    2. Lisinopril 5 mg orally once a day
    3. Digoxin 1.25 mg orally once a day
    4. Isosorbide dinitrate 20 mg orally twice a day

19. The RN is supervising a student nurse caring for a patient with hypertension. The health care provider prescribed enalapril 2.5 mg orally twice a day. The student tells the nurse that the patient has swelling around the eyes and lips. What does the nurse tell the student is the **first** best action?
    1. Assess the patient's ability to speak and breathe.
    2. Apply ice to the patient's eyes and lips.
    3. Check the patient's white blood cell count.
    4. Check the patient's vital signs.

20. A patient with hypertension is prescribed atenolol 25 mg orally once a day. Which change would be **most** important for the nurse to report to the health care provider after the patient begins taking this drug?
    1. Heart rate of 58 beats/min
    2. Cold hands and feet
    3. Patient report of depression
    4. Patient report of tiredness

21. The assistive personnel (AP) reports to the nurse that a patient with hypertension is experiencing a blood pressure decrease when sitting up after receiving his morning medications. The patient received furosemide 20 mg, a multivitamin, and quinapril 10 mg orally. What side effect does the nurse recognize?
    1. Hypokalemia
    2. Hyponatremia
    3. Photosensitivity
    4. Postural hypotension

 Answer Key for this chapter begins on p. 207

22. The nurse is providing patient teaching for an older adult about spironolactone. Which key points would the nurse include? **Select all that apply.**
    1. Avoid the use of salt substitutes.
    2. Do not consume excessive amounts of foods that are high in potassium.
    3. Be prepared for a decrease in your urine output.
    4. This drug works by conserving sodium and excreting potassium.
    5. Older adults may be more sensitive to the action of this drug.
    6. As an older adult, you are more likely to experience side effects from this drug.

23. The RN is preparing to administer drugs to a group of patients. Which drug is **most** important for the nurse to discuss with the health care provider before administering?
    1. Albuterol for a patient with chronic obstructive pulmonary disease
    2. Hydrochlorothiazide for a patient with hypertension
    3. Ibuprofen for a patient with osteoarthritis
    4. Methimazole for a patient with hypothyroidism

24. A patient has been taking prednisone 20 mg orally each day for 10 days for a severe allergic skin reaction. The patient tells the nurse that she no longer needs to take the prednisone because she is feeling better and the reaction has cleared up. What is the nurse's **best** response?
    1. "After taking this drug for over 1 week, it must be slowly decreased to allow the adrenal glands to begin making cortisol."
    2. "When the health care provider (HCP) visits, I will ask if he will write an order prescribing that this drug be discontinued."
    3. "You may need to continue taking the prednisone for another week or two to be sure that the skin allergic reaction is under control."
    4. "Because you have taken prednisone for 10 days, it will be necessary for the HCP to order a topical form of the drug for use as needed."

25. A child with an ear infection is prescribed liquid amoxicillin 20 mg/kg every 8 hours. The child weighs 12 kg (26.5 lb). How many milligrams of amoxicillin will the nurse give with each dose?
    _____ mg

26. A patient visits the urgent care clinic with a bacterial respiratory infection. The nurse will anticipate the need for patient teaching about which medication?
    1. Azithromycin
    2. Amantadine
    3. Fluconazole
    4. Ethambutol

27. A patient diagnosed with overactive bladder is prescribed oxybutynin 5 mg orally twice a day. The nurse is providing patient teaching about the side effects of this drug. Which side effects would be included? **Select all that apply.**
    1. Diarrhea
    2. Dry mouth
    3. Dizziness
    4. Headache
    5. Rash
    6. Constipation

28. A patient is prescribed 3000 units of heparin subcutaneously. The drug is available in vials of 5000 units/1 mL. How many milliliters will the nurse administer?
    _____ mL

29. The nurse is providing care for a patient with chronic kidney disease who receives hemodialysis 3 days a week. As the nurse prepares to administer the patient's dose of epoetin alfa subcutaneously, the patient asks why the shot is necessary. What is the nurse's **best** response?
    1. "It will help stimulate production of white blood cells to protect you from infection."
    2. "It will help stimulate production of platelets to improve your ability to form clots."
    3. "It will help stimulate production of phagocytes to engulf and kill bacteria."
    4. "It will help stimulate production of red blood cells (RBCs) to increase your RBC count."

30. The patient is experiencing nausea as a result of Ménière disease. For which drug is the nurse **most** likely to plan patient teaching?
    1. Promethazine
    2. Prochlorperazine
    3. Meclizine
    4. Granisetron

31. The patient is experiencing nausea and vomiting for which the health care provider has prescribed promethazine 12.5 mg orally four times a day as needed. Which patient care task would the nurse appropriately delegate to the assistive personnel (AP) before giving this drug?
    1. Check the patient's temperature, blood pressure, and heart rate.
    2. Auscultate the patient's abdomen for active bowel sounds.
    3. Examine the patient's abdomen for any distention.
    4. Ask the patient about constipation or difficulty swallowing.

32. The nurse assigns an LPN/LVN to administer pro-chlorperazine 10 mg orally to an older adult patient experiencing nausea. Which specific instruction would the nurse give the LPN/LVN regarding monitoring this patient after the drug has been given?
    1. "You should expect the patient's bowel sounds to decrease after he takes this drug."
    2. "Be sure to monitor his level of consciousness and watch for sedation."
    3. "Apply oxygen by nasal cannula in case his respiratory rate decreases."
    4. "The patient should be able to ambulate on his own to the bathroom."

33. The health care provider prescribes a bisacodyl 10 mg suppository rectally for an older adult who has not had a bowel movement for over 5 days. Which actions are accurate when the nurse administers this drug rectally? **Select all that apply.**
    1. Explain the procedure and include how long the drug must be held in the rectum.
    2. Bring the drug, some lubricant, and a pair of disposable gloves to the bedside.
    3. Place the patient in a prone position.
    4. Provide privacy by closing doors or pulling the curtains.
    5. Remove the suppository wrapping and coat the blunt end with lubricant.
    6. Have the patient take a deep breath and push the suppository 1 inch (2.5 cm) into the rectum.

34. A patient with diarrhea has been prescribed loperamide 2 mg orally after each unformed stool. Which laboratory value will be **most** important for the nurse to monitor for this patient?
    1. Serum sodium
    2. Serum potassium
    3. Urine protein
    4. Urine nitrogen

35. The RN is preparing to administer drugs to a group of patients with gastrointestinal disorders. Which drug is **most** important to discuss with the health care provider before administering?
    1. Omeprazole for the patient with peptic ulcer disease (PUD)
    2. Famotidine for the patient with gastroesophageal reflux disease (GERD)
    3. Diphenoxylate with atropine for the patient with constipation
    4. Ondansetron for the patient with nausea because of chemotherapy

36. The RN is caring for a patient in the emergency department with severe chest pain for which the health care provider has prescribed morphine 2 mg IV push. Morphine is available in prefilled syringes with 4 mg/

mL. How many milliliters does the nurse administer?
_____ mL

37. During a check-up at the health care provider's (HCP's) office, a male patient tells the nurse that he is having difficulty getting and keeping an erection. The HCP diagnoses the patient with erectile dysfunction and prescribes sildenafil 50 mg orally once daily 30 minutes to 1 hour before sexual activity. Which are key teaching points about this drug? **Select all that apply.**
    1. The drug will have no effect without sexual stimulation.
    2. Notify the HCP if the patient experiences an erection lasting longer than 2 hours.
    3. If a prolonged and painful erection occurs, be sure to notify the HCP.
    4. The action of sildenafil last up to 36 hours.
    5. The patient should not take sildenafil while taking nitrate drugs.
    6. Consuming high-fat meals may delay the maximum effectiveness of this drug.

38. A patient with pulmonary edema is prescribed furosemide 60 mg IV push. The drug comes in a 10-mL vial with a concentration of 10 mg/mL. How many milliliters will the nurse administer?
_____ mL

39. The health care provider prescribes IV remdesivir for a client who is positive for COVID-19. For which side effects will the nurse monitor? **Select all that apply.**
    1. Nausea and vomiting
    2. Bleeding
    3. Elevated blood pressure
    4. Diarrhea
    5. Bradycardia
    6. Abnormal liver function tests

40. Medical marijuana has been used for many conditions but little research has been done on the use of this drug. What is the major reason for the lack of research?
    1. The U.S. Drug Enforcement Administration (DEA) considers marijuana a drug, likely to be abused and lacking in medical value.
    2. The U.S. Food and Drug Administration (FDA) has only approved its use for the treatment of two rare and severe forms of epilepsy.
    3. Marijuana contains some of the same chemicals found in tobacco and there is concern that smoking it can harm the lungs.
    4. The U.S. FDA doesn't oversee medical marijuana like it does other prescription drugs.

Answer Key for this chapter begins on p. 207

41. Enhanced Multiple Response _____

Question

Medical marijuana is legal in more than half of the United States and the District of Columbia. Which of the conditions listed on the right has this drug been used to treat?

Instructions: Read the question on the left then circle or highlight the numbers that best answer the question. **Select all that apply.**

1. Loss of appetite
2. Chronic pain
3. Constipation
4. Nausea and vomiting
5. Acute kidney disease
6. Decrease spasticity from multiple sclerosis
7. Osteoarthritis
8. Chronic obstructive pulmonary disease
9. PTSD (post-traumatic stress disorder)

42. Enhanced Multiple Response _____

Case Study and Question

The nurse is providing care for an 83-year-old patient with type 2 diabetes, hypertension, renal insufficiency, mild chronic obstructive pulmonary disease, and peripheral vascular disease.
Which findings increase the patient's risk for development of HHS?

Vital signs:
Temperature 98.7°F (37.06°C)
Pulse 98 beats/min
Respirations 27 breaths/min
Blood pressure 168/94 mm Hg
AM glucose greater than 600 mg/dL (33.3 mmol/L)

Medications:
Hydrochlorothiazide (HCTZ)
metformin
albuterol inhaler as needed

Morning assessment findings: The patient describes a weight gain of 6 lb (2.7 kg) over the past month and adequate urine output but states she drinks very little liquid after dinner. The patient describes bowel movements every 1 to 2 days.

Instructions: Read the case study on the left then circle or highlight the numbers that best answer the question. **Select all that apply.**

1. HCTZ prescribed to control blood pressure
2. Weight gain of 6 lb (2.7 kg) over the past month
3. Patient avoiding taking in liquids during the evenings
4. Blood pressure 168/94 mm Hg
5. Urine output of 50 to 75 mL/hr
6. Glucose greater than 600 mg/dL (33.3 mmol/L)
7. Patient is overhydrated.
8. Patient has type 2 diabetes
9. Ketone levels are absent or low

Answers

1. **Ans: 2** Urine output should exceed 0.5 mL/kg/hr to prevent hyperkalemia. This patient's weight is 80 kg so he should minimally put out 40 mL of urine per hour. His total urine output for the past 24 hours was 550 mL, which equals around 22.9 mL/hr. The health care provider must be notified of this. The patient's sodium level is low normal, placement of a new IV would not interfere with giving the IV potassium, and a positive Chvostek sign is an indicator of hypoparathyroidism. **Focus:** Prioritization.

2. **Ans: 1** Hydrochlorothiazide is a thiazide diuretic often used to treat hypertension. An adverse effect of these diuretics is that when sodium (Na^+) reabsorption is blocked by thiazide diuretics, this increases Na^+ delivery to the cortical collecting duct and increases Na^+ reabsorption in this segment of the nephron. Because Na^+ reabsorption is coupled to potassium (K^+) secretion in the cortical collecting duct, these drugs can lead to excessive K^+ secretion and hypokalemia (where the K^+ in extracellular fluid is too low). The same is true of loop diuretics (e.g., furosemide). Thiazide and loop diuretics may be combined with potassium-sparing diuretics (e.g., spironolactone) to counteract this possibility. The other actions are also appropriate for this patient but are not as urgent. **Focus:** Prioritization. **Test-Taking Tip:** Remember that most diuretics affect serum potassium levels so it is essential to follow this lab value whenever a patient is prescribed a diuretic. Thiazide and loop diuretics decrease potassium. Potassium-sparing diuretics may increase potassium.

3. **Ans: 3** A drug's plasma half-life depends on how quickly the drug is eliminated from the plasma. The half-life of a given medication is how long it takes for the body to get rid of half of the dose. If a drug with a long half-life is given too often or at too short of intervals, its level can become so high that it is toxic. **Focus:** Prioritization.

4. **Ans: 3** LPN/LVNs are licensed and therefore responsible for their own practice. Their scope of practice includes administration of medications. The RN team leader is responsible for supervision as well as for making assignments for LPN/LVNs (team leaders also make assignments for other RNs on the team). Delegation of checking and recording vital signs is appropriate for the APs. The LPN/LVN could perform the dressing change, but the RN would assign, not delegate, the task. **Focus:** Assignment.

5. **Ans: 4** When mixing two different types of insulin in the same syringe, inject both bottles with the amount of air equal to the dose of that insulin, then draw up the short-acting insulin first. Regular insulin is short acting. NPH insulin is an intermediate-acting insulin. Take care not to inject any regular insulin into the NPH bottle. **Focus:** Prioritization.

6. **Ans: 2** Glyburide is a sulfonylurea antidiabetic drug. Its action is to lower blood glucose levels by triggering the beta cells of the pancreas to release the small amount of preformed insulin present in the beta cells. Acarbose is an alpha-glucosidase inhibiting drug. Its action is to slow the digestion of dietary starches and other carbohydrates by inhibiting an enzyme that breaks them down into glucose. The result of this action is that blood glucose does not rise as far or as fast after a meal. Drugs from this class do not cause hypoglycemia when taken as the only therapy for diabetes. **Focus:** Prioritization.

7. **Ans: 1** Miglitol is an alpha-glucosidase inhibiting drug. Make sure the patient's meal is actually on the unit before giving the drug. Give the drug with the first bite of the meal. The action of the drug is quick and brief. If the drug is taken too long before the meal is eaten, it will not prevent the carbohydrates from being absorbed, and the patient's blood glucose level will rise. The other teaching is also appropriate for diabetics but is not specific to the effectiveness of miglitol. **Focus:** Prioritization.

8. **Ans: 2** Prefilled insulin syringes, cartridges, and pens should be stored upright rather than lying flat. The needle must point upward. **Focus:** Prioritization.

9. **Ans: 2** Glipizide is a second-generation sulfonylurea antidiabetic drug. These drugs are contraindicated for breastfeeding mothers because they enter the milk and increase the infant's risk for hypoglycemia. **Focus:** Prioritization.

10. **Ans: 2.5 mg/min** 5 mg in 5 mL = 5 mL / 2 min = 2.5 mL/min. **Focus:** Prioritization.

11. **Ans: 1, 2, 4, 5, 6** Amlodipine is a calcium channel blocker with side effects that include peripheral and pulmonary edema, weight gain, decreased heart rate (bradycardia), and decreased blood pressure (hypotension). The nurse would be sure to get a baseline for each of these parameters and then assess for each regularly after administering the drug. Although respirations and body temperature are parts of vital sign assessment, they are not as high a priority because they are not usually affected by antihypertensive drugs. **Focus:** Prioritization.

12. **Ans: 2, 3, 5, 6** After the first dose of most antihypertensive drugs, dizziness is a common side effect. The patient should call for help when getting out of bed, and the call light should be within easy reach. The patient should rise slowly, sitting on the side of the bed before standing, and then can be assisted to the bathroom. The AP's scope of practice includes these actions. Patients are not restricted to bed rest or kept in a supine (flat) position, and side rails are not all kept up for safety of the patient. Assessment is not within the scope of

practice for an AP. Nevertheless, the RN could instruct the AP to ask the patient about dizziness before and during ambulation and then report any dizziness immediately to the RN. **Focus:** Delegation. **Test-Taking Tip:** The nurse must be aware of the scope of practice for an AP to understand which patient care tasks may be delegated. Remember that the nurse may not delegate tasks such as assessment, teaching, evaluating, or administering drugs to an AP.

13. **Ans: 2** Salmeterol is a LABA and is used to prevent episodes of shortness of breath. When a patient becomes suddenly short of breath, the drug of choice would be a SABA such as albuterol. Statements 1, 3, and 4 all demonstrate correct understanding of how to use an aerosol inhaler. An older adult may be more sensitive to the cardiac effects of these drugs and should check the heart rate before and after each dose. **Focus:** Prioritization. **Test-Taking Tip:** The nurse must know the differences between SABA and LABA drugs, including how they work and why they are prescribed, to be able to assess the patient's understanding of these drugs and determine if additional teaching is required.

14. **Ans: 3** Side effects of inhaled anti-inflammatory drugs include leaving a bad taste in the mouth after use and an increased risk for oral candidiasis (thrush). Rinsing with water or mouthwash helps remove the drug from the mouth and reduces the bad taste and oral infection risk. 1, 2, and 4 are all actions that are within the scope of practice for the RN. Assisting the patient with rinsing the mouth after administration of these drugs is within the scope of practice for an AP. **Focus:** Delegation.

15. **Ans: 4** Patients who are prescribed statin drugs such as atorvastatin can develop the adverse effect of rhabdomyolysis. Signs and symptoms include general muscle soreness, muscle pain, weakness, vomiting, stomach pain, and brown urine. When a patient develops these signs and symptoms, the drug needs to be discontinued and another type of antilipidemic drug should be prescribed. Upset stomach and constipation are common side effects of statin drugs but are not adverse effects. Bloating is a more common side effect of the bile acid sequestrant type of antilipidemic drug. **Focus:** Prioritization.

16. **Ans: 1** Apixaban is a direct thrombin inhibitor. Bleeding from the gums is a side effect of these drugs. The nurse should be notified of any bleeding so that she or he can assess this effect. Instructing and teaching are not within the scope of practice for an AP, but the AP can remind patients about what the RN has taught. Apixaban does not require laboratory monitoring. **Focus:** Supervision.

17. **Ans: 2, 3, 6** Antacids can interfere with absorption of clopidogrel (an antiplatelet drug) and many other drugs. Clopidogrel does not interfere with absorption of antacids. Side effects of antiplatelet drugs include nausea and upset stomach, which can be minimized by given the drug with or just after a meal. Antiplatelet

drugs should be given 2 hours after or 1 hour before an antacid. **Focus:** Assignment.

18. **Ans: 3** Digoxin maintenance doses are very low (0.1 to 0.375 mg/day orally). This dosage is 10 times what a maintenance dose should be and could cause adverse, and even life-threatening, effects. Options 1, 2, and 4 all include dosages within the normal limits. **Focus:** Prioritization.

19. **Ans: 1** Enalapril is an angiotensin-converting enzyme (ACE) inhibitor. Swelling of the eyes, mouth, and tongue may indicate angioedema, which is an adverse effect of ACE inhibitors. This can lead to swelling of the trachea, which interferes with breathing and can be life threatening. After the nurse assesses the patient's breathing, the health care provider should be notified. Ice may help reduce swelling but is not a priority at this time. Checking the white blood cell count, especially neutrophils, is important if neutropenia is suspected. Checking vital signs is a good idea but not the highest priority in this situation. **Focus:** Prioritization.

20. **Ans: 3** Atenolol is a beta-blocker. Depression is a side effect of beta-blockers. These drugs may cause first-time depression or may cause existing depression to worsen. Decreased heart rate and blood pressure are expected responses to beta-blockers. Bradycardia, cold hands and feet, and tiredness are expected side effects of beta-blockers and should be monitored but are not as urgent and often do not require changes in the treatment plan. **Focus:** Prioritization.

21. **Ans: 4** Furosemide is a loop diuretic, and quinapril is an angiotensin-converting enzyme inhibitor. Both lower blood pressure, and patients may experience a decrease in blood pressure when sitting or standing, which is a classic sign of postural hypotension. Signs of low potassium include dry mouth, muscle cramps, and irregular heartbeat, and signs of low sodium include confusion, seizures, decreased mental activity, and weakness or fatigue. Photosensitivity is a side effect of furosemide, but it involves increased sensitivity to sunlight. **Focus:** Prioritization.

22. **Ans: 1, 2, 5, 6** Spironolactone is a potassium-sparing diuretic, so patients should avoid excessive intake of foods high in potassium such as bananas, broccoli, and spinach. Salt substitutes should also be avoided because the sodium is replaced with potassium. Urine output should increase, not decrease. The drug works by increasing excretion of water and sodium, but not potassium, in urine. Older adults are more sensitive to the action of this drug and are also more likely to experience side effects. **Focus:** Prioritization.

23. **Ans: 4** Methimazole is a thyroid-suppressing drug, which would make hypothyroidism worse. An appropriate drug for hypothyroidism would be a thyroid replacement drug such as levothyroxine. Options 1, 2, and 3 include appropriate drugs for the conditions listed. **Focus:** Prioritization.

24. **Ans: 1** Prednisone is a corticosteroid drug that is similar to the natural cortisol secreted by the adrenal glands. The amount of cortisol made each day is influenced by the amount circulating in the blood. When a patient takes this drug, the adrenal glands reduce production of cortisol. After taking the drug for more than 1 week, it is necessary to taper the drug before stopping it to give the adrenal glands time to produce more cortisol. The HCP would not suddenly discontinue the drug or continue it at the same level when it is no longer needed. A topical form of the drug would not be needed. **Focus:** Prioritization.

25. **Ans: 240 mg** 20 mg/kg × 12 kg = 240 mg. **Focus:** Prioritization.

26. **Ans: 1** Azithromycin is an antibacterial drug. Amantadine is an antiviral, fluconazole is an antifungal, and ethambutol is an antitubercular. **Focus:** Prioritization.

27. **Ans: 2, 3, 4, 6** Oxybutynin is an anticholinergic drug used to treat overactive bladder. It inhibits the neurotransmitter acetylcholine, which results in decreased secretions and can cause the side effects of dry mouth and eyes, headaches, dizziness, and constipation. Diarrhea and rash are not common side effects of this drug. **Focus:** Prioritization.

28. **Ans: 0.6 mL** Need 3000 units/X mL: Have 5000 units/1 mL = 3/5 = 6/10 = 0.6 mL. **Focus:** Prioritization.

29. **Ans: 4** Epoetin alfa is a colony-stimulating factor, an erythropoiesis-stimulating agent that helps stimulate production of RBCs, and is often used for patients who have chronic kidney disease, anemia from chemotherapy, or need to increase their RBC count before surgery. Another type of colony-stimulating factor is oprelvekin, a thrombopoiesis-stimulating agent that helps increase platelet counts. Both types of colony-stimulating factors are used to decrease the need for transfusion of blood and blood products. **Focus:** Prioritization.

30. **Ans: 3** Meclizine is an antihistamine antiemetic drug that is prescribed for labyrinth disorders, including motion sickness and Ménière disease. Promethazine and prochlorperazine are phenothiazine antiemetic drugs with sedating effects that help to control sensations of nausea. Granisetron is a $5HT_3$-receptor antagonist antiemetic drug commonly used to manage nausea and vomiting associated with cancer chemotherapy. **Focus:** Prioritization.

31. **Ans: 1** Checking and recording vital signs for patients is within the scope of practice for an AP. Auscultating, examining, and asking questions about patient history remain within the scope of practice for a nurse and should not be delegated to an AP. **Focus:** Delegation.

32. **Ans: 2** Prochlorperazine is a phenothiazine antiemetic drug. These drugs commonly have sedation as a side effect, and the sedation (especially in older adults) is what helps control the sensation of nausea when they are given to a patient. Bowel sounds should not change after this drug. Although the nurse should monitor for respiratory depression, oxygen is not necessary unless the patient experiences respiratory difficulties. Because of the sedation effects of this drug, a patient should be instructed to call for help and be assisted to ambulate to the bathroom at least until the effects of the drug on a patient are known. **Focus:** Assignment, Supervision.

33. **Ans: 1, 2, 4, 6** Statements 1, 2, 4, and 6 are accurate with regard to administering a rectal suppository. The best position to place a patient in for administering a suppository is left Sims. Only a small amount of lubricant should be used to coat the pointed end of the suppository, and a small amount of lubricant should also be used to coat the end of the finger that the nurse will use to insert the suppository. **Focus:** Prioritization.

34. **Ans: 2** Patients with diarrhea have increased water in bowel movements as well as increased volume and frequency of stools. A common side effect of diarrhea is electrolyte imbalance, especially low potassium (hypokalemia), so the nurse must monitor this laboratory value. Even small changes in potassium level may cause potentially life-threatening problems such as dysrhythmias. **Focus:** Prioritization.

35. **Ans: 3** Diphenoxylate with atropine is an antimotility drug commonly used to treat diarrhea. The actions of this drug would not relieve a patient's constipation but would likely make it much worse. Omeprazole is a proton pump inhibitor often used to treat PUD and GERD, famotidine is a histamine₂ blocker used to treat GERD and PUD, and ondansetron is a 5H3-receptor antagonist used to treat nausea caused by chemotherapy. Appropriate drugs to treat constipation include emollient stool softeners (e.g., docusate), stimulants (e.g., bisacodyl), and osmotic laxatives (e.g., lactulose). **Focus:** Prioritization.

36. **Ans: 0.5 mL** Need 2 mg/X mL: Have 4 mg/1 mL = 2/4 = 1/2 = 0.5 mL. **Focus:** Prioritization.

37. **Ans: 1, 3, 5, 6** Sildenafil requires sexual stimulation to work. The HCP should be notified about erections lasting longer than 4 hours as well as painful, prolonged erections (priapism). The action of sildenafil lasts about 4 hours (vardenafil's action can last up to 36 hours). Use of nitrate drugs along with sildenafil can lead to severe hypotension, and consuming high-fat meals can cause a delay in the maximum effect of this drug. **Focus:** Prioritization.

38. **Ans: 6 mL** Need 60 mg/X mL: Have 10 mg/1 mL = 6/1 = 6 mL. **Focus:** Prioritization.

39. **ANS: 1, 4, 6** Remdesivir is an intravenous antiviral drug. Common side effects include: nausea and vomiting, low blood pressure, rash, and abnormal liver function tests. Focus: Prioritization.

40. **Ans: 1** A major reason that more research has not been done on medical marijuana is because the U.S.

DEA still considers marijuana to be a Schedule I drug (like heroin, lysergic acid diethylamide [LSD], and ecstasy). These are drugs that are considered to be likely to be abused and have little medical value. To study medical marijuana, researchers need a special license. **Focus:** Prioritization.

41. **Ans: 1, 2, 4, 6, 9** Medical marijuana uses the plant or chemicals from the plant to treat a number of conditions including Alzheimer disease, loss of appetite, cancer, Crohn disease, eating disorders (e.g., anorexia), epilepsy, glaucoma, schizophrenia, PTSD, multiple sclerosis, nausea, pain, and wasting syndrome. Many of these conditions have little research to support the efficacy of marijuana as a treatment. The conditions with the most research evidence include reduction of chronic pain, nausea, and vomiting (e.g., chemotherapy) and decrease of spasticity from multiple sclerosis. **Focus:** Prioritization.

42. **Ans: 1, 3, 6, 8, 9** HHS often occurs in older adults with type 2 diabetes. Risk factors include taking diuretics and having an inadequate fluid intake. Serum glucose is greater than 600 mg/dL (33.3 mmol/L). Patients with HHS are dehydrated, and ketones are absent or low. Weight loss (not weight gain) would be a symptom. Although the patient's blood pressure is high, this is not a risk factor. A urine output of 50 to 75 mL/hr is adequate. **Focus:** Prioritization.

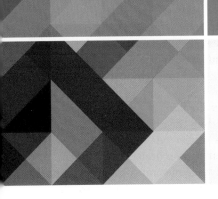

Questions

1. The hospital administration issues a statement that surge capacity is likely to be exceeded because state-wide measures have not been successful in "flattening the curve" of COVID-19 (coronavirus) cases. How is this information **most** likely to affect the nursing staff?
   1. Nurses will be expected to revise infection control policies, as needed.
   2. Nurses will be asked to work extra shifts or keep working beyond end-of-shift.
   3. Nurses will be given priority usage for personal protective equipment.
   4. Nurses can temporarily practice outside scope of practice, as needed.

2. An emergency department clinical nurse specialist is training staff in how to don and doff personal protective equipment (PPE) when caring for patients with infections such as Ebola. Which staff member has demonstrated the **most** grievous error during the practice session?
   1. A triage nurse forgets to perform hand hygiene and inspect PPE before donning.
   2. An assistive personnel performs self-inspection, then begins to doff PPE.
   3. A health care provider forgets to wipe shoes with disinfectant after doffing shoe covers.
   4. An emergency medical technician doffs both pairs of gloves first.

3. The charge nurse in an emergency department (ED) must assign two staff members to cover the triage area. Which team is **best** for this assignment?
   1. An advanced practice nurse and an experienced RN
   2. An experienced LPN/LVN and an inexperienced RN
   3. An experienced RN and an inexperienced RN
   4. An experienced RN and an experienced assistive personnel (AP)

4. The nurse is working in the triage area of an emergency department, and the following four patients approach the triage desk at the same time. List the order in which the nurse will assess these patients.
   1. An ambulatory, dazed 25-year-old man with a bandaged head wound
   2. An irritable newborn with a fever, petechiae, and nuchal rigidity
   3. A 35-year-old jogger with a twisted ankle who has a pedal pulse and no deformity
   4. A 50-year-old woman with moderate abdominal pain and occasional vomiting

   _____, _____, _____, _____

5. When a primary survey of a trauma patient is conducted, which action would be performed **first**?
   1. Obtain a complete set of vital sign measurements.
   2. Palpate and auscultate the abdomen.
   3. Perform a brief neurologic assessment.
   4. Check the pulse oximetry reading.

6. A 56-year-old patient comes to the triage area with left-sided chest pain, diaphoresis, and dizziness. What is the **priority** action?
   1. Initiate continuous electrocardiographic monitoring.
   2. Notify the emergency department health care provider.
   3. Administer oxygen via nasal cannula.
   4. Draw blood and establish IV access.

7. The patient's blood alcohol level is 0.45%. Based on this information, what is the **priority** nursing concept that underlies emergency medical and nursing interventions for this patient?
   1. Cognition
   2. Addiction
   3. Gas Exchange
   4. Functional Ability

8. According to the Emergency Nurses' Association (ENA), what are the main issues when providing emergency care for patients with mental health problems or psychiatric disorders? **Select all that apply.**
   1. Seeking and ruling out medical causes for psychiatric behaviors and problems
   2. Ensuring safety for patients, staff, and others related to restraints, aggressive behavior, and agitation
   3. Improving length of stay in the emergency department (ED) related to lack of resources and providers' decisions about disposition
   4. Establishing ongoing care after triage by dedicated psychiatric emergency nurses
   5. Providing additional education for psychiatric nursing assistants to include care of mental health patients in the ED
   6. Improving communication to describe symptoms and findings in hand-off, disposition, and follow-up care

9. It is the summer season, and patients with signs and symptoms of heat-related illness come to the emergency department. Which patient needs attention **first**?
   1. Older adult who reports dizziness and syncope after standing in the sun for several hours to view a parade
   2. Marathon runner who reports severe leg cramps and nausea and presents with tachycardia, diaphoresis, pallor, and weakness
   3. Healthy homemaker who reports that air conditioner has been broken for days; she has tachypnea, hypotension, fatigue, and profuse diaphoresis
   4. Homeless person who displays altered mental status, poor muscle coordination, and hot, dry, ashen skin; duration of heat exposure is unknown

10. The nurse responds to a call for help from the emergency department waiting room. An older adult patient is lying on the floor. List the order in which the nurse must carry out the following actions.
    1. Perform the chin lift or jaw thrust maneuver.
    2. Establish unresponsiveness.
    3. Initiate cardiopulmonary resuscitation (CPR).
    4. Call for help and activate the code team.
    5. Instruct assistive personnel to get the crash cart.

    _____, _____, _____, _____, _____

11. Emergency medical services has transported a patient with severe chest pain. As the patient is being transferred to the emergency stretcher, the nurse notes unresponsiveness, cessation of breathing, and no palpable pulse. Which task is appropriate to delegate to the assistive personnel (AP)?
    1. Performing chest compressions
    2. Initiating bag-valve mask ventilation
    3. Assisting with oral intubation
    4. Placing the defibrillator pads

12. Although the incidence of tetanus has decreased through routine immunization, there is still a danger. Which patient represents the group that is **most** vulnerable for risk?
    1. Child who helps on the family's farm and sustained scratches while feeding the animals
    2. Newborn who is delivered in the emergency department; mother had no prenatal care
    3. Older adult who lives alone and sustained a minor cut while cleaning the basement
    4. Young adult who works in an auto repair shop and sustained a deep cut on a metal edge

13. A healthy but anxious 24-year-old college student reports tingling sensations, palpitations, and sore chest muscles. Deep, rapid breathing and carpal spasms are noted. Which action is the **priority**?
    1. Notify the health care provider immediately.
    2. Administer supplemental oxygen.
    3. Have the student breathe into a paper bag.
    4. Obtain a prescription for an anxiolytic medication.

14. An experienced traveling nurse has been assigned to work in the emergency department (ED); however, this is the nurse's first week on the job. Which area of the ED would be the **best** assignment for this nurse?
    1. Trauma team
    2. Triage
    3. Ambulatory or fast-track clinic
    4. Pediatric medicine team

15. The nurse and her friends are at the lake. Suddenly, someone says, "Look across the lake! It looks like someone might be drowning out there!" What is the nurse's **first** action?
    1. Determine who is the strongest swimmer in the group.
    2. Direct someone to locate a cell phone and call 911.
    3. Find a boat, raft, or some type of flotation device.
    4. Use a pair of binoculars and look across the lake.

16. In the care of a patient who has experienced sexual assault, which task is **most** appropriate for an LPN/LVN to perform?
    1. Assessing the patient's immediate emotional state and physical injuries
    2. Collecting hair samples, saliva specimens, and scrapings from beneath fingernails
    3. Providing emotional support and supportive communication
    4. Ensuring that the chain of custody of evidence is maintained

17. The LPN/LVN is performing care for a patient who sustained an amputation of the first and second digits in a chainsaw accident. What instructions would the RN give to the LPN/LVN?
    1. Clean the amputated digits and the hand with a povidone-iodine and normal saline solution, then wrap with gauze.
    2. Clean the amputated digits, wrap them in gauze, and place cleansed digits directly into an ice slurry.
    3. Clean the amputated digits with saline, wrap in moist gauze, seal in a plastic bag, and place in an ice slurry.
    4. Clean the digits with sterile normal saline and submerge the digits in sterile normal saline in a sterile cup.

18. According to the World Health Organization (WHO), Violence Against Women: Guidelines for Health Sector Response, which group of patients should be screened for intimate partner violence (IPV)?
    1. All females that enter the health care system regardless of risk for IPV
    2. All persons, male and female, that seek health care (universal screening for IPV)
    3. Any female patient that has a risk factors for IPV, such as pregnancy
    4. Any patient that presents with conditions suspected to have been caused by IPV

19. The nurse is giving discharge instructions to a woman who was treated for contusions and bruises sustained during an episode of domestic violence. Which intervention is the **priority** for this patient?
    1. Discuss the option of going to a safe house.
    2. Make a referral to a counselor.
    3. Advise the patient about contacting the police.
    4. Make an appointment to follow up on the injuries.

20. A newly graduated nurse overhears a senior emergency department nurse making sarcastic remarks toward a medical student and refusing to help the student find the equipment for a nonemergent patient procedure. What should the new nurse do **first**?
    1. Step in and offer to assist the medical student because the other nurse is unwilling.
    2. Confront the senior nurse and indicate that an apology is the right thing to do.
    3. Observe the situation and then report the behaviors of both parties to the charge nurse.
    4. Watch and observe the dynamics; the scenario is probably typical of unit norms.

21. The nurse notifies the emergency department (ED) health care provider (HCP) about a patient who has abdominal pain, nausea and vomiting, and fever. The abdomen is distended, rigid, and boardlike, and there is rebound tenderness. Later the nurse sees that the patient is to be discharged with a follow-up appointment in the morning. The nurse reexamines the patient and the symptoms seem worse. What should the nurse do **first**?
    1. Contact the nursing supervisor and express concerns.
    2. Express findings and concerns to the HCP.
    3. Discharge the patient but stress the importance of following up.
    4. Follow the discharge orders and write an incident report.

22. A confused patient admits to frequently drinking alcohol. The emergency department health care provider (HCP) makes a preliminary diagnosis of Wernicke encephalopathy. Which medication does the nurse anticipate that the HCP will prescribe **first**?
    1. Glucagon IV
    2. Naltrexone intramuscularly
    3. Thiamine IV
    4. Naloxone IV

23. When an unexpected death occurs in the emergency department, which task is **most** appropriate to delegate to the assistive personnel (AP)?
    1. Escorting the family to a place of privacy
    2. Accompanying the organ donor specialist to talk to the family
    3. Assisting with postmortem care
    4. Helping the family to collect belongings

24. After emergency endotracheal intubation, tube placement must be verified before securing the tube. Which bedside assessment is the **most** accurate and can be performed immediately after the tube is placed?
    1. Visualize the movement of the thoracic cage.
    2. Auscultate the chest during assisted ventilation.
    3. Confirm that the breath sounds are equal and bilateral.
    4. Check exhaled carbon dioxide levels with capnography.

25. A man with a known history of alcohol abuse has been in police custody for 48 hours. Initially, anxiety, sweating, and tremors were noted. Now disorientation, hallucination, and hyperreactivity are observed. The medical diagnosis is delirium tremens. Which nursing concept is the **priority** in planning interventions for this emergency condition?
    1. Safety
    2. Psychosis
    3. Thermoregulation
    4. Addiction

 Answer Key for this chapter begins on p. 219

26. The nurse is assigned to telephone triage. A patient who was just stung by a common honeybee calls for advice. Which question would the nurse ask **first**?
    1. "Is this the first time you have been stung by a bee or wasp?"
    2. "Do you have access to and know how to use an epinephrine autoinjector?"
    3. "What type of first aid measures have you tried?"
    4. "Are you having any facial swelling, wheezing, or shortness of breath?"

27. A victim of heat stroke arrives in the emergency department. His skin is hot and dry; his body temperature is 105°F (40.6°C). He is confused and demonstrates bizarre behavior. His blood pressure is 85/60 mm Hg, pulse is 130 beats/min, and respirations are 40 breaths/min. Which task should be assigned to an experienced LPN/LVN?
    1. Insert a rectal probe to measure core body temperature.
    2. Administer aspirin or another antipyretic.
    3. Insert an indwelling urinary drainage catheter.
    4. Assess respiratory effort, hemodynamics, and mental status.

28. The nurse is assessing a patient who has sustained a cat bite to the left hand. The cat's immunizations are up to date. The date of the patient's last tetanus shot is unknown. What is the **priority** concern?
    1. Treating an infection specific to cat bites
    2. Suturing the puncture wounds
    3. Administering the tetanus vaccine
    4. Maintaining mobility of finger joints

29. The following patients come to the emergency department triage desk reporting acute abdominal pain. Which patient has the **most** severe condition?
    1. A 35-year-old man reporting severe intermittent cramps with three episodes of watery diarrhea 2 hours after eating
    2. An 11-year-old boy with a low-grade fever, right lower quadrant tenderness, nausea, and anorexia for the past 2 days
    3. A 23-year-old woman reporting dizziness and severe left lower quadrant pain who states she is possibly pregnant
    4. A 50-year-old woman who reports gnawing midepigastric pain that is worse between meals and during the night

30. Which combination of employees would be **best** to include in a committee to address the issue of violence against emergency department (ED) personnel?
    1. ED health care providers and charge nurses
    2. Experienced RNs and experienced paramedics
    3. RNs, LPNs/LVNs, and assistive personnel
    4. At least one person from all ED groups

31. The nurse is caring for a patient with multiple injuries sustained during a head-on car collision. Which assessment finding takes **priority**?
    1. A deviated trachea
    2. Unequal pupils
    3. Ecchymosis in the flank area
    4. Irregular apical pulse

32. A patient involved in a one-car rollover comes in with multiple injuries. List in order of **priority** the interventions that must be initiated for this patient.
    1. Secure two large-bore IV lines and infuse normal saline.
    2. Use the chin lift or jaw thrust maneuver to open the airway.
    3. Assess for spontaneous respirations.
    4. Give supplemental oxygen via mask.
    5. Obtain a full set of vital sign measurements.
    6. Remove or cut away the patient's clothing.

    _____, _____, _____, _____, _____, _____

33. A young woman is brought to the emergency department (ED) by emergency medical services (EMS) because she has been depressed and threatening to commit suicide. On arrival to the ED, the woman is confused, her speech is slurred, and there is vomit on her clothes. EMS found several empty prescription bottles at the house. Which intervention is the **priority** for this patient?
    1. Identify toxic substances by history and analysis of blood, urine, and gastric contents.
    2. Initiate supportive care, such as checking the airway and giving oxygen and IV fluids.
    3. Reduce absorption by giving activated charcoal or performing gastric lavage.
    4. Promote poison removal using drugs to facilitate excretion or by starting hemodialysis.

34. The nurse is caring for a patient who is on the cardiac monitor because of these symptoms: syncope, dizziness, and intermittent episodes of palpitations. Below is a display of what the nurse sees on the cardiac monitor. What should the nurse do **first**?

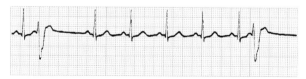

    1. Call the rapid response team.
    2. Obtain the automated external defibrillator.
    3. Assess the patient and take vital signs.
    4. Check the adherence of the gel pads on the chest.

35. A group of people arrive at the emergency department by private car. They all have extreme periorbital swelling, coughing, and tightness in the throat. There is a strong odor emanating from their clothes. They report exposure to a "gas bomb" that was set off in their house. Which action is the **priority**?
    1. Measure vital signs and listen to lung sounds.
    2. Direct patients to the decontamination area.
    3. Alert security about possible terrorism activity.
    4. Direct patients to cold or clean zones for immediate treatment.

36. In the work setting, what is the nurse's **primary** responsibility in preparing for the management of disasters, including natural disasters and bioterrorism incidents?
    1. Knowing the agency's emergency response plan
    2. Being aware of the signs and symptoms of potential agents of bioterrorism
    3. Knowing how and what to report to the Centers for Disease Control and Prevention
    4. Making ethical decisions about exposing self to potentially lethal substances

37. List in order of **priority** the actions that should be taken by emergency department staff in the event of a biochemical incident.
    1. Report to the public health department or Centers for Disease Control and Prevention per protocol.
    2. Decontaminate the affected individuals in a separate area.
    3. Protect the environment for the safety of personnel and nonaffected patients.
    4. Don personal protective equipment.
    5. Perform triage according to protocol.
    _____, _____, _____, _____, _____

38. According to the Joint Commission, hospitals are required to form emergency management committees to periodically exercise the disaster operations plan. Hospital administration has selected various health care providers (HCPs) to join the committee. Members from which other key departments should be included? **Select all that apply.**
    1. Security and communications
    2. Nursing and assistive personnel
    3. Laboratory and diagnostic services
    4. Medical records and information technology
    5. Maintenance and engineering
    6. Quality improvement and occupational therapy

39. A newly hired emergency department (ED) clinical nurse specialist (CNS) is reviewing the hospital's disaster plan and finds that it has not been reviewed or revised for 3 years. Which finding will be **most** important for the CNS to address related to the status of the disaster plan?
    1. Stockpiles of antibiotics and resuscitation equipment may be depleted.
    2. Current staff is unlikely to have training and practice in using the plan.
    3. Resources within and outside of the hospital are likely to have changed.
    4. Surrounding communities are at an increased risk for technologic disasters.

40. The nurse is talking to a group of people about an industrial explosion in which many people were killed or injured. Which individual has the **greatest** risk for psychiatric difficulties, such as post-traumatic stress disorder, related to the incident?
    1. Individual who repeatedly watched television coverage of the event
    2. Person who recently learned that her son was killed in the incident
    3. Individual who witnessed the death of a co-worker during the explosion
    4. Person who was injured and trapped for several hours before rescue

41. Identify the five **most** critical elements in performing disaster triage for multiple victims.
    1. Obtain past medical and surgical histories.
    2. Check airway, breathing, and circulation.
    3. Assess the level of consciousness.
    4. Visually inspect for gross deformities, bleeding, and obvious injuries.
    5. Note the color, presence of moisture, and temperature of the skin.
    6. Check vital signs, including pulse and respirations.
    _____, _____, _____, _____, _____

 Answer Key for this chapter begins on p. 219

⚡ **42.** Drag and Drop _____

Scenario: The nurse is working in a small rural community hospital. There is a fire in a local church, and six people have arrived at the hospital. Emergency medical services report that approximately 250 people were in the church when the fire started. Many other victims are expected to arrive soon, and other hospitals are 5 hours away.

Using disaster triage principles, in which order would the patients receive attention?

Instructions: Patients are listed in the left-hand column. In the right-hand column, indicate the order in which the patients will receive care; 1 being the first and 6 being the last.

Patients who have arrived at the emergency department	Order of care
A. 52-year-old man in full cardiac arrest has been receiving continuous cardiopulmonary resuscitation (CPR) for the past 90 minutes	
B. 35-year old firefighter is confused and combative has respiratory stridor	
C. 60-year old woman has full-thickness burns to the hands and forearms	
D. 16-year old adolescent has a crushed leg that is very swollen; he is anxious, pulse is 130 beats/min	
E. 3-year-old child is lethargic; with slow, shallow respirations and burns over more than 70% of the anterior body	
G. 12-year-old child has wheezing and very labored respirations which are unrelieved by an asthma inhaler	

⚡ **43.** Cloze _____

Scenario: A patient presents to the emergency department with nausea, vomiting, colicky abdominal pain, fever, and tachycardia. The health care provider informs the nurse that the patient probably has a strangulated intestinal obstruction with perforation.

Instructions: Complete the sentences by choosing the most probable option for the missing information that corresponds with the same numbered list of options provided.

____1____, and ____2____, are administered followed by ____3____ to decompress the stomach and intestine. ____4____ and ____5____ are performed as soon as possible to detect location of the obstruction and guide surgical decisions. The patient is prepared for ____6____.

Option 1 and 2	Option 3	Option 4 and 5	Option 6
IV broad-spectrum antibiotics	Nasogastric (NG) tube insertion	Barium enema examination	Transfer to the intensive care unit
PO Polyethylene Glycol 3350 solution	Paracentesis of the abdomen	Abdominal radiography	Discharge with clinic appointment in the am
IV normal saline	Rectal tube insertion	Capsule endoscopy	Transfer to the medical-surgical unit
Acetaminophen 650 mg PO for fever	Percutaneous endoscopic gastrostomy tube insertion	CT scan	Emergency surgery

⚡ **44.** Matrix

Scenario: The nurse knows that intimate partner violence (IPV) occurs in all socioeconomic and cultural groups, but she feels that the population served by a large urban clinic has many risk factors. While assessing her patients, the nurse is vigilant for evidence of IPV, which are divided in to four categories: physical violence, psychological violence, sexual violence and control behaviors.

Instructions: For each patient statement, place an X in the box to indicate whether it is physical violence, psychological violence, sexual violence, or control behavior.

Patient Statements	Physical violence	Psychological violence	Sexual violence	Control behavior
"When my boyfriend wants sex, it's easier just to give in; once it's over he leaves me alone."				
"I have moved 3 times in the past year; she always manages to track me down."				
"He slapped me last week; I kicked at him, but that just made him mad."				
"She keeps saying she'll just take the kids and disappear if I don't pay more attention to her."				
"If I go anywhere, even to the grocery store, he's calling me to come back home."				
"He said I was fat and ugly and if he threw me out, nobody else would want me."				
"I don't like it, but he says that rectal intercourse is exciting for him."				
"She said that if I ever left her, she would kill herself."				
"He has all of the money in an account in his name; I need his permission to buy things."				
"Things just build up. After he hits me, he apologizes; then we go back to normal."				

45. An active shooter incident occurs in the triage area of a large busy emergency room. What is the **priority** action for the triage nurse to take?
1. Assist vulnerable patients, who are in the line of fire, to drop to the floor.
2. Locate a safe path and run to a safe place; take others if possible.
3. Find a secure place, such as a barricaded room, to hide self and others.
4. Aggressively fight off the attacker using any means available.

Answer Key for this chapter begins on p. 219

PART 2   Common Health Scenarios

46. Drag and Drop

Scenario: The Joint Commission recommends hospital preparedness for an active shooter incident. It is expected that law enforcement would be involved in the planning. A communication plan is required. Patient and employee safety must be established. Employees need training and drills. Post-event actions must be outlined.

Which person or group is **best** to assign each task that is part of the active shooter incident?

Instructions: The person or group who would be involved in the active shooter incident plan are listed in the left column. In the right column write in the letter to indicate the best person or group for each task. **Note that all responses will be used only once.**

Person or Group:

A. Emergency department RNs
B. Public relation officer
C. Hospital Incident Commander
D. Hospital liaison officer
E. Emergency department clinical nurse specialist
F. Local law enforcement officers
G. Emergency medical service personnel
H. Hospital security officers
I. Employee Assistance staff

Tasks

1. _____ Functions as primary contact during incident between hospital personnel and law enforcement
2. _____ Participates in community based-drills
3. _____ Uses a predetermined script to relay information to family and public
4. _____ Subdues any individual who is killing or attempting to kill people in a confined space
5. _____ Recognizes the early warning signs of potential threat or violence
6. _____ Operationalizes the lockdown of the facility to control and prevent walk-in traffic
7. _____ Assists staff, post-event, to access mental health resources
8. _____ Organizes video and classroom training for emergency department staff
9. _____ Is responsible for the overall activities related to an incident

Answer Key for this chapter begins on p. 219

Answers

1. **Ans: 2** Nurses are likely to be asked to work additional shifts/hours as the patient load increases. When the surge capacity of a hospital is exceeded, a sudden and unexpectedly large number of patients overwhelm the resources and capabilities to provide care. By "flattening the curve," there are fewer infections, so patients enter the health care system at slower and more controlled rate. Infection control policies have been affected by the pandemic, but revision of the policies and guidance for nurses would have occurred in anticipation of the surge, as part of disaster preparedness planning. While nurses should be among those who get personnel protective equipment, other staff members, patients, and visitors may receive first priority. Nurses cannot legally practice outside scope of practice even in emergency situations. **Focus:** Prioritization; **Test-Taking Tip:** Recommendations for management of COVID-19 are likely to evolve as we learn more about the disease process and how to safely care for patients and protect selves and others. National Council of State Boards of Nursing currently has self-paced courses related to the care of COVID-19 patients at https://catalog.icrsncsbn.org/

2. **Ans: 4** All team members have made errors, but removing both pairs of gloves puts the emergency medical technician at the greatest risk because the outer surfaces of the remaining PPE are considered contaminated. According to the latest recommendations from the Centers for Disease Control and Prevention, the flow of donning (for N95 respirator option) is as follows: a trained observer arrives to oversee the inspection process; team members remove personal clothing/items, inspect their PPE, put on boot covers, and then don, in this order, inner gloves, gown, N95 respirator, hood, outer gloves, and face shield. Afterward, team members inspect themselves and are inspected by the trained observer. The flow of doffing (for N95 respirator option) starts with an inspection by the team member and by the trained observer. Afterward, team members disinfect outer gloves; remove their apron if used; inspect the apron for cuts or tears; disinfect, inspect, and remove outer gloves; inspect and disinfect inner gloves; remove face shield; disinfect inner gloves; remove hood; disinfect inner gloves; remove gown; disinfect inner gloves; remove boot covers; disinfect and change inner gloves; remove N95 respirator; disinfect inner gloves; disinfect washable shoes; disinfect and remove inner gloves; and then practice hand hygiene. After all that, team members inspect themselves one more time and are inspected by the trained observer. **Focus:** Supervision; **Test-Taking Tip:** The Centers for Disease Control and Prevention is a good source for information relating to infection control. For addition information about donning and doffing PPE, see https://www.cdc.gov/hai/pdfs/ppe/ppe-sequence.pdf.

3. **Ans: 1** Triage requires at least one experienced RN. Advanced practice nurses can perform medical screening exams, and this expedites treatment and decreases overall time spent in the ED. Pairing an experienced RN with an inexperienced RN provides opportunities for mentoring. This would be the second-best choice. Pairing an experienced RN with an experienced AP is an option if licensed staff is unavailable because the AP can measure vital signs and assist in transporting. An LPN/LVN should not perform the initial patient assessment or decision making, and the expertise of the LPN/LVN could be used elsewhere in a busy ED. **Focus:** Assignment.

4. **Ans: 2, 1, 4, 3** An irritable newborn with fever and petechiae should be further assessed for other signs of meningitis. The patient with the head wound needs additional assessment because of the risk for increased intracranial pressure. The patient with moderate abdominal pain is in discomfort, but her condition is not unstable at this point. For the ankle injury, medical evaluation could be delayed for 24 to 48 hours if necessary, but the patient should receive the appropriate first aid. **Focus:** Prioritization; **Test-Taking Tip:** Use knowledge of growth and development and remember that newborns have immature immune systems that are readily overwhelmed by infection. Any temperature elevation in a neonate is considered a life-threatening emergency.

5. **Ans: 3** A brief neurologic assessment to determine level of consciousness and pupil reaction is part of the primary survey. Measuring vital signs, assessing the abdomen, and checking pulse oximetry readings are considered part of the secondary survey. **Focus:** Prioritization.

6. **Ans: 3** The priority goal is to increase myocardial oxygenation. The other actions are also appropriate and should be performed immediately after administering oxygen. **Focus:** Prioritization; **Test-Taking Tip:** Remember to use the ABCs (airway, breathing, and circulation) in determining priorities. This is especially important when the patient is in critical distress.

7. **Ans: 3** At a blood alcohol level of 0.45%, the patient would demonstrate respiratory depression, stupor, and coma. At 0.05%, the patient would display euphoria and decreased inhibitions; at 0.20%, reduced motor skills and slurred speech occur; and at 0.30%, altered perception and double vision occur. **Focus:** Prioritization.

8. **Ans: 1, 2, 3, 4, 6** The ENA has summarized current issues for managing behavioral health problems in the ED. For patients that present to the ED with behavioral problems, underlying medical causes must be ruled out first. Ongoing care of these patients is best accomplished by psychiatric emergency nurses who have the expertise to assess behavior problems that may include psychosis and agitation and who can intervene to prevent harm to self or others. Length of stay is an issue that is related to lack of services, lack of specialists, and long waits for treatment and disposition. Communication in hand-off, disposition, and follow-up care needs to be improved to decrease length of stay. Education for psychiatric mental health assistants is not currently one of the issues. **Focus:** Prioritization.

9. **Ans: 4** The homeless person has symptoms of heat stroke, a medical emergency that increases the risk for brain damage. The care includes arterial blood gases; possible endotracheal intubation; IV fluids; blood for electrolytes, cardiac and liver enzymes, and complete blood count; muscle relaxants (benzodiazepines) if the patient begins to shiver; the monitoring of urine output and specific gravity to determine fluid needs; cooling interventions; and the discontinuation of cooling interventions when core body temperature is reduced to 102°F (38.9°C). The older adult patient is at risk for heat syncope and should be educated to rest in a cool area and avoid future similar situations. The runner is having heat cramps, which can be managed with rest and fluids. The housewife is experiencing heat exhaustion, and management includes administration of fluids (IV or oral) and cooling measures. **Focus:** Prioritization.

10. **Ans: 2, 4, 1, 3, 5** Establish unresponsiveness first. (The patient may have fallen and sustained a minor injury.) If the patient is unresponsive, get help and activate the code team. Performing the chin lift or jaw thrust maneuver opens the airway. The nurse is then responsible for starting CPR. A pocket mask or bag-valve mask (a second rescuer must be present for the bag-valve mask to be used effectively) is used to deliver rescue breaths. CPR should not be interrupted until the patient recovers or it is determined that all heroic efforts have been exhausted. A crash cart should be at the site when the code team arrives; however, basic CPR can be effectively performed until the code team arrives. **Focus:** Prioritization.

11. **Ans: 1** APs are trained in basic cardiac life support and can perform chest compressions. The use of the bag-valve mask requires practice, and usually a respiratory therapist will perform this function. The nurse or the respiratory therapist should provide assistance as needed during intubation. The defibrillator pads are clearly marked; however, placement should be done by the RN or health care provider because of the potential for skin damage and electrical arcing. **Focus:** Delegation.

12. **Ans: 3** Older adults are the most likely to be nonvaccinated or undervaccinated. Tetanus usually occurs when a minor wound gets contaminated by wood, metal, or other organic material. In addition, most people would not seek medical treatment for minor wounds. Farm work offers many opportunities for injuries, but most children are usually immunized before entering elementary school (the nurse should always ask). People with deep cuts from industrial accidents are more likely to present to the emergency department for treatment. Neonatal tetanus is more likely to occur in underdeveloped countries and is related to poor hygienic conditions during birth. **Focus:** Prioritization.

13. **Ans: 3** The patient is hyperventilating secondary to anxiety, and breathing 6 to 12 natural breaths into a paper bag will allow rebreathing of carbon dioxide. Have the patient remove the bag, breath normally, repeat breathing into the bag as needed. Also, encouraging slow breathing will help. Other treatments such as oxygen administration and medication may be needed if other causes are identified. **Focus:** Prioritization.

14. **Ans: 3** The fast-track clinic deals with patients in relatively stable condition. The triage, trauma, and pediatric medicine areas should be staffed with experienced nurses who know the hospital routines and policies and can rapidly locate equipment. **Focus:** Assignment.

15. **Ans: 4** First, the nurse would gather as much data as possible. In this case, data might include the number of potential victims; distance from shore; hazards or barriers that may affect rescue (e.g., water temperature, roughness of waves, wind, or lightning); and the resources available to victim(s) or rescuers (e.g., boat, pier, closer rescuers). These data can be reported to the 911 dispatcher and used to decide whether a rescue attempt is reasonably safe for the nurse and the bystanders. **Focus:** Prioritization; **Test-Taking Tip:** The first step in the nursing process is assessment. In this case, the nurse must assess the multiple factors that affect the safety of potential victims and rescuers. The data are then used to weigh harms and benefits.

16. **Ans: 3** An LPN/LVN can listen and provide emotional support for patients. The other tasks are the responsibility of an RN, or preferably, a sexual assault nurse examiner who has received training in assessing, collecting, and safeguarding evidence and caring for assault victims. **Focus:** Assignment.

17. **Ans: 3** The correct intervention is to gently cleanse the digits with normal saline, wrap them in sterile gauze moistened with saline, and place them in a plastic bag or container. The container is then placed in an ice slurry. **Focus:** Supervision, Knowledge.

18. **Ans: 4** WHO recommends screening patients that present with conditions that are suspected to have been caused by IPV. This includes assessment findings that suggest physical or psychologic abuse. WHO further recommends that the health care team be knowledgeable and trained to detect IPV and intervene.

Universal screening is currently not recommended. **Focus:** Prioritization.

19. **Ans: 1**   Safety is a priority for this patient, and she should not return to a place where violence could recur (nevertheless, she retains the right to choose where she goes). The other options are important for the long-term management of this case. **Focus:** Prioritization.

20. **Ans: 1**   First, the new nurse should step in and take action to protect and address the needs of the vulnerable people: the medical student who is being bullied and the patient who needs the procedure. The next step would be to take the senior nurse aside and discuss the behaviors and how they impact team morale and overall patient care. It is difficult to approach someone who is more senior, but the new nurse can use "I" statements, which are less accusatory. For example, "I overheard the interaction with the medical student. I stepped in to help him because I felt uncomfortable." Observing the dynamics of the scenario is appropriate, and those observations can be shared with the charge nurse or unit manager so that steps can be taken to create a climate of interprofessional collaboration. **Focus:** Prioritization.

21. **Ans: 2**   First, the nurse tries to express concerns to the HCP. The ED can be very hectic, and the ED staff should work as a team and watch out for each other as well as for the patients. If the HCP refuses to consider concerns, then the nurse may have to contact the nursing supervisor and write an incident report. This patient has signs of peritonitis. If the patient dies or has a poor outcome, the nurse is liable for failing to intervene. **Focus:** Prioritization.

22. **Ans: 3**   Wernicke encephalopathy is caused by a thiamine deficiency and manifests as confusion, nystagmus, and abnormal ocular movements. It can be reversed with thiamine. IV glucagon is given if change of mental status is caused by severe hypoglycemia. Naltrexone is used to decrease the craving for alcohol. Naloxone is used to reverse opioid overdose. **Focus:** Prioritization.

23. **Ans: 3**   Postmortem care requires turning, cleaning, lifting, and so on, and the AP is able to assist with these duties. The RN should take responsibility for the other tasks to help the family begin the grieving process. In cases of questionable death, belongings may be retained for evidence, so the chain of custody must be maintained. **Focus:** Delegation.

24. **Ans: 4**   Checking exhaled carbon dioxide levels is the most accurate way of immediately verifying placement. Observing chest movements and auscultating and confirming equal bilateral breath sounds are considered less accurate. (Note to student: You may possibly see the health care team auscultating the chest; this is a long-time practice that is quick to perform and doesn't harm the patient if used in conjunction with other verification methods.) Radiographic study will verify and document correct placement. **Focus:** Prioritization.

25. **Ans: 1**   The patient demonstrates neurologic hyperreactivity and is on the verge of a seizure. Patient safety is the priority. The patient needs medications such as chlordiazepoxide to decrease neurologic irritability and phenytoin for seizures. Thiamine is given to correct underlying nutritional deficiency. An antipsychotic medication such as haloperidol may be prescribed. **Focus:** Prioritization.

26. **Ans: 4**   First, the nurse would try to determine if the patient is having a severe allergic reaction to the bee sting. Facial swelling, wheezing, or shortness of breath can rapidly progress to a life-threatening airway obstruction. If these signs and symptoms are occurring, the nurse would instruct the patient to call 911 and to use the epinephrine autoinjector if it is available. If the patient is not having a life-threatening reaction, the nurse could ask other questions to determine appropriate interventions. **Focus:** Prioritization.

27. **Ans: 3**   Inserting an indwelling urinary catheter is within the scope of practice of an experienced LPN/LVN. Experienced assistive personnel should be directed to insert the rectal probe to monitor the core temperature. Initial assessment of new patients and critically ill patients should be performed by the RN. Aspirin and other antipyretics are not given because they won't work to decrease the body temperature and may be harmful. The care of this patient would also include arterial blood gases; possible endotracheal intubation; IV fluids; blood for electrolytes, cardiac and liver enzymes, and complete blood count; muscle relaxants (benzodiazepines) if the patient begins to shiver; the monitoring of urine output and specific gravity to determine fluid needs; cooling interventions; and the discontinuation of cooling interventions when core body temperature is reduced to 102°F (38.9°C). **Focus:** Assignment.

28. **Ans: 1**   Cats' mouths contain a virulent organism, *Pasteurella multocida,* which can lead to septic arthritis or bacteremia. Appropriate first aid includes rigorous washing of the wound site with soap and water to combat infection. Puncture wounds, especially those caused by bites, are usually not sutured. There is also a risk for tendon damage and loss of joint mobility caused by deep puncture wounds, but an orthopedic surgeon would be consulted after initial emergency care is started. A tetanus shot can be given before discharge. **Focus:** Prioritization.

29. **Ans: 3**   The woman with lower left quadrant pain could have an ectopic pregnancy. This is a life-threatening condition. The 11-year-old boy needs evaluation to rule out appendicitis. The 35-year-old man has food poisoning, which is usually self-limiting. The woman with midepigastric pain may have an ulcer, but follow-up diagnostic testing and teaching of lifestyle modification can be scheduled with the primary care provider. **Focus:** Prioritization.

30. **Ans: 4** At least one representative from each group should be included because all employees are potential targets for violence in the ED. **Focus:** Assignment.

31. **Ans: 1** A deviated trachea is a symptom of tension pneumothorax, which will result in respiratory arrest if not corrected. All of the other symptoms are potentially serious but are of lower priority. **Focus:** Prioritization.

32. **Ans: 3, 2, 4, 1, 5, 6** For a trauma patient with multiple injuries, many interventions (e.g., assessing for spontaneous respirations, performing techniques to open the airway such as chin lift or jaw thrust, and applying oxygen) may occur simultaneously as team members assist in the resuscitation. A quick assessment of respiratory status precedes intervention. Opening the airway must precede the administration of oxygen because, if the airway is closed, the oxygen cannot enter the air passages. Starting IV lines for fluid resuscitation is part of supporting circulation. (Emergency medical service personnel will usually establish at least one IV line in the field.) Assistive personnel can be directed to obtain and report vital signs and remove or cut away clothing. **Focus:** Prioritization.

33. **Ans: 2** Maintaining airway, oxygenation, and circulation are the priorities. The other steps are also important in managing patients who have ingested toxic substances. **Focus:** Prioritization.

34. **Ans: 3** The nurse recognizes that the monitor is showing sinus rhythm with occasional premature ventricular contractions (PVCs). The patient is likely to be alert and in no distress. Sometimes people do report the subjective sensation of "skipped beats." The nurse would ask the patient about subjective symptoms and assess for any signs of decreased cardiac output or problems related to decreased perfusion. The nurse would continue to observe the patient. Increase in frequency or duration of PVCs can precede ventricular tachycardia or dysthymias. **Focus:** Prioritization.

35. **Ans: 2** Decontamination in a specified area is the priority. Performing assessments delays decontamination and does not protect the total environment. Personnel should don personal protective equipment before assisting with decontamination or assessing the patients. The patients must undergo decontamination before entering cold or clean areas. The nurse should notify the charge nurse or nurse manager about communicating with security regarding potential terrorist activities. **Focus:** Prioritization.

36. **Ans: 1** In preparing for disasters, the RN should be aware of the emergency response plan. The plan gives guidance that includes the roles of team members, responsibilities, and mechanisms of reporting. Signs and symptoms of exposure to many agents will mimic common complaints, such as flulike symptoms. Discussions with colleagues and supervisors may help the individual nurse to sort through ethical dilemmas related to potential danger to self. **Focus:** Prioritization.

37. **Ans: 3, 4, 2, 5, 1** The first priority is to protect personnel, unaffected patients, bystanders, and the facility. Personal protective gear should be donned by staff before victims are assessed or treated. Decontamination of victims in a separate area is followed by triage and treatment. The incident should be reported according to protocol as information about the number of people involved, history, and signs and symptoms becomes available. **Focus:** Prioritization.

38. **Ans: 1, 2, 3, 4, 5** When the disaster plan is activated, the expectation is that a large number of patients will arrive who need triage and various levels of care. Security and communications are essential to the flow of people and information in and out of the facility. HCPs, nurses, and assistive personnel are assigned to care for patients. Laboratory and diagnostic services are required for ongoing patient care. Accurate records and patient tracking are essential during a disaster. Maintenance and engineering are responsible for the ongoing integrity of the facility's structure. In fact, all hospital personnel are needed in the immediate period after a disaster, but members of departments such as quality improvement, physical therapy, volunteer services, and occupational therapy are less likely to be performing their usual functions. **Focus:** Assignment.

39. **Ans: 2** The ED CNS would be most concerned that the staff has not had any training or practice opportunities for at least the past 3 years because training staff members is the direct responsibility of the CNS. The Joint Commission recommends biannual training practice and rehearsal; training exercises also provide data that can be used to revise and update the plan. The CNS should also alert hospital administration about the need to inventory stockpiles, to conduct an internal and external resource analysis, and to contact public health officials about increased risk in surrounding communities. **Focus:** Prioritization.

40. **Ans: 4** Any of these people may need or benefit from psychiatric counseling. Obviously, there will be variations in previous coping skills and support systems; however, a person who experienced a threat to his or her own life is at the greatest risk for psychiatric problems after a disaster incident. **Focus:** Prioritization.

41. **Ans: 2, 3, 4, 5, 6** Quickly assessing respiratory effort, level of consciousness, obvious injuries, appearance of skin (indicative of peripheral perfusion), and vital signs are appropriate for disaster triage. Other information, such as medical and surgical history, medication history, support systems, and last tetanus booster, would be collected when the staff has more time and resources. **Focus:** Prioritization.

42. **Ans: 1F, 2B, 3D, 4C, 5E, 6A** In disaster triage, the goal is to provide the greatest good for the greatest number with limited resources. Ethical considerations include prognosis, years of life saved, and age of patient. Treat the 12-year-old child with asthma first by initiating an albuterol treatment. This action is quick

to initiate, and the child or parent can be instructed to hold the apparatus while the nurse attends to other patients. The firefighter is next. The firefighter is in greater respiratory distress than the 12-year-old child; however, managing a strong combative patient is difficult and time consuming (e.g., the 12-year-old could die if too much time is spent trying to control the firefighter). Next, attend to the adolescent with a crush injury. Anxiety and tachycardia may be caused by pain or stress; however, the swelling suggests hemorrhage. The woman with burns on the forearms needs cleaning, dressings, and pain management. The child with burns over more than 70% of the anterior body should be given pain relief, comfort measures, and emotional support; however, the prognosis is very poor. The prognosis for the patient in cardiac arrest is also very poor because CPR efforts have been prolonged. This patient is likely to be unresponsive. **Focus:** Prioritization.

43. **Ans: Option 1, IV normal saline; Option 2, IV broad-spectrum antibiotics; Option 3, nasogastric (NG) tube insertion; Option 4, Abdominal radiography; Option 5, CT scan; Option 6, emergency surgery.** Strangulated intestinal obstruction is a surgical emergency. IV fluids are needed to maintain fluid and electrolyte balance. IV broad-spectrum antibiotics would be ordered because perforation can cause peritonitis. The NG tube is for decompression of the intestine. Abdominal radiography is the most useful diagnostic aid; CT scan is also a common diagnostic test. A barium enema examination is not ordered if perforation is suspected. The images and data from capsule endoscopy require lengthy processing and interpretation, thus this diagnostic tool is not used when results are urgently needed. An abdominal paracentesis can be used to diagnosis infection but would not be the first choice for this patient. Methylprednisolone is a steroid that could be used to decrease inflammation in gastrointestinal disorders, such as ulcerative colitis. After emergency surgery, the patient will be transferred from the post-anesthesia care unit to the intensive care unit or the medical-surgical unit. **Focus:** Prioritization.

44. **Ans:** While physical and sexual violence may be detected by physical examination, psychological abuse and controlling behaviors will go unnoticed unless the nurse is attuned to patients' verbal and nonverbal behaviors. According to the Emergency Nurses Association: Clinical Practice Guideline for Intimate Partner Violence, examples of physical violence include hitting, slapping, kicking, and beating. Examples of sexual violence include forced or coerced sexual activity. Examples of psychological abuse include insults, belittling, intimidation, humiliation, harmful threats or threats to take away children. Examples of controlling behavior includes isolation from friends and family; stalking; or restricting access to finances, education, employment or health care. **Focus:** Prioritization.

Patient Statements	Physical violence	Psychological violence	Sexual violence	Control behavior
"When my boyfriend wants sex, it's easier just to give in; once it's over he leaves me alone."			X	
"I have moved 3 times in the past year; she always manages to track me down."				X
"He slapped me last week; I kicked at him, but that just made him mad."	X			
"She keeps saying she'll just take the kids and disappear if I don't pay more attention to her."		X		
"If I go anywhere, even to the grocery store, he's calling me to come back home."				X
"He said I was fat and ugly and if he threw me out, nobody else would want me."		X		
"I don't like it, but he says that rectal intercourse is exciting for him."			X	
"She said that if I ever left her, she would kill herself."		X		
"He has all of the money in an account in his name; I need his permission to buy things."				X
"Things just build up. After he hits me, he apologizes; then we go back to normal."	X			

45. **Ans: 2** The city of Houston in conjunction with Homeland Security developed the most well-known response "Run-Hide-Fight" for individuals who are involved in an active shooter incident. If a safe path is located, running to a safe place and taking others if possible is the first action. Hiding in a safe place, such as a barricaded room, is the second option. Aggressively fighting the attacker is the last resort. **Focus:** Prioritization.

46. **Ans: 1D, 2G, 3B, 4F, 5A, 6H, 7I, 8E, 9C** In the hospital, the most common site of active shooter incidents is in the emergency department. The Joint Commission recommends that hospitals develop a plan that includes: 1) involving local law enforcement in the planning stages to develop an action plan and to co-ordinate drills, 2) planning communication to decrease confusion between the hospital and law enforcement and to relay information to the public and families, 3) establishing procedures for patient and staff safety, such as accounting for patients and personnel, continuing care for critically ill patients, and evacuating if necessary, 4) creating training and hands-on drills for hospital employees and first responders and separate drills for command team security officers and hospital administrators, and 5) planning for post-event activities to include debriefings or hot washes after drills and incidents to improve the plan. Post-event, mental health resources should be available through the hospital's Employee Assistance Program. **Focus:** Prioritization.

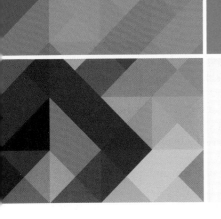

CHAPTER 22

Psychiatric/Mental Health Problems

Note: In this chapter, the term "psychiatric nursing assistant" (PNA) is used, rather than the more familiar "assistive personnel" (AP). Different facilities and localities use different titles for APs. The key point to remember in assigning tasks or making patient assignments is that APs who routinely work on a medical-surgical unit will have different skill sets than PNAs, who usually work on a psychiatric unit.

1. Which patient is the **most** likely candidate for outpatient depot antipsychotic therapy?
   1. Older man with psychosis secondary to dementia who lives with his daughter
   2. Homeless veteran with schizophrenia who occasional sleeps in a nearby shelter
   3. Housewife with bipolar disorder who has psychotic features during the manic phase
   4. Student with recently diagnosed schizophrenia who lives at home with his parents

2. What is the nurse's **most** important role in helping patients, who have schizophrenia, to benefit from a comprehensive approach that includes medication and multidisciplinary nondrug therapies?
   1. Help identify patients who would benefit from conventional psychotherapy.
   2. Refer patients to a psychiatric nurse specialist for education about the disease.
   3. Suggest that patients talk to vocational specialists for additional training.
   4. Establish a therapeutic relationship with patients and encourage participation.

3. A patient with a mental health disorder is brought to the emergency department by the police. In determining hospitalization versus discharge back into the community, which consideration is given the **highest priority**?
   1. Willingness of person to follow the treatment plan
   2. Potential for harm to self or others
   3. Availability of family or social support
   4. Ability of person to meet own basic physical needs

4. A patient who was recently diagnosed with conversion disorder is experiencing a sudden loss of vision after witnessing a violent fight between her husband and adult-age son. What is the **priority** therapeutic approach to use with this patient?
   1. Reassure her that her blindness is temporary and will resolve with time.
   2. Gently point out that she can see well enough to function independently.
   3. Encourage expression of feelings and link emotional trauma to the blindness.
   4. Teach ways to cope with blindness, such as methodically arranging personal items.

5. The charge nurse is reviewing the assignment sheet for an acute psychiatric unit. Which experienced team member should be reassigned?
   1. Male LVN assigned to an older male patient with chronic depression and excessive rumination
   2. Young male psychiatric nursing assistant assigned to a female adolescent with anorexia nervosa
   3. Female RN assigned to a newly admitted female patient who has command hallucinations and delusions of persecution
   4. Older female RN with medical-surgical experience assigned to a male patient with Alzheimer disease

6. The nurse arrives home and finds that a neighbor's (Jane's) house is on fire. A fireman is physically restraining Jane as she screams and thrashes around to get free to run back into the house. What is the nurse's **best** action?
   1. Make eye contact and encourage Jane to verbalize feelings.
   2. Physically restrain Jane so that the fireman can resume his job.
   3. Use a firm tone of voice and give Jane simple commands.
   4. Use a gentle persuading tone and ask Jane to be calm.

7. There is a patient on the rehabilitation unit who has been there for several months. He is hostile, rude, and belligerent, and no one likes to interact with him. How should the charge nurse handle the assignment?
   1. Rotate the assignment schedule so that no one has to care for him more than once or twice a week.
   2. Pair a float nurse and a nursing student and assign this team to care for the patient; they will have a fresh perspective.
   3. Identify several experienced nurses as primary caregivers and develop a plan that includes psychosocial interventions.
   4. Assign self as primary caregiver and role-model how patients should be treated.

8. After reviewing medication prescriptions on an acute psychiatric unit, which prescription is the nurse **most** likely to question?
   1. Fluoxetine for a middle-aged patient with depression
   2. Chlorpromazine for a young patient with schizophrenia
   3. Loxapine for an older adult patient with dementia and psychosis
   4. Lorazepam for a young patient with generalized anxiety disorder

9. A patient diagnosed with paranoid schizophrenia says, "Dr. Smith has killed several other patients, and now he is trying to kill me." What is the **best** response?
   1. "I have worked here a long time. No one has died. You are safe here."
   2. "What has Dr. Smith done to make you think he would like to kill you?"
   3. "All of the staff, including Dr. Smith, are here to ensure your safety."
   4. "Whenever you are concerned or nervous, talk to me or any of the nurses."

10. Which patient needs assessment **first**?
    1. A patient who is having command hallucinations
    2. A patient who is demonstrating clang associations
    3. A patient who is verbalizing ideas of reference
    4. A patient who is using neologisms

11. The nurse is talking to the primary caregiver of Martha, who was diagnosed 8 years ago with Alzheimer disease. The caregiver says, "We love Martha, but my daughter needs help with her kids, and my husband's health is poor. I really need help." Which member of the health care team should the nurse consult **first**?
    1. Health care provider to review long-term prognosis and new treatments for Alzheimer disease
    2. Psychiatric clinical nurse specialist to design behavioral modification therapies for Martha
    3. Clinical psychologist to assess caregiver for major depression and need for treatment
    4. Social worker to identify and arrange placement for Martha in an acceptable nursing home

12. The patient has a panic disorder and is having difficulty controlling his anxiety. Which symptoms are cause for **greatest** concern?
    1. His heart rate is increased, and he reports chest tightness.
    2. He demonstrates tachypnea and carpopedal spasms.
    3. He is pacing to and fro and pounding his fists together.
    4. He is muttering to himself and is easily startled.

13. The nurse is interviewing a patient with suicidal ideations and a history of major depression. Which comment is cause for **greatest** concern?
    1. "I have had problems with depression most of my adult life."
    2. "My father and my brother both committed suicide."
    3. "My wife is having health problems, and she relies on me."
    4. "I am afraid to kill myself, and I wish I had more courage."

14. A patient comes into the walk-in clinic and tells the nurse that he would like to be admitted to an alcohol rehabilitation program. Which question is the **most** important to ask?
    1. "What made you decide to enter a program at this time?"
    2. "How much alcohol do you usually consume in a day?"
    3. "When was the last time you had a drink?"
    4. "Have you been in a rehabilitation program before?"

15. The nurse is working with a health care provider (HCP) who recently started treating patients with depression. Which action by the HCP would prompt the nurse to intervene?
    1. Tells the patient and family that it may take 4 to 8 weeks before the antidepressant medication begins to relieve symptoms
    2. Prescribes 3 months of antidepressants for a patient newly diagnosed with depression and gives a 3 month follow-up appointment
    3. Instructs the patient that the initial dose is low but will gradually be increased to reach a maintenance dosage
    4. Tells the patient and the family to watch for and immediately report anxiety, agitation, irritability, or suicidal thoughts

16. A patient on the acute psychiatric unit develops neuroleptic malignant syndrome. Which task would be delegated to the psychiatric nursing assistant (PNA)?
    1. Wiping the patient's body with cool moist towels
    2. Monitoring and interpreting vital signs every 15 minutes

3. Attaching the patient to the electrocardiogram (ECG) monitor
4. Transporting the patient to the medical intensive care unit (ICU)

17. A newly graduated nurse has just started working at the acute psychiatric unit. Which patient would be the **best** to assign to this nurse?
    1. Patient who is frequently admitted for borderline personality disorder and suicidal gestures
    2. Patient admitted yesterday for disorganized schizophrenia and psychosis
    3. Patient newly admitted to determine differential diagnosis of depression, dementia, or delirium
    4. Patient newly diagnosed with major depression and rumination about loss and suicide

18. Which task can be delegated to a medical-surgical assistive personnel (AP) who has been temporarily floated to the acute psychiatric unit to help?
    1. Performing one-to-one observation of a patient who is suicidal
    2. Assisting the occupational therapist to conduct a craft class
    3. Accompanying an older adult patient who wanders on a walk outside
    4. Assisting the medication nurse who is having problems with a patient

19. The nurse has identified a patient who may be a candidate for substance addiction treatment. Which health care team member should the nurse contact to increase the likelihood of a successful long-term outcome?
    1. Call a social worker who can locate an immediately available treatment program.
    2. Call admissions to obtain the patient's voluntary consent to enter a treatment program.
    3. Consult a pharmacist about medication therapy to counter addiction.
    4. Contact the health care provider to initiate admission to a medical detoxification unit.

20. The team must apply restraints to a combative patient to prevent harm to others or to self. Which action requires the charge nurse's intervention?
    1. Psychiatric nursing assistant uses a quick-release knot to tie restraints.
    2. Health care provider (HCP) secures the restraint to the side rail.
    3. RN checks the pulses distal to the restraints.
    4. LPN/LVN explains to the patient why he is being restrained.

21. A well-known celebrity is admitted to the psychiatric unit. Several RNs from other units drop by and express an interest in seeing the patient. What is the **best** response?

1. "Please be discreet and do not interrupt the workflow."
2. "How did you find out that the patient was admitted to this unit?"
3. "Please wait. I need to call the nursing supervisor about this request."
4. "I'm sorry; the patient has asked that only family be allowed to visit."

22. An LPN/LVN complains to the charge nurse that she is always assigned to the same patient with chronic depression. What should the charge nurse do?
    1. Look at the assignment sheet and see if there is any way to switch assignments with another LPN/LVN.
    2. Tell her to care for the patient today but that her request will be considered for future assignments.
    3. Remind her that continuity of care and patient-centered care are the primary goals.
    4. Explain that patients with chronic conditions are more likely to fall under the LPN/LVN scope of practice.

23. Which person is displaying behaviors that **most** strongly suggest the need for additional screening for possible substance abuse?
    1. Person with cancer progressively needs more pain medication to achieve relief
    2. College student reports occasionally smoking marijuana during semester break
    3. Stay-at-home mom reports drinking when her kids are in school or in bed asleep
    4. Person with a fractured leg reports taking opioids and tapering off when pain subsides

24. The emergency department (ED) nurse is calling to report on a patient who will be admitted to the acute psychiatric unit. He has a history of bipolar disorder and was in an altercation that resulted in the death of another. He has contusions, abrasions, and minor lacerations. What is the **priority** question that the receiving nurse should ask?
    1. "When will the patient be transferred?"
    2. "Will a police officer be with him while he is on the unit?"
    3. "Why isn't the patient being admitted to the trauma unit?"
    4. "What is the patient's current mood and behavior?"

25. An adolescent girl is juuling all of the time with her friends. Her mother is distraught, because, "She won't stop and I know it's harming her." Which substance abuse problem will the nurse assess for?
    1. Opioid abuse
    2. Nicotine addiction
    3. Alcohol abuse
    4. Cannabinoid hyperemesis syndrome

Answer Key for this chapter begins on p. 232

26. A 23-year-old man with no known health problems says, "Well, I was a little nervous, so I smoked four or five cigarettes right before I came into the clinic." Which vital signs would be consistent with the patient's use of cigarettes?
    1. Blood pressure of 90/60 mm Hg; pulse of 60 beats/min
    2. Temperature of 100.6°F (38.1°C); respirations of 40 breaths/min
    3. Blood pressure of 140/90 mm Hg; pulse of 120 beats/min
    4. Temperature of 97.4°F (36.3°C); respirations of 30 breaths/min

27. A patient is displaying muscle spasms of the tongue, face, and neck, and his eyes are locked in an upward gaze. He has been prescribed haloperidol. Which action will the nurse take **first**?
    1. Maintain eye contact and stay with him until the spasms pass.
    2. Place the patient on aspiration precautions until the spasms subside.
    3. Obtain a prescription for intramuscular or IV diphenhydramine.
    4. Obtain a prescription for and administer an anti-seizure medication.

28. Several patients are taking antipsychotic medications and are having medication side effects. Place the following patients in **priority** order for additional assessment and appropriate interventions, with 1 being the **most** critical and 4 being the least.
    1. A patient who is taking trifluoperazine and has a temperature of 103.6°F (39.8°C) with tachycardia, muscular rigidity, and dysphagia
    2. A patient who is taking fluphenazine and has dry mouth and dry eyes, urinary hesitancy, constipation, and photosensitivity
    3. A patient who is taking loxapine and has a protruding tongue with lip smacking and spastic facial distortions
    4. A patient who is taking clozapine and reports a sore throat, fever, malaise, and flulike symptoms that began about 6 weeks ago after starting the new antipsychotic medication; white blood cell count is 2000/mm³ (2.0 × 10⁹/L)
    _____, _____, _____, _____

29. The patient tells the nurse that he drinks three or four servings of alcohol every day. He also reports frequently taking acetaminophen for stress-related headaches. Based on this information, which laboratory test results are the **most** important to follow up on?
    1. Renal function tests
    2. Liver function tests
    3. Cardiac enzymes
    4. Serum electrolytes

30. The nurse is caring for a young patient with type 1 diabetes who has sustained injuries when she tried to commit suicide by crashing her car. Her blood glucose (BG) level is 700 mg/dL (38.8 mmol/L), but she refuses insulin; however, she wants the pain medication. What is the **best** action?
    1. Notify the charge nurse and make arrangements to transfer to intensive care.
    2. Explain the significance of BG and insulin and call the health care provider (HCP).
    3. Withhold the pain medication until she agrees to accept the insulin.
    4. Give her the pain medication and document the refusal of the insulin.

31. The health care provider recently prescribed rivastigmine twice daily for a 62-year-old patient who lives at home with his wife. Based on this information, which additional assessment would the home health nurse plan to perform **first**?
    1. Assess for psychotic features, such as hallucinations.
    2. Perform a comprehensive pain assessment.
    3. Assess for cognitive deficits and memory loss.
    4. Observe for fine and gross motor deficits.

32. Which behavior would be the **most** problematic and require vigilance to prevent danger to self or others?
    1. Avolition
    2. Echolalia
    3. Motor agitation
    4. Stupor

33. A patient frequently comes to the clinic with repeated complaints of nausea, constipation, and "excruciating stomach pain." Multiple diagnostic tests have consistently yielded negative results. What is the **priority** nursing intervention for this patient?
    1. Advocate for the patient to have a psychiatric consultation.
    2. Make an appointment as soon as possible with the same health care provider (HCP) for continuity of care.
    3. Perform a physical assessment to identify any physical abnormalities.
    4. Assess for concurrent symptoms of depression or anxiety.

34. An older man was admitted for palliative care of terminal pancreatic cancer. His wife stated, "We don't want hospice; he wants treatment." The patient requested discharge and home health visits. Several hours after discharge, the man committed suicide with a gun. Which people should participate in a root cause analysis of this sentinel event? **Select all that apply.**
    1. The wife and all immediate family members
    2. Only the health care provider (HCP) who discharged the patient
    3. Any nurse who cared for the patient during hospitalization

4. The case manager who arranged home visits for the patient
5. Only the nurse who discharged the patient
6. All HCPs who were involved in the care of the patient

35. An adolescent girl is admitted to the medical-surgical unit for diagnostic evaluation and nutritional support related to anorexia nervosa. She is mildly dehydrated, her potassium level is 3.5 mEq/L (3.5 mmol/L), and she has experienced weight loss of more than 25% within the past 3 months. What is the **primary** collaborative goal?
   1. Assist her to increase feelings of control.
   2. Decrease power struggles over eating.
   3. Resolve dysfunctional family roles.
   4. Restore normal nutrition and weight.

36. In caring for a patient who is admitted to a medical surgical unit for treatment of anorexia nervosa, which task can be delegated to assistive personnel (AP)?
   1. Sitting with the patient during meals and for 1 to 1½ hours after meals
   2. Observing for and reporting ritualistic behaviors related to food
   3. Obtaining special food for the patient when she requests it
   4. Weighing the patient daily and reinforcing that she is underweight

37. Nurse B frequently asks to be assigned to care for patients who require opioids for pain; drug counts involving Nurse B frequently show discrepancies. Nurse A suspects that Nurse B may have a substance abuse problem. Based on the ethical principle of negligence, what should Nurse A do **first**?
   1. Talk to Nurse B and give counsel about the ethical issues of taking patients' medications.
   2. Continue to assess Nurse B's behavior for other signs and symptoms of abuse.

3. Work closely with Nurse B to give support and help to reduce stress of workload.
4. Report facts (e.g., date, time, circumstance) about Nurse B's behavior to the nursing supervisor.

38. A male-to-female transgender patient (transwoman) is admitted to an acute care psychiatric unit for depression and suicidal ideations. On her arrival, several other patients display suspicion and contempt and verbal harassment is directed toward the woman. What should the charge nurse do **first**?
   1. Isolate the patient and explain that the action is meant for her safety and privacy.
   2. Make a general announcement to patients and staff that bullying is not tolerated.
   3. Assess the patient's reaction to the comments and nonverbal behaviors.
   4. Gently suggest that the patient could temporarily adopt natal gender appearance.

39. For several years, a patient diagnosed with hypochondriasis has undergone multiple diagnostic tests for "cancer," with no evidence of organic disease. Today he declares, "I know I have a brain tumor. My appointment is tomorrow, but I can't wait!" What is the **most** therapeutic response?
   1. Present reality: "Sir, you have been seen many times in this clinic and had many diagnostic tests. The results have always been negative."
   2. Encourage expression of feelings: "Let me spend some time with you. Tell me about what you are feeling and why you think you have a brain tumor."
   3. Set boundaries: "Sir, I will take your vital signs, but then I am going to call your case manager so that you can discuss the scheduled appointment."
   4. Respect the patient's wishes: "Sir, sit down and I will make sure that you see the health care provider right away. Don't worry; we will take care of you."

Answer Key for this chapter begins on p. 232

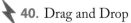 **40.** Drag and Drop

Scenario: Two patients had to be restrained and isolated for an episode of physical aggression. The patients and staff were upset by the incident. The disruption of the milieu prompted the charge nurse to conduct a staff in-service that included, the principles of "least restrictive" interventions to be used when patients are in danger of harming self or others.

Based on the principles of "least restrictive", what is the correct order for interventions that are designed to prevent patients from harming self or others?

Instructions: Place the interventions in the correct order from the least restrictive to the most restrictive. In the left column are interventions that the staff can use. In the right column, write the number (1-9) to indicate the correct order: 1 being the least restrictive and 9 being the most restrictive.

Interventions to prevent patients from harming self or others	Order of interventions
a. Escort the patient to a quiet room for a time out.	
b. Restrain the patient's arms and legs with wrist and ankle restraints.	
c. Verbally instruct the patient to stop the unacceptable behavior (i.e., yelling)	
d. Accompany the patient out into the garden courtyard.	
e. Observe and quickly identify signs of escalating aggression (e.g., pacing, loud comments)	
f. Restrain the patient's upper extremities with wrist restraints.	
g. Place the patient in isolation room with psychiatric nursing assistant observing.	
h. Calmly tell the patient the expected action that he/she should take (e.g., move to another part of the day room)	
i. Use distraction (e.g., talk to the person, or engage him/her in an activity)	
j. Address the person by name	
k. Document behaviors, type of intervention, response to each intervention.	

41. Enhanced Hot Spot

Scenario: A parent reports that her 19-year-old son started to have episodes of frustration and anxiety about 1 year ago. His grades declined and he withdrew from school activities and socializing with friends. After high school graduation, he had no interest in going to college or getting a job. Lately, he wants to go to the Antarctic, to get away from the voices that are always telling him what to do. He believes that eating pure Antarctic snow/foods will make him feel better. He has lost weight, because he rejects "unpure" food that his mother offers him.

Instructions: Underline or highlight the factors that indicate the patient may have a thought disorder, such as schizophrenia.

Vital signs:
Temperature 98.7° F (37°C)
Pulse 80 beats/min
Respirations 14 breaths/min
Blood pressure 115/78 mmHg

Assessment findings: Height 5' 9" (1.75 meters), Weight 125 lb (56.7 kg). Clothes are dirty and disheveled. Affect is flat. Displays poverty of speech and thought.

Which information (signs, symptoms, and history) supports the nurse's hypothesis that the 19-year old may have a thought disorder, such as schizophrenia?

42. Drag and Drop

Scenario: A patient needs clonazepam 0.25 mg PO. The pharmacy delivers lorazepam 2-mg tablets. A nursing student asks the supervising nurse if clonazepam and lorazepam are interchangeable or if they are the same drug.

What is the correct sequence of the steps that the nurse will teach the student to help decrease or prevent medication errors?

Instructions: Steps are listed in the left column. In the right column write in the number to indicate the correct sequence of steps to prevent medication errors; 1 being the first step and 9 being the last step.

Steps to prevent medication errors	Sequence of steps
a. Advise the pharmacy of any corrections (if necessary).	
b. Recognize that "look-alike, sound-alike" drugs increase the chances of error.	
c. Consult a medication book or electronic resource to verify the purpose of the drugs and generic and brand names.	
d. Check the original medication prescription to verify what was prescribed.	
e. Write an incident report if a system error is occurring.	
f. Call the health care provider (HCP) for clarification of the prescription (if necessary).	
g. Verify (if unsure) that the patient has a condition that would require the prescribed medication.	
h. Enter HCP's new prescription (if necessary) into the record as a phone order.	
i. Document notification of the HCP and pharmacy (if necessary) into the medical record.	

    Answer Key for this chapter begins on p. 232

Answers

1. **Ans: 2** Depot antipsychotic therapy uses long-acting injectable medications. These medications are used for long-term maintenance for schizophrenia for patients who may have some difficulties with adherence to taking medications. The homeless veteran has the least amount of social support and stability, which are factors in medication adherence. For the older adult patient with dementia and psychosis, identifying underlying factors and then behavioral therapies would be recommended first. Psychotic features in the manic phase of bipolar disorder would be treated as an acute episode. The student has the support of family, and the health care team will try to work with the patient and the family to build behaviors that support lifetime adherence to therapy. **Focus:** Prioritization.

2. **Ans: 4** The nurse and the psychiatric nursing assistant spend more time with the patients than any of the other members of the health care team; thus establishing a good therapeutic relationship is essential to building trust; increasing social skills; encouraging medication adherence; and suggesting participation in educational, socialization, and vocational opportunities. Conventional psychotherapy is generally not used with patients with schizophrenia. **Focus:** Prioritization.

3. **Ans: 2** Potential for harm to self or others would be the priority; however, the other options are also important in planning for long-term outcomes. **Focus:** Prioritization.

4. **Ans: 4** Patients with conversion disorders are experiencing symptoms, even though there is no identifiable organic cause; therefore the patient should be assisted in learning ways to cope and live with the disability. The patient may physically be able to see, but pointing this out is not helpful. Encouraging the expression of feelings is okay, but it is premature to expect the patient to link the fight to her blindness. It is likely that the sudden onset of blindness will resolve, but the priority therapeutic approach is teaching her ways to cope in the meantime. **Focus:** Prioritization.

5. **Ans: 2** Adolescents, in general, are self-conscious in the presence of members of the opposite sex, and teenagers with anorexia are overly concerned with their appearance; therefore it would be better to assign this patient to a mature female staff member. An experienced LVN is able to set boundaries and to assist patients with chronic health problems. An experienced RN should be assigned to new admissions and to patients with acute safety issues. An RN with medical-surgical experience would be well acquainted with care issues related to dementia. **Focus:** Assignment.

6. **Ans: 3** Jane is experiencing a panic level of anxiety, and initially she needs firm, simple, and direct instructions. It may be very difficult for the nurse to safely restrain Jane. Speaking softly and gently and encouraging her to express feelings are appropriate when her anxiety is more under control. **Focus:** Prioritization.

7. **Ans: 3** This patient has trouble with interpersonal interactions, so consistent caregivers who use psychosocial interventions have the best chance of developing a functional nurse-patient relationship. Rotating the assignment sheet to give the staff a break and using float staff are frequent strategies that are used, but these are not necessarily the best for the patient. Taking the patient may seem like the easiest solution for the charge nurse, but in the long run, strengthening and supporting the staff are better strategies. **Focus:** Assignment.

8. **Ans: 3** Conventional (first-generation) antipsychotics are usually not prescribed for older adult patients with psychosis secondary to dementia because of the increased incidence of death, usually from cardiac problems or infection. Fluoxetine for depression, chlorpromazine for schizophrenia, and lorazepam for generalized anxiety disorder are viable options. **Focus:** Prioritization. **Test-Taking Tip:** In general, older adults patients have more complex issues related to medications. While studying for the NCLEX® Examination, pay attention to information that highlights the care of older adults.

9. **Ans: 4** The nurse can acknowledge the patient's fears without agreeing or disagreeing with his accusation. Directing him to talk to the nursing staff provides a source of emotional support and an action that he can use to decrease his anxiety. Telling the patient that no one has died and that the staff will ensure safety is presenting reality; however, he has a delusional belief and arguments should be avoided. Asking him to explain his rationale for his beliefs encourages him to elaborate on his delusion. **Focus:** Prioritization.

10. **Ans: 1** During command hallucinations, the patient may be getting a command to harm self or others; content must be assessed. Ideas of reference occur when an ordinary thing or event (e.g., a song on the radio) has personal significance (e.g., belief that the lyrics were written for him or her). Ideas of reference could escalate into aggression if delusions of persecution are present; content must be assessed. Clang association is a meaningless rhyming of words, and neologisms are new words created by patients. These communication patterns create frustration for staff and patients, but there is no need for immediate intervention.

Focus: Prioritization. **Test-Taking Tip:** Safety is a priority concern for all patients. In identifying safety issues for patients with active psychosis, the potential concern is frequently harm to self or to others.

11. **Ans: 4** The caregiver needs assistance to identify and locate an alternative care situation for Martha. The family has been coping and caring for Martha for a long time, but family circumstances and a patient's condition will change over time. The nurse may do additional assessment to see if the caregiver needs to be referred for depression, guilt, or anxiety related to having to make this change for Martha. New treatments and behavioral modification can be attempted, but currently there are no therapies that reverse the gradual decline. **Focus:** Prioritization.

12. **Ans: 3** All of these symptoms signal an increase of anxiety; however, physically aggressive behavior signals a danger to others and to self. Verbal intervention is still possible, but the pacing and fist pounding are a step above the other symptoms. Tachycardia and chest tightness are assessed, but should abate as the patient becomes less anxious. Carpopedal spasms occur during hyperventilation; assisting the patient to breathe in a paper bag will help. Muttering to self can be interrupted by using a normal conversational tone and topic. **Focus:** Prioritization.

13. **Ans: 2** The patient has a strong family history of completed suicide, which is an increased risk factor. The patient may believe that other family members have successfully used suicide to solve their problems. A long history of depression suggests that the problem is chronic; assess for treatment history, risk factors, and coping strategies. Having a feeling of responsibility toward others and feeling fear are protective factors that can be used in the treatment plan. **Focus:** Prioritization.

14. **Ans: 3** Before someone enters an alcohol rehabilitation program, there should be a medically supervised detoxification. This patient has walked in off the street; therefore the nurse must determine whether he is at risk for withdrawal symptoms. Withdrawal from alcohol can be life threatening. The other questions are relevant and are likely to be included in the interview. **Focus:** Prioritization.

15. **Ans: 2** Patients with depression are at high risk for suicide, and antidepressants can be used to commit suicide. For the patient who was recently diagnosed with depression and prescribed antidepressants, the nurse intervenes because a small number of doses should be prescribed and dispensed, and follow-up should be weekly to allow for close monitoring and assessment. The other options are correct information to share with patients and family members. **Focus:** Prioritization.

16. **Ans: 1** A PNA can perform this simple cooling measure with minimal instruction. Neuroleptic malignant syndrome is a rare but potentially fatal reaction to antipsychotic medication. Symptoms include fever, altered mental status, muscle rigidity, and autonomic instability. The RN should continuously interpret vital signs, although taking vital signs can be delegated. Assistive personnel in the ICU and emergency department will be familiar with how to attach ECG leads, but PNAs will rarely have occasion to use this equipment; therefore the RN should perform this task. The RN (or health care provider) should accompany the patient to the ICU, although the PNA could assist. **Focus:** Delegation. **Test-Taking Tip:** In assigning, delegating, or supervising tasks to ancillary personnel, be familiar with state laws that relate to the scope of practice for these individuals. Because it is impossible to list every task and every circumstance, you must learn to analyze the situation and the skills of available personnel. This will help you to determine if the task is within their scope of practice.

17. **Ans: 4** Although the patient is ruminating about suicide, in the early phase of major depression the patient has minimal energy to act. The danger for suicide will increase as the medication and therapy begin to help. A new nurse lacks experience with therapeutic boundary setting that is necessary for patients with borderline personality disorder. Psychotic patients can seem very threatening to new nurses and it takes experience to interpret psychotic behavior. Depression, dementia, and delirium have some behavior and symptom overlap; this patient should be assigned to an experienced nurse until the delirium is treated or ruled out. **Focus:** Assignment.

18. **Ans: 3** Medical-surgical APs assist patients to ambulate, and they frequently care for older confused patients. Performing one-to-one suicide watch requires experience to recognize behaviors and to immediately alert the nurse and intervene. Assisting the occupational therapist or medication nurse may be possible, but the medical-surgical AP is unlikely to be familiar with the behavioral interventions required in these situations. **Focus:** Assignment.

19. **Ans: 1** Early treatment contributes to success; however, one of the greatest barriers in addiction treatment is locating a treatment program that can immediately accept a patient. Limited finances and lack of comprehensive programs make locating a program even more difficult. Medication therapy is one important aspect. Medical detoxification is also important, but it is only one step in a long treatment process. Patients' voluntary participation and consent are ideal, but pressure and support from family, friends, or employers can increase the likelihood of success. **Focus:** Prioritization.

20. **Ans: 2** The restraints must be tied to a stationary portion of the bed. HCPs are usually less familiar with how the beds function. Quick-release knots are for safety in case the restraints need to be quickly

removed. Distal pulses should be checked. The HCP or RN is usually responsible for explaining the restraint procedure; however, restraining a combative patient is rarely a planned event, and the caregiver who has the best relationship with the patient may be the best spokesperson. **Focus:** Supervision.

21. **Ans: 2** Determine how the nurses found out about the patient's admission. This is a serious Health Insurance Portability and Accountability Act violation, and information disclosure must be immediately stopped. Unfortunately for these RNs, administration will have to be notified, but as a professional courtesy, it would be better if they went directly to the supervisor and admitted the error rather than immediately calling the supervisor and reporting them. **Focus:** Prioritization.

22. **Ans: 2** Switching the assignments at shift change or midshift creates delays for everyone, so politely ask her to continue for the day. Nevertheless, her request is not unreasonable; dealing with depressed patients can be very exhausting, so consider her request for future assignments. Although many patients benefit from having the same caregiver, a chronically depressed patient might benefit from stimulation by various caregivers. Explaining scope of practice and continuity of care is probably not necessary and may seem condescending. **Focus:** Assignment, Supervision.

23. **Ans: 3** A woman who is drinking when her children are out of sight is displaying substance use that is not based on medical needs or social norms. The college student is using an illegal substance, but at this point, the frequency does not suggest that it is a compulsive problem. The person with cancer and person with a fracture are using medications for pain as indicated. **Focus:** Prioritization.

24. **Ans: 4** Knowing the current mood and behavior is the priority so that the nurse can prepare for physical or chemical restraints, isolation or a private room, and allocation and assignment of staff members. The other questions are also relevant; however, the nurse should be aware that challenging the appropriateness of the psychiatric unit versus the trauma unit requires contacting the nursing supervisor because the ED nurse will not be able to resolve this issue. **Focus:** Prioritization.

25. **Ans: 2** The nurse would assess for signs/symptoms of nicotine addiction. Juul is a type of e-cigarette that is popular among children and teenagers. It comes in flavors (e.g., fruity or minty). The device may look like a pen or a USB flash drive. It is easy to use and produces no odor. There is a higher concentration of nicotine compared with other electronic nicotine device systems. (For additional information see http://www.center4research.org/the-dangers-of-juuling/). **Focus:** Prioritization.

26. **Ans: 3** Nicotine promotes the release of norepinephrine and epinephrine. This can result in

vasoconstriction, which elevates the pulse rate and the blood pressure. **Focus:** Prioritization.

27. **Ans: 3** IV administration of diphenhydramine will rapidly alleviate the symptoms. The patient is experiencing medication side effects. This condition is frightening and uncomfortable for the patient, but it is not usually harmful. Swallow precautions will not harm the patient, but waiting for the spasms to pass delays the most appropriate intervention. **Focus:** Prioritization.

28. **Ans: 1, 4, 3, 2** The highest priority is patient 1, who has symptoms of neuroleptic malignant syndrome, which is rare but potentially fatal. This patient should be transferred to a medical unit. Patient 4 may have agranulocytosis. The mortality rate is high, and interventions include discontinuing the medication, aggressively treating the infection, and ensuring that the patient is not exposed to others with infections. Patient 3 has symptoms of tardive dyskinesia, which should be reported to the health care provider. A new medication, valbenazine (Ingrezza) was recently approved for the treatment of tardive dyskinesia. Side effects include somnolence and possible QT prolongation. Patient 2 is showing anticholinergic effects, which can be treated symptomatically (i.e., provide sips of water or hard candy, encourage use of artificial tears, place a warm towel on the abdomen, give stool softeners, and encourage the use of sunglasses). **Focus:** Prioritization.

29. **Ans: 2** Regular, even moderate, consumption of alcohol and excessive use of acetaminophen (maximum dose is 4000 mg/day) can cause fatal liver damage. Some authorities recommend that people who drink moderately should limit the total daily dose of acetaminophen to 2 g/day. **Focus:** Prioritization.

30. **Ans: 2** Explain that insulin is a priority because life-threatening ketoacidosis may already be in progress. If she is already aware of the dangers of an elevated BG level, then her refusal suggests ongoing suicidal intent and the HCP should be notified so that steps can be taken to override her refusal (potentially a court order). A BG level of over 600 mg/dL (33.3 mmol/L) can be criterion for transfer to intensive care, but making arrangements for transfer is time consuming, and treatment of the elevated BG should begin as soon as possible. Withholding pain medication is unethical, and merely documenting refusal of insulin is inappropriate because of the elevated BG and possible ongoing suicidal intent. **Focus:** Prioritization.

31. **Ans: 3** Rivastigmine is prescribed for mild to moderate cognitive impairment that occurs in Alzheimer disease. The medication does not improve cognition but may slow the decline. It is likely that the nurse will also assess the other areas to establish baseline information. Severe Alzheimer disease will eventually affect motor activity. Psychosis can occur in patients who have dementia. Later in the disease course,

the patient may not be able to verbally express pain. **Focus:** Prioritization.

32. **Ans: 3** All unusual behavior requires ongoing assessment, intervention, and documentation; however, motor agitation presents the greatest safety issue because excessive physical activity such as running about or flailing the arms and legs creates a risk for injury to self and others or exhaustion (to the point of death). Avolition is a lack of energy in initiating activities. Echolalia is pathologically repeating other people's words or phrases. Stupor is a state in which the patient may remain motionless for a prolonged period. **Focus:** Prioritization.

33. **Ans: 3** The health care team must always be vigilant for actual physical disease; however, the patient most likely has an undiagnosed somatoform disorder, which is a chronic and severe psychological condition in which the patient experiences physical symptoms but without apparent organic cause. Depression and anxiety are common among patients with somatoform disorders. After physical disease has been ruled out, the diagnosis of somatoform disorder should be verified. Having emotional support from a consistent HCP is often the most effective approach for somatoform disorders. Thus all of the options would be included in the care plan. **Focus:** Prioritization.

34. **Ans: 3, 4, 6** Everyone who was involved in the direct care of the patient should be invited to participate. The purpose of this root cause analysis is to review the event to identify behaviors, signs, or signals of risk for suicide. This information would be used to increase the staff's awareness to prevent future similar events. Inviting the wife and family is not appropriate because the performance of the staff is internally reviewed to improve performance. The purpose is not to fix blame or to create a situation that engenders guilt or conflict for the wife or family (or the staff). Likewise, the purpose of the analysis is not to provide psychotherapy or emotional support for the wife or family. (Referrals should be made for this.) **Focus:** Assignment.

35. **Ans: 4** If the patient meets the criteria for admission to a medical-surgical unit, nutritional restoration is the primary concern. Concurrently, the health care team will assist the patient to achieve success in the other areas. **Focus:** Prioritization.

36. **Ans: 1** The AP should be instructed to observe the amount of food eaten and ensure that the patient is not throwing out the food. After meals, observation is necessary to ensure that the patient does not induce vomiting. Ritualistic behaviors can be subtle or difficult to define. Observation for these behaviors cannot be delegated. Requests for special foods could be delaying tactics or attempts to manipulate the staff. The AP should not be responsible for deciding if food requests are appropriate. Daily weights may not be ordered, because this could increase the patient's emotional focus on weight. In addition, repeatedly telling

the patient that she is underweight is counterproductive because she does not believe she is underweight. **Focus:** Delegation.

37. **Ans: 4** Nurse A should report factual events to the nursing supervisor. The other actions may be well intended, but they serve to enable Nurse B's behavior by delaying confrontation and resolution of the suspected substance abuse. Negligence is failure to meet the standard of care. Intentional or unintentional actions that increase risk or harm to patients are considered negligence. Reporting suspicious behaviors is for the safety of patients and coworkers. **Focus:** Prioritization.

38. **Ans: 3** The charge nurse would first assess the patient's reaction to what is happening. The patient is in a fragile state and should be encouraged to verbalize feelings and preferences. Based on the assessment findings, the nurse can plan interventions to help the patient feel safe and comfortable. **Focus:** Prioritization.

39. **Ans: 3** The case manager has a relationship with the patient, knows the specific details of agreements made with the patient, and is the most capable of helping him to decrease anxiety and preoccupation with physical symptoms. In general, presenting reality does not have an impact on patients with hypochondriasis. Encouraging expression of feelings and following the patient's wishes contribute to secondary gains of maintaining the sick role. **Focus:** Prioritization.

40. **Ans: 1e, 2j, 3c, 4h, 5i, 6d, 7a, 8g, 9f, 10b, 11k** The least restrictive method starts with the quick identification of escalating aggression to initiate early intervention. Addressing the person by name is the best way to make a therapeutic connection with a confused, agitated, or highly anxious patient. Clear and concise directions are given to stop the undesirable behavior and then the person is directed to independently do an alternative and acceptable behavior. Distraction is a step up from independent behavior because a staff member is selecting and guiding the patient's actions. The patient should be allowed to stay in public areas if possible, and then progressively moved to more isolated spaces. After exhausting less restrictive methods, the patient can be physically (or chemically) restrained for safety. All interventions and patient responses should be carefully documented to validate progression from least restrictive to most restrictive. **Focus:** Prioritization.

41. **Ans:** A parent reports that her **19-year-old** son started to have episodes of **frustration and anxiety** about 1 year ago. His **grades declined** and he **withdrew from school activities and socializing with friends**. After high school graduation, he had **no interest** in going to college or getting a job. Lately, he wants to go to the Antarctic to get away from **the voices that are always telling him what to do**. He believes that eating pure Antarctic snow/foods will make him feel better. His mother reports, he has **lost**

weight, because he rejects the **"unpure" food** that his mother offers him. Vital signs: T 98.7° F (37°C), P 80, R 14, BP 115/78 mmHg. Assessment: Height: 5' 9" (1.75 meters), Weight: **125 lbs (56.7 kg). Clothes are dirty and disheveled. Affect is flat. Displays poverty of speech and thought.** Schizophrenia often starts in adolescence or young adulthood. For this patient, the nurse considers the onset and gradual progression of the symptoms. Early signs/symptoms are frustration and anxiety that worsen to a progressive loss of function in school, work or social activities. There is a gradual decline of hygiene and ability to meet basic needs. The negative symptoms of avolition, flat affect, poverty of thought and speech and decreased emotional expression further contribute to the person's ability to interact with his/her environment. Positive symptoms include hallucinations (auditory being the most common) and delusions (fixed false belief). There are other thought disorders that have similar symptoms, such as, delusional disorder, schizoaffective disorders, schizophreniform disorder and brief psychotic disorder. **Focus:** Prioritization.

42. **Ans: 1b, 2d, 3c, 4g, 5f, 6h, 7a, 8i, 9e**   The first step is to maintain an awareness of the ways that medication errors can occur. Check the original prescription for legibility and clarification. (If the prescription is handwritten, these two drugs could easily be mistaken if the handwriting is not legible.) Consult a drug reference to determine the purpose of the prescribed medication; check to see if clonazepam and lorazepam are interchangeable or different names for the same drug. (Note: Medications become familiar with clinical practice and experience. Experienced nurses will recognize that clonazepam and lorazepam are not the same drug and therefore may not consult a reference; however, all nurses should continue to look up any new or unfamiliar drugs.) The patient should have a condition that warrants the prescribed medication (if unsure the student would be directed to go and look at the patient's medical records). The HCP is notified if the prescription is not clear or if the medication does not seem appropriate for the patient's condition. (HCPs can also mistake drug names.) If the HCP gives a new prescription, this is immediately entered onto the order sheet as a phone prescription. Advise the pharmacy about any errors or changes so that the correct medication is delivered. Documentation in the nurses' notes would include a brief explanation about HCP and pharmacy notification (e.g., Dr. S contacted for clarification of clonazepam; pharmacy notified about prescription change). An incident report is submitted to evaluate circumstances and prevent system errors in the future. **Focus:** Prioritization.

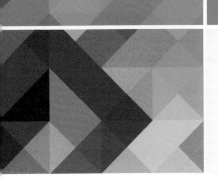

CHAPTER 23

NCLEX Next Generation

Questions

1. Drag and Drop

Scenario: An older patient with early stage Alzheimer's disease sustained a hip fracture after falling. He has been discharged and is returning home to live with his wife. He qualifies for home health visits through Medicare. The home health team includes: RN, LPN, physical therapist, social worker and a home health aide.

Which member of the home health team is best to assign or delegate for each intervention?

Instructions: Staff members are listed in the left-hand column. In the right-hand column, in the space provided, write in the letter for the best member of the home health team for each intervention. Note that all responses will be used and may be used more than once.

Staff Member	Intervention
a. RN	1. _____ Assist the patient to take a bath
b. LPN/LVN	2. _____ Administer prescribed medications
c. Home health aide	3. _____ Assess patient's memory and level of cognitive function
d. Physical therapist	4. _____ Teach patient and wife about memory aids (e.g., post-a-notes)
e. Social worker	5. _____ Assist wife to organize pill box for routine medications
	6. _____ Assess patient's strength, balance and movement.
	7. _____ Accompany the patient for short walks in the garden
	8. _____ Teach patient how to use a walker and the bathroom handrails
	9. _____ Advise patient and family about community resources
	10. _____ Help patient and family to understand Medicare benefits
	11. _____ Assess wife's risk for caregiver stress
	12. _____ Monitor for safety issues related to changes in behavior or safety risks in the environment

⚡ **2.** Cloze

Scenario: The nurse is caring for a 57-year-old African American man who came to the ophthalmologist for his annual eye examination. The patient is aware that_____1_____ is the leading cause of blindness among African Americans. If the patient has the most common type, the first symptom is likely to be _____2_____. To assist the ophthalmologist in making the diagnosis, the nurse will prepare the patient for _____3_____.

Instructions: Complete the sentences by choosing the most probable option for the missing information that corresponds with the same numbered list of options provided.

Option 1	Option 2	Option 3
Retinal detachment	Excruciating pain in or around the eye	Amsler grid
Glaucoma	Loss and compromise of peripheral vision	Snellen visual acuity chart
Macular degeneration	Curtain-like obstruction across the visual field	Ultrasound
Cataracts	Blurred and darkened vision with blind spots	Intraocular pressure measurements

⚡ **3.** Enhanced Hot Spot

Scenario: A 72-year-old woman is brought to the emergency department by her daughter, who reports, "Mom seems more confused and irritable than usual. She is not eating or drinking very much. She is unusually restless during the day and doesn't sleep throughout the night. She is spending a lot of time in the bathroom, but she gets mad when I ask her what she is doing in there. Her underwear has a strong urine odor and pink-tinged stains. She has mild dementia and she takes a blood pressure medication and a pill for diabetes."

Instructions: Underline or highlight information (signs, symptoms, verbal reports, history, assessment findings) that indicates to the nurse that the patient may have a UTI with a possible risk for urosepsis.

Vital signs:
Temperature 99.3° F (37.38°C)
Pulse 100 beats/min
Respirations 24 breaths/min
Blood Pressure 130/78 mmHg
Oxygen Saturation 96%
Blood glucose (fingerstick) 160mg/dL (8.9 mmol/L)

Assessment findings: Alert, oriented to self, speech clear. Follows simple instructions but is irritable and distractable. PERRLA (pupils equal, round, reactive to light and accommodation). Breath sounds clear and equal bilaterally. Respirations even and unlabored. Skin turgor poor, mucous membranes dry. Denies pain at any source. Assisted to the toilet and voids a small amount of dark amber urine with a strong odor. Becomes anxious and is reluctant to leave the bathroom. The nurse reviews the signs and symptoms, history, assessment findings and the daughter's observations. Which information leads the nurse to suspect that the patient has a urinary tract infection (UTI) and is at risk for urosepsis?

Answer Key for this chapter begins on p. 246

4. Matrix

Scenario: In order to maximize efficiency and safely accomplish care for a group of patients, the charge nurse must assign or delegate patient care interventions to the nursing staff. Available staff includes an RN, LPN/LVN, and an AP. All of these staff members are experienced and familiar with the routines of the unit.

Instructions: For each intervention place an X in the box to indicate whether the action is best delegated or assigned to the RN, LPN/LVN, or AP.

Intervention	RN	LPN/LVN	AP
Take vital signs every 4 hours or as directed			
Check color and temperature of fingers for a patient with a forearm cast.			
Change linens for patients as needed.			
Assist patients to ambulate in the hallway, as ordered by the HCP.			
Report if any patient has pain or discomfort.			
Assist older patient with weakness to turn every 2 hours.			
Give preoperative teaching to a patient about patient-controlled analgesia pump and measures to prevent postoperative complications			
Assess for pain on a patient who has a kidney stone			
Assess relief of heat application for patient with lower back pain			
Perform admission assessment on a patient admitted for chest pain and shortness of breath			
Evaluate patient's ability to independently perform colostomy care			

5. Extended Multiple Response

Scenario: The charge nurse on a medical-surgical unit is making patient assignments for the day. The team for 10 patients includes 3 experienced staff members: RN, LPN/LVN and an assistive personnel (AP).

Which patients can be assigned to the LPN/LVN who will function under the supervision of an RN?

Instructions: Place an X, in the space provided, or highlight each patient that can be assigned to an LPN/LVN who will function under the supervision of an RN or charge nurse. **Select all that apply**.

1. _____ Patient underwent a toe amputation and has diabetic neuropathic pain.
2. _____ Patient has a leg cast and needs neuro-circ checks and as needed (PRN) hydrocodone.
3. _____ Patient with terminal cancer has severe pain but is refusing pain medication.
4. _____ Patient reports abdominal pain after being kicked, punched, and beaten.
5. _____ Patient with arthritis needs scheduled pain medications and heat applications.
6. _____ Patient needs preoperative teaching about pain management and chest tube.
7. _____ Patient transferred from long-term care for evaluation of change of mental status.
8. _____ Patient with hemiplegia needs oral antibiotics and a dressing change for pressure injury.
9. _____ Patient has dementia and was treated for pneumonia and is awaiting transfer back to a memory care unit
10. _____ Patient with chronic renal failure needs teaching about dialysis and transplant

Answer Key for this chapter begins on p. 246

6. Cloze _____

Scenario: A 54-year-old male is admitted to the ED with a severe headache, nausea, vomiting, and blurred vision. He has a history of hypertension and smokes 2 packs of cigarettes a day. He is prescribed Lisinopril.

Vital Signs:
Temperature 98.6°F (37°C)
Oxygen saturation 95% on room air
Respirations 20 breaths/min
Mean arterial pressure (MAP) 160

Assessment findings: Alert, oriented, restless and states he is frightened. Chest sounds clear bilateral, diminished in the bases. Cardiac monitor shows sinus tachycardia with infrequent PVC's. Bounding radial and femoral pulses are present bilateral. Auscultation of the heart reveals an S3. Pedal edema is 2+ pitting.

The nurse suspects the patient's problem is ____1____. The first nursing action is to____2____ in order to ____3____. The nurse anticipates the healthcare provider (HCP) will order____4____.

Instructions: Complete the sentences below by choosing the most probable option for the omitted information that corresponds with the same numbered list of options provided.

Option 1	Option 2	Option 3	Option 4
Left sided heart failure	Assess pupil reaction	Maintain oxygenation	Furosemide 40mg intravenously
Right sided heart failure	Insert a saline lock	Decrease intracranial pressure	Hydrocodone 5mg oral
Panic attack	Place in a semi-fowlers position	Provide access for medication	Ativan 0.5mg oral
Asthma	Apply 2 liters of oxygen by nasal cannula	Assess for intracranial hemorrhage	Labetalol 20mg Intravenously
Hypertensive emergency			

7. Cloze _____

Scenario: 34-year-old-patient with a history of depression is brought to the Emergency Department (ED) in a wheelchair by his wife. He is obtunded with sonorous respirations. The wife states she found him sitting at the foot of the stairs and that he may have ingested 10 opioid pain pills that she received after dental surgery.

Vital signs:
Temperature 99° F (37.2°C)
Pulse 90 beats/min
Respirations 6 breaths/min
Blood Pressure 80/60 mmHg
Oxygen Saturation 84%
Blood glucose (fingerstick) 80 mg/dL (3.3 mmol/L)

Assessment findings: Glasgow coma scale= 11 (E=3,V=3,M=5) Pupils are constricted. Breath sounds diminished and equal bilaterally. Respirations labored and sonorous. Skin cool and pale.

The first action the nurse will take is ____1____ followed by____2____. After administration of ____3____, a successful resuscitation with stable vital signs was achieved. The patient is at risk for____4____ so the nurse anticipates the health care provider (HCP) will request ____5____.

Instructions: Complete the sentences below by choosing the most probable option for the omitted information that corresponds with the same numbered list of options provided.

Option 1	Option 2	Option 3	Option 4	Option 5
Apply personal protective gear (PPE)	Rapid Intubation	Naloxone 0.4 mg intravenously	Infection	Complete Blood Count
Head tilt Chin lift maneuver	Bag Valve Mask 12-16 breaths per minute with 100%oxygen	Dextrose 50% 10 ml intravenously	Anxiety	Drug Screen
Jaw thrust maneuver	Glucagon 1mg Intramuscular	Activated charcoal via nasogastric tube	Suicide	Inpatient admission
Apply 100% oxygen via non rebreather mask	Intravenous Normal Saline 1000 ml over 15 minutes		Drug addiction	Hemoglobin A1-C
Insert an intravenous saline lock	Insertion of a nasogastric tube		Hypoglycemia	Drug counseling

 8. Drag and Drop _____

Scenario: The nurse is assisting at the scene of a mass casualty. How would the nurse triage each victim?

Instructions: Place the letter that indicates the correct triage tag before the number of each victim. Note that all options will be used and may be used more than once.

Triage Tags	Victims
A. Black	1. _____ Teenager walking around the field holding his forearm.
B. Red	2. _____ Unresponsive middle age man with brain matter observed.
C. Yellow	3. _____ Responsive young woman with pale, moist skin breathing rapidly.
D. Green	4. _____ Unresponsive male with sonorous respirations that improve with a jaw thrust.
	5. _____ Elderly male who is alert, complaining of pain, has an open fracture of the left forearm.
	6. _____ Young female with a faint rapid pulse, respirations of 26/min and a fractured femur.
	7. _____ Middle aged male with a deformed shoulder and humerus who is alert with mild tachycardia and respirations of 24

9. Extended Multiple Response _____

Scenario: The Emergency Department (ED) triage nurse is caring for a 10-year-old female child who recently migrated from the Dominican Republic with cold symptoms, inflammation of the conjunctiva, small white spots inside her cheek and a flat red rash on her forehead. She has never been immunized and has no allergies.

Vital signs:
Temperature 102°F (38.8°C)
Pulse 100 beats/min
Respirations 24 breaths/min
Blood Pressure 100/80mmHg
Oxygen Saturation 95%

Which of the following actions should the nurse take?

Instructions: Place an X, in the space provided, or highlight each action that the nurse should take for this patient. **Select all that apply.**

1. _____ Refer the patient to urgent care
2. _____ Directly admit the patient to the pediatric unit
3. _____ Admit the patient to an airborne infection isolation room
4. _____ Don an N95 respirator
5. _____ Administer an MMR vaccine to the patient
6. _____ Administer intramuscular Immune Globulin
7. _____ Administer 20,000IU of vitamin A by mouth
8. _____ Increase fluid intake
9. _____ Administer oseltamivir 60mg by mouth
10. _____ Administer aspirin by mouth for pain and fever
11. _____ Contact the infection control nurse

PART 2 Common Health Scenarios

10. Matrix _____

Scenario: The RN assigned to the medical surgical unit is assessing a female patient, age 35, admitted with thyroid disease. The patient complains of palpitations and tachycardia, dyspnea, extreme fatigue, and increasing acne. She is sweating despite being dressed in light clothing. Her LMP (Last menstrual period) was 1 month ago but they have been scant and irregular for the last 3 months.

Instructions: For each potential prescription listed below, check to specify whether the prescriptions anticipated, non-essential or contraindicated.

Vital signs:
Temperature 98.7F° (37°C)
Pulse 110 beats/min
Respirations 24 breaths/min
Blood Pressure 154/88mmHg
Oxygen Saturation 95% (on room air)

Past history: Asthma controlled with montelukast 10mg every day and a bronchodilating inhaler as needed. Moderate acne for which she uses tretinoin 0.025% gel and tetracycline 250mg a day. Surgeries include an appendectomy at age 10. She has no known drug allergies. Family history includes a mother who is alive and a father who died of a myocardial infarction at age 50.

Potential Prescriptions	Anticipated	Nonessential	Contraindicated
12 lead EKG			
Cardiac troponins T and I			
Vital Signs q4hrs			
Estrogen level			
Increase tetracycline to 500mg/day			
Thyroid Scan			
TSH, T3 and T4 levels			
Monitor Intake and Output			
Propranolol 20mg every 6 hours			

11. Cloze _____

Instructions: Choose the most likely options for the information missing from the statements below by selecting from the lists of options provided.

Scenario A: The nurse is working with an AP to provide care for a bedridden patient. The patient is unable to move or turn in bed without assistance. The nurse may delegate the AP to _____1_____ and _____2_____ the patient every _____3_____.

Scenario A

Option 1	Option 2	Option 3
Weigh	Offer bedpan	Every 2 hours
Turn	Elevate head of bed	Once a shift
Lower head of bed	Offer fluids	Every 4 hours
Feed	Reposition	Every 6 hours

Scenario B: The AP informs the nurse that the patient has a rapid respiratory rate of 40 breaths per minute and the breaths are shallow. The nurse would first _____1_____, such as_____2_____, and then would ____3____, and ____4____.

Scenario B

Option 1	Option 2	Option 3	Option 4
Assess the patient	Draw arterial blood gases	Elevate head of bed	Start a new IV
Apply oxygen	Call a code	Notify Healthcare provider (HCP)	Call respiratory therapist
Suction the patient	Check pulse oximetry	Instruct patient to cough	Instruct AP to provide mouth care
Notify rapid response team	Ask patient to take slow deep breaths	Assist patient up to chair	Apply oxygen

Answer Key for this chapter begins on p. 246

12. Extended Multiple Response _____

Scenario: The nurse is providing care for an 81-year-old patient with type 2 diabetes, hypertension, and peripheral vascular disease.

Vital signs:
Temperature 98.7°F (37.06°C)
Pulse 98 beats/min
Respirations 27 breaths/min
Blood Pressure 168/94 mmHg
Morning glucose greater than 600 mg/dL (33.3 mmol/L)

Prescribed drugs: Hydrochlorothiazide (HCTZ); metformin; Albuterol inhaler as needed

Assessment findings: During morning assessment, the patient describes a weight gain of 6 lb. (2.7 kg) over the past month, adequate urine output but drinks very little liquids after dinner. The patient describes bowel movements every 1-2 days.

Which findings increase the patient's risk for development of hyperglycemic-hyperosmolar syndrome (HHS)?

Instructions: Place an X, in the space provided, or highlight each finding that increases the patient's risk for development of HHS. **Select all that apply.**

1. _____ Hydrochlorothiazide (HCTZ) prescribed to control blood pressure
2. _____ Weight gain of 6 lb. (2.7 kg) over the past month
3. _____ Patient avoids taking in liquids during the evenings
4. _____ Blood pressure 168/94mm Hg
5. _____ Urine output of 50 to 75 mL/hr
6. _____ Glucose greater than 600 mg/dL (33.3 mmol/L)
7. _____ History of hypertension
8. _____ Patient is an older adult

13. Extended Multiple Response _____

Scenario: The nurse is admitting an 88-year-old patient from long-term care to an acute care medical/surgical unit. The patient was alert until recently and has become confused. His history includes smoking cigarettes for 55 years but he quit at age 70. He has a history of post-traumatic stress disorder (PTSD) and has had surgery for appendicitis and gall bladder removal. Over the past 36 hours the patient developed headache, muscle aches, cough with thick clear sputum, and chest discomfort.

Admission Vital signs:
Temperature 101.4° F (38.°C)
Pulse 104 beats/min
Respirations 30 breaths/min
Blood Pressure 108/62 mmHg

Admission assessment findings: warm dry skin, crackles bilaterally with wheezes, tachycardia with normal heart sounds, and pulse oximetry reading of 89% on oxygen at 2 L by nasal cannula. The patient does not tolerate lying flat in bed.

Admission Lab: Complete blood count (CBC) reveals elevate white blood cell (WBC) Count. Electrolytes: Na⁺ 135mEq/L (135 mmol/L), K⁺ 3.8mEq/L (3.8 mmol/L), Cl⁻ 98 mEq/L (98 mmol/L)

Which of the following findings with this patient, are factors that increase the risk for a diagnosis of pneumonia?

Instructions: Place an X, in the space provided, or highlight each finding that increases the patient's risk for development of pneumonia. **Select all that apply.**

1. _____ Patient age
2. _____ History of PTSD
3. _____ Smoked cigarettes 55 years
4. _____ Thick clear sputum
5. _____ Crackles and wheezes
6. _____ Elevated WBC count
7. _____ Altered level of consciousness
8. _____ Admission electrolyte values

PART 2

Common Health Scenarios

 Answer Key for this chapter begins on p. 246

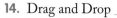

14. Drag and Drop _____

Scenario: The nurse is admitting a 55-year-old patient with a history of a hiatal hernia and peptic ulcers to the medical unit.

Instructions: Indicate which staff member listed in the left-hand column is appropriate for each intervention. Note that all responses may be used more than once.

Staff Member	Intervention
A. RN	1. _____ Check vital signs every 8 hours
B. LPN/LVN	2. _____ Assist patient up to bathroom
C. Assistive Personnel (AP)	3. _____ Administer Famotidine 150 mg orally every 12 hours
D. Dietician	4. _____ Schedule esophagogastroduodenoscopy (EGD)
E. Health Care Provider	5. _____ Teach patient to avoid foods that decrease lower esophageal pressure (LES)
	6. _____ Teach patient to avoid smoking and alcohol
	7. _____ Instruct patient to consume 4 to 6 small meals per day and discuss strategies for this change.
	8. _____ Remind the patient to use a large wedge-style pillow for sleep
	9. _____ Ask patient about episodes of sleep apnea
	10. _____ Explain risks associated with EGD procedure

15. Enhanced Hot Spot _____

Scenario: The nurse is orienting a new RN to the coronary care unit. They are providing care for a 64-year-old patient who is at risk for heart problems. She was admitted with chest pain and shortness of breath. Which findings will the nurse teach the new RN to recognize as factors that increase the patient's risk for development of heart problems?

Instructions: Underline or highlight or underline each factor that increases the patient's risk for heart problems.

Patient has a history of 35 pack-years smoking cigarettes. Patient states she would like to quit smoking. Patient was exposed to second-hand smoke during childhood and teen years. Patient started smoking at age 12 but would like to quit. Patient is overweight and was diagnosed with type 2 diabetes 5 years ago. She leads a sedentary lifestyle with her job and home life. Her gallbladder was removed 15 years ago. Her mother and grandfather both died after heart attacks. She is married and has 2 grown daughters who live nearby.

16. Matrix

Scenario: A 71-year-old woman is admitted to the long-term care facility for confusion, wandering and frequent falls. She is alert, conversant and shows an immediate interest in exploring the facility. The daughter says, "Mom does many things for herself. She likes morning walks, and she prefers to wear long flowing clothes and high heels. She has eyeglasses and a cane, but she forgets or sometimes denies the need for those items. She has fallen several times, but she rejects help or suggestions; she has always been very independent."

Additional history: hypertension, early stage Alzheimer, wrist fracture 2 years ago secondary to a fall, with subsequent diagnosis of osteoporosis. Medications include chlorothiazide, captopril, donepezil, vitamin D, calcium, and alendronate

The RN and LPN/LVN plan initial interventions to prevent falls for this resident. Which team member is the **best** to assign or delegate for each intervention?

Instructions: For each intervention, place an X in the box to indicate whether the RN, LPN/LVN or AP is the best team member to perform the task. *Hint: There is one intervention that all team members are responsible for.*

Potential Interventions	RN	LPN/LVN	AP
Assist resident to don slip-resistant and safe footwear			
Perform frequent rounding to evaluate resident's receptiveness to fall prevention interventions			
Remind resident to sit slowly and dangle before getting out of bed in the morning			
Help resident to dress in comfortable, well-fitting clothing			
Conduct medication reconciliation			
Monitor resident's ongoing abilities to perform activities of daily living			
Assess baseline cognitive status			
Obtain admission and weekly vital signs to include orthostatic blood pressure measurements			
Perform initial gait testing, such as the Timed Up and Go test			
Perform hourly environmental checks, such as: call bell and personal items within reach and walkways free of clutter			
Observe resident's daily abilities: gait, balance and independent ambulation			
Check blood pressure prior to administering medications that may cause orthostatic hypotension			
Discuss fall prevention goals and interventions with resident and family			
Monitor resident's location at all times			
Assist resident to locate eyeglasses and cane before attempting to ambulate			
Direct team members to observe for and report barriers to fall prevention			

 Answer Key for this chapter begins on p. 246

Answers

1. **Ans: 1c, 2b, 3a, 4a, 5b, 6d, 7c, 8d, 9e, 10e, 11a, 12b** In home health, every team member must be experienced and be able to work with relative independence to fulfill their roles. The RN is responsible for the initial assessment of psychosocial, physical, and environmental problems. Initial and ongoing assessment of cognitive functions would be particularly important for a patient with Alzheimer's. Teaching the patient and family to cope with the behavioral and cognitive changes is also an RN responsibility. The RN maintains responsibility for total patient care and must be available to team members for offsite consultation and periodic onsite visits. The LPN/LVN is trained in medication administration and can assist the wife to create a system for routine medication doses. The LPN/LVN is also responsible to monitor for new behavioral changes or ongoing safety issues. The physical therapist is responsible for assessing functions that are related to mobility and movement and then designing and teaching interventions to the patient and family to maximize mobility and strength. The social worker can assist with locating community resources and help them to understand Medicare benefits. The home health aide assists the patient and family to accomplish activities of daily living in the home setting. The aide must receive instructions specific to the patient (e.g., special skin care products, and safety and mobility issues). **Focus:** Assignment, Delegation, Supervision.

2. **Ans: Option 1, glaucoma; Option 2, loss and compromise of peripheral vision; Option 3, intraocular pressure measurements.** Glaucoma is the leading cause of blindness for African Americans and the second leading cause of blindness in the United States. Primary open-angle glaucoma is the most common type and it has a slow and insidious progression. The patient is frequently asymptomatic until there is severe compromise of peripheral vision. Patients are encouraged to have frequent intraocular pressure measurements. Slit lamp microscopy is also used to examine the angle where the iris meets the cornea; this is the place of aqueous outflow. Excruciating pain in or around eye occurs with acute angle-closure glaucoma. Curtain-like obstruction across the visual field is an associated with retinal detachment. An ultrasound can be used to examine the area of detachment if the cornea, lens or vitreous is hazy. Blurred and darkened vision with blind spots occurs with macular degeneration and Amsler grid is used to define the area. With cataracts, the patient may have decreased vision or glare. The Snellen chart and other visual acuity instruments are used in the diagnosis. **Focus:** Prioritization. **Test Taking Tip:** As you study for NCLEX, pay attention to common serious conditions that are preventable with early detection and treatment.

3. **Ans:** A **72-year old woman** is brought to the emergency department by her daughter, who reports, "Mom seems **more confused and irritable than usual.** She is **not eating or drinking very much.** She is **unusually restless during the day and doesn't sleep throughout the night.** She is spending **a lot of time in the bathroom,** but she gets mad when I ask her what she is doing in there. Her underwear has a **strong urine odor and pink-tinged stains.** She has mild **dementia** and she takes a blood pressure medication and a pill for **diabetes.**" Vital signs: **Temperature 99.3° F (37.38°C), Pulse 100 beats/min,** Respirations 24 breaths /min, Blood Pressure 130/78 mmHg, Oxygen Saturation 96%, **Blood glucose (fingerstick) 160mg/dL (8.9 mmol/L).** Assessment findings: Alert, oriented to self, speech clear. Follows simple instructions, but is **irritable and distractible.** PERRLA (pupils equal, round, reactive to light and accommodation). Breath sounds clear and equal bilaterally. Respirations even and unlabored. **Skin turgor poor, mucous membranes dry.** Denies pain at any source. Assisted to the toilet and voids **a small amount of dark amber urine with a strong odor. Becomes anxious and is reluctant to leave the bathroom.**

   Older females have a risk for urinary tract infections because of a short urethra, tissue fragility and decreased lubrication of mucous membranes. Changes in behavior and usual patterns for eating, drinking and sleeping can accompany infection, especially in older patients. The change in toileting habits, anxiety related to toileting, and the presence of strong odor and pink staining are consistent with a UTI. Dementia increases the risk for infection because patients may have difficulty recognizing or articulating problems. Diabetes also increases the risk for infection. Temperature of 99.3° F (37.38°C) may seem insignificant, but older people often have baseline subnormal temperatures due to lower metabolism. Increased pulse and blood glucose may also signal infection. Poor skin turgor and dry mucous membranes indicate fluid volume deficit which would worsen a UTI. **Focus:** Prioritization. **Test Taking Tip:** This question tests your ability to analyze information in a clinical situation. First recognize that most of the information relates to a urinary tract infection. Other key information relates to the changes in this older patient's baseline behavior.

4. **Ans:** Taking vital signs, changing linens, assisting with ambulation, reporting discomfort or pain, and turning patients are within the scope of practice

of the AP. The LPN/LVN would assess the patient's forearm; casts can interfere with circulation and there is a risk for compartment syndrome. The LPN/LVN would also assess pain relief after pharmacological or non-pharmacological interventions. The RN should perform teaching about the PCA pump, perform admission assessments and evaluate patient outcomes. **Focus:** Assignment, Delegation.

Intervention	RN	LPN/LVN	AP
Take vital signs every 4 hours or as directed			X
Check color and temperature of fingers for a patient with a forearm cast.		X	
Change linens for patients as needed.			X
Assist patients to ambulate in the hallway, as ordered by the HCP.			X
Report if any patient has pain or discomfort.			X
Assist older patient with weakness to turn every 2 hours.			X
Give preoperative teaching to a patient about patient-controlled analgesia pump and measures to prevent postoperative complications	X		
Assess for pain on a patient who has a kidney stone		X	
Assess relief of heat application for patient with lower back pain		X	
Perform admission assessment on a patient admitted for chest pain and shortness of breath	X		
Evaluate patient's ability to independently perform colostomy care	X		

5. **Ans: 1, 2, 5, 8, 9** The patients with the cast, toe amputation, arthritis, hemiplegia and awaiting transfer to a memory care unit are in stable condition. These patients need ongoing assessment, medications, comfort measures and therapies that are within the scope of practice of an LPN/LVN under the supervision of an RN. An RN takes responsibility for preoperative teaching and for teaching about dialysis, transplant and self-care issues related to renal failure. The patient with terminal cancer needs a comprehensive assessment to determine the reason for refusal of medication. The patient with trauma is not considered stable; serial assessments to detect occult trauma are required. Change in mental status could be related to infection, decreased brain perfusion secondary to respiratory or cardiac problems, metabolic disturbance, neurologic event, or trauma. This patient would not be assigned to an LPN/LVN until the cause is determined and patient is stable. **Focus:** Assignment.

6. **Ans: Option 1, hypertensive emergency; Option 2, place in a semi-fowlers position; Option 3, decrease intracranial pressure; Option 4, labetalol 20mg intravenously.** Hypertensive emergency signs; severe headache, nausea, vomiting, blurred vision and mild confusion with a history of suspected uncontrolled hypertension and bounding pulses indicate a high blood pressure (MAP of 160 or BP 200/140) and are highly suspect for a hypertensive crises which can be life threatening. A hypertensive emergency if not treated rapidly and appropriately can cause stroke, myocardial infarction, renal failure, aneurysms and end organ failure. The nursing action is to place the patient in a semi fowlers position. Doing so protects helps protect the airway in a confused patient, decreases intracranial pressure and decreases blood pressure. Oxygen and an IV placement are not considered to be nursing interventions but rather medical interventions. **Focus:** Prioritization.

7. **Ans: Option 1, jaw thrust maneuver; Option 2, Bag valve mask 12-16 breaths per minute with 100% oxygen; Option 3, Naloxone 0.4mg; Option 4, suicide; Option 5, inpatient admission.** Airway is always the first priority. The patient is obtunded and has sonorous respirations indicating an obstructed airway. His airway should be opened using a jaw thrust maneuver because he was found at the base of the stairs indicating a risk for C-spine injury. Once the airway is open and clear, a bag valve mask resuscitation with 12-16 breaths a minute with 100% oxygen is administered. Rapid intubation is not necessary as the patient is being oxygenated and breaths are being delivered with the bag valve mask resuscitator. The dose of naloxone will reverse the negative effects of the opioid and the patient will begin breathing on his own making intubation unnecessary and possibly dangerous. Neither glucagon nor dextrose is necessary for a blood sugar of 80 mg/dL 3.3 mmol/L. According to the Center for Disease Control (CDC) patients with mental health conditions such as depression are more prone to overdose than other patients. These patients are at risk for suicide and suicidal attempts which is the priority for this patient so an inpatient admission with mental health consult is anticipated. **Focus:** Prioritization.

8. **Ans: 1D, 2A, 3B, 4B, 5C, 6B, 7C** Red: Immediate threat to life; patients 3 and 6 are exhibiting signs of

shock and patient 4 has an airway issue that if taken care of will prevent immediate death. Green: Non urgent does not need immediate treatment; patient 1 is considered walking wounded and holding his forearm even if it broken is not an immediate threat to life. Black: Expected to die; patient 2 is expected to die with exposed brain matter. Yellow: Urgent treatment; patient 5 is stable but needs urgent treatment because an open fracture of the forearm has a high-risk of infection. Patient 7 is also urgent because he is at risk for shoulder deformity and permanent dysfunction. **Focus:** Prioritization.

9. **Ans: 3, 4, 7, 8, 11**   The child has measles which is a highly contagious disease that has recently resurged in the United States. According to the Center for Disease Control (CDC), measles is spread through airborne contact so the child must be isolated immediately and for 4 days after the appearance of the rash. Health care personnel who come in contact with the child should wear an N95 respirator. Vitamin A is administered to children with the measles because vitamin A deficiency is a risk factor for developing severe measles infections. Fluids should be increased to minimize fluid loss from fever. Aspirin should never be given to children with viral diseases. They could develop Reye's disease. The infection control nurse should be contacted so post exposure prophylaxis can begin with the child's family and others who may have come in contact with the child. Most health care professionals have been vaccinated but if they have not, they should have a measles, mumps, rubella (MMR) vaccination within 72 hours and intramuscular immune globulin as post-exposure prophylaxis within 6 days. **Focus:** Prioritization.

10. **Ans:**   A 12 lead EKG is prescribed to establish a baseline and rule out arrythmias that are common in hyperthyroidism. Cardiac troponin levels are not essential as the patient does not have symptoms indicative of a myocardial infarction. Vital signs are prescribed every 4 hours with an emphasis on temperature. A rise in temperature of 1 degree should be reported to the health care provider (HCP) at once because this could be indicative of a thyroid storm which is a medical emergency. Estrogen levels are not essential because changes in menstruation are normal for hyperthyroidism. A pregnancy test should be done prior to administering tetracycline or completing the thyroid scan as both are contraindicated in pregnancy. TSH, T3 and T4 levels need to be drawn. There is no indication for intake an output for this patient. Propranolol is contraindicated in patients who have asthma. A selective beta blocker like atenolol could be ordered to control increased pulse and blood pressure instead. **Focus:** Priority.

Potential Prescriptions	Anticipated	Nonessential	Contraindicated
12 lead EKG	X		
Cardiac troponins T and I		X	
Vital Signs q4hrs	X		
Estrogen level		X	
Increase tetracycline to 500mg/day			X
Thyroid Scan			X
TSH, T3 and T4 levels	X		
Monitor Intake and Output		X	
Propranolol 20mg every 6 hours			X

11. **Ans: A. Option 1, turn; Option 2, reposition; Option 3, every 2 hours.**   Turning and repositioning patients is within the scope of practice for an AP and is appropriate for the professional nurse to delegate to an AP.
Ans B. Option 1, assess the patient; Option 2, check pulse oximetry; Option 3, notify HCP; Option 4, apply oxygen. The nurse should first assess the patient and gather more information because this will enable answering questions from the HCP. Once this step is complete, the next step is to notify the HCP (for oxygen order). Alternately the nurse could notify the rapid response team (RRT). Applying oxygen per order (by HCP, RRT, or unit standing order) would be important. The patient is breathing and not yet in need of a ventilator. **Focus:** Prioritization.

12. **Ans: 1, 3, 6, 8**   HHS often occurs in older adults with type 2 diabetes. Risk factors include taking diuretics and inadequate fluid intake. Serum glucose is greater than 600 mg/dL (33.3 mmol/L). Weight loss (not weight gain) would be a symptom. Although the patient's blood pressure is high, this is not a risk factor. A urine output of 50 to 75 mL/hr is adequate. Hypertension is not a risk factor for HHS. **Focus:** Prioritization.

13. **Ans: 1, 3, 5, 6, 7** Older patients are at an increased risk for pneumonia in the community and health care settings. A history of smoking is also a risk factor. Assessment findings include the presence of crackles over areas with interstitial fluid and wheezes are heard if inflammation or exudate narrows the airways. An elevated WBC count is a common finding in older adults as are changes in level of consciousness. PTSD would not be a risk factor for pneumonia. Generally, sputum is purulent, blood-tinged, or rust colored. The electrolytes listed in this case study are all within normal limits. **Focus:** Prioritization.

14. **Ans: 1c, 2c, 3b, 4a, 5d, 6a, 7d, 8c, 9a, 10e** As a member of the health care team, it is essential to be familiar with the roles and scopes of practice of other members of the team. The RN could complete all tasks except #10, but the question asks which team member is most appropriate for each action so the RN must be aware of the scope of practice for each member of the team. **Focus:** Assignment, Delegation.

15. **Ans:** Patient has a history of **35 pack-years smoking cigarettes.** Patient states she would like to quit smoking. Patient was **exposed to second-hand smoke** during childhood and teen years. Patient started smoking at age 12 but would like to quit. **Patient is overweight** and was diagnosed with **type 2 diabetes** 5 years ago. She leads a **sedentary lifestyle** with her job and home life. Her gallbladder was removed 15 years ago. Her **mother and grandfather both died after heart attacks.** She is married and has 2 grown daughters who live nearby. Smoking history, second-hand exposure to smoke, overweight, type 2 diabetes, death of close relatives from myocardial infarction, and lack of exercise (sedentary lifestyle) are all risk factors for heart problems. **Focus:** Prioritization, Supervision.

16. **Ans:**

Potential Interventions	RN	LPN/LVN	AP
Assist resident to don slip-resistant and safe footwear.			X
Perform frequent rounding to evaluate resident's receptiveness to fall prevention interventions.	X		
Remind resident to sit slowly and dangle before getting out of bed in the morning.			X
Help resident to dress in comfortable, well-fitting clothing.			X
Conduct medication reconciliation.	X		
Monitor resident's ongoing abilities to perform activities of daily living.		X	
Assess baseline cognitive status.	X		
Obtain admission and weekly vital signs to include orthostatic blood pressure measurements.			X
Perform initial gait testing, such as the Timed Up and Go test.	X		
Perform hourly environmental checks, such as: call bell and personal items within reach and walkways free of clutter.			X
Observe resident's daily abilities: gait, balance, and independent ambulation		X	
Check blood pressure before administering medications that may cause orthostatic hypotension.		X	
Discuss fall prevention goals and interventions with resident and family.	X		
Monitor resident's location at all times.	X	X	X
Assist resident to locate eyeglasses and cane before attempting to ambulate.			X
Direct team members to observe for and report barriers to fall prevention.	X		

PART 2 Common Health Scenarios

The RN is responsible for the initial admission assessment that includes medication reconciliation, cognitive status, and gait and balance testing. The RN discusses the goals and interventions with the resident and family. Frequent rounding on newly admitted residents provides opportunities for formative evaluation, so that the care plan can be revised as needed. Barriers should be quickly identified and reported to the RN. For example, the AP can suggest safe shoes, clothing, and the use of the eyeglasses and cane, but if the resident refuses, the AP must report this to the RN. The LPN/LVN performs daily assessments and those associated with administering oral medications. APs provide much of the care for residents in long-term care facilities, such as assisting with dressing, morning care, ambulation, and basic environmental safety checks. APs can also obtain vital signs for stable residents. Finally, wandering creates a safety issue and all team members are expected to observe for and be aware of the resident's location. **Focus:** Assignment, Delegation.

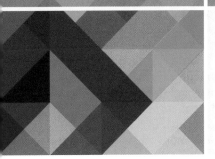

CASE STUDY 1

Chest Pressure, Indigestion, and Nausea

Questions

Ms. S is a 58-year-old African-American woman who was admitted to the coronary care unit (CCU) from the emergency department (ED) with reports of chest pressure and indigestion associated with nausea. She started feeling ill about 10 hours before she called her daughter, who brought her to the ED for admission. She told the nurse that she tried drinking water and took some bismuth subsalicylate that was in her bathroom medicine cabinet. She also tried lying down to rest, but none of these actions helped. She states, "It just gets worse and worse." Ms. S has been under a health care provider's (HCP's) care for the past 12 years for management of hypertension and swelling in her ankles. She was a smoker for 43 years but quit 1 year ago. Her past medical history includes gall bladder disease and gastroesophageal reflux disease (GERD).

In the ED, admission laboratory tests, including levels of cardiac markers, were performed, and a 12-lead electrocardiogram (ECG) was taken.

Ms. S's CCU vital sign values on admission are as follows:

Blood pressure	174/92 mm Hg
Heart rate	120 to 130 beats/min, irregular
O_2 saturation	91% on room air
Respiratory rate	30 to 34 breaths/min
Temperature	99.8°F (37.7°C) (oral)

1. Based on Ms. S's admission vital signs, which HCP orders would the nurse expect? **Select all that apply.**
   1. Continuous cardiac monitoring
   2. Blood pressure checks every 10 minutes
   3. Oxygen at 2 L per nasal canula
   4. Instruct patient to breathe and rebreathe into a paper bag.
   5. Acetaminophen 650 mg as needed for temperature greater than 99°F (37.2°C)
   6. Check apical heart rate with each set of vital signs

2. Extended Multiple Response

   Instructions: Based on Mrs. S's history (see above), circle all of the correct responses in the right column that answer the question in the left column.

Question	
Which risk factors from Ms. S's history would suggest a possible cardiac problem to the nurse?	1. Hypertension for 12 years
	2. Smoked for 43 years; quit smoking 1 year ago
	3. Surgery for gallbladder removal 1 year ago
	4. Ms. S's father died at age 42 years from a heart attack
	5. Patient's weight is 278 lb (126 kg)
	6. Diet includes fast foods three to five times a week
	7. Patient is an African-American female
	8. History of gastroesophageal reflux disease
	9. Report of chest pressure and indigestion associated with nausea

3. Which action is **best** for the nurse to delegate to a new assistive personnel (AP) orienting to the CCU when caring for Ms. S?
   1. Placing the patient on a cardiac telemetry monitor
   2. Drawing blood to test cardiac marker levels and sending it to the laboratory
   3. Obtaining a 12-lead ECG
   4. Checking and recording the patient's intake and output

4. Which action prescribed by the health care provider (HCP) for Ms. S takes **first priority** at this time?
   1. Measure vital signs every 2 hours.
   2. Obtain a 12-lead ECG every 6 hours.
   3. Place the patient on a cardiac monitor.
   4. Check levels of cardiac markers every 6 hours.

5. Ms. S's cardiac telemetry monitor shows a rhythm of sinus tachycardia with frequent premature ventricular contractions (PVCs) and short runs of ventricular tachycardia (more than 3 PVCs in a row). Which drug should the nurse be prepared to administer **first**?
   1. Amiodarone IV push
   2. Nitroglycerin sublingually
   3. Morphine sulfate IV push
   4. Atenolol IV push

6. All of these laboratory values were obtained for Ms. S in the emergency department. Which value would be of **most** concern to the nurse and have immediate implications for the care of the patient?
   1. Potassium level of 3.5 mEq/L (3.5 mmol/L)
   2. Troponin T level of more than 0.20 ng/mL (0.2 μg/L)
   3. Glucose level of 123 mg/dL (6.83 mmol/L)
   4. Slight elevation of white blood cell count

7. Ms. S tells the nurse that she has worsening chest discomfort. The cardiac monitor shows ST-segment elevation, and the nurse notifies the HCP. Which prescribed action takes the **highest priority** at this time?
   1. Administer morphine sulfate 2 mg IV push.
   2. Schedule an ECG.
   3. Draw blood for coagulation studies.
   4. Administer ranitidine 75 mg PO every 12 hours.

8. Enhanced Multiple Response

Instructions: Circle all of the correct responses in the right column that answer the question in the left column.

Question:
Because Ms. S continues to experience chest discomfort and has elevated levels of cardiac markers, the following interventions have been prescribed by the health care provider. Which interventions should the nurse delegate to an experienced AP? **Select all that apply.**

1. Measuring vital signs every 2 hours
2. Accurately recording intake and output
3. Administering tenecteplase IV push
4. Drawing blood for coagulation studies
5. Assessing the cardiac monitor every 4 hours
6. Assisting the patient to the bedside commode
7. Helping the patient with morning care and partial bed bath
8. Assessing the patient's pain level
9. Reminding the patient to report any episodes of chest discomfort

9. The patient is scheduled for an emergent cardiac catheterization with possible percutaneous coronary intervention (PCI). Ms. S asks the nurse what is involved with this procedure. What is the nurse's **best** response?
   1. "It is a procedure that is usually done on patients who have heart attacks to diagnose blockages in the arteries that feed the heart."
   2. "The cardiologist will use a catheter to inject dye and locate narrowed arteries, then may inflate a balloon to open the artery and place a stent to keep it open."
   3. "Cardiac catheterization is usually performed on an outpatient basis to determine whether or not you have had a heart attack."
   4. "After the cardiac catheterization, you will come back to the coronary care unit, where you will be on bed rest for 6 to 8 hours, and we will check your vital signs often."

Complex Health Scenarios

PART 3

10. Ms. S has returned to the CCU after a cardiac catheterization and a percutaneous coronary intervention procedure. Which follow-up care orders should the nurse assign to an experienced LPN/LVN? **Select all that apply.**
    1. Reminding the patient to remain on bed rest with the insertion site extremity straight
    2. Preparing a teaching plan that includes activity restrictions and risk factor modification
    3. Measuring the patient's vital signs every 15 minutes for the first hour
    4. Assessing the catheter insertion site for bleeding or hematoma formation
    5. Monitoring peripheral pulses, skin temperature, and skin color with each measurement of vital signs
    6. Administering two tablets of acetaminophen for back pain

11. Which information is **most** important to prevent recurrence of reocclusion of the coronary artery, chest discomfort, or myocardial infarction?
    1. Remain on bed rest for the next 24 hours.
    2. Patient will be prescribed dual antiplatelet therapy (DAT).
    3. Patient should do no heavy lifting for 48 hours.
    4. HCP will prescribe a beta-blocker.

12. Ms. S's daughter asks the nurse why her mother did not receive a "clot-buster" drug. What is the nurse's **best** response?
    1. "Thrombolytic agents, also called clot busters, are most effective when administered within the first 6 hours of a coronary event."
    2. "Thrombolytic drugs are much more effective when used for patients who have had a recent stroke."
    3. "Thrombolytic drugs work better for patients who have a heart attack at a much younger age."
    4. "Contraindications for these drugs include recent surgeries, and your mother had gallbladder surgery a year ago."

13. Ms. S's condition is stable, and she has been transferred to the cardiac step-down unit. What should the step-down nurse instruct the AP to report immediately?
    1. Temperature of 99°F (37.2°C) with morning vital sign monitoring
    2. Chest pain episode occurring during morning care
    3. Systolic blood pressure increase of 8 mm Hg after morning care
    4. Heart rate increase of 10 beats/min after ambulation

14. The nurse delegates to the AP the task of taking Ms. S's vital signs every 4 hours and recording the vital sign values in the electronic chart. Later the nurse checks the patient's chart and discovers that vital sign measurements have not been recorded. What is the nurse's **best** action?
    1. Take the vital signs because the AP is not competent to complete this task.
    2. Notify the nurse manager immediately.
    3. Reprimand the AP at the nurses' station.
    4. Speak to the AP privately to determine why the values were not recorded.

15. The HCP prescribes captopril 12.5 mg orally twice daily and hydrochlorothiazide (HCTZ) 25 mg orally daily. Which information would the nurse be sure to include when teaching Ms. S about these drugs?
    1. "Take your HCTZ in the morning."
    2. "If you miss a dose of captopril, take two tablets next time."
    3. "Avoid foods that are rich in potassium, such as bananas and oranges."
    4. "You should expect an increase in blood pressure with these drugs."

16. The HCP orders dual antiplatelet therapy (DAT) for Ms. S. What is the nurse's **highest priority** concern for this patient?
    1. Reminding the patient to do no heavy lifting while hospitalized
    2. Assessing the progression of walking in the halls
    3. Teaching the patient to apply oxygen for any shortness of breath
    4. Monitoring the patient for any form of bleeding

17. The HCP prescribes atenolol 50 mg each morning for Ms. S. Which instruction would the nurse provide for the LPN/LVN assigned to give this drug?
    1. Hold the drug if the patient's blood pressure is higher than 100/80 mm Hg.
    2. Give the drug if the patient's respiratory rate is greater than 30 breaths/min.
    3. Hold the drug if the patient's heart rate is less than 55 beats/min.
    4. Give the drug if the patient's blood pressure is less than 90/50 mm Hg.

18. Which activities could the nurse delegate to AP assisting Ms. S during phase 1 of cardiac rehabilitation? **Select all that apply.**
    1. Assist with Ms. S's morning bath as needed.
    2. Refer Ms. S to a monitored cardiac rehab program.
    3. Ambulate with Ms. S to the bathroom.
    4. Administer Ms. S's morning doses of captopril and HCTZ.
    5. Assist with progressive ambulation in the hall.
    6. Assess Ms. S for additional chest pain or pressure.

Answer Key for this chapter begins on p. 255

19. Before discharging Ms. S, the HCP orders an electrocardiogram (ECG). This test reveals normal sinus rhythm with a heart rate of 87 beats/min. What is the nurse's **best** action at this time?

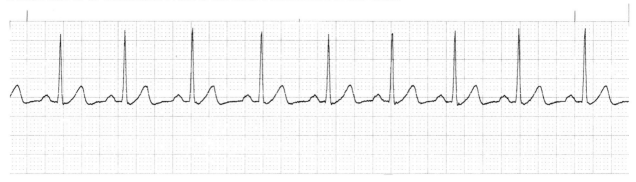

1. Delay the patient's discharge until she is seen by the HCP.
2. Administer the patient's next dose of atenolol 3 hours early before she goes home.
3. Contact the HCP and ask about drawing an additional set of cardiac markers.
4. Document this finding as the only action and prepare for discharge.

Answers

1. **Ans: 1, 3, 6** Because the patient's heart rate is rapid and irregular, she should be on a continuous cardiac monitor and her apical pulse should be monitored. Her O_2 saturation is low normal and her heart rate is rapid and irregular, so supplemental oxygen will be useful to her heart. Although her blood pressure is high and needs to be monitored, every 10 minutes would not allow for patient rest (it would be sensible in an emergency but not routinely). Adding oxygen to increase myocardial oxygen levels may help restore Ms. S's respiratory rate to normal. Using a bag is a strategy for a patient who is hyperventilating and is not appropriate in this case. Acetaminophen is usually ordered for a higher temperature. Also, the HCP would likely want to discover the reason for any very elevated temperature so it could be treated. **Focus:** Prioritization.

2. **Ans: 1, 2, 4, 5, 6, 7, 9** Risk factors for cardiac problems include hypertension, family history, obesity, and high-fat diets (which may cause elevation of cholesterol). African-Americans have higher rates of high blood pressure, high cholesterol, obesity, and diabetes, which are major risk factors for heart disease. Symptoms of chest pressure with indigestion and nausea are signs that suggest a heart problem. Gallbladder surgery and GERD would not be risk factors. Quitting smoking would be a risk factor, and the years that the patient smoked would be a strong risk factor. **Focus:** Prioritization.

3. **Ans: 4** Monitoring and recording intake and output are within the scope of practice for APs. Initiating telemetry, performing venipuncture, and obtaining ECGs require additional education and training and would not be delegated to a new AP. Attaching ECG leads may be done by APs in some facilities, as may venipuncture and ECG recording. The APs performing these tasks, however, would require additional specialized training. These actions are generally considered to be within the scope of practice of licensed nurses. **Focus:** Delegation.

4. **Ans: 3** Cardiac monitoring is the highest priority because the patient's heart rate is rapid and irregular, and the patient is experiencing chest pressure. The patient is at risk for life-threatening dysrhythmias such as frequent premature ventricular contractions. Measuring vital signs every 2 hours, checking levels of cardiac markers, and recording a 12-lead ECG every 6 hours are important to accomplish, but cardiac monitoring takes first precedence at this time. **Focus:** Prioritization.

5. **Ans: 1** With frequent PVCs, the patient is at risk for life-threatening dysrhythmias such as ventricular tachycardia or ventricular fibrillation. The patient is already showing short runs of ventricular tachycardia (greater than three PVCs in a row). Amiodarone is an antidysrhythmic drug used to control ventricular dysrhythmias. Nitroglycerin and morphine can be given for chest pain relief. Atenolol is a beta-blocker, which can be used to control heart rate and decrease blood pressure. **Focus:** Prioritization. **Test-Taking Tip:** When a question asks for what to do first or what takes priority, the nurse should consider what is the most serious danger for the patient. In this case, that danger is related to life-threatening dysrhythmias.

6. **Ans: 2** A troponin T level of more than 0.20 ng/mL (0.2 µg/L) is an elevated level and indicates myocardial injury or infarction (heart attack). Although the other laboratory values are all abnormal except the potassium, which is low normal, none of them is life threatening. The low normal potassium level would be the second highest concern and might require supplementation to keep it within normal limits. **Focus:** Prioritization. **Test-Taking Tip:** Remember that hypokalemia can also be a risk for dysrhythmias.

7. **Ans: 1** Morphine sulfate has been ordered to relieve the chest discomfort that is common when a patient has an acute myocardial infarction. Relief from the chest pain is the highest priority at this time. Ranitidine is a histamine$_2$ blocker used to prevent gastric ulcers. Scheduling an ECG or drawing blood for coagulation studies, although important, will not help relieve chest discomfort. **Focus:** Prioritization.

8. **Ans: 1, 2, 6, 7** Measuring vital signs, recording intake and output, and assisting patients with activities of daily living (e.g., morning care, partial or complete bed bath, bedside commode) are all within the scope of practice of the AP. Administration of IV drugs, venipuncture for laboratory tests, interpreting ECG's, and assessments are beyond the scope of practice of APs and are applicable to the practice scope of the professional nurse. In some facilities, APs may receive additional training to perform venipuncture, but the RN would need to assess the AP's ability to safely perform this skill before delegation. **Focus:** Delegation.

9. **Ans: 2** The nurse's best response should be attentive to and answer the patient's question. For the cardiac catheterization, the patient is taken to a special lab where the cardiologist uses an invasive catheter with injectable dye to locate and diagnose narrowed sections of coronary arteries. For percutaneous coronary intervention, a catheter is placed with a balloon, which can be inflated to open the narrowed section, and a stent (an expandable metal mesh device) can be left in place to keep the artery opened. Options 1, 3, and 4 do

PART 3 Complex Health Scenarios

not accurately answer the patient's question about the procedure. **Focus:** Prioritization.

10. **Ans: 1, 3, 4, 5, 6** All of these interventions are within the scope of practice of an experienced LPN/LVN. The LPN/LVN would be instructed when to notify the RN or the HCP of any abnormal findings. Preparing a teaching plan requires additional education and is more suited to the RN's scope of practice. Taking vital signs and reminding the patient about bed rest could also be delegated to the AP. **Focus:** Assignment, Supervision.

11. **Ans: 2** Without stent placement, the artery often re-occludes because of the artery's normal elasticity and memory. Patients who undergo percutaneous coronary intervention are required to take DAT consisting of aspirin and a platelet inhibitor to prevent recurrence of artery blockage, chest pain, and MI. Patients are not kept on bed rest for 24 hours; rather, they are instructed to do no heavy lifting for several days after this procedure, and they are often prescribed a beta-blocker to slow heart rate and lower blood pressure. **Focus:** Prioritization.

12. **Ans: 1** Thrombolytic therapy using fibrinolytics dissolves thrombi in the coronary arteries and restores myocardial blood flow. Intracoronary fibrinolytics may be delivered during cardiac catheterization. Thrombolytic agents are most effective when administered within the first 6 hours of a coronary event. They are used in men and women, young and old. **Focus:** Prioritization.

13. **Ans: 2** Chest pain can be an indicator of additional myocardial muscle damage. Additional episodes of chest pain significantly affect the patient's plan of care. Small increases in heart rate and blood pressure after activity are to be expected. The patient's temperature, only 0.2°F (0.1°C) higher than at admission, is not a priority at this time, but it will need continued monitoring. **Focus:** Prioritization, Delegation, Supervision.

14. **Ans: 4** Measuring and recording vital sign values are within the scope of practice of the AP. When the AP makes a mistake, it is best to communicate specifically, stressing the importance of recording vital sign values after they have been obtained. Supervision should be done in a supportive rather than confrontational manner. Notifying the nurse manager is not appropriate at this time. Reprimanding the AP in front of others also is not appropriate. **Focus:** Delegation, Supervision.

15. **Ans: 1** HCTZ is a thiazide diuretic used to correct edema and lower blood pressure, and it should

be taken in the morning so that its diuretic effects do not keep the patient up during the night. A side effect of HCTZ is loss of potassium, and patients may require potassium supplementation. Captopril is an angiotensin-converting enzyme inhibitor that lowers blood pressure. It is never appropriate to take twice the dose of this drug. **Focus:** Prioritization.

16. **Ans: 4** DAT is suggested for all patients with acute coronary syndrome, incorporating aspirin and either clopidogrel or ticagrelor. The major side effect for each of these agents is bleeding. Observe for bleeding tendencies, such as nosebleeds or blood in the stool. Medications will need to be discontinued if evidence of bleeding occurs. **Focus:** Prioritization. **Test-Taking Tip:** With DAT, the patient is prescribed two drugs that increase the risk for bleeding, so bleeding is the priority assessment when a patient is prescribed this therapy.

17. **Ans: 3** Atenolol is a beta-blocker drug. Do not give beta-blockers if the pulse rate is below 55 or the systolic blood pressure is below 100 mm Hg without first checking with the HCP. The beta-blocking agent may lead to persistent bradycardia or further reduction of systolic blood pressure, leading to poor peripheral and coronary perfusion. **Focus:** Assignment, Supervision.

18. **Ans: 1, 3, 5** Cardiac rehabilitation is the process of actively assisting the patient with cardiac disease in achieving and maintaining a vital and productive life while remaining within the limits of the heart's ability to respond to increases in activity and stress. It can be divided into three phases. Phase 1 begins with the acute illness and ends with discharge from the hospital. Activities during this phase that could be delegated to an AP include assisting with morning care such as a bath, assisting a patient to the bathroom, and assisting with progressive ambulation in the hall. The nurse would be sure to instruct to AP to stop any activity that caused chest pain or pressure and report this at once. Referrals, administering drugs, and assessing patients require additional educational preparation and are suitable for professional nurses. **Focus:** Delegation, Supervision.

19. **Ans: 4** Normal sinus rhythm with a rate of 87 beats/min is a normal finding. There is no need to delay the patient's discharge, give early medications, or draw additional cardiac markers. The nurse would document this as a normal finding and prepare the patient for discharge. **Focus:** Prioritization.

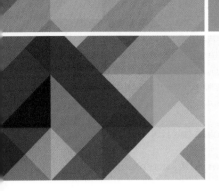
Dyspnea and Shortness of Breath

Questions

Mr. W is an 83-year-old man who was brought to the hospital from a long-term care facility by emergency medical services after reporting severe dyspnea and shortness of breath. He has been experiencing cold-like symptoms for the past 2 days. He has a productive cough with thick yellowish sputum. When Mr. W awoke in the nursing home, it was found that he was having difficulty breathing even after using his albuterol metered-dose inhaler (MDI). He appears very anxious and is in respiratory distress. His history includes chronic obstructive pulmonary disease (COPD) related to smoking two packs of cigarettes per day since he was 15 years old; he quit smoking 2 years ago when he was admitted to the long-term facility. Mr. W has been incontinent of urine and stool for the past 2 years.

In the emergency department (ED), Mr. W undergoes chest radiography, and admission laboratory tests are performed, including serum electrolyte levels and a complete blood count. A sputum sample is sent to the laboratory for culture and sensitivity testing and Gram staining.

Mr. W's vital sign values are as follows:

Blood pressure	154/92 mm Hg
Heart rate	118 beats/min, regular
O_2 saturation	88% on 1 L/min oxygen by nasal cannula
Respiratory rate	38 breaths/min
Temperature	100.9°F (38.3°C) (oral)

 1. Matrix

Instructions: For each nursing action listed below, check to specify whether the action is essential, non-essential or contraindicated.

Nursing Action	Essential	Nonessential	Contraindicated
Place on cardiac monitor			
Get a baseline set of vital signs			
Draw admission laboratory tests			
Place a saline lock			
Change adult pad			
Send for a chest x-ray			
Order a lunch tray			
Increase oxygen 2 L per nasal cannula as ordered by the ED health care provider.			
Keep head of bed elevated at least 45 degrees.			
Place a urinary catheter with a drainage bag			

2. What is the **priority** nursing concern for this patient?
   1. Skin care because of incontinence
   2. Clearance of thick secretions
   3. Rapid heart rate
   4. Elevated temperature

3. The RN assesses Mr. W in the ED. Which assessment findings are consistent with a diagnosis of COPD? **Select all that apply.**
   1. Enlarged neck muscles
   2. Forward bent posture
   3. Respiratory rate 15 to 25 breaths/min
   4. Inspiratory and expiratory wheezes
   5. Blue-tinged dusky appearance
   6. Symmetrical lung expansion

4. The health care provider's (HCP's) prescribed actions for this patient include all of the following. Which intervention should the nurse complete **first**?
   1. Send an arterial blood gas (ABG) sample to the laboratory.
   2. Schedule pulmonary function tests.
   3. Repeat chest radiography each morning.
   4. Administer albuterol via MDI 2 puffs every 4 hours.

Mr. W's ABG results include the following: pH, 7.37; arterial partial pressure of carbon dioxide ($Paco_2$), 55.4 mm Hg; arterial partial pressure of oxygen (Pao_2), 51.2 mm Hg; and bicarbonate (HCO_3^-) level, 38 mEq/L (38 mmol/L).

5. What is the nurse's interpretation of these results?
   1. Compensated metabolic acidosis with hypoxemia
   2. Compensated metabolic alkalosis with hypoxemia
   3. Compensated respiratory acidosis with hypoxemia
   4. Compensated respiratory alkalosis with hypoxemia

6. Based on the patient's ABG results, what are the nurse's **priority** actions at this time? **Select all that apply.**
   1. Administer oxygen at 2 L/min via nasal cannula.
   2. Initiate a rapid response.

3. Teach the patient how to cough and deep breathe.
4. Begin IV normal saline at 100 mL/hr.
5. Arrange a transfer to the intensive care unit (ICU).
6. Remind the patient to practice incentive spirometry every hour while awake.

7. Which intervention would the RN assign to an experienced LPN/LVN?
   1. Drawing a sample for ABG determination
   2. Administering albuterol by handheld nebulizer
   3. Measuring vital signs every 2 hours
   4. Increasing oxygen flow rate from 1 to 2 L/min by nasal cannula

After the rapid response, the respiratory therapist (RT) provides the patient with a handheld nebulizer treatment, and Mr. W is stable enough to be admitted to the acute care unit.

8. Which interventions would the acute care RN delegate to an experienced assistive personnel (AP)? **Select all that apply.**
   1. Changing the patient's incontinence pad as needed
   2. Performing pulse oximetry every shift
   3. Teaching the patient to cough and deep breathe
   4. Reminding the patient to use incentive spirometry every hour while awake
   5. Assessing the patient's breath sounds every shift
   6. Encouraging the patient to drink adequate oral fluids

9. Mr. W's ED lab values include a serum potassium of 2.8 mg/dL (2.8 mmol/L). What is the **priority** nursing action at this time?
   1. Teach the patient about potassium-rich foods.
   2. Provide the patient with oxygen at 2 L per nasal cannula.
   3. Contact and notify the HCP immediately.
   4. Initiate 0.9% saline at 20 mL/hr.

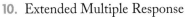

10. Extended Multiple Response _____

Instructions: Circle all of the correct responses in the right column that answer the question in the left column.

Question:

Mr. W is receiving an IV dose of potassium 10 mEq/100 mL (10 mmol/100 mL) normal saline to run over 1 hour. The AP asks the nurse why it takes so long to infuse such a small amount of fluid. What should the nurse explain to the AP? **Select all that apply.**	1. "IV potassium is very irritating to the veins and can cause phlebitis." 2. "Tissue damaged by potassium can become necrotic." 3. "Oral potassium can cause nausea, so IV potassium is preferred." 4. "The maximum recommended infusion rate for IV potassium is 5 to 10 mEq/hr (5 to 10 mmol/hr)." 5. "That's a good question, and I will ask the HCP if I can give the drug IV push." 6. "The goal is to prevent infiltration into the tissue." 7. "The patient is not taking in sufficient dietary potassium to keep the level within normal limits." 8. "Giving the potassium slowly will give use time to teach the patient about dietary sources of potassium."

11. During morning rounds, the nurse notes all of these assessment findings for Mr. W. Which finding indicates a **worsening** of the patient's condition?
1. Barrel-shaped chest
2. Clubbed fingers on both hands
3. Crackles bilaterally
4. Frequent productive cough

12. The nurse reports the morning assessment findings **(see question 11)** to the HCP. Which prescribed intervention is **most** directly related to the nurse's assessment findings?
1. Administer furosemide 20 mg IV push now.
2. Keep accurate records of intake and output.
3. Administer potassium 20 mEq (20 mmol) orally every morning.
4. Weigh the patient every morning.

13. Which assessment finding would the nurse instruct the AP to report **immediately**?
1. Incontinence of urine and stool
2. 1-lb (0.45-kg) weight loss since admission
3. Patient cough productive of greenish-yellow sputum
4. Eating only half of breakfast and lunch

14. The AP checks morning vital signs and immediately reports the following values to the nurse. Which takes **priority** when notifying the HCP?
1. Heart rate of 96 beats/min
2. Blood pressure of 160/90 mm Hg
3. Respiratory rate of 34 breaths/min
4. Oral temperature of 103.5°F (39.7°C)

15. An LPN/LVN tells the RN that the patient is now receiving oxygen at 2 L/min via nasal cannula and his pulse oximetry reading is 91%, but he still has crackles in the bases of his lungs. What intervention should the RN assign to the LPN/LVN?
1. Begin creating a plan for discharging the patient.
2. Administer furosemide 20 mg orally each morning.
3. Get a baseline weight for the patient now.
4. Administer cefotaxime IV piggyback every 6 hours.

16. The RN administers the patient's first dose of IV cefotaxime. Within 15 minutes, Mr. W develops a rash with fever and chills. What is the nurse's **first** action at this time?
1. Discontinue the IV infusion.
2. Administer two tablets of acetaminophen.
3. Measure the area of the rash.
4. Check for numbness and tingling.

17. The RN observes the patient's use of the albuterol MDI. The patient takes two puffs from the inhaler in rapid succession. Which intervention takes **priority** at this time?
1. Call the pharmacy to request a spacer for the patient.
2. Notify the provider that the patient will need to continue receiving nebulizer treatments.
3. Ask the AP to help get the patient into a chair.
4. Instruct the patient about proper techniques for using an MDI.

PART 3 Complex Health Scenarios

18. Mr. W has lost 15 lb (6.8 kg) over the past year. On assessment, he tells the nurse that his appetite is not what it used to be, and he becomes short of breath while eating. Which interventions should be included in his nursing care plan? **Select all that apply.**
    1. Initiate a dietary consult.
    2. Stress that he must eat all of his meals or he'll become malnourished.
    3. Monitor serum prealbumin levels.
    4. Suggest four to six small meals per day.
    5. Instruct the patient to use his bronchodilator 30 minutes before meals.
    6. Encourage dry foods to avoid coughing.

19. The AP tells the nurse that Mr. W is unable to complete his morning care without assistance and wonders if he is being lazy. What is the nurse's **best** response?
    1. "Encourage the patient to do as much as he can as quickly as he can."
    2. "If the patient is short of breath, increase his oxygen flow."
    3. "Remind the patient to take his time and not to rush his morning care."
    4. "He may not need as much help as he is asking for, so try to get him to do more."

20. Mr. W is to be transferred back to the long-term care facility after lunch. Which nursing care intervention would be **best** for the RN to assign to the experienced LPN/LVN?
    1. Administer the patient's 12:00 PM oral medications.
    2. Check and record a set of vital signs at 12:00 PM.
    3. Pack the patient's personal items to be taken with him.
    4. Change Mr. W's incontinence pad before he is transferred.

Answer Key for this chapter begins on p. 261

Answers

1. **Ans:** Baseline data that are essential to decisions for the care of this patient take priority at this time. These include vital signs, cardiac rhythm, lab values, and chest x-ray findings. Placement of a saline lock is essential for administration of fluids and emergency drugs. The patient's oxygen saturation is only 88% on 1 L, so increasing it to 2 L may improve oxygenation, as may elevating the head of the patient's bed. Changing the patient's incontinence pad is important to protect his skin but is not urgent. In addition, this could require placing him in a supine position, which would make breathing more difficult and force him to struggle to move into an upright position for easier breathing. Ordering a lunch tray may be premature because the interventions for this patient's care are undecided when he is first admitted to the ED. Placing a urinary catheter may lead to a urinary tract infection. **Focus:** Prioritization.

Nursing Action	Essential	Nonessential	Contraindicated
Place on cardiac monitor	X		
Get a baseline set of vital signs	X		
Draw admission laboratory tests	X		
Place a saline lock	X		
Change adult pad			X
Send for a chest x-ray	X		
Order a lunch tray		X	
Increase oxygen 2 L per nasal cannula as ordered by the ED health care provider.	X		
Keep head of bed elevated at least 45 degrees.	X		
Place a urinary catheter with a drainage bag			X

2. **Ans: 2** The patient's major problems at this time relate to airway and breathing including thick sputum, difficulty breathing, and respiratory distress. The patient's skin care, blood pressure, and elevated temperature will need to be followed up on soon but are not as urgent at this time as his respiratory status. **Focus:** Prioritization.

3. **Ans: 1, 2, 4, 5** The presence of wheezing, enlarged neck muscles, bluish dusky appearance, and forward bent posture are all classic manifestations in a patient with COPD. The respiratory rate is usually higher than normal and during an exacerbation can be as high as 30 to 40 breaths/min. Lung expansion in patients with COPD is usually asymmetrical. **Focus:** Prioritization.

4. **Ans: 1** Baseline ABG results are important in planning the care of this patient. The unit clerk can schedule the pulmonary function tests and chest radiography. The albuterol therapy is a routine order and the patient may need this after the ABG is drawn. **Focus:** Prioritization.

5. **Ans: 3** The pH is on the low side of normal, and the $Paco_2$ is elevated, which indicates an underlying respiratory acidosis. The HCO_3^- level is elevated, which indicates compensation and since the pH is within normal limits it is completed compensation. Both the Pao_2 and the oxygen saturation levels are low, which points to hypoxemia. These blood gas results are typically expected when a patient has a chronic respiratory problem such as COPD. **Focus:** Prioritization. **Test-Taking Tip:** The nurse must remember and apply physiologic concepts learned in school to patient care (e.g., normal ABG values).

6. **Ans: 1, 2, 3, 6** The patient's major problem at this time is impaired gas exchange with hypoxemia based on the ABG results. Strategies to compensate include administration of low-flow oxygen as well as interventions to improve gas exchange, such as having the patient cough and take deep breaths and perform incentive spirometry. These strategies may improve the patient's condition and prevent the need to initiate a code, transfer to the ICU, or both. A rapid response is for hospitalized patients with early signs of deterioration on non-ICUs to prevent respiratory or cardiac arrest. The team includes members that may not be routinely in the ER (e.g. RT, pharmacist, ICU nurse). The patient's symptoms call for initiation of a rapid response to treat him now and prevent the need for a code. A saline lock is a good idea, but giving the patient too much fluid may worsen his condition by producing a fluid overload. Transfer to the ICU at this point is not warranted because the patient is unstable. **Focus:** Prioritization.

PART 3 Complex Health Scenarios

7. **Ans: 4**   Increasing oxygen flow for a patient based on an HCP's prescription is within the scope of practice of LPN/LVNs. APs may measure vital signs. Arterial draws for laboratory tests are not within the LPN/LVN's scope of practice unless they have had additional special training. The RN would need to assess the LPN/LVN's skill before assigning this task. Handheld nebulizers are usually operated by RTs. **Focus:** Assignment, Supervision.

8. **Ans: 1, 2, 4, 6**   Assisting patients with activities of daily living such as toileting is within the scope of practice of APs. After licensed nurses or RTs have taught the patient to use incentive spirometry, the AP can play a role in reminding the patient to perform it. APs can participate in encouraging patients to drink adequate fluids. Assessing and teaching are not within the scope of practice of APs. Performing pulse oximetry is appropriate for experienced APs after they have been taught how to use the pulse oximetry device to gather additional data. Before delegating this task, the nurse would be sure to assess the AP's skills. **Focus:** Delegation, Supervision.

9. **Ans: 3**   A low serum potassium places the patient at risk for cardiac dysrhythmias, which can be life threatening. The HCP should be notified immediately and will likely order IV or oral potassium supplements to move the patient's level back into the normal range. Later, before discharge, the nurse would certainly want to teach the patient about potassium-rich foods, but this is not urgent. Oxygen is essential for the patient's respiratory problem but will not correct the low potassium, nor will IV normal saline. **Focus:** Prioritization.

10. **Ans: 1, 2, 4, 6**   A dilution no greater than 1 mEq (1 mmol) of potassium to 10 mL of solution is recommended for IV administration. The maximum recommended infusion rate is 5 to 10 mEq/hr (5 to 10 mmol/hr); this rate is never to exceed 20 mEq/hr (20 mmol/hr) under any circumstances. In accordance with National Patient Safety Goals, potassium is not given by IV push to avoid causing cardiac arrest. Oral potassium can cause nausea and vomiting (give it with food to prevent this), but this does not answer the AP's question. Lack of dietary intake and teaching about dietary sources of potassium do not answer the AP's question. **Focus:** Prioritization, Supervision.

11. **Ans: 3**   Barrel chest and clubbed fingers are signs of chronic COPD. The patient had a productive cough on admission to the hospital. Bilateral crackles are a new finding and indicate fluid-filled alveoli and pulmonary edema. Fluid in the alveoli affects gas exchange and can result in worsening ABG concentrations. **Focus:** Prioritization.

12. **Ans: 1**   Furosemide is a loop diuretic. The uses of this drug include treatment of pulmonary edema, which is **most** directly related to the new finding. Intake and output records and daily weights are important

in documenting the effectiveness of the medication. A side effect of this drug is hypokalemia, and some patients are also prescribed a potassium supplement when taking this medication. **Focus:** Prioritization.

13. **Ans: 3**   The patient's temperature was elevated on admission, and his cough was productive. The changes in Mr. W's sputum could indicate an ongoing infection. The HCP needs to be notified and an appropriate treatment plan started. All of the other pieces of information are important but not urgent. The patient's incontinence is not new. **Focus:** Supervision, Prioritization.

14. **Ans: 4**   The heart rate and blood pressure are slightly increased from admission, and the respiratory rate is slightly decreased. The continued elevation in temperature indicates a probable respiratory tract infection that needs to be recognized and treated. **Focus:** Prioritization. **Test-Taking Tip:** Always consider an infectious process when a patient has an elevated temperature and be sure to notify your nurse preceptor and/or the HCP so that appropriate actions can be taken to treat the infection.

15. **Ans: 2**   Discharge planning and IV administration of antibiotics are more appropriate to the scope of practice of the RN. Nevertheless, in some states, LPN/LVNs with special training may administer IV antibiotics. (Be aware of state regulations and nursing practice laws in your state.) Administering oral medications is appropriate to assign to LPN/LVNs, and in this case, furosemide may help clear up the crackles. Although the LPN/LVN could weigh the patient, this intervention is also appropriate to the scope of practice of the AP. **Focus:** Assignment, Supervision. **Test-Taking Tip:** Even when the LPN/LVN is permitted to give IV drugs, the RN should administer the first dose of medications, such as IV antibiotics, because these drugs can cause an allergic reaction that may require emergency intervention.

16. **Ans: 1**   Serious side effects of cefotaxime include rashes, fever, and chills, as well as diarrhea, bruising, numbness, tingling, and bleeding. If the patient is taking this drug as an outpatient, the HCP should be notified immediately. Because the drug is being given IV, the first step would be to stop the infusion. The HCP should be notified, and the patient should be assessed for additional symptoms of a serious reaction to the drug. The HCP will prescribe a different antibiotic for the patient. **Focus:** Prioritization.

17. **Ans: 4**   The patient is demonstrating improper use of the MDI by taking two puffs in rapid succession, which can lead to incorrect dosage and ineffective action of the albuterol. Teaching is the first priority. The patient is taught to wait for at least 1 minute between MDI puffs. As the nurse works with this patient, it may be determined that he would benefit from the use of a spacer. Sitting up in a chair may also be useful, but

these interventions are not the first priority. Notifying the provider that the patient needs to continue with nebulizer treatments is not within nursing scope of practice and does not address the problem, which is that the patient does not know how to properly use his MDI. **Focus:** Prioritization.

18. **Ans: 1, 3, 4, 5**   A dietitian can help with the selection of foods that are easy to chew, do not form gas, and are high in calories and protein. Serum prealbumin levels are a good indicator of nutritional status and should be monitored. Small meals can help prevent meal-related dyspnea. Using a bronchodilator before meals will reduce bronchospasm. The second response does not demonstrate respect for the patient's role in his care. Dry foods stimulate coughing. **Focus:** Prioritization.

19. **Ans: 3**   The patient with COPD often has chronic fatigue and needs help with activities. Teaching the patient not to rush through activities is important because rushing increases dyspnea, fatigue, and hypoxemia. Reminding a patient of what has already been taught is within the scope of practice for an AP. Patients with COPD should be kept on low-flow oxygen because their stimulus to breathe is a low arterial oxygen level. **Focus:** Supervision, Delegation, Prioritization.

20. **Ans: 1**   The scope of practice for an experienced LPN/LVN includes administering oral medications. Although the LPN could certainly check the patient's vital signs, pack his personal belongings, and change his incontinence pad, these interventions are also within the scope of practice for an AP. **Focus:** Assignment, Supervision. **Test-Taking Tip:** The nurse must be familiar with the scope of practice for LPN/LVNs and APs. LPN/LVNs have additional educational preparation in areas such as pharmacology and medication administration.

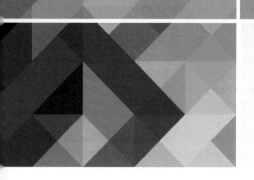

Multiple Patients on a Medical-Surgical Unit

Questions

The RN is the leader of a team providing care for six patients. The team includes the RN, an experienced LPN/LVN, and a newly educated assistive personnel (AP) who is in his fourth week of orientation to the acute care unit. (Note to student: Use the information from the shift change report below to make brief notes about these six patients and refer to the notes as you work through the case study.) The patients are as follows:

- Mr. C, a 68-year-old man with unstable angina who needs reinforcement of teaching for a cardiac catheterization scheduled this morning

- Ms. J, a 45-year-old woman who had chest pain during the night and is now experiencing chest pain. She is scheduled for a graded exercise test later today.
- Mr. R, a 75-year-old man who had a left-hemisphere stroke 4 days ago
- Ms. S, an 83-year-old woman with heart disease, a history of myocardial infarction, and mild dementia
- Mr. B, a 93-year-old newly admitted man from a long-term care facility, with decreased urine output, altered level of consciousness, and an elevated temperature of 99.5°F (37.5°C)
- Mr. L, a 59-year-old man with mild shortness of breath (SOB) and chronic emphysema

 1. Drag and Drop

Scenario: The charge nurse is delegating and assigning patient care to his or her team members for the shift.

Instructions: Staff members are listed in the left-hand column. In the right-hand column, in the space provided, write in the number for the best member of the patient care team for each intervention. Note that all responses may be used more than once.

Staff Member	Intervention
a. LPN/LVN	1. _____ Check and record vital signs for each patient.
b. AP (assistive personnel)	2. _____ Administer docusate sodium, 50 mg orally to a patient passing hard stool.
c. RN	3. _____ Bathe bedridden confused patient.
	4. _____ Complete an assessment on a newly admitted patient for altered level of consciousness.
	5. _____ Measure output and empty patient's urinary catheter bag at end of shift.
	6. _____ Place a urinary catheter as ordered by the health care provider (HCP).
	7. _____ Teach a rehab patient to call for help when getting out of bed to the bathroom.
	8. _____ Check fingerstick blood glucose and administer sliding scale insulin as ordered if glucose is elevated.

2. During the shift change report, the night RN informs the team that Ms. S is to be transferred back to her long-term care facility after lunch. What action should be taken for this patient?
   1. Instruct the AP to awaken her for vital signs and breakfast.
   2. Allow her to sleep for an hour or two while the other patients are assessed.
   3. Assign the LPN/LVN to immediately pack up the patient's belongings.
   4. Call the nursing home to find out if the transfer can wait until tomorrow.

3. Which patients should the team leader assign to the LPN/LVN for nursing care under the RN's supervision? **Select all that apply.**
   1. Mr. C (unstable angina)
   2. Ms. J (chest pain)
   3. Mr. R (stroke)
   4. Ms. S (heart disease and dementia)
   5. Mr. B (decreased urine output, altered level of consciousness)
   6. Mr. L (SOB and chronic emphysema)

4. Which patient should the RN assess **first**?
   1. Mr. C (unstable angina)
   2. Ms. J (chest pain)
   3. Mr. B (decreased urine output, altered level of consciousness)
   4. Mr. L (SOB and chronic emphysema)

5. The RN is assessing Ms. J's chest pain. Which questions would the RN be sure to ask the patient? **Select all that apply.**
   1. "When did you first notice the chest pain?"
   2. "Did your pain start suddenly or gradually?"
   3. "How long has the chest pain lasted?"
   4. "Have you experienced confusion or loss of memory with the pain?"
   5. "Can you grade your pain on a scale of 0 to 10, with 10 being the worst pain ever?"
   6. "What were you doing when the chest pain started?"

6. The HCP's prescribed actions for Ms. J, who is currently experiencing chest pain, are as follows. Which intervention should be completed **first**?
   1. Administer nitroglycerin 0.6 mg sublingually as needed for chest pain.
   2. Administer morphine 2 mg IV push as needed for chest pain.
   3. Check blood pressure and heart rate.
   4. Complete lab tests including cardiac markers and daily electrocardiogram.

7. Which tasks should the nurse delegate to the newly hired AP? **Select all that apply.**
   1. Asking Ms. S memory-testing questions
   2. Teaching Ms. J about treadmill exercise testing
   3. Checking vital signs on all six patients
   4. Recording oral intake and urine output for Mr. B
   5. Assisting Mr. L to walk to the bathroom
   6. Helping Mr. R with morning care

8. Which key point would the nurse be sure to include when teaching Mr. C about the postprocedural care for cardiac catheterization?
   1. "There are no restrictions after the procedure."
   2. "You will be able to get out of bed within 2 hours after the procedure."
   3. "You will have to stay almost flat in bed with limited position changes for 4 to 6 hours."
   4. "Family visitors will be restricted until the next day."

9. The cardiac lab calls to have Ms. J sent for her graded exercise test (GXT). What is the nurse's best action?
   1. Instruct the AP to put the patient in a wheelchair and take her to the lab.
   2. Call the cardiac lab and ask to delay the test until later in the day.
   3. Contact the HCP to ask if the patient should still have the GXT.
   4. Ask the patient if she is continuing to have chest pain.

10. The AP is delegated the task of measuring morning vital signs for all six patients. Which finding would the nurse instruct the AP to report immediately?
    1. Oral temperature higher than 102°F (38.9°C)
    2. Blood pressure higher than 140/80 mm Hg
    3. Heart rate lower than 65 beats/min
    4. Respiratory rate lower than 18 breaths/min

11. The AP asks the RN why it is important to notify someone whenever a patient with heart problems reports chest pain. What is the RN's best response?
    1. "It's important to keep track of the chest pain episodes so we can notify the HCP."
    2. "The patient may need morphine to treat the chest pain."
    3. "Chest pain may indicate coronary artery blockage and heart muscle damage that will need treatment."
    4. "Our unit policy includes specific steps to take in the treatment of patients with chest pain."

12. The HCP's prescribed interventions for Mr. R, who had a stroke 4 days ago, include assisting the patient with meals. Which staff member would be best to assign this task?
    1. Physical therapist
    2. AP
    3. LPN/LVN
    4. Occupational therapist

Answer Key for this chapter begins on p. 268

13. The LPN/LVN reports to the RN that Mr. R was unable to take his oral medications because of difficulty swallowing. The RN assesses Mr. R and finds that he is having dysphagia. What is the RN's best instruction for the LPN/LVN?
    1. "Keep Mr. R NPO, and I will contact his HCP."
    2. "Try giving his medications with applesauce or pudding."
    3. "Check with the pharmacy to find out if they have liquid forms of Mr. R's medications."
    4. "Assess Mr. R's ability to speak and move his tongue."

14. The AP reports to the RN that Mr. L, the patient with chronic emphysema, says he is feeling short of breath after walking to the bathroom. What action should the RN take **first**?
    1. Notify the HCP.
    2. Increase oxygen flow to 6 L/min via nasal cannula.
    3. Assess oxygen saturation by pulse oximetry.
    4. Remind the patient to cough and deep breathe.

15. The oral temperature of Mr. B, the patient newly admitted from a long-term care facility with decreased urine output and altered level of consciousness, is now 102.6°F (39.2°C). What is the nurse's best action?
    1. Notify the HCP.
    2. Administer acetaminophen 2 tablets orally.
    3. Assign the LPN/LVN to give an acetaminophen suppository.
    4. Remove extra blankets from the patient's bed.

16. Which factor does the nurse suspect **most** likely precipitated Mr. B's elevated temperature?
    1. Bladder infection
    2. Increased metabolic rate
    3. Kidney failure
    4. Nosocomial pneumonia

17. The RN is working on a care plan for Mr. B. Which care intervention is **most** appropriate to delegate to the AP?
    1. Checking the patient's level of consciousness every shift
    2. Assisting the patient with ambulation to the bathroom to urinate
    3. Teaching the patient the side effects of antibiotic therapy
    4. Administering sulfamethoxazole–trimethoprim orally every 12 hours

18. The AP reports that Mr. L's heart rate, which was 86 beats/min in the morning, is now 98 beats/min. What would be the **most** appropriate question for the nurse to ask Mr. L?
    1. "Have you just returned from the bathroom?"
    2. "Did you recently use your albuterol inhaler?"
    3. "Are you feeling short of breath?"
    4. "How much do you smoke?"

19. The LPN/LVN reports to the RN that Ms. S will not leave the chest leads for her cardiac monitor in place and asks if the patient can be restrained. What is the RN's best response?
    1. "Yes, this patient had a heart attack, and we must keep her on the cardiac monitor."
    2. "Yes, but be sure to use soft restraints so that the patient's circulation is not compromised."
    3. "No, we must have an HCP's order before we can apply restraints in any situation."
    4. "No, but try covering the lead wires with the sheet so that the patient does not see them."

20. Mr. C has returned from the cardiac catheterization lab and requires close monitoring after the procedure. Which postprocedural tasks would be best assigned to the LPN/LVN? **Select all that apply.**
    1. Check bilateral pedal pulses every 15 minutes during the first hour.
    2. Check right groin area for bleeding every 15 minutes during the first hour.
    3. Continue IV fluids normal saline at 50 mL/hr.
    4. Assist patient to bathroom as needed during first 6 hours after the procedure.
    5. Administer morphine sulfate 2 mg IV push as needed for pain.
    6. Give patient's daily multivitamin and stool softener on return to medical unit.

21. Near the end of the shift, the LPN/LVN reports that the AP has not totaled the patients' intake and output for the past 8 hours. What is the nurse's best action?
    1. Confront the AP and instruct him to complete this assignment at once.
    2. Assign this task to the LPN/LVN.
    3. Ask the AP if he needs assistance completing the intake and output records.
    4. Notify the nurse manager to include this on the AP's evaluation.

22. Cloze _____

Instructions: Choose the correct words or phrases to complete the sentences and write the number for the words in the appropriate space.

Case Study A

The LPN/LVN is working with an AP to provide care for Ms. S before her transfer back to the long-term care facility. In preparation for the transfer, the LPN/LVN may delegate the AP to assist this patient with/by (a)_____, (b)_____, and (c)_____, as needed.

A Options

1. getting out of bed
2. washing her hands and face
3. feeding the patient rapidly and giving her fluids from her tray after every bite
4. notifying the long-term care facility that the patient is ready for transfer
5. instructing her to pack her belongings as soon as possible
6. ambulating to the bathroom

Case Study B

The AP informs the LPN/LVN that the patient now has a rapid heart rate of 118 per minute and that she states her chest hurts a little. The LPN/LVN would first (a)_____. Then the priority would be to (b)_____ and (c)_____. The next priori would be to (d)_____ and (e)_____.

B Options

1. notify the HCP
2. apply oxygen
3. assess the patient
4. check pulse oximetry
5. gather more information
6. notify the RN

23. Enhanced Multiple Response _____

Instructions: Read the case study on the left and circle the numbers that best answer the question.

Case Study

Near the end of the shift the RN is admitting Mr. E, an 88-year-old patient, from long-term care to the acute care medical/surgical unit. The patient was alert until early this morning and has become confused. His history includes smoking cigarettes for 55 years, but he quit at age 70. He has a history of post-traumatic stress disorder (PTSD) and has had surgery for appendicitis and gallbladder removal. Over the past 36 hours the patient developed headache, muscle aches, cough with thick clear sputum, and chest discomfort.

Vital signs:
Temperature 101.4 °F (38.6 °C)
Pulse 104 beats/min
Respirations 30 breaths/min
Blood pressure 108/62 mmHg

Assessment findings: Warm dry skin, crackles bilaterally with wheezes, tachycardia with normal heart sounds, and a pulse oximetry reading of 89 on oxygen at 2 L by nasal cannula. The patient does not tolerate lying flat in bed.

Admission Lab: Complete blood count reveals elevated white blood cell (WBC) count. Electrolytes (Na^+ 135, K^+ 3.8, Cl^- 98)

Question

Which of the following findings with this patient are factors that increase the risk for a diagnosis of pneumonia? **Select all that apply.**

1. Patient age
2. PTSD
3. Smoked cigarettes 55 years
4. Thick, clear sputum
5. Crackles and wheezes
6. Elevated WBC count
7. Altered level of consciousness
8. Electrolyte values
9. Temperature 101.4 °F (38.6 °C)

Answer Key for this chapter begins on p. 268

Answers

1. **Ans: 1b; 2a; 3b; 4c; 5b; 6a; 7c; 8a** The RN could complete all of these tasks, but the question asks which team member is most appropriate for the RN to delegate or assign to complete each task. The RN must be aware of the scope of practice for each member of the team. The AP can do personnel care (e.g., bathing, feeding, vital signs, turning and repositioning, intake and output) so delegation of these types of functions by the RN to an AP is appropriate. Experienced APs may be taught special tasks such as checking fingerstick glucose level or pulse oximetry. The RN must ensure that the AP has been taught and is skilled before delegating these tasks. An RN can assign care to other RNs and LPN/LVNs (who are licensed professionals). The LPN/LVN can be assigned to pass oral and subcutaneous medications (and in some states or facilities IV meds with extra training). They can also perform tasks within their scope of practice (e.g., placement of urinary catheters and checking fingerstick glucose). They can perform shift assessments (usually checked by an RN in the acute care unit). RNs are responsible for higher-level patient care including assessment, care planning, evaluation, and reevaluation of patient care. **Focus:** Delegation, Assignment.

2. **Ans: 2** Because Ms. S is not scheduled to be transferred until after lunch, it is not urgent to get her ready at this time. Allowing her to rest while the staff takes care of other patients whose needs are more urgent is acceptable. The RN could instruct the AP to keep the patient's breakfast tray and warm it up when she is ready to eat. **Focus:** Prioritization, Supervision.

3. **Ans: 1, 3, 4, 6** It is important to recognize that the RN continues to be accountable for the care of all patients by the team. Appropriate patient assignments for the LPN/LVN include patients whose conditions are stable and not complex. Ms. J is currently experiencing chest pain, and Mr. B is a complex new admission. These patients will benefit from the advanced skills of the RN. **Focus:** Assignment, Supervision.

4. **Ans: 2** Although it is important that the nurse see all of these patients, Ms. J's assessment takes priority. Her chest pain may indicate coronary artery blockage and acute heart attack. None of the other patients' needs are life threatening. **Focus:** Prioritization. **Test-Taking Tip:** A question like this asks the nurse to prioritize in order to make a decision about which patient most urgently needs to be evaluated. The patient is having chest pain, and the risk is life threatening for coronary artery blockage and heart attack.

5. **Ans: 1, 2, 3, 5, 6** The RN should thoroughly evaluate the nature of the patient's pain. Asking the patient when the pain started focuses on the onset. Asking if the pain was sudden or slow in onset deals with the manner of onset. Asking how long the pain has lasted speaks to the duration of symptoms. Having the patient grade the pain on a scale of 0 to 10 evaluates the intensity. Asking the patient what he or she was doing when the pain started helps delineate factors that can lead to pain onset. Patients do not usually experience confusion or memory loss with cardiac pain. **Focus:** Prioritization.

6. **Ans: 3** When the patient experiences chest pain, vital signs should be checked immediately to establish a baseline. Nitroglycerin is usually tried every 5 minutes for three doses before morphine to relieve the chest pain. Hypotension is a side effect of nitroglycerin. Blood pressure and heart rate are monitored after each dose of nitroglycerin is administered. When nitroglycerin fails to relieve chest pain, IV morphine is the next action, and the HCP should be notified. **Focus:** Prioritization. **Test-Taking Tip:** This question asks the nurse to apply knowledge about common side effects of medications. Checking blood pressure and heart rate is essential when evaluating a patient for the common side effect of nitroglycerin, which is hypotension.

7. **Ans: 3, 4, 5, 6** Assessment and teaching are more appropriate to the educational preparation of licensed nursing staff. Checking vital signs, monitoring and recording intake and output, assisting patients to the bathroom, and helping patients with morning care are all within the educational scope of the AP. **Focus:** Delegation, Supervision.

8. **Ans: 3** Cardiac catheterization is usually accomplished by inserting a large-bore needle into the femoral vein or artery (or both). Patients are routinely restricted to bed rest, with the affected extremity kept straight, for 4 to 6 hours after the procedure to prevent hemorrhage. Family members are usually permitted to visit as soon as the patient returns to the room. **Focus:** Prioritization.

9. **Ans: 3** The patient had chest pain during the night and this morning. She may be experiencing acute coronary syndrome, a term used to describe patients who have either unstable angina or an acute myocardial infarction. In this situation, the best action by the RN is to contact the HCP and ask if the patient's GXT should be cancelled. Sending her to take the GXT would increase the risk of cardiac damage and should not be done. Asking if the patient is still having chest pain is important and may reinforce the need to cancel the test. **Focus:** Prioritization.

10. **Ans: 1** A temperature elevation to 102°F (38.9°C) is likely an indicator of an infectious process. The other criterion parameters are near normal, and assessment

or evaluation would instead be based on abnormalities from each patient's baseline. **Focus:** Delegation, Supervision.

11. **Ans: 3** Acute chest pain can indicate myocardial ischemia, coronary artery blockage, or myocardial damage. The AP's question should be answered with the most accurate response. Although the unit may have protocols that the AP should be familiar with, option 4 is not the most accurate response. **Focus:** Prioritization, Supervision.

12. **Ans: 2** Assisting patients with activities of daily living such as feeding is most appropriate to the scope of practice of the AP. The RN would be sure to instruct the AP to avoid rushing the patient and to report any difficulty with swallowing. **Focus:** Delegation, Supervision.

13. **Ans: 1** The patient who has difficulty chewing or swallowing foods and liquids (dysphagia) is at risk for aspiration pneumonia. At this time, the best action is to keep the patient NPO and contact the HCP. Attempting to give him oral foods, drugs, or fluids increases his risk for aspiration. Assessing his speech and tongue movement is important but not as urgent as keeping him NPO. The patient likely will require screening or use of an evidence-based bedside swallowing screening tool to determine if dysphagia is present. A referral to a speech-language pathologist for a swallowing evaluation per stroke protocol is needed. If dysphagia is present, develop a collaborative plan of care to prevent aspiration and support nutrition and prevent constipation or dehydration. **Focus:** Prioritization.

14. **Ans: 3** The nurse should gather more information before notifying the HCP. A pulse oximetry assessment provides information about the patient's gas exchange and oxygenation status. Patients with chronic obstructive pulmonary disease (COPD) usually receive low-dose oxygen (1 to 3 L) because their stimulus for breathing is a low oxygen level. Coughing and deep breathing help mobilize secretions and can be helpful, but these are not the first priority. **Focus:** Prioritization.

15. **Ans: 1** This patient's temperature elevation is most likely caused by an infection. The HCP must be notified to modify the patient's plan of care. Administering acetaminophen and removing extra blankets may decrease the patient's temperature, but they will not treat the infection. **Focus:** Prioritization.

16. **Ans: 1** The patient's temperature elevation indicates an infectious process. For older adult patients, changes in level of consciousness are frequently an early sign of bladder or urinary tract infections. **Focus:** Prioritization.

17. **Ans: 2** Assisting patients with activities of daily living (including ambulation to the bathroom) is appropriate to the educational preparation and scope of practice of the AP. An LPN/LVN could administer the oral drug. Teaching, assessing, and administering medications fall within the scope of practice for licensed nurses. **Focus:** Delegation, Supervision.

18. **Ans: 2** A common side effect of beta-adrenergic agonists such as albuterol is increased heart rate. Drugs such as albuterol are commonly prescribed for patients with COPD to use as needed to dilate the airways when experiencing shortness of breath. Although the other factors are important and may be related to the patient's COPD, they may not have contributed to the increase in heart rate. **Focus:** Prioritization.

19. **Ans: 4** Standards of practice for the use of restraints require that nurses attempt alternative strategies before asking that a patient be restrained. An HCP's written order is required for continued use of restraints but can be obtained after the fact if the patient's actions endanger his or her well-being. Remember that when a patient is restrained, a flow sheet should be at the bedside and the restraints frequently assessed (every 1 to 2 hours) and released (every 2 hours). **Focus:** Prioritization, Assignment, Supervision. **Test-Taking Tip:** This question asks the nurse to apply the standards of practice associated with the use of restraints. Nurses are expected to try alternatives before making use of restraints.

20. **Ans: 1, 2, 3, 6** The LPN/LVN is experienced and post cardiac catheterization care would be familiar to her. Basic assessments such as checking peripheral pulses, watching for bleeding, and monitoring IV fluid flow, as well as administering oral drugs are within his or her scope of practice. Most IV drugs are administered by RNs; however, some LPN/LVNs may administer these drugs with additional training. The patient would most likely be on bed rest, keeping the affected extremity straight for 4 to 6 hours after the procedure. **Focus:** Assignment.

21. **Ans: 3** The AP is new to the unit and may need assistance or instruction regarding the completion of this assignment. **Focus:** Delegation, Supervision.

22. **A. Ans: a1; b2; c6** Assisting patients with getting out of bed, performing morning care, and ambulating to the bathroom are within the scope of practice for an AP and are appropriate for the LPN/LVN to delegate to an AP. If the patient needed assistance with feeding, it would be best to go slowly at the patient's speed. Because this patient is confused, asking her to pack her belongings may be confusing, so it would be better to assist her in packing. The RN would be responsible for giving the report on the patient and letting them know when she is to be transferred. **Focus:** Delegation.

B. Ans: a6; b3; c5; d1; e2 The first action would be to notify the RN who would then assess the patient and gather more information. Next it would be essential to notify the HCP and follow orders including application of oxygen, which will help in the delivery of oxygen to the myocardium. Alternately the nurse could notify the rapid response team (RRT) if that were a choice. Applying oxygen per order (by HCP, RRT, or unit standing order) would be important. The patient is breathing and not yet in need of a ventilator. **Focus:** Prioritization.

23. **Ans: 1, 3, 5, 6, 7, 9**   Older patients are at increased risk for pneumonia in the community and in health care settings. A history of chronic lung disease is also a risk factor. Assessment findings include the presence of crackles over areas with interstitial fluid, and wheezes are heard if inflammation or exudate narrows the airways. Elevated WBC count is a common finding in older adults as are changes in level of consciousness. PTSD would not be a risk factor for pneumonia. Generally, with pneumonia, sputum is purulent, blood-tinged, or rust colored. The electrolytes listed in this case study are all within normal limits. **Focus:** Prioritization.

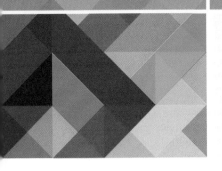

Shortness of Breath, Edema, and Decreased Urine Output

Questions

Ms. J is a 63-year-old Hispanic woman who is being admitted directly to the medical unit after visiting her health care provider (HCP) because of shortness of breath and increased swelling in her ankles and calves. She is being admitted with a diagnosis of chronic kidney disease (CKD). Ms. J states that her symptoms have become worse over the past 2 to 3 months and that she uses the bathroom less often and urinates in small amounts. Her medical history includes hypertension (30 years), coronary artery disease (18 years), type 2 diabetes (14 years), an appendectomy at age 28, cataract surgery to the left eye 2 years ago and right eye 1 year ago, and four pregnancies with healthy births. She also has gastroesophageal reflux disease (GERD), which is controlled with over-the-counter (OTC) famotidine 20 mg as needed.

Ms. J's vital sign values on admission were as follows:

Blood pressure	162/96 mm Hg
Heart rate	88 beats/min
O$_2$ saturation	89% on room air
Respiratory rate	28 breaths/min
Temperature	97.8°F (36.6°C)

The patient is to be placed on oxygen at 2 L/min via nasal cannula. Admission laboratory tests for which patient samples are to be collected on the unit include serum electrolyte levels, kidney function tests, complete blood count, and urinalysis. A 24-hour urine collection for the determination of creatinine clearance has also been ordered.

1. The LPN/LVN rechecks Ms. J's O$_2$ saturation after she has been on oxygen at 2 L/min per nasal cannula and finds the reading is now 93%. What is the LPN/LVN's best action?
   1. Increase the oxygen to 3 L/min per nasal cannula.
   2. Ask the respiratory therapist to start Ms. J on incentive spirometry.
   3. Teach Ms. J to take 10 deep breaths every hour while awake.
   4. Notify the team leader RN and record the finding.

2. Which patient admission tasks should the nurse delegate to the experienced assistive personnel (AP)? **Select all that apply.**
   1. Check vital signs every 4 hours.
   2. Record accurate intake and output.
   3. Place a saline lock in left forearm.
   4. Check oxygen saturation by pulse oximetry.
   5. Teach the patient the importance of keeping oxygen in place.
   6. Check and record the fingerstick blood glucose before lunch.

3. During admission assessment, Ms. J has all of these findings. For which finding should the nurse notify the HCP **immediately**?
   1. Bilateral pitting ankle and calf edema rated + 2
   2. Crackles in both lower and middle lobes
   3. Dry and peeling skin on both feet
   4. Faint but palpable pedal and post-tibial pulses

4. Which task associated with the patient's 24-hour urine collection is appropriate for the nurse to delegate to the AP?
   1. Instructing Ms. J to collect all urine with each voiding
   2. Teaching Ms. J the purpose of collecting urine for 24 hours
   3. Ensuring that all of Ms. J's urine collected for the test is kept on ice
   4. Assessing Ms. J's urine for color, odor, and sediment

5. The results of Ms. J's 24-hour urine collection reveal a creatinine clearance of 65 mL/min (1.09 mL/sec). How does the nurse best interpret this finding?
   1. Creatinine clearance is lower than normal.
   2. Creatinine clearance is higher than normal.
   3. Creatinine clearance is within normal range.
   4. Creatinine clearance indicates adequate kidney function.

6. Enhanced Multiple Response _____

Instructions: Based on Ms. J's history (see above), circle all of the correct responses in the right column that answer the question in the left column.

Question:

Which risk factors in Ms. J's history indicate increased risk for CKD?

Responses:

1. GERD
2. Hypertension
3. Four pregnancies
4. Type 2 diabetes
5. Patient is Hispanic
6. Coronary artery disease (CAD)
7. Cataracts
8. Long-term use of OTC ranitidine

7. The RN reviews Ms. J's laboratory results. Which laboratory finding is of greatest concern?
1. Serum potassium level of 7.1 mEq/L (7.1 mmol/L)
2. Serum creatinine level of 7.3 mg/dL (645 µmol/L)
3. Blood urea nitrogen level of 180 mg/dL (64.3 mmol/L)
4. Serum calcium level of 7.8 mg/dL (1.95 mmol/L)

8. Which medication should the nurse be prepared to administer to lower the patient's potassium level?
1. Furosemide 40 mg IV push
2. Epoetin alfa 300 units/kg subcutaneously
3. Calcium 1 tablet PO
4. Sodium polystyrene sulfonate 15 g PO

9. Ms. J states that she feels increasingly short of breath. The nurse team leader is supervising an LPN/LVN and an AP. Which nursing care action for Ms. J is the **most** appropriate to assign to the LPN/LVN?
1. Checking for residual urine with the bedside bladder scanner
2. Planning restricted fluid amounts to be given with meals
3. Assessing breath sounds for increased bilateral crackles
4. Discussing renal replacement therapies with the patient

10. The team leader RN observes the AP perform all of these actions for Ms. J. For which actions must the RN intervene? **Select all that apply.**
1. Assisting the patient to replace her oxygen nasal cannula
2. Checking vital signs after the patient has had something cold to drink
3. Ambulating with the patient to the bathroom and back
4. Increasing the patient's oxygen flow rate by nasal cannula from 2 to 4 L/min
5. Washing the patient's back, legs, and feet with warm water
6. Reminding Ms. J to perform prescribed incentive spirometry every hour while awake

11. The RN team leader assigns the LPN/LVN to give Ms. J's 9:00 AM oral medications. Which key instruction or action will be **most** important regarding the action of Ms. J's atenolol 50-mg tablet?
1. Give this drug with just a few swallows of water.
2. Ask the patient if she has been taking a diuretic at home.
3. Instruct the patient to use the bedside commode.
4. Check the patient's heart rate and blood pressure.

12. Enhanced Multiple Response _____

Instructions: Circle all of the correct responses in the right column that answer the question in the left column.

Question:

Ms. J's care plan includes the nursing concern, excess fluid volume. What interventions are appropriate for this nursing concern?

Responses:

1. Measure weight daily.
2. Monitor daily intake and output.
3. Restrict sodium intake with meals.
4. Restrict fluid to 1500 mL plus urine output.
5. Assess for crackles in the lungs at least once per shift.
6. Check for peripheral edema and note any increase.
7. Assess level of consciousness and cognition.
8. Ask patient about headache or blurred vision.

13. The RN is delegating and assigning care for Ms. J related to her type 2 diabetes. Which action by the RN indicates that the team leader needs to intervene?
    1. RN delegates fingerstick glucose check to newly hired AP.
    2. RN assigns administering morning dose of metformin to the LPN/LVN.
    3. RN refers the patient to a dietitian for education about a diabetic diet.
    4. RN assesses the condition of the patient's feet daily.

14. After discussing renal replacement therapies with the HCP and nurse, Ms. J is considering hemodialysis (HD). Which statement indicates that Ms. J needs additional teaching about HD?
    1. "I will need surgery to create an access route for HD."
    2. "I will be able to eat and drink what I want after I start dialysis."
    3. "I will have a temporary dialysis catheter for a few months."
    4. "I will be having dialysis three times every week."

15. The RN is precepting a new nurse orientating to the unit, who is providing care for Ms. J after her return from surgery to create a left forearm access for dialysis. Which action by the orienting nurse requires that the preceptor intervene?
    1. Monitoring the patient's operative site dressing for evidence of bleeding
    2. Obtaining a blood pressure reading by placing the cuff on the right arm
    3. Drawing blood for laboratory studies from the temporary dialysis line
    4. Administering acetaminophen with codeine PO for moderate postoperative pain

16. Assessment of Ms. J after dialysis reveals all of these findings. Which assessment finding necessitates the immediate notification of the HCP?
    1. Weight decrease of 4.5 lb (2 kg)
    2. Systolic blood pressure decrease of 14 mm Hg
    3. Decreased level of consciousness
    4. Small blood spot near the center of the dressing

17. Six months later, Ms. J is readmitted to the unit. She has just returned from HD. Which nursing care action should the nurse delegate to the AP?
    1. Measuring vital signs and postdialysis weight
    2. Assessing the HD access site for bruit and thrill
    3. Checking the access site dressing for bleeding
    4. Instructing the patient to request assistance getting out of bed

18. Ms. J is preparing for discharge. The RN is supervising a student nurse, who is teaching the patient about her discharge medications. For which statement by the student nurse will the RN intervene?
    1. "Sevelamer prevents your body from absorbing phosphorus."
    2. "Take your folic acid after dialysis on dialysis days."
    3. "The docusate is to prevent constipation that may be caused by ferrous sulfate."
    4. "You must take the epoetin alfa three times a week by mouth to treat anemia."

Ms. J is admitted for a kidney transplantation 6 months later. Her son is the kidney donor.

19. The RN is caring for Ms. J on the first day postoperatively after a kidney transplant. On assessment, her temperature is 100.4°F (38°C), her blood pressure is 168/92 mm Hg, and the patient tells the RN she has pain around the transplant site. What is the **best** interpretation of these findings?
    1. Hyperacute rejection
    2. Acute rejection
    3. Chronic rejection
    4. Transplant site infection

20. What intervention is required at this time?
    1. Increased doses of immunosuppressive drugs
    2. IV antibiotics
    3. Conservative management including dialysis
    4. Immediate removal of the transplanted kidney

21. While making the rounds, the RN finds Ms. J in tears and sobbing. She states, "I just don't want to have to go back to dialysis 3 days a week!" What is the nurse's best response?
    1. "Would you like me to call someone to come in and sit with you?"
    2. "You can always get on the list for another kidney transplant."
    3. "Tell me some more about how you are feeling."
    4. "Let me call your HCP to come in and speak with you."

Answer Key for this chapter begins on p. 274

PART 3   Complex Health Scenarios

Answers

1. **Ans: 4**   An oxygen saturation of 93% on 2 L/min is acceptable, and the best action is to notify the team lead and record the value. **Focus:** Prioritization.

2. **Ans: 1, 2, 4, 6**   Checking vital signs and recording intake and output fall within the scope of practice for any AP. An experienced AP will have been taught to use pulse oximetry to check oxygen saturation and to use a glucometer to check a patient's fingerstick blood glucose. In Canada, however, glucose monitoring is considered an advanced skill and would not be performed by an AP. Placing an IV line and teaching require additional education and training that are more within the scope of practice for a licensed nurse. **Focus:** Delegation, Supervision.

3. **Ans: 2**   All of these findings are important, but only the presence of crackles in both lungs is urgent because it signifies fluid-filled alveoli and interruption of adequate gas exchange and oxygenation, worsening of the patient's condition, and possibly pulmonary edema. The patient's peripheral edema is not new. The faint pulses are most likely caused by the presence of peripheral edema. The dry and peeling skin is a result of chronic diabetes and merits careful monitoring to prevent infection, but it is not immediately urgent. **Test-Taking Tip:** Always consider new assessment findings and if they indicate worsening of a patient's condition, be sure to notify the HCP. **Focus:** Prioritization.

4. **Ans: 3**   Teaching, instructing, and assessing are all functions that require additional education and preparation appropriate to the scope of practice for professional nurses. Providing the patient with ice for the urine collection and reminding the patient to collect her urine fit the scope of practice of the AP. Remember that the AP can remind a patient about anything that has already been taught. **Focus:** Delegation, Supervision.

5. **Ans: 1**   The normal creatinine clearance is 107 to 139 mL/min for men (1.78 to 2.32 mL/sec) and 87 to 107 mL/min (1.45 to 1.78 mL/sec) for women tested with a 24-hour urine collection. A low result indicates that the kidneys are functioning at a lower than expected level. The patient has CKD. **Focus:** Prioritization. **Test-Taking Tip:** The nurse should be familiar with the normal values of frequently ordered lab tests, as well as main causes and risks of high and low levels.

6. **Ans: 2, 4, 5, 6**   Major risk factors for CKD include hypertension and diabetes. CAD has a related pathophysiology to hypertension. Hispanics and African-Americans have an increased risk for CKD over Caucasian patients. Pregnancy, cataracts, long-term use of famotidine, and GERD are not risk factors for CKD. **Focus:** Prioritization.

7. **Ans: 1**   A patient with a serum potassium level of 7 to 8 mEq/L (7 to 8 mmol/L) or higher is at risk for electrocardiographic changes and fatal dysrhythmias. The HCP should be notified immediately about this potassium level. Although the serum creatinine and blood urea nitrogen levels are high, these levels are commonly reached before patients experience symptoms of CKD. The serum calcium level is low but not life threatening. **Focus:** Prioritization. **Test-Taking Tip:** Keep in mind that there is an inverse relationship between calcium and phosphorus, so when calcium is low, expect phosphorus to be high.

8. **Ans: 4**   Sodium polystyrene sulfonate removes potassium from the body by exchanging sodium for potassium in the large intestine. Diuretics such as furosemide generally do not work well in chronic kidney failure. The patient may need a calcium supplement and subcutaneous epoetin alfa; however, these drugs do nothing to decrease potassium levels. **Focus:** Prioritization.

9. **Ans: 1**   Checking residual urine with a bedside bladder scanner is within the scope of practice of the LPN/LVN, who would remain under the supervision of the RN. Planning care and discussing options such as renal replacement therapies require additional education and training, which are within the scope of practice for the professional RN. Although in many acute care hospitals, LPN/LVNs auscultate breath sounds as a part of their observations, RNs follow up for overall assessment and synthesis of data. Because Ms. J is a potentially unstable patient with respiratory changes that may indicate worsening of her condition, the more appropriate person to assess her lung sounds would be the RN. **Focus:** Assignment, Supervision.

10. **Ans: 2, 4**   Checking vital signs usually includes measuring oral body temperature. Because the patient just finished drinking fluids, an oral temperature measurement would be inaccurate at this time. If the fluids were cold, the temperature would be falsely low; if the fluids were hot, the temperature would be falsely high. Changing the oxygen flow rate without prescription or instruction is not acceptable practice. All of the other actions are appropriate and within the scope of practice of the AP. An AP's scope of practice includes reminding patients of content that has already been taught. **Focus:** Delegation, Supervision.

11. **Ans: 4**   Atenolol is a beta-blocker drug with actions that slow the heart rate and decrease the blood pressure. HCPs often have blood pressure (BP) and heart rate (HR) guidelines (e.g., low BP and/or HR) for

when to give and when to hold these drugs. The nurse should instruct the patient to call for help getting out of bed when the drug is newly prescribed or if the drug results in dizziness and syncope symptoms. The other instructions and actions may be included in the patient's care but will not affect the administration of atenolol. **Focus:** Prioritization.

12. **Ans: 1, 2, 3, 5, 6, 7, 8** The usual fluid restriction for patients with chronic kidney failure is 500 to 700 mL plus urine output. All of the other actions are appropriate for a patient with fluid overload. Remember that it is essential for the nurse to compare findings with previous shifts and days to determine if symptoms are worsening. **Focus:** Prioritization.

13. **Ans: 1** The newly hired AP would need to be taught how to use a glucometer and perform a fingerstick before having this task delegated to him or her. In addition, the RN would need to ensure that the APs had learned the skill before performing it independently. All of the other care tasks are appropriate to the staff members. **Focus:** Delegation, Assignment, Supervision.

14. **Ans: 2** Even after beginning HD, patients are still required to restrict fluid intake. In addition, patients on HD have nutritional restrictions (e.g., protein, potassium, phosphorus, sodium restrictions). All of the other patient statements indicate an appropriate understanding of HD. **Focus:** Prioritization.

15. **Ans: 3** Temporary dialysis lines are to be used only for HD. The preceptor nurse would stop the new nurse before the temporary HD system is interrupted. Breaking into the system increases the risk for complications such as infection. The blood pressure should always be assessed on the nondialysis arm. Postoperative patients should always be monitored for bleeding. Acetaminophen with codeine, when ordered by the HCP, is an appropriate analgesic for moderate to severe pain. **Focus:** Assignment, Supervision. **Test-Taking Tip:** It's essential that the nurse know the key principles for care of a patient after a surgical procedure. In this case, with a temporary HD line in place, the most important aspect is preventing infection, which is a risk whenever the system is interrupted.

16. **Ans: 3** Changes in level of consciousness during or after HD can signal dialysis disequilibrium syndrome, a life-threatening situation that requires early recognition and treatment with anticonvulsants. This should be immediately reported to the HCP so that appropriate treatment can be prescribed. Decreases in weight and blood pressure are to be expected as a result of dialysis therapy. A small amount of drainage is common after HD. **Focus:** Prioritization.

17. **Ans: 1** Measuring vital signs and weighing the patient are within the education and scope of practice of the AP. The AP could remind the patient to request assistance when getting out of bed after the RN has instructed the patient to do so. Assessing the HD access site for bleeding, bruit, and thrill require additional education and skill and are appropriately performed by a licensed nurse. **Focus:** Delegation, Supervision.

18. **Ans: 4** Epoetin alfa is used to treat anemia and is given two to three times a week; however, it is given by either the IV or subcutaneous route, not by mouth. Most commonly epoetin alfa is given subcutaneously. All of the other statements about medications for patients with CKD are accurate. **Focus:** Delegation, Supervision.

19. **Ans: 1** Hyperacute rejection occurs within 48 hours after transplant surgery. Increased temperature, increased blood pressure, and pain at the transplant site are manifestations. **Focus:** Prioritization.

20. **Ans: 4** The treatment for hyperacute rejection is immediate removal of the transplanted kidney and a return to dialysis until another kidney becomes available. Increased doses of immunosuppressant drugs are used to treat acute rejection, conservative management is used for chronic rejection, and IV antibiotics are administered for infections. **Focus:** Prioritization.

21. **Ans: 3** The RN should be supportive and nonjudgmental. Listening and encouraging the patient to verbalize her concerns (e.g., grief, feeling of failure) are essential at this time. Asking someone else to come in to talk with the patient is not responding to her concern. Suggesting that she can get on the transplant list again is not acknowledging Ms. J's grief for losing the transplanted kidney. **Focus:** Prioritization.

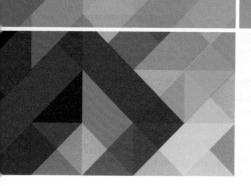

Questions

Mr. D, a 19-year-old premed student, has been brought to the emergency department (ED) by his roommate, who is a medical student and a family friend. Mr. D reports abdominal pain, polyuria, vomiting, and thirst. He appears flushed, and his lips and mucous membranes are dry and cracked. His skin turgor is poor. He has deep, rapid respirations, and there is a fruity odor to his breath. He has type 1 diabetes and "may have skipped a few doses of insulin because of cramming for finals." He is alert and conversant but is having trouble focusing on the nurse's questions.

Mr. D's vital signs and blood glucose are as follows:

Blood glucose level (fingerstick)	*685 mg/dL (38.1 mmol/L)*
Blood pressure	*100/60 mm Hg*
Heart rate	*120 beats/min*
Respiratory rate	*32 breaths/min*
Temperature	*100.8°F (38.2°C)*

1. To clarify pertinent data, which questions would the nurse ask Mr. D? **Select all that apply.**
   1. "When did your symptoms start?"
   2. "How many times have you vomited?"
   3. "When were you diagnosed with diabetes?"
   4. "Where does your abdomen hurt?"
   5. "Did you take any insulin today?"
   6. "Do you have any allergies?"

2. The nurse has completed the triage assessment and history taking. Which action is the **priority**?
   1. Page the ED health care provider (HCP) to come to triage.
   2. Call the patient's parents for permission to treat.
   3. Notify the patient's primary HCP.
   4. Take the patient immediately to a treatment room.

3. Based on the patient's history and clinical presentation, the HCP says that the probable medical diagnosis is diabetic ketoacidosis (DKA). In DKA, which abnormalities would the health care team expect to see and treat? **Select all that apply.**
   1. Ketosis
   2. Metabolic acidosis
   3. Dehydration
   4. Hyperglycemia
   5. Glycosuria
   6. Cardiac dysrhythmias
   7. Hyperosmolarity

4. Which nursing concept is the **priority** in planning the initial emergency interventions for Mr. D?
   1. Gas exchange
   2. Acid-base balance
   3. Fluid and electrolyte balance
   4. Adherence

5. Which tasks can be delegated to an experienced assistive personnel (AP)? **Select all that apply.**
   1. Measuring and reporting Mr. D's vital signs every 15 minutes
   2. Taking and reporting Mr. D's blood glucose level
   3. Bagging and labeling Mr. D's belongings
   4. Updating the roommate regarding Mr. D's status
   5. Measuring emesis and cleaning the basin as needed
   6. Obtaining an infusion pump from the supply room

6. For the initial emergency care of Mr. D, which collaborative treatment goal is the **priority**?
   1. Correction of hyperglycemia with IV insulin
   2. Correction of acid-base imbalance using IV bicarbonate
   3. Correction of fluid imbalance with IV fluids
   4. Correction of potassium imbalance with IV potassium

7. In the initial emergency care for Mr. D, which HCP prescriptions would the nurse question? **Select all that apply.**
   1. Start a peripheral IV line with a large-bore catheter.
   2. Obtain a urine specimen with a small-bore straight catheter.
   3. Administer regular insulin subcutaneously.
   4. Maintain the patient in a semi-Fowler position.
   5. Initiate continuous electrocardiographic (ECG) monitoring.
   6. Encourage intake of oral fluids as tolerated.

8. According to evidence-based practice, which IV solution will the HCP prescribe **first** for the initial fluid replacement?
   1. Normal saline (0.9% sodium chloride)
   2. Half-strength saline (0.45% sodium chloride)
   3. 5% dextrose in water and half-strength saline
   4. Normal saline with potassium chloride

9. The HCP instructs the nurse to give 1 L of IV fluid over the next hour. The available IV pump delivers fluid in mL/hr and allows three digits for programming the flow rate. Which action would the nurse take **first**?
   1. Try to find a pump that will accurately deliver the fluid.
   2. Program the IV pump for 1 L/hr and start the infusion.
   3. Ask the HCP to revise the rate to accommodate the available equipment.
   4. Program the IV pump for 999 mL/hr and start the infusion.

The arterial blood gas (ABG) results for Mr. D are:

pH	7.25
PaO$_2$	97 mm Hg
Paco$_2$	25 mm Hg
Bicarbonate	19 mEq/L (19 mmol/L)

10. Which physical assessment finding is **most** likely to accompany these laboratory results?
    1. Kussmaul respirations
    2. Dilated pupils
    3. Increased urination
    4. Elevated blood pressure

11. The nurse is reviewing the potassium values that were obtained when Mr. D first arrived in the ED. Which serum potassium level is **most** concerning?
    1. 3.5 mEq/L (3.5 mmol/L)
    2. 2 mEq/L (2 mmol/L)
    3. 5.8 mEq/L (5.8 mmol/L)
    4. 6 mEq/L (6 mmol/L)

12. An insulin infusion is ordered for Mr. D to begin at 0.1 units/kg/hr. Mr. D weighs 155 lb. The pharmacy delivers a premixed bag of 100 units of regular insulin in 100 mL of normal saline. Nurse A has calculated the infusion pump setting as 10 mL/hr. What would the charge nurse do?
    1. Tell Nurse A to obtain a pump and start the infusion as calculated.
    2. Advise Nurse A to recalculate the infusion rate.
    3. Call the HCP and ask for the exact pump setting to be clarified.
    4. Allow Nurse A to administer the infusion using her own judgment.

13. Which complication, secondary to the treatment of DKA, is **most** common?
    1. Cerebral edema
    2. Pulmonary venous congestion
    3. Chloremic acidosis
    4. Hypokalemia

14. Which action would the nurse take **first** to follow up on the patient's report of abdominal pain?
    1. Assess for paralytic ileus, which is expected with DKA.
    2. Assess pain and obtain a prescription for pain medication.
    3. Perform assessments for a possible abdominal infection.
    4. Wait for pain to resolve after treatment of DKA.

15. Mr. D says to the nurse, "Please don't call my mother. If she knows I'm in the hospital, she'll make me quit school and move back home. I messed up, but I really don't want to move back in with my parents." Which response is the **most** therapeutic?
    1. "None of the staff will say anything, but you should tell her yourself."
    2. "Your mom loves you, and she is just concerned about your well-being."
    3. "It sounds like you want to be independent and responsible for yourself."
    4. "You are an adult, and you have a right to make your own decisions."

16. The nurse overhears the AP talking to someone on the phone. The AP says, "Yes, Mr. D is doing much better than when he first got here. I will tell him that you called, and I will give him your message." Which action would the nurse take **first**?
    1. Ask the AP about the phone conversation that was just overheard.
    2. Remind the AP that release of information is outside her scope of practice.
    3. Report the AP to the nurse manager for a patient privacy violation.
    4. Give positive feedback for trying to help the patient and the caller.

Answer Key for this chapter begins on p. 280

PART 3 Complex Health Scenarios

17. An IV potassium infusion needs to be started. Which information, related specifically to the potassium infusion, is the **most** important to give to the intensive care unit (ICU) nurse who will assume the care of the patient?
    1. Mental status and cognition have improved with therapy.
    2. Urinary output is 60 mL/hr, and urine is a clear yellow color.
    3. Admitting blood pressure (BP) was 100/60 mm Hg; last BP is 125/76 mm Hg.
    4. There are two existing peripheral IV lines, and both flush easily.

18. The ED nurse is preparing the SBAR (situation, background, assessment, recommendation) report before the ICU transfer. Which detail would be **most** important to include as background to ensure that Mr. D's right to privacy is maintained?
    1. Patient is a premed student who was studying for finals, and this interfered with his normal routine.
    2. Roommate is a medical student and a family friend, and he brought Mr. D to the ED.
    3. Patient has not informed family that he is in the hospital, and he is reluctant to allow notification.
    4. Patient arrived alert and conversant, but he initially had trouble focusing on questions.

19. The ED nurse is trying to call a report to the ICU but is told, "We were not notified about the admission." What should the nurse do **first**?
    1. Call the admissions office supervisor to resolve the delay.
    2. Ask the unit secretary to call the admissions office now.
    3. Write an incident report; a delay violates Joint Commission guidelines.
    4. Ask the ICU nurse to take the report regardless of the clerical omission.

20. As the nurse is getting ready to transfer Mr. D to the ICU, the unit secretary hands the nurse the last blood glucose result, which is 150 mg/dL (8.33 mmol/L). What should the nurse do **first**?
    1. Proceed with the transfer because blood glucose is trending toward the normal value.
    2. Stop the insulin infusion, proceed with the transfer, and inform the ICU nurse on arrival.
    3. Immediately notify the HCP and anticipate an order for IV fluid of 5% or 10% glucose.
    4. Slow the insulin infusion and obtain an order to have the blood glucose redrawn.

21. Which member of the health care team is demonstrating a behavior that is an example of a barrier to interprofessional collaboration?
    1. ICU nurse asks the ED nurse to hold the patient for 30 minutes until the shift change is over.

2. Admitting endocrinology specialist directs the ED nurse to change the rate of all IV fluids.
3. ED provider reviews the triage nurse's admission notes before completing the provider summary.
4. ED nurse tells the charge nurse that the AP failed to record vital signs in a timely fashion.

22. Which tasks can the nurse direct an experienced AP to perform to facilitate Mr. D's transfer to the ICU? **Select all that apply.**
    1. Giving Mr. D's roommate directions to the ICU waiting room
    2. Independently transporting Mr. D to the ICU
    3. Collecting and organizing the chart and laboratory reports
    4. Obtaining a portable oxygen tank and cardiac monitor
    5. Connecting Mr. D's ECG leads to the portable cardiac monitor
    6. Obtaining the last set of vital sign values

23. The nurse is preparing to transfer Mr. D to the ICU and notices the cardiac monitor display. Which ECG pattern is cause for **greatest** concern?
    1.

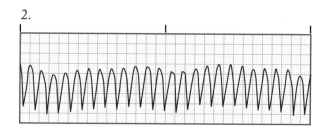

    2.

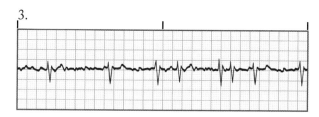

    3.

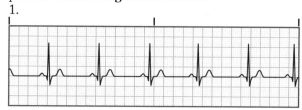

    4.

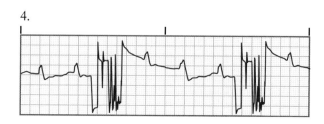

24. Enhanced Multiple Response

Scenario: In caring for Mr. D, the nurse is vigilant for signs and symptoms of hypokalemia. Early detection and treatment are necessary to prevent complications, such as lethal cardiac arrhythmias.

Which signs and symptoms are characteristic of hypokalemia?

Instructions: Place an X, in the space provided, or highlight signs or symptoms that accompany hypokalemia. **Select all that apply.**

1. _____ Fatigue
2. _____ Cold, clammy skin
3. _____ Muscle weakness
4. _____ Hypotension
5. _____ Weak pulse
6. _____ Shallow respirations
7. _____ Paralytic ileus
8. _____ Nausea and vomiting
9. _____ Abdominal distention
10. _____ Irritability

25. Enhanced Multiple Response

Scenario: Many hospital employees have legitimate reasons to be in and out of the ED. In addition, most larger hospitals allow system-wide electronic access to patient records. Furthermore, most patients have family and friends who are concerned about the well-being of their loved one and they would like to be informed about the condition, treatments, and outcomes.

Which people would have access to Mr. D's medical records?

Instructions: Place an X, in the space, provided or highlight each person who would be allowed to have access to Mr D's medical records. **Select all that apply.**

1. _____ ED health care provider who is managing the care in the ED
2. _____ ICU nurse who will receive Mr. D upon transfer to ICU
3. _____ Nursing student who wants to write a paper about DKA
4. _____ Roommate of Mr. D who is a medical student and a family friend
5. _____ Labor and delivery nurse who is Mr. D's girlfriend
6. _____ Clinical nurse specialist who is conducting research on insulin compliance for her doctoral degree
7. _____ ED nurse who is caring for Mr. D in the ED
8. _____ Hospital chaplain who offers to speak with Mr. D's family if needed
9. _____ Discharge nurse who will provide instructions and referrals at discharge
10. _____ Quality assurance nurse who is performing documentation audits for all ED patients

Answer Key for this chapter begins on p. 280

PART 3   Complex Health Scenarios

Answers

1. **Ans: 1, 2, 4, 5, 6** The onset of symptoms and the amount of fluid loss help to determine acuity. Pain assessment of the abdomen should be performed to obtain a baseline; his pain is probably associated with diabetic ketoacidosis, but infection or trauma also cause pain. If Mr. D had insulin today, this could affect treatment. Information about allergies should be obtained for all patients regardless of the presenting problem. Knowing when the patient was diagnosed with diabetes does not alter the priority actions at this point. **Focus:** Prioritization.

2. **Ans: 4** Mr. D should be taken to a treatment room for immediate evaluation and treatment. Paging the ED provider to come to the triage area is not necessary unless the patient becomes unresponsive in the triage area. Calling the parents is not necessary because Mr. D is old enough to provide consent for himself. (If Mr. D were under age, the treatment would not be delayed if the parents were unavailable in an emergency situation.) Calling the primary HCP is usually done by the ED provider after the preliminary workup is completed. (Policies for calling primary HCPs vary among institutions; be familiar with facility policies.) **Focus:** Prioritization.

3. **Ans: 1, 2, 3, 4, 5, 7** Hyperglycemia, ketosis, and metabolic acidosis are hallmark characteristics of DKA. Hyperglycemia results in glucosuria. This causes osmotic diuresis and fluid and electrolytes are lost through urination. Hyperosmolality of the blood draws water from the cells, causing cellular dehydration. Lack of insulin causes the body to metabolize fats at a higher rate and this leads to ketosis. Metabolic acidosis occurs as a result of the acidic byproducts of fat metabolism. Polyuria is expected and urine output is closely monitored because severe hypovolemia can cause acute renal failure. There is a risk for cardiac dysrhythmias, but they are not expected. Electrolytes must be closely monitored and corrected; electrolyte imbalances (especially potassium) can cause cardiac dysrhythmias. **Focus:** Prioritization.

4. **Ans: 3** Mr. D is severely dehydrated and is at risk for hypovolemic shock and electrolyte imbalance. Although he is demonstrating Kussmaul respirations, this breathing pattern is the body's attempt to compensate for the acidosis. Acid-base imbalance is usually corrected by administering fluids, electrolytes, and insulin. Adherence is relevant but can be addressed after Mr. D's condition is stabilized. **Focus:** Prioritization.

5. **Ans: 1, 2, 3, 5, 6** Taking vital signs, bagging up belongings, obtaining equipment, measuring output, and assisting with hygienic needs (e.g., cleaning emesis basin) are within the scope of duties for the AP. Checking the blood glucose level is accomplished with a fingerstick. APs, particularly in specialty areas such as the ED, will usually receive training to do this task, but this may vary by state and facility. Information should not be released by the AP because of confidentiality issues. Release of information to friends and family varies by facility policies, but typically the RN would escort the family in to see the patient as soon as possible. **Focus:** Delegation.

6. **Ans: 3** Fluid replacement is the first priority. Furthermore, the fluid dilutes the glucose levels, which helps to correct osmotic diuresis. The serum potassium level may not reflect the total body potassium. Hypokalemia occurs because of loss of potassium in the urine and transcellular movement of fluid; however, potassium levels are closely monitored, and supplements are given accordingly. Insulin is given to slowly lower the blood glucose level, but this occurs after rehydration and evaluation of potassium levels. Bicarbonate is rarely given unless acidosis becomes life threatening; acidosis usually resolves with fluids, electrolytes, and insulin. **Focus:** Prioritization.

7. **Ans: 2, 3, 6** The nurse would question the insertion of a straight catheter to obtain a urine specimen for a patient who is alert and able to use a urinal or commode because there is currently an emphasis on reducing catheter-associated urinary tract infections. (Note to student: The HCP may order an indwelling catheter for critically ill patients because hourly urinary output reflects cardiac output and kidney perfusion.) Subcutaneous insulin requires time to absorb; IV insulin is preferred. The patient is likely to be on food and fluid restrictions until the vomiting resolves. In addition, intra-abdominal conditions (e.g., appendicitis) should be ruled out before allowing oral fluids. At least one peripheral IV is needed for fluid replacement during the acute period. Semi-Fowler position is preferred to reduce the risk for aspiration. ECG monitoring is appropriate for all critical care patients. In this case, electrolyte imbalances increase the risk for dysrhythmias. **Focus:** Prioritization. **Test-Taking Tip:** If the nurse is questioning the HCP, the plan of care, or the interventions, the question is asking you to identify the incorrect options.

8. **Ans: 1** Normal saline (0.9% sodium chloride) is the first fluid used to correct dehydration in most adults with DKA. Half-strength saline (0.45% sodium chloride) can be used for children and adults at risk for volume overload. Potassium supplements are added to correct potassium deficit before starting insulin. Solutions of 5% dextrose are added to the therapy

when the blood glucose level approaches 250 mg/dL (13.9 mmol/L). **Focus:** Prioritization.

9. **Ans: 4** Many pumps only allow three digits for programming flow, so the nurse knows to use the available IV pump and program the rate to 999 mL/hr. It would not be possible to change the pump to deliver in L/hr. **Focus:** Prioritization.

10. **Ans: 1** The ABG results indicate metabolic acidosis. The pH is low (reference range, 7.35–7.45). $Paco_2$ is decreased (reference range 38–42 mmHg) because the deep and rapid Kussmaul respirations are the body's attempt to lower the pH by blowing off carbon dioxide. Bicarbonate level is the metabolic component of the ABG; in metabolic acidosis the bicarbonate is low (reference range, 21–28 mEq/L [21–28 mmol/L]). PaO_2 is normal (reference range 80–100 mmHg) because gas exchange is not impaired in metabolic acidosis. **Focus:** Prioritization.

11. **Ans: 2** Initially in patients with DKA, the serum potassium level is expected to be within normal limits or elevated (reference range, 3.5–5 mEq/L[3.5–5 mmol/L]); regardless of the laboratory value, there is an overall potassium deficit. After insulin therapy, hypokalemia is expected as the potassium shifts back into the cells; therefore, if the potassium level is initially low, it will be even lower after therapy. **Focus:** Prioritization. **Test-Taking Tip:** Potassium imbalances can cause lethal cardiac dysrhythmias. It is likely that the NCLEX Examination will include questions about potassium levels. It is worthwhile to memorize the reference range (reference range, 3.5–5 mEq/L[3.5–5 mmol/L]).

12. **Ans: 2** The calculations are incorrect. The pump should be set at 7 mL/hr.

155 / 2.2 = 70.4 kg; round to 70 kg
70 kg / x units : 1 kg / 0.1 units = 7 units
100 units / 100 mL = 1 unit / 1 mL : 7 units / x mL = 7 mL

Calling the HCP is inappropriate; the nurse is responsible for calculating the pump settings. Insulin is a high-alert drug, and calculations must always be double-checked. When discrepancies are discovered, the source of the error must be determined and corrected. **Focus:** Prioritization, Supervision. Test-Taking Tip: When weight is given in pounds and medications or fluids are prescribed per kilogram, the first step is to convert pounds to kilograms.

13. **Ans: 4** Hypokalemia and hypoglycemia are the most common complications associated with the treatment of DKA. In DKA, the initial serum potassium level may be normal or elevated, but this is because of diuresis and fluid shift within the cells; the body could have an overall potassium deficit. Insulin causes intracellular movement of potassium and bicarbonate therapy and can contribute to hypokalemia. Hypokalemia can be avoided by carefully monitoring the potassium and

glucose levels and then adding dextrose and potassium to IV fluids as needed. Chloremic acidosis has been associated with excessive fluid resuscitation. Cerebral edema is seen in children and is related to rapid fluid resuscitation. Pulmonary venous congestion is a potential complication, but this has not been validated by research findings. **Focus:** Prioritization.

14. **Ans: 3** Abdominal pain is a common symptom of DKA; however, an infection can also trigger DKA. An intra-abdominal infection, such peritonitis or appendicitis, would also cause abdominal pain. The nurse would continue to assess the abdomen. Worsening pain with tenderness and rigidity and unresolved elevation of temperature would be reported to the HCP. Paralytic ileus is not expected in DKA, but is a sign of hypokalemia, which is a common complication of therapy. Administering pain medication would not be the first action. The pain should resolve after treatment if the metabolic disturbance is the cause; however, the nurse would perform ongoing pain assessments. **Focus:** Prioritization.

15. **Ans: 3** Acknowledging and reflecting underlying feelings is therapeutic. Options 1 and 4 give unsolicited advice, and option 2 is a platitude that is not supported by firsthand knowledge of the mother–son relationship. **Focus:** Prioritization. **Test-Taking Tip:** To provide a therapeutic answer, the patient is first encouraged to express feelings, then the nurse and patient can define the needs and work on problem solving. In this case, the nurse uses reflection to help Mr. D to expand on his emotional concerns.

16. **Ans: 1** First, the situation should be assessed to determine if a privacy violation has occurred. Patient information should be released only to facilitate continuity of care (e.g., in a shift report) and only to those who are directly involved in the care. If Health Insurance Portability and Accountability Act rules were violated, the incident would be reported to the nurse manager for potential complaints related to the AP's actions and so that the AP could receive the proper remediation. Giving positive feedback for sincere efforts to assist patients and families is appropriate, but guidelines must be recognized and followed. **Focus:** Prioritization, Supervision.

17. **Ans: 2** Before potassium is administered, it is important to know that the kidneys are functioning. The other information is important but has less relevance to the potassium infusion. **Focus:** Prioritization.

18. **Ans: 3** The nursing staff is likely to encourage the patient to inform his family, but the ICU staff should be aware that he is resistant to notifying his family. (Note to student: Policies vary greatly, but some facilities do not allow staff to confirm or deny the admission or discharge of patients. In such cases, the patient may be asked to provide a list of people that can visit or phone in.) **Focus:** Prioritization.

19. **Ans: 2** Ask the secretary to correct the omission by calling the admissions office right away. If the ED

nurse has a good relationship with the ICU nurse, she or he will probably take the report; however, the ED nurse retains responsibility for the patient's care until the admission procedure and transfer are completed. After the patient's needs are met, the nurse could investigate the situation to determine if the admitting process can be improved. Writing an incident report would be appropriate, because the Joint Commission has a Core measure that addresses waiting times in the ED. **Focus:** Prioritization, Supervision.

20. **Ans: 3** Hyperglycemia should be reduced gradually, and in the critical phase if the blood glucose falls below 250 mg/dL (13.9 mmol/L), 5% or 10% IV glucose solution is added, and the insulin is continued. **Focus:** Prioritization.

21. **Ans: 4** Before going straight to the charge nurse, the nurse should speak directly to the AP about the vital signs to problem solve and find a solution. This action builds trust and team building. The ICU nurse and the ED nurse are negotiating, which is fundamental to collaboration. For patients with DKA, fluids, rates of fluids, and medications are continuously adjusted according to the patient's condition. By reading the nurse's notes, the ED provider demonstrates respect and trust that the nurse has gathered valuable information that should be included in the overall summary of care. **Focus:** Prioritization, Supervision.

22. **Ans: 1, 4, 5, 6** The AP can direct family and visitors to appropriate waiting areas, obtain equipment, and measure vital signs. An RN or HCP should accompany Mr. D to the ICU; the AP can help but should not independently transport patients to the ICU. The unit secretary usually prepares the papers, but the RN is responsible for ensuring that everything is in order. In specialty areas such as the ED, APs may receive additional training to connect patients' cardiac leads to the cardiac monitor; however, the RN is responsible for ensuring the lead placement and for assessing the cardiac rhythm. **Focus:** Delegation.

23. **Ans: 2** Option 2 shows ventricular tachycardia, which can be associated with an electrolyte imbalance, such as hypokalemia. This is a significant cause of death in patients with DKA. Option 1

shows normal sinus rhythm; note that one P wave normally precedes every QRS complex. Option 3 shows atrial fibrillation (AF). Patients with AF should be assessed for decreased cardiac output. Patients may tolerate AF, but this finding should be reported to the HCP because there is an increased risk for emboli. Option 4 shows artifact, which is usually caused by loose leads or patient movement. **Focus:** Prioritization. **Test-Taking Tip:** Rhythm interpretation takes a lot of practice, but ventricular dysrhythmias are among the most dangerous. Learn to differentiate normal from abnormal ECG findings and then focus your study on the most serious cardiac dysrhythmias.

24. **Ans: 1, 3, 4, 5, 6, 7, 8, 9, 10** All of these signs and symptoms are associated with hypokalemia, except cold, clammy skin which occurs with hypoglycemia or decreased perfusion. Hypokalemia is a low level of potassium in the blood (normal: 3.5–5.0 mEq/L or 3.5-5 mmol/L). Potassium plays an important in nerve conduction and muscle contraction. The most serious complications are cardiac dysrhythmias with the potential for cardiac arrest. **Focus:** Prioritization.

25. **Ans: 1, 2, 7, 9, 10** For protection of medical information, access is restricted to staff who are involved in the direct care of the patient. By job description, the quality assurance nurse has access to patient records for the purpose of reviewing the direct care and documentation provided by the nursing staff. Friends and family do not have access to medical records without specific consent of the patient. Students are allowed some access to medical records but only if they are involved in the direct care of patients. People conducting research may have access to patient records, but this involves a formal process to obtain research approval. Hospital employees, such as the chaplain, social worker, or nutritionist, may have access to some (or all) portions of the patient's record but would not freely access the record unless they became involved in the patient's care. **Focus:** Assignment, Supervision.

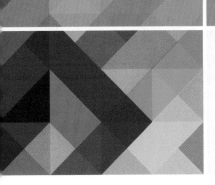

Home Health

Questions

The managing RN is assigning home visits to a registered nurse under her supervision for six patients:

1. *Ms. A:*
   - *Diagnosis: Chronic obstructive pulmonary disease (COPD)*
   - *Data: Called reporting increased dyspnea; has been increasing home oxygen flow rate*
2. *Mr. D:*
   - *Diagnoses: Diabetes, chronic leg infection*
   - *Data: Needs weekly assessment of leg infection; daily home health aide visits*
3. *Ms. F:*
   - *Diagnosis: Chronic kidney disease with peritoneal dialysis*
   - *Data: Daughter assists patient with dialysis*
4. *Mr. I:*
   - *Diagnosis: Lung cancer*
   - *Data: Last chemotherapy 1 week ago; needs to have blood drawn today at nadir for complete blood count (CBC) with differential*
5. *Ms. R:*
   - *Diagnosis: Coronary artery disease with percutaneous coronary angioplasty and stenting*
   - *Data: Hospital discharge yesterday; needs home health admission assessment*
6. *Mr. W:*
   - *Diagnosis: Schizophrenia*
   - *Data: Receives risperidone injection every 4 weeks; risperidone dose scheduled today*

1. Drag and Drop

Scenario: The managing RN of a home health agency is assigning several responsibilities to the home health team.

Instructions: In the left-hand column is a list of team members. Place the letter of the team member that would be most appropriate for the assigned task in the right-hand column, in the space provided. **Letters may be used more than once.**

Team Members	Tasks
a. RN b. LPN/LVN c. AP	1. _____ Bed bath, reposition, and take and record vital signs on a homebound patient with a laryngectomy.
	2. _____ Perform a manual digital evacuation of stool on a homebound patient with a spinal cord injury.
	3. _____ Assist a severely arthritic patient with bathing and taking morning medications.
	4. _____ Clean, rebandage, and document the condition of a healing leg wound.
	5. _____ Place medications in a pill organizer for a patient with dementia.
	6. _____ Assist a family member with application of an artificial limb on a patient with a right leg amputation.

2. After receiving the six patient assignment from the nurse manager, the registered nurse learns about a required in-service scheduled for 2:00 PM, which will leave time for only four home visits. Which four patients should be scheduled for today?
   1. Ms. A
   2. Mr. D
   3. Ms. F
   4. Mr. I
   5. Ms. R
   6. Mr. W

3. After adjusting the schedule to see these four patients, which patient should be seen **first**?
   1. Ms. A, the patient who has COPD and increased shortness of breath
   2. Mr. I, the patient receiving chemotherapy who will need blood drawn
   3. Ms. R, the patient with coronary artery disease who will need an initial assessment
   4. Mr. W, the patient with schizophrenia who will need a risperidone injection

4. When the nurse calls Ms. R to schedule a visit, the patient says that she doesn't have much time today but will be available for a longer visit tomorrow. What is the **best** response?
   1. "The visit will not take very long, so I will plan on seeing you today."
   2. "I have rescheduled other patients because it is essential that I assess you today."
   3. "Perhaps you are feeling that you do not really need any help at home."
   4. "Because of the recent angioplasty and stenting, I would like to visit as soon as possible."

After obtaining Ms. R's consent for a visit later today, the nurse arrives at Ms. A's home. Her husband answers the door and says that Ms. A was very short of breath and restless last night, but now she is sleeping deeply and completely relaxed. The nurse finds that Ms. A is very difficult to awaken and that her speech is slurred. The flow meter on her home oxygen unit is set at 6 L/min.

5. Which nursing action should the nurse take next?
   1. Auscultate Ms. A's anterior and posterior lung sounds.
   2. Check Ms. A's oxygen saturation using pulse oximetry.
   3. Continue to stimulate Ms. A until she can respond to you.
   4. Notify the health care provider (HCP) about Ms. A's change in status.

6. The oxygen saturation is 99% per pulse oximeter. Which action is appropriate next?
   1. Discontinue the patient's oxygen.
   2. Draw a sample for arterial blood gas analysis.

3. Call the HCP and obtain an order to transport Ms. A to the hospital.
4. Remind the patient's husband about the reasons for using oxygen at low flow rates.

The nurse calls the HCP to discuss Ms. A's status and then arranges for her admission to the hospital for further evaluation.

The nurse receives a phone call from Mr. D's home health aide, who reports that Mr. D is experiencing generalized aches and pains. His morning blood glucose level was 306 mg/dL (16.98 mmol/L), and his temperature is 100.1°F (37.8°C).

7. Which action by the nurse is **most** appropriate?
   1. Suggest that Mr. D take acetaminophen to treat pain and fever.
   2. Arrange to see Mr. D as the first patient on tomorrow's schedule.
   3. Reorganize today's schedule so that Mr. D can be seen and assessed.
   4. Reassure the aide that these findings are normal for patients with diabetes.

8. Because Mr. D will be visited today, which of the three patients that are scheduled for today is best to reschedule for tomorrow?
   1. Mr. I, who is receiving chemotherapy and needs a blood specimen drawn
   2. Ms. R, who needs an initial home health visit after coronary artery stenting
   3. Mr. W, who is scheduled for an injection of risperidone to treat schizophrenia

9. The nurse arrives at Ms. R's home as arranged, and the patient is waiting at the door. Her respiratory effort seems a little labored, and she looks anxious. The nurse asks Ms. R how she has been feeling since her discharge from the hospital yesterday. Which response indicates a need for immediate intervention?
   1. "I have been a bit short of breath."
   2. "I feel some left-sided chest pressure."
   3. "I don't understand why I need to take all these pills."
   4. "I am confused about why you are here to see me."

10. Five minutes after taking a nitroglycerin sublingual tablet, Ms. R says that the chest pressure is "almost gone." Which action should the nurse take next?
    1. Proceed with assessing her and completing the admission documentation.
    2. Have her rest for another 5 minutes and then reassess the chest pressure.

3. Check her blood pressure and administer another nitroglycerin tablet.
4. Call the HCP, anticipating an order to readmit her to the hospital.

After taking a second nitroglycerin tablet, Ms. R says that the chest pressure and shortness of breath are completely gone, and the nurse proceeds with the admission assessment. Ms. R lives alone, but her daughter lives nearby and is with Ms. R today.

Ms. R's blood pressure is 126/72 mm Hg, pulse is 82 beats/min, and respirations are 20 breaths/min. She has felt chest pressure twice since her discharge yesterday but says, "I just waited and it went away after an hour or so." She has not been taking her prescribed medications because "I can't remember which ones I have taken, and I don't want to take an overdose." She has many questions about her medications, which include:
- *Nitroglycerin 0.4 mg sublingually as needed for chest pain*
- *Transdermal nitroglycerin 0.2 mg/hr every morning*
- *Metoprolol succinate 25 mg PO daily*
- *Clopidogrel 75 mg PO daily*
- *Aspirin 81 mg PO daily*
- *Enalapril 2.5 mg PO daily*

11. Which action should the nurse take next?
    1. Schedule the next home visit with the patient.
    2. Assist the patient to take the prescribed medications.
    3. Call the HCP to report the patient's condition.
    4. Remind the patient about the importance of medication compliance.

12. Which activities in the patient's care plan will the nurse delegate to a home health aide? **Select all that apply.**
    1. Setting up Ms. R's medications in a multidose pill box twice a week
    2. Instructing the daughter how to set up Ms. R's daily medications
    3. Teaching Ms. R and her daughter the purpose of each medication
    4. Assisting Ms. R with a bath and personal hygiene every day
    5. Measuring vital signs daily
    6. Weighing the patient daily
    7. Checking for any peripheral edema weekly

13. When will the nurse schedule the next home visit with Ms. R?
    1. Later today because Ms. R's condition is very unstable, and she may require hospital readmission
    2. Tomorrow because Ms. R's assessment indicates that she needs frequent evaluation or interventions
    3. In 3 days because the home health aide will see Ms. R every day and will call if there are any further problems
    4. Early next week so that there will be enough time to evaluate the effect of the medications on Ms. R's symptoms

14. The nurse still has visits to make to Mr. D and Mr. I before the mandatory in-service session. Which patient should be visited **first**?
    1. Mr. D, who has diabetes and has an elevated glucose and fever
    2. Mr. I, who has lung cancer and is receiving chemotherapy

While driving to the next home visit, the nurse receives a telephone call from the home health manager about a newly referred 70-year-old patient with emphysema who will need an initial visit today to evaluate the need for home oxygen therapy.

15. Which staff member will the nurse suggest as the **best** person to make the initial home visit for this new patient?
    1. An experienced and knowledgeable LPN/LVN who has worked for 10 years in home health
    2. A respiratory therapist who regularly works with patients who are receiving home oxygen therapy
    3. An RN who usually works in the maternal-child division of the public health agency
    4. An on-call RN who works in the home health agency for a few days each month on an as-needed basis

16. When the nurse arrives at Mr. I's condominium, his wife says that Mr. I is very lethargic and a little confused today. Usually he is well oriented and cheerful despite his diagnosis of right-sided lung cancer. Which information noted during the assessment is the **best** indicator that rapid nursing action is needed?
    1. Breath sounds are decreased on the right posterior chest.
    2. Mr. I says that his appetite has not been very good recently.
    3. Mr. I's oral temperature is 101°F (38.3°C).
    4. The oral mucosa is pale and dry.

17. The nurse calls the oncologist to discuss Mr. I's condition and receives directions to have the patient transported to the hospital emergency department (ED) for evaluation. Which information is **most** important to communicate when calling a report to the ED?
    1. Mr. I has lung cancer and decreased breath sounds.
    2. Mr. I's appetite and oral intake are decreased.
    3. Mr. I needs a CBC today.
    4. Mr. I is receiving chemotherapy and has a fever.

Answer Key for this chapter begins on p. 287

Complex Health Scenarios

PART 3

In preparation for the final visit of the day to Mr. D, the nurse checks the patient data that the home health aide has entered into the electronic record for this week:

Day	Temperature	Heart Rate (beats/min)	Respiratory Rate (breaths/min)	Blood Pressure (mm Hg)	Weight (kg)	Capillary Blood Glucose Level
Monday	98°F (36.7°C)	78	22	152/72	77	142 mg/dL (7.88 mmol/L)
Tuesday	97.9°F (36.6°C)	82	20	140/66		140 mg/dL (7.77 mmol/L)
Wednesday	99.5°F (37.5°C)	74	18	148/72	77.2	256 mg/dL (14.21 mmol/L)
Thursday	100.5°F (38°C)	76	22	144/80		300 mg/dL (16.65 mmol/L)
Friday	101.2°F (38.4°C)	88	24	146/78	77.5	326 mg/dL (18.09 mmol/L)

18. Which data in the table are **most** important to report to the HCP? **Select all that apply.**
    1. Temperature
    2. Heart rate
    3. Respiratory rate
    4. Blood pressure
    5. Weight
    6. Glucose level

The nurse assesses Mr. D, finding that the wound on his left heel is dry appearing and pale pink, with no wound drainage.

There are scattered coarse crackles and wheezes over the left posterior chest. Mr. D says he feels short of breath with activity, but "my breathing is fine when I rest." He has been coughing up some thick green mucus for the last few days. He has been voiding the usual amounts with no problems. He is using regular insulin with sliding-scale dosing as prescribed for elevated blood glucose levels.

19. After communicating Mr. D's findings to the HCP, in which order will the nurse implement the prescribed interventions?
    1. Give ciprofloxacin 500 mg orally now and instruct the patient to take the medication every 12 hours.
    2. Obtain blood specimens for culture from two separate sites.
    3. Check the oxygen saturation level.
    4. Teach the patient about the use of antibiotics and to increase fluid intake to 2000 mL/day.

20. The assistive personnel (AP) reports to the RN the next day that Mr. D has swelling, tenderness, and stiffness of his right elbow. What is the best action for the RN to take?
    1. Return to the home and assess Mr. D's right elbow as soon as possible today.
    2. Inform the HCP of the change.
    3. Instruct the AP to apply warm packs alternating with cool packs every 20 minutes.
    4. Instruct the AP to discourage Mr. D from playing fetch with his dog.

Complex Health Scenarios   PART 3

Answers

1. **Ans: 1c, 2a, 3c, 4b, 5b, 6c**   Personal care and vital signs can be assigned to the AP. An RN should perform the manual evacuation of stool on a recently injured spinal cord patient because digital extraction of bowel contents could initiate a parasympathetic response through vagal nerve stimulation, causing bradycardia and hypotension. An AP cannot administer medications; however, they may assist the patient with safe self-administration by opening the bottles and assisting the patient with hand to mouth placement of the pills. An LPN/LVN should clean, rebandage, and document the condition of a wound. An LPN/LVN can place medications in a pill organizer, which is a better use of resources than assigning this task to an RN. An AP can assist the family member with application of the artificial limb. **Focus:** Assignment.

2. **Ans: 1, 4, 5, 6**   Ms. A's dyspnea and increased use of oxygen require rapid assessment. Mr. I's sample for a CBC must be drawn when the bone marrow is most suppressed to accurately assess the impact of chemotherapy on bone marrow function. Ms. R should be seen as soon as possible after discharge to determine the plan of care. Mr. W needs to receive the scheduled dose of risperidone. Mr. D and Ms. F do not have urgent needs, and these visits can be rescheduled for the following day. **Focus:** Prioritization.

3. **Ans: 1**   Ms. A's increased shortness of breath indicates a need for rapid assessment. In addition, high oxygen flow rates can cause an increase in the partial pressure of carbon dioxide ($Paco_2$) and suppression of respiratory drive in patients with COPD, so Ms. A should be seen as soon as possible. The other patients can be scheduled according to criteria such as location or patient preference about visit time. **Focus:** Prioritization.

4. **Ans: 4**   In the home health setting, the patient is in control of health management, so enlisting the patient's cooperation for the visit is essential. In this response, the nurse indicates that the patient has a choice about whether the visit is scheduled for today but educates the patient about why it is important that the visit occur as soon as possible. Because the initial visit requires a multidimensional assessment, it is usually quite lengthy. The patient's comments do not indicate a lack of need or desire for home health services. **Focus:** Prioritization.

5. **Ans: 2**   The patient has symptoms and risk factors that could indicate that her oxygen saturation is either excessively high or too low, so checking oxygen saturation is the first action that should be taken. The other actions may also be appropriate, but assessment of oxygen saturation will determine which action should occur next. **Focus:** Prioritization.

6. **Ans: 1**   Since the goal for oxygen saturation for a patient with COPD is usually 90% to 94% (0.90 to 0.94), because high oxygen levels can decrease respiratory drive and lead to increases in $Paco_2$, the nurse's first action should be to discontinue the oxygen for this patient. The next step is to notify the HCP, who may want to admit the patient to the hospital or order arterial blood gas analysis. It will be important to discuss appropriate home oxygen use with the patient and her husband but not until the immediate situation is resolved. **Focus:** Prioritization. **Test-Taking Tip:** Remember that some patients with COPD may have a decrease in respiratory drive if oxygen saturations are elevated. Although administration of a high oxygen percentage may be necessary if the patient is hypoxemic, you will need to monitor the patient's oxygen saturation carefully and adjust the oxygen flow rate down as the patient's oxygen saturation improves.

7. **Ans: 3**   Generalized aches and pains, an elevated temperature, and an elevated glucose level are signs of infection in patients with diabetes, indicating a significant change in the patient's status and need for further assessment. Acetaminophen may be indicated for discomfort but will not treat infection. Because diabetes decreases immune function and increases the risk for serious infections, the nurse should not wait another day before seeing the patient. **Focus:** Prioritization.

8. **Ans: 3**   Although the risperidone is scheduled for today, the medication is absorbed gradually, and rescheduling the dose for tomorrow will not have an adverse impact on control of the patient's schizophrenia. The other patients have more urgent needs and should receive visits today. **Focus:** Prioritization.

9. **Ans: 2**   The chest pressure indicates that Ms. R may be experiencing myocardial ischemia and requires immediate assessment and intervention (e.g., administration of sublingual nitroglycerin). The shortness of breath requires further investigation and is likely to be related to the chest pressure and myocardial ischemia. The other responses also indicate the need for further assessment and interventions such as teaching but do not require immediate action. **Focus:** Prioritization. **Test-Taking Tip:** Report of chest pain or chest pressure in a patient with known coronary artery disease is a red flag that requires immediate assessment and intervention. Do not minimize this finding or allow the patient to minimize the symptom. Remember that angina signifies coronary ischemia, and the goal for treatment is that chest discomfort is completely absent (0 on a 1–10 scale).

10. **Ans: 3**   National guidelines for patients with coronary artery disease indicate that, if the chest pain is

improving after nitroglycerin administration, giving another nitroglycerin tablet is the first action to take. Completing the admission assessment, having her rest, and notifying the HCP about her chest pain are also appropriate actions, but administration of another nitroglycerin tablet and resolution of the chest discomfort are the priorities. **Focus:** Prioritization.

11. **Ans: 2**   Because the patient has not taken the prescribed medications to control coronary artery disease and angina, the nurse's first action will be to ensure that the medications are taken. Scheduling the next home visit, educating about the medications, and communicating with the HCP are all appropriate but can be done later in the visit. **Focus:** Prioritization. **Test-Taking Tip:** In taking a test, carefully read all information that is supplied. If you missed this answer, go back and read the information that precedes the question and the answer will be clear.

12. **Ans: 4, 5, 6**   Home health aide education and scope of practice include assisting with personal hygiene and obtaining routine data such as vital sign values and daily weights. It is the RN's responsibility to evaluate these data and plan individualized care using the data. Assessments, medication preparation, and patient teaching about medications require more education and a broader scope of practice and should be performed by the RN. **Focus:** Delegation.

13. **Ans: 2**   The focus in home health nursing is on empowering the patient and family members by teaching self-care. Ms. R's condition is not so unstable that she needs to be reassessed today because her chest pain did resolve after she took two nitroglycerin tablets, she has taken her medications, and her daughter will be available. The patient's symptoms of chest discomfort and confusion about how to take her medications do indicate a need for reassessment the next day. Although the home health aide will visit, the education and role of the home health aide do not include evaluating the patient's response to prescribed therapies and planning changes in care based on the evaluation. **Focus:** Prioritization.

14. **Ans: 2**   Because Mr. I is in the nadir period after his chemotherapy, he is at high risk for infection. Avoidance of any cross-contamination from Mr. D's leg infection is essential. **Focus:** Prioritization.

15. **Ans: 4**   The initial assessment and development of the plan of care, including interventions such as oxygen therapy, are the responsibility of RN staff members. The RN with the most experience in caring for patients with emphysema is the on-call part-time RN. Some patient care activities are assigned to staff members from other disciplines, such as LPN/LVNs and respiratory therapists, after the plan of care is developed by the RN. **Focus:** Assignment.

16. **Ans: 3**   Chemotherapy decreases the patient's ability to mount a fever in response to infection, so even a minor increase in temperature (especially in combination with symptoms such as lethargy and confusion) can be an indicator of a serious infection, including sepsis. The decreased right-sided breath sounds are consistent with the patient's diagnosis of lung cancer. The poor appetite and dry oral mucous membranes also require assessment and intervention, but infection is one of the most serious complications of chemotherapy. **Focus:** Prioritization.

17. **Ans: 4**   Mr. I's immunosuppression, fever, and possible sepsis diagnosis indicate that he should be assessed and treated immediately when he arrives in the ED. The other information will also be helpful but will not ensure that Mr. I is assessed and that treatment with antibiotics is initiated rapidly. **Focus:** Prioritization.

18. **Ans: 1, 4, 6**   The elevated temperatures and blood glucose levels suggest a possible infectious process and should be reported to the HCP so that interventions can be quickly implemented to prevent complications such as sepsis, diabetic ketoacidosis, or hyperglycemic hyperosmolar nonketotic coma. The blood pressures should also be reported because current national guidelines indicate that blood pressure for patients with diabetes should be maintained at a level of less than 130/80 mm Hg to decrease cardiovascular risk. The pulse, respiratory rate, and weight are stable and in the appropriate range. **Focus:** Prioritization. **Test-Taking Tip:** Diabetes and hypertension are two of the most common diagnoses that you will encounter (both on the NCLEX and in your career). It is important to be familiar with normal values and national guidelines to help in decision making about how to manage patients with these problems.

19. **Ans: 3, 2, 1, 4**   Mr. D's assessment suggests that he has an acute lower respiratory tract infection such as pneumonia. Because his oxygenation may be compromised, the first action should be to determine his oxygen saturation. National guidelines indicate that initiation of antibiotics is a priority whenever patients have an infection, but if cultures are prescribed, they should be obtained before starting antibiotic therapy. Teaching about self-care can be done after the other interventions are implemented. **Focus:** Prioritization.

20. **Ans: 1**   Mr. D is likely having an adverse side effect from the ciprofloxacin. Serious side effects from taking fluoroquinolones include tendinitis and tendon rupture. As the AP is not qualified to make an assessment, the RN should return to the home and thoroughly assess the patient before contacting the HCP. **Focus:** Prioritization.

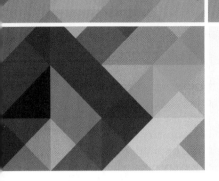

CASE STUDY 7

Spinal Cord Injury

Questions

Mr. M is a 32-year-old man brought to the emergency department (ED) by paramedics after a fall from the second-story roof of his home. He was placed on a spinal board with a cervical collar to immobilize his spine. After spinal radiographs are obtained, the health care provider (HCP) determines that he has a vertebral compression injury at the C4 to C5 level.

1. Drag and Drop
Instructions: Mechanism of injury, level of injury, or degree of injury are listed in the left-hand column. In the right-hand column, in the space provided, write in the letter next to the most appropriate description.

Mechanism of injury, level of injury, or degree of injury	Descriptions
a. Cervical injury	1. _____ Displacement of vertebrae
b. Hyperextension injury	2. _____ Paralysis of four extremities occurs
c. Complete cord involvement	3. _____ Total loss of sensory and motor function below the level of injury
d. Compression fracture	4. _____ Forward dislocation, ruptured posterior ligaments, and damage to the spinal cord
e. Thoracic injury	
f. Flexion injury	5. _____ Paralysis and loss of sensation in the legs
g. Incomplete cord involvement	6. _____ Ruptured anterior ligament compressed ligament
h. Flexion-rotation injury	7. _____ Fractured vertebrae, compression of the spinal cord

2. Which questions would the nurse ask the paramedics to obtain a history of the patient's acute spinal cord injury (SCI)? **Select all that apply.**
   1. What was the location and position of the patient immediately after the injury?
   2. Did the patient experience symptoms before the injury?
   3. Have any changes occurred since the injury?
   4. What type of stabilization devices were used to stabilize the patient?
   5. Were any other people injured at the same time at the patient?
   6. What treatments were given at the injury scene and en route to the ED?

3. What is the nurse's **priority** concern during admission to the ED?
   1. Spinal immobilization to prevent additional injuries to the patient
   2. Airway status because of interruption of spinal innervation to the respiratory muscles
   3. Potential for injuries related to the patient's decreased sensation
   4. Dysrhythmias caused by disruption of the autonomic nervous system

4. The ED nurse assists the ED HCP in testing Mr. M's deep tendon reflexes (DTRs), which are all absent. What does the nurse suspect is the likely cause of the absent DTRs?
   1. Spinal shock
   2. Stabilization devices
   3. Lack of oxygen to the nerves
   4. Neurogenic shock

5. Enhanced Multiple Response

Question: Mr. M is stabilized and moved to the neurologic intensive care unit (ICU) with a diagnosis of SCI at level C4 to C5. As the admitting RN working with an experienced assistive personnel (AP), when frequent respiratory assessments are performed, which actions can the RN delegate to the AP?

Instructions: Circle or highlight the numbers that best answer the question. **Select all that apply.**
1. Auscultating breath sounds every hour to detect decreased or absent ventilation
2. Ensuring that oxygen is flowing at 5 L/min via the nasal cannula
3. Teaching the patient to breathe slowly and deeply and use incentive spirometry
4. Checking the patient's oxygen saturation by pulse oximetry every 2 hours
5. Assessing the patient's chest wall movement during respirations
6. Reminding the patient to use his or her spirometry every hour while awake
7. Checking the patient's respiratory rate every 2 hours
8. Monitoring the patient's intravenous fluid rate

6. An hour later, the AP informs the RN that Mr. M's oxygen saturation has dropped to 88%, and his respirations are rapid and shallow at 34 breaths/min. On auscultation, he has decreased breath sounds bilaterally. What is the nurse's **best** action at this time?
1. Increase the oxygen flow to 10 L/min.
2. Suction the patient's airway for oral secretions.
3. Notify the HCP immediately.
4. Call the respiratory therapist for a nonrebreather mask.

7. Which instructions would the RN give the experienced AP with regard to Mr. M's care at this time? **Select all that apply.**
1. Check and record vital signs every 15 minutes.
2. Use pulse oximetry to check oxygen saturation with each set of vital signs.
3. Increase oxygen flow rate by 2 L/min when oxygen saturation is more than 91%.
4. Empty the patient's urinary catheter bag and record the output.
5. Teach the patient how to perform coughing and deep breathing.
6. Immediately report decrease in oxygen saturation or increase in respiratory rate.

The HCP prescribes that Mr. M receive endotracheal (ET) intubation and be placed on mechanical ventilation; his oxygen saturation increases to 96%, and respirations decrease to 18 breaths/min (10 ventilator breaths per minute). On auscultation, he has breath sounds present in all lung lobes bilaterally.

8. The nurse is caring for Mr. M when the ventilator's high-pressure alarm goes off. What intervention is the patient likely to need at this time?
1. Assessment of all ventilator tubing for disconnection
2. Evaluation of the patient's ET tube for a cuff leak
3. Suctioning of the patient for an increased amount of secretions
4. Notification of the respiratory therapist to assess the machine

9. Mr. M has stabilized and has been weaned off the ventilator. The neurologic ICU nurse is to remove the ET tube. Which actions will the nurse take before removing the tube? **Select all that apply.**
1. Set up an oxygen delivery system.
2. Bring emergency equipment for reintubation to the bedside.
3. Hyperoxygenate the patient.
4. Rapidly deflate the ET tube cuff.
5. Instruct the patient to cough while the tube is being removed.
6. Administer oxygen by face mask.

10. The patient's cervical injury has been immobilized with cervical tongs and traction to realign the vertebrae, facilitate bone healing, and prevent further injury. Which occurrence necessitates the nurse's immediate intervention?
1. The traction weights are resting on the floor after the patient is repositioned.
2. The traction ropes are located within the pulley and are hanging freely.
3. The insertion sites for the cervical tongs are cleaned with hydrogen peroxide.
4. The patient is repositioned every 2 hours by using the logrolling technique.

11. Mr. M's care plan has a nursing concern of impaired mobility. Which actions should the RN delegate to the nursing student providing care for this patient on the neurology unit? **Select all that apply.**
    1. Administering 50 mg of IV famotidine in 50 mL of normal saline to prevent gastric ulcers
    2. Monitoring traction ropes and weights while the patient is repositioned
    3. Assessing the patient's neurologic status for changes in movement and strength
    4. Providing pin site care using hydrogen peroxide and normal saline
    5. Adding a nursing concern to the care plan for the patient of risk for depression
    6. Checking vital signs and oxygen saturation

12. Which action to prevent complications associated with Mr. M's nursing concern of impaired mobility should the RN delegate to the experienced AP?
    1. Assisting with turning and repositioning the patient in bed every 2 hours
    2. Inspecting the patient's skin for reddened areas
    3. Performing physical therapy exercises every 8 hours
    4. Administering enoxaparin subcutaneously every 12 hours

13. The nursing student asks the nurse how best to assess Mr. M's motor function. What is the nurse's best response?
    1. "Apply resistance while the patient plantar flexes his feet."
    2. "Apply resistance while the patient lifts his legs from the bed."
    3. "Apply downward pressure while the patient shrugs his shoulders upward."
    4. "Make sure the patient is able to grasp objects firmly and form a fist."

14. The AP reports that Mr. M's blood pressure is 178/98 mm Hg; his heart rate is 50 beats/min; he is sweating around his face, neck, and shoulders; and he reports a severe headache. What does the nurse suspect when assessing this patient?
    1. Spinal shock
    2. Autonomic dysreflexia
    3. Neurogenic shock
    4. Venous thromboembolism

15. Which actions should the nurse take in caring for Mr. M at this time? **Select all that apply.**
    1. Place the patient in bed in the prone position.
    2. Notify the HCP.
    3. Check the patient's bladder for urinary retention.
    4. Place an incontinence pad on the patient.
    5. For bladder distention, catheterize the patient.
    6. Monitor blood pressure and heart rate every 10 to 15 minutes.

16. Mr. M's condition has stabilized. His cervical injury is now immobilized with a halo fixation device with jacket. He has regained the use of his arms and partial movement in his legs. Which instruction should the nurse give the AP about providing help to Mr. M in activities of daily living?
    1. "Feed, bathe, and dress the patient so that he does not become fatigued."
    2. "Encourage the patient to perform all of his own self-care."
    3. "Allow the patient to do what he can and then assist with what he can't."
    4. "Let the patient's wife do the bathing and dressing."

17. Mr. M is very upset and tells the nurse that he is afraid his wife will divorce him because he is "no longer a man." What is the nurse's best response at this time?
    1. "Have you spoken with your wife about this yet?"
    2. "Let me call your health care provider to talk with you about this."
    3. "Do you have any children with your wife?"
    4. "Can you tell me more so I can understand how you are feeling?"

18. Mr. M is experiencing incontinence. The nurse plans to establish a bladder retraining program for him. Which actions are important points for this program? **Select all that apply.**
    1. Remove the indwelling urinary catheter.
    2. Encourage the patient to limit fluid intake to 1000 mL/day.
    3. Gradually increase intervals between catheterizations.
    4. Teach the patent to initiate voiding by tapping on his bladder every 4 hours.
    5. Teach the patient to perform self-catheterization if necessary.
    6. Administer bethanechol chloride 20 mg orally twice a day.

19. Mr. M is to be transferred to a rehabilitation facility. Which statement indicates that the patient needs additional teaching?
    1. "After rehabilitation, I may be able to achieve control of my bladder."
    2. "With rehabilitation, I will regain all of my motor functions."
    3. "Rehabilitation will help me to become as independent as possible."
    4. "After rehabilitation, I hope to return to gainful employment."

Answer Key for this chapter begins on p. 292

PART 3 Complex Health Scenarios

Answers

1. **Ans: 1h, 2a, 3c, 4f, 5e, 6b, 7d**   Classification of spinal cord injury is by the mechanism of injury (e.g., flexion, hyperextension, compression injury, flexion-rotation injury), level of injury or skeletal level of injury (e.g., cervical, thoracic, lumbar, sacral), and the degree of injury (e.g., complete or incomplete [partial] cord involvement). **Focus:** Prioritization. **Test-Taking Tip:** The higher the level of spinal cord injury, the more damage and impairment.

2. **Ans: 1, 3, 4, 6**   When obtaining a history from a patient with an acute SCI, gather as much data as possible about how the accident occurred and the probable mechanism of injury after the patient is stabilized. Questions asked by the nurse should include:
   - Location and position of the patient immediately after the injury
   - Symptoms that occurred immediately with the injury
   - Changes that have occurred since the injury
   - Type of immobilization devices used and whether problems occurred during stabilization and transport to the hospital
   - Treatment given at the scene of injury or in the ED (e.g., medications, IV fluids)
   - Medical history, including osteoporosis or arthritis of the spine, congenital deformities, cancer, and previous injury or surgery of the neck or back
   - History of respiratory problems especially if the patient has experienced a cervical SCI

   Focus: Prioritization.

3. **Ans: 2**   The priority at the time of admission to the ED with an SCI at the C4 to C5 level is airway and respiratory status. The cervical spine nerves C3 to C5 innervate the phrenic nerve, which controls the diaphragm. Careful and frequent assessments are necessary, and ET intubation may be required to prevent respiratory arrest. The other three concerns are appropriate but are not as urgent as airway and respiratory status. **Focus:** Prioritization. **Test-Taking Tip:** Remember that priorities for care are those aspects that are most urgent. In this case, with such a high SCI, the patient is at risk for airway and respiratory problems.

4. **Ans: 1**   The HCP tests DTRs, including the biceps (C5), triceps (C7), patella (L3), and ankle (S1). It is not unusual for these reflexes, as well as all mobility or sensory perception, to be absent immediately after the injury because of spinal shock. When spinal shock has resolved, the reflexes may return if the lesion is incomplete. Complete but temporary loss of motor, sensory, reflex, and autonomic function often lasts less than 48 hours but may continue for several weeks. Spinal shock is not the same as neurogenic shock. Neurogenic shock results from hypotension and sometimes occurs with bradycardia. It can be caused by severe damage in the central nervous system, which includes the brain and cervical and thoracic spinal cord. The trauma or injury brings sudden loss of sympathetic stimulation of the blood vessels, causing blood vessels to relax and leading to a rapid decrease in blood pressure. **Focus:** Prioritization.

5. **Ans: 2, 4, 6, 7**   An experienced AP can make sure that the oxygen flow setting is correct and that the cannula is in place after instructed by the RN. The experienced AP would also know how to measure oxygen saturation by pulse oximetry. Reminding a patient about what has already been taught by the RN (e.g., to use incentive spirometry) is within the scope of practice for an AP. The nurse retains responsibility for ensuring that the patient's oxygen flow rate is correct and interpreting oxygen saturation measurements. AP's scope of practice includes checking vital signs. Assessments, including auscultation, and patient teaching require additional education, training, and skill and are appropriate to the scope of practice of the RN. Monitoring IV fluids also requires the skills of a nurse. **Focus:** Delegation, Supervision.

6. **Ans: 3**   The nurse should notify the HCP immediately. The patient's symptoms indicate the strong possibility of impending respiratory arrest. This patient probably needs endotracheal (ET) intubation and mechanical ventilation. **Focus:** Prioritization.

7. **Ans: 1, 2, 4, 6**   Checking vital signs and recording urine output are both within the AP's scope of practice. He or she would also know how to empty the patient's catheter bag. Instructing the AP to report an increase in respiratory rate or a decrease in oxygen saturation is essential because these findings indicate worsening of the patient's condition. An experienced AP would also have the skill and knowledge to operate a pulse oximetry device. An oxygen saturation of 91% would be acceptable and would not require increasing the oxygen flow rate. Teaching would require additional skills included within the scope of practice for the professional RN. **Focus:** Delegation, Supervision.

8. **Ans: 3**   The high-pressure ventilator alarm commonly is an indication that the patient has increased secretions and needs to be suctioned. The nurse could auscultate for coarse crackles over the trachea because this is also a very common indication that suctioning is needed. Tubing disconnection or cuff air leak would set off the low-pressure alarm. The nurse should assess the patient first and then the machine to discover the problem. If he or she cannot determine the problem, then the RN should manually ventilate the patient while the respiratory therapist is notified and determines the problem. **Focus:** Prioritization.

9. **Ans: 1, 2, 3, 4**   Before extubation (tube removal), oxygen would be set up, emergency equipment would be brought to the bedside, the patient would be hyperoxygenated, and the tube cuff would be deflated. The patient would not be asked to cough, and oxygen would not be applied by face mask or nasal cannula until after the tube had been removed. **Focus:** Prioritization.

10. **Ans: 1**   The traction weights must be hanging freely at all times to maintain the cervical traction and prevent further injury. The other options are appropriate for the care of a patient with cervical tongs. **Focus:** Prioritization. **Test Taking Tip:** A question like this is asking the nurse to recognize actions or findings that can be harmful to the patient. In this case, when the weights do not hang freely, there is no traction to keep the patient's spine aligned.

11. **Ans: 1, 4, 6**   A nursing student can administer medications and simple treatments such as cervical tong pin care under the supervision of an RN. He or she can also check and record vital signs and oxygen saturation. The nursing student should be mentored by the nurse when monitoring traction during patient repositioning and performing neurologic assessments. The nurse should also mentor the student with regard to adding to the patient's care plan because planning care is within the scope of practice for the professional RN. **Focus:** Delegation, Supervision.

12. **Ans: 1**   The experienced AP has been taught how to reposition patients while maintaining proper body alignment. The nurse remains responsible for ensuring that this action is performed correctly. Inspecting a patient's skin and administering medications require additional education and skill and are appropriately performed by licensed nurses. Performing physical therapy exercises also requires additional education and skill and is appropriate to the scope of practice of licensed nurses and physical therapists. However, some APs are given extra training and are able to perform range-of-motion exercises for patients. The skill level and job descriptions of AP team members should be checked to determine their ability to perform range-of-motion exercises. **Focus:** Delegation, Supervision.

13. **Ans: 3**   Mr. M has a level C4 to C5 spinal injury. The best way to assess motor functions in a patient with this type of injury is to apply downward pressure while the patient shrugs his shoulders upward. Testing plantar flexion assesses S1-level injuries. Applying resistance when the patient lifts the legs assesses injuries at the L2 to L4 level. Having a patient grasp and form a fist assesses C8-level injuries. **Focus:** Prioritization.

14. **Ans: 2**   Autonomic dysreflexia is a possibly life-threatening condition in which noxious visceral or cutaneous stimuli cause a sudden, massive, uninhibited reflex sympathetic discharge in patients with high-level SCI. Symptoms include elevated blood pressure, bradycardia, profuse diaphoresis, flushing, blurred vision, spots in the visual field, and a severe throbbing headache. **Focus:** Prioritization.

15. **Ans: 2, 3, 5, 6**   The patient's symptoms indicate the possibility of autonomic dysreflexia, which can be life threatening. Immediate interventions for this patient include placing him in a sitting position or previous safe position, notifying the HCP, checking for urinary retention, and providing catheterization if the patient does not already have a catheter. The nurse would check an indwelling catheter's tubing for kinks or obstruction. Vital signs should be checked at least every 10 to 15 minutes. Other actions that could be taken include checking for fecal impaction or worsening of an existing pressure ulcer. If the HCP prescribes drugs, nifedipine or a nitrate may be administered. An incontinence pad is not necessary at this time. **Focus:** Prioritization.

16. **Ans: 3**   The patient should be encouraged to perform as much self-care as he is able to do, and the AP should help with the care the patient is unable to complete. The patient's wife should also be taught to encourage the patient to do as much as possible for himself. **Focus:** Prioritization, Delegation, Supervision.

17. **Ans: 4**   Patients experiencing an SCI often have significant behavioral and emotional problems as a result of changes in functional ability, body image, role performance, and self-concept. Assess patients for their reaction to the injury and provide opportunities to listen to their concerns. Be realistic about their abilities and projected function but offer hope and encouragement. Options 1, 2, and 3 do not acknowledge the patient's immediate concern so are not the best way to respond. With option 4, the nurse indicates that he or she hears what the patient is saying and is listening in a supportive and nonjudgmental manner. The nurse needs to assist the patient to verbalize feelings and fears about body image, self-concept, role performance, self-esteem, and sexuality. After understanding the patient's concerns, the nurse may be able to refer the patient to a sexuality or intimacy counselor. **Focus:** Prioritization. **Test-Taking Tip:** When a patient indicates to the nurse that he or she is upset and concerned, the most immediately important role of the nurse is to listen, gather more information, and offer support in a nonjudgmental manner.

18. **Ans: 1, 3, 4, 5, 6**   Patients should be taught to drink 2000 to 2500 mL of fluid each day to prevent urinary tract infections and calculus formation. They may be taught to decrease the amount of fluid intake after 6:00 to 7:00 PM to decrease the need to void or to self-catheterize in the middle of the night. The other points are appropriate for a bladder training program. **Focus:** Prioritization.

19. **Ans: 2**   The first, third, and fourth statements are reasonable patient goals for rehabilitation. The second statement likely represents an unrealistic expectation, and the patient needs additional teaching about setting realistic goals for rehabilitation. **Focus:** Prioritization.

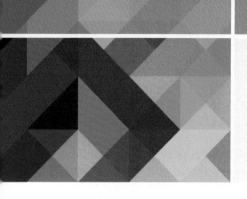

Multiple Patients With Adrenal Gland Disorders

Questions

Ms. B is a 68-year-old woman admitted to the medical unit through the emergency department (ED) after being hit in the abdomen by an automobile while walking home. An 18-gauge IV catheter was inserted in the left forearm, and normal saline was started at 100 mL/hr. ED vital signs were a blood pressure (BP) of 118/80 mm Hg, a heart rate of 82 beats/min, respiratory rate of 26 breaths/min, and oral temperature of 98.4°F (36.9°C). Ms. B has a small dressing to a wound on her right side with a small amount of serosanguinous drainage present.

The assistive personnel (AP) checks her vital signs while she is lying down with the head of her bed elevated and reports that the patient's BP is now 92/58 mm Hg, and she describes feelings of weakness, fatigue, and abdominal pain. When the nurse assesses Ms. B, it is also discovered that she is nauseated and has just vomited 560 mL of greenish fluid and undigested food from breakfast.

Laboratory values from the ED were as follows:

Aldosterone level	3 ng/dL (low) (0.083 nmol/L)
Cortisol level	2 mcg/dL (low) (55.18 nmol/L)
Potassium level	5.2 mEq/L (5.2 mmol/L)
Sodium level	136 mEq/L (136 mmol/L)

1. Based on the assessment of Ms. B, what is the nurse's **first** action?
   1. Administer an antiemetic.
   2. Measure abdominal girth.
   3. Notify the health care provider (HCP).
   4. Start another IV and hang another bag of normal saline.

2. The AP informs the RN that Ms. B's BP is now 84/50 mm Hg. Which prescribed action by the HCP would the nurse implement **first**?
   1. Infuse normal saline at 250 mL/hr.
   2. Type and cross-match for 2 units of packed red blood cells.
   3. Insert a second large-bore IV catheter.
   4. Administer prednisone 10 mg PO.

3. What are three key components of emergency management of a patient with adrenocortical insufficiency? **Select all that apply.**
   1. Hormone replacement with hydrocortisone
   2. Administration of potassium-sparing diuretics
   3. Hypoglycemia management with IV glucose
   4. Subcutaneous insulin before meals and at bedtime
   5. Hyperkalemia management with a potassium-binding and potassium-excreting resin
   6. Fluid restrictions to maintain body weight and prevent edema

⚡ **4.** Enhanced Multiple Response

Question: When providing care for Ms. B, which actions will the nurse delegate to the AP?

Instructions: Circle or highlight the numbers that best answer the question. **Select all that apply.**
1. Encouraging the patient to take in adequate oral fluids
2. Measuring vital signs every 15 minutes
3. Recording intake and output accurately every hour
4. Getting a baseline weight to guide therapy
5. Administering oral antinausea medication
6. Assisting the patient up to the bathroom
7. Assessing the patient's abdomen for bowel sounds every 4 hours
8. Providing oral care every morning before breakfast
9. Changing the patient's dressing

5. Which patient care action would the nurse assign to an experienced LPN/LVN?
1. Interpret Ms. B's lab values.
2. Change Ms. B's dressing on her right side.
3. Prepare a nursing care plan for Ms. B.
4. Administer IV promethazine for nausea.

6. Ms. B develops diaphoresis, an increased heart rate (124 beats/min), and tremors. She also reports an increasing headache. Which action should the nurse take **first**?
1. Check the fingerstick glucose level.
2. Check the serum potassium level.
3. Place the patient on a cardiac monitor.
4. Decrease IV fluids to 100 mL/hr.

Ms. H is admitted to the acute medical-surgical unit for a workup for Cushing disease.

7. Which vital sign value reported to the RN by the AP is of **most** concern for a patient with Cushing disease (hypercortisolism)?
1. Heart rate of 102 beats/min
2. Respiratory rate of 26 breaths/min
3. BP of 156/88 mm Hg
4. Oral temperature of 101.8°F (38.8°C)

8. Which factor reported by Ms. H to the nurse supports the diagnosis of Cushing disease?
1. Cessation of menses at age 33 years
2. Increased craving for salty foods
3. Weight loss of 25 lbs
4. Nausea, diarrhea, and loss of appetite

⚡ **9.** Enhanced Multiple Response

Question
The RN is supervising a nursing student who will assess Ms. H. Which findings will the RN teach the student nurse to expect in a patient with Cushing disease?

Instructions: Circle or highlight the numbers that best answer the question. **Select all that apply.**
1. Truncal obesity
2. Weight loss
3. Bruising
4. Hypertension
5. Thickened skin
6. Dependent edema
7. Moon face
8. Petechiae
9. Hair loss
10. Darkened skin

10. Which laboratory values would the nurse expect to find for Ms. H? **Select all that apply.**
1. Elevated serum cortisol level
2. Decreased serum sodium level
3. Elevated serum glucose level
4. Decreased lymphocyte count
5. Increased serum calcium level
6. Decreased urine androgen level

11. Cushing disease is diagnosed in Ms. H because of hypercortisolism (increased secretion of cortisol), and she is scheduled for an adrenalectomy. Which preoperative actions should the nurse assign to the LPN/LVN? **Select all that apply.**
1. Assessing the patient's cardiac rhythm
2. Reviewing the patient's laboratory results
3. Checking the patient's fingerstick glucose results
4. Administering insulin on a sliding scale as needed
5. Discussing goals and outcomes of care with the patient
6. Giving the patient oral preoperative medications

Answer Key for this chapter begins on p. 297

PART 3   Complex Health Scenarios

12. A nursing concern of risk for infection related to immunosuppression and inadequate primary defenses has been identified for Ms. H. Which nursing care actions should the RN delegate to the AP? **Select all that apply.**
    1. Providing the patient with a soft toothbrush
    2. Instructing the patient to avoid activities that may result in skin trauma
    3. Reminding the patient to change positions in bed every 2 hours
    4. Assessing the patient's skin for reddened areas, excoriation, and edema
    5. Ensuring that the patient has tissues and a bag for disposal of used tissues
    6. Teaching the patient to avoid crowded areas and people with cold symptoms

13. The RN is teaching an AP about fluid retention when a patient such as Ms. H is diagnosed with Cushing disease. Which method does the RN instruct the AP is best for indicating fluid retention?
    1. Strict intake and output measures
    2. Measuring urine-specific gravity
    3. Checking daily weights with the same scale
    4. Comparing ankle swelling on a day-by-day basis

14. Ms. H had a complete adrenalectomy, and the nurse is preparing to teach her about cortisol replacement therapy. Which key points should be included in the teaching plan? **Select all that apply.**
    1. "Take your medication in divided doses, with the first dose in the morning and the second dose between 4:00 and 6:00 PM."
    2. "Take your medications on an empty stomach to facilitate absorption."
    3. "Weigh yourself daily using the same scale and wearing the same amount of clothes."
    4. "Never skip a dose of medication."
    5. "Call your doctor if you experience persistent nausea, severe diarrhea, or fever."
    6. "Report any rapid weight gain, round face, fluid retention, or swelling to your doctor."

Ms. L is a 59-year-old woman who is admitted after experiencing intermittent episodes of high BP accompanied by headaches, diaphoresis, and chest pain. She tells the admitting nurse that she gets frightened and feels a "sense of doom" when these episodes occur. The endocrinologist has ordered hospitalization to rule out pheochromocytoma.

15. Which assessment action should the nurse **avoid** when admitting Ms. L?
    1. Palpating the patient's abdomen
    2. Checking the patient's extremity reflexes
    3. Testing the pupillary reaction to light
    4. Measuring baseline weight with the patient standing

16. The HCP orders a 24-hour urine collection for vanillylmandelic acid (VMA), metanephrine, and catecholamine testing. Which instruction given to Ms. L by a nursing student would cause the nurse to intervene?
    1. "You will be on a special diet for 2 to 3 days before the urine collection for this test."
    2. "You should not drink caffeinated beverages or eat citrus fruits, bananas, or chocolate."
    3. "You will take your usual medications, including the aspirin and the beta-blocker for your high BP."
    4. "In 2 to 3 days, you will begin the 24-hour urine collection after discarding the first void in the morning."

17. In providing nursing care for Ms. L, which action should the nurse delegate to the AP?
    1. Working with the patient to identify stressful situations that may lead to a hypertensive crisis
    2. Reminding the patient not to smoke, drink caffeinated beverages, or change positions suddenly
    3. Assessing the patient's hydration status and reporting manifestations of dehydration or fluid overload
    4. Telling the patient to limit activity and remain in a calm, restful environment during headaches

18. As the charge nurse, which patients would be appropriate to assign to a newly graduated RN who has just completed orientation to the unit? **Select all that apply.**
    1. Ms. L with pheochromocytoma, who is scheduled for an adrenalectomy and needs preoperative teaching
    2. Ms. B with adrenal gland hypofunction, whose BP is dropping and who is experiencing Addisonian crisis
    3. Ms. H with Cushing disease, who is very anxious and fearful about her scheduled adrenal surgery
    4. Mr. J with hyperaldosteronism, whose current serum potassium level is 3.2 mEq/L (3.2 mmol/L)
    5. Mr. M with rule-out Addison disease, who is newly admitted with muscle weakness, weight loss, and hypotension
    6. Ms. A, who was admitted 2 days ago to rule out hyperaldosteronism

Answers

1. **Ans: 3** The patient's signs and symptoms indicate a possible adrenal crisis (Addisonian crisis), or acute adrenocortical insufficiency, a life-threatening event in which the need for cortisol and aldosterone is greater than the available supply. It often occurs in response to a stressful event (e.g., surgery, trauma, severe infection), especially when the adrenal hormone output is already reduced. The other actions are important and will likely be implemented rapidly because a common cause of acute adrenal gland hypofunction is hemorrhage, but the first priority is that the HCP be notified immediately. **Focus:** Prioritization.

2. **Ans: 1** The patient is hypotensive and most likely hypovolemic. Because the patient already has an IV line, the IV fluids should be started first to address the primary problem. The second IV line and typing and cross-matching need to be accomplished rapidly, and the blood sample may be drawn at the same time that the second IV line is inserted. The patient needs cortisol replacement, but with nausea and vomiting present, the oral route is not the best option and an IV form of the drug should be considered. **Focus:** Prioritization. **Test-Taking Tip:** A question like this asks the nurse to prioritize what action must be taken first. To best answer, consider what is most life threatening to the patient. In this case, the threat is severe hypovolemia and severe hypotension, which can be life threatening.

3. **Ans: 1, 3, 5** With acute adrenal insufficiency, the nurse must be aware of three major areas of concern for treatment, which are hormone replacement, hyperkalemia management, and hypoglycemia management. **Focus:** Prioritization.

4. **Ans: 2, 3, 4, 6, 8** The patient is experiencing nausea and vomiting, so oral fluids are not appropriate at this time. The AP can take frequent vital sign measurements, record intake and output, weigh the patient, provide oral care, and assist the patient to the bathroom. The nurse should instruct the AP about which variations in vital signs must be reported. Administration of medications is appropriate to the scope of practice of licensed nurses. This could be assigned to an LPN/LVN. Assessments and dressing changes should be completed by the nurse. **Focus:** Delegation, Assignment, Supervision.

5. **Ans: 2** Interpreting lab values, preparing care plans, and administering IV drugs are within the scope of practice for the professional RN. In some states, an LPN/LVN may administer some IV drugs with additional training (although administration of IV drugs to unstable patients is best done by RN staff who have education and scope of practice to evaluate patient response). Be sure to check the scope of practice in your state and at your facility. Changing a simple dressing is within the scope of practice for an LPN/LVN, although the RN would want to be sure to assess the wound site. **Focus:** Assignment, Supervision.

6. **Ans: 1** The manifestations the patient has developed are classic signs of hypoglycemia, a complication of adrenal gland hypofunction. The nurse should check the patient's glucose level first. If it is low, the patient should receive some form of glucose, most likely dextrose 50% IV. **Focus:** Prioritization.

7. **Ans: 4** A patient with Cushing disease is immunosuppressed because excess cortisol reduces the number of circulating lymphocytes and inhibits production of cytokines and inflammatory chemicals such as histamine. These patients are at greater risk for infection. Therefore it is essential that the nurse be told about any temperature elevation with this patient. **Focus:** Prioritization, Supervision, Delegation. **Test-Taking Tip:** To answer a question such as this one, the nurse needs to understand basic pathophysiology and then apply that knowledge to the patient's situation. In this case, the patient is immunosuppressed and is at risk for infection, so the nurse would be extra alert for any signs of infection.

8. **Ans: 1** Women with Cushing disease may report a history of early cessation of menses. Increased androgen production can interrupt the normal hormone feedback mechanism for the ovaries, which decreases the production of estrogens and progesterone and results in oligomenorrhea (scant or infrequent menses). **Focus:** Prioritization.

9. **Ans: 1, 3, 4, 6, 7** A patient with Cushing disease typically has paperlike thin skin and weight gain as a result of an increase in total body fat caused by slow turnover of plasma fatty acids. Weight loss, hair loss and darkened skin are to be expected in a patient with hypocortisolism (e.g., Addison disease). The other findings are typical of a patient with Cushing disease. **Focus:** Supervision, Prioritization.

10. **Ans: 1, 3, 4, 5** A patient with Cushing disease would have lab values that include increased serum, salivary, and urinary cortisol levels. Other lab value expectations include increased blood glucose level, decreased lymphocyte count, increased serum sodium, and decreased serum calcium. In a 24-hour urine collection, there would also be increased levels of cortisol and androgens. **Focus:** Prioritization.

11. **Ans: 3, 4, 6** The educational preparation of the LPN/LVN includes fingerstick glucose monitoring and administering oral and subcutaneous medications. Assessing cardiac rhythms and reviewing laboratory

PART 3 · Complex Health Scenarios

results require additional education and skill and are appropriate to the RN's scope of practice. **Focus:** Assignment, Supervision.

12. **Ans: 1, 3, 5**   The AP can provide articles for self-care (e.g., toothbrushes, tissues, small trash bags) and reinforce what the RN has already taught the patient. The AP can also remind the patient about changing positions once the nurse has instructed the patient to do this. Instructing and assessing are within the scope of practice of the professional nurse. **Focus:** Delegation, Supervision.

13. **Ans: 3**   Fluid retention may not be visible. Rapid weight gain is the best indicator of fluid retention. The best and most accurate way to detect fluid retention is to weigh the patient on a daily basis. Weigh the patient at the same time daily (before breakfast) using the same scale. Have the patient wear the same type of clothing for each weight check. **Focus:** Prioritization, Supervision, Delegation.

14. **Ans: 1, 3, 4, 5, 6**   Cortisol replacement drugs should be taken with meals or snacks because the patient can develop gastrointestinal irritation when the drugs (e.g., cortisone, hydrocortisone, prednisone, fludrocortisone) are taken on an empty stomach. All of the other teaching points are appropriate. **Focus:** Prioritization.

15. **Ans: 1**   When a patient with possible pheochromocytoma is assessed, the abdomen should not be palpated because this action could cause a sudden release of catecholamines and severe hypertension. None of the other assessments should have an adverse effect on this patient. **Focus:** Prioritization.

16. **Ans: 3**   During the 3- to 4-day VMA testing period, medications usually withheld include aspirin and antihypertensive agents. Beta-blockers are avoided because these drugs may cause a rebound rise in BP. All of the other instructions are appropriate for this diagnostic test. **Focus:** Delegation, Supervision.

17. **Ans: 2**   The AP should remind the patient about elements of the care regimen that the nurse has already

taught the patient. Assessing, instructing, and identifying stressful situations that may trigger a hypertensive crisis require additional education and skill appropriate to the scope of practice of the professional RN. **Focus:** Delegation, Supervision.

18. **Ans: 1, 4, 6**   The newly graduated RN who has just completed orientation should be assigned patients whose conditions are relatively stable and not complex. The new graduate should be familiar with adrenal surgery after completing his or her orientation and should be able to provide any teaching the patient needs. The patient with a low potassium level will need some form of potassium supplementation, which the new nurse should be able to administer. The patient who was admitted 2 days ago to rule out hyperaldosteronism would be stable and not in need of complex nursing care. Patients with significant changes would benefit from care by experienced RNs. The patient in Addisonian crisis and the fearful, anxious patient would also benefit from being cared for by an experienced nurse. The newly admitted patient may have many questions and would also benefit from care with an experienced RN. **Focus:** Assignment.

19. **Ans: 1, 2, 3, 5, 6**   When surgery for hyperaldosteronism (adrenalectomy) cannot be performed, spironolactone (a potassium-sparing diuretic) therapy is continued to control hypokalemia and hypertension. Patients are advised to avoid potassium supplements and foods rich in potassium. Hyponatremia can occur with spironolactone therapy, and the nurse should monitor for and report manifestations such as dry mouth, thirst, lethargy, and drowsiness. Headaches are a common manifestation of hyperaldosteronism, so acetaminophen may be prescribed as a treatment. Side effects of spironolactone should also be taught to the patient. Examples include gynecomastia and erectile dysfunction, as well as diarrhea, hives, hirsutism, and amenorrhea. **Focus:** Prioritization.

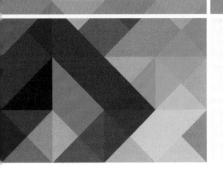

Questions

An RN is the leader of a team caring for patients with gastrointestinal disorders on a medical-surgical unit. The team includes a newly graduated RN who has recently completed hospital orientation, an experienced assistive personnel (AP), and a nursing student. The following information about the six assigned patients is included in the hand-off report. (Note to student: Use the information from the hand-off report to make brief notes about these six patients and refer to the notes as you work through the case study. This gives you practice in identifying important information and simulates how you would use the notes to remember and keep track of six patients over the course of a shift.)

- *Ms. H, a 42-year-old woman, has right upper quadrant pain that radiates to the right shoulder. She has a history of gallstones. She was admitted through the emergency department last night with acute cholecystitis. The night shift nurse reports, "She had a good night."*
- *Ms. D, a 60-year-old woman, was admitted with vomiting and pain in the midabdomen related to a bowel obstruction. She reports abdominal pain that has gradually improved since the insertion of a nasogastric (NG) tube. She is receiving IV fluids and is currently NPO.*

- *Ms. T, a 29-year-old woman, was admitted for an acute exacerbation of ulcerative colitis. She appears wasted and malnourished. She has severe diarrhea and reports predefecation abdominal pain and generalized tenderness to palpation. The plan is to start administering total parenteral nutrition (TPN) through a central line this morning.*
- *Mr. A, a 26-year-old man, will be discharged in the afternoon. He is homeless and frequently sleeps in a nearby shelter. He had discharge teaching from the enterostomal therapist yesterday regarding his infected wound secondary to a ruptured appendix; he wants a review of the wound care instructions before he leaves.*
- *Mr. K, an 85-year-old man, is frail but alert and oriented to person and place. He was transferred from an extended-care facility to receive a percutaneous endoscopic gastrostomy (PEG) tube that was placed 5 days ago. He has a large family. They ask a lot of questions and argue continuously among themselves and with the staff. His vital signs are stable.*
- *Mr. R, a 57-year-old man, has periumbilical pain. The pain is very severe, despite medication, and radiates to the back. Mr. R was admitted with acute pancreatitis. He is NPO and has an NG tube and IV line. He is belligerent and confused. His white blood cell (WBC) count and blood glucose level are increased.*

1. The night shift nurse has just finished giving the RN team leader a report on the six patients. Which patient has the **highest** acuity level and the **greatest** risk for shock?
   1. Ms. H (acute cholecystitis)
   2. Ms. D (bowel obstruction)
   3. Ms. T (ulcerative colitis)
   4. Mr. A (appendectomy)
   5. Mr. K (PEG tube)
   6. Mr. R (acute pancreatitis)

2. Which patients would be **best** to assign to the new RN? **Select all that apply.**
   1. Ms. H (acute cholecystitis)
   2. Ms. D (bowel obstruction)

   3. Ms. T (ulcerative colitis)
   4. Mr. A (appendectomy)
   5. Mr. K (PEG tube)
   6. Mr. R (acute pancreatitis)

3. Which tasks can be delegated to the AP? **Select all that apply.**
   1. Assisting Ms. T with perineal care after diarrheal episodes
   2. Measuring vital signs every 2 hours for Mr. R
   3. Transporting Ms. H off the unit for a procedure
   4. Gently cleansing the nares around Ms. D's NG tube
   5. Removing Mr. A's dressing
   6. Helping Mr. K brush his teeth

4. Which reporting tasks are appropriate to delegate to the AP? **Select all that apply.**
   1. Reporting on the condition of Ms. T's perineal area after application of ointment
   2. Reporting the quality and color of NG drainage for Ms. D
   3. Reporting whether Mr. R's blood pressure is below 100/60 mm Hg
   4. Reporting if any of the patients are complaining of pain
   5. Reporting if Mr. A is seen leaving the unit to smoke a cigarette
   6. Reporting that Mr. K's family has questions

5. The night nurse gives a brief and incomplete report. Which question should the oncoming RN team leader pose to the night shift nurse to help determine the **priority** actions for Ms. H, who was admitted for acute cholecystitis?
   1. "What are her vital signs?"
   2. "Is she going to surgery or radiology this morning?"
   3. "Is she still having pain?"
   4. "Does she need any morning medications?"

6. It is confirmed that Ms. H needs to have an endoscopic retrograde cholangiopancreatography (ERCP) this morning. While preparing the patient to go to the procedure, the nurse discovers the following information. Which finding is the **most** urgent to report to the health care provider (HCP)?
   1. Ms. H reveals that she is supposed to be taking medication for high blood pressure.
   2. Ms. H has several sudden episodes of vomiting large amounts of green bile emesis.
   3. Ms. H has been hesitant to sign the consent form and the form is still unsigned.
   4. Ms. H reports that she had "some type of reaction" to contrast media in the past.

7. Ms. H decided to have the ERCP. The procedure was successfully performed without incident and she returns to the medical-surgical unit. What is the **priority** assessment in the immediate postprocedural care?
   1. Signs/symptoms of perforation
   2. Signs/symptoms of pancreatitis
   3. Signs/symptoms of an allergic reaction
   4. Signs/symptoms of biliary colic

8. Ms. H's (acute cholecystitis) ERCP shows a decreased bile flow with gallbladder disease and obstruction. Because of the obstruction, the nurse is vigilant for the complication of biliary colic. What are the key signs and symptoms that the nurse will watch for?
   1. Rebound tenderness and a sausage-shaped mass in the right upper quadrant (RUQ)

2. Flatulence, dyspepsia, and eructation after eating or drinking
3. RUQ abdominal pain that radiates to the right shoulder or scapula
4. Severe abdominal pain with tachycardia, pallor, diaphoresis, and prostration

9. The HCP told Ms. H (acute cholecystitis) that she would probably need a laparoscopic cholecystectomy; however, the ERCP and laboratory results are still pending. Ms. H asks, "What should I expect?" What is the **best** intervention at this point?
   1. Describe the surgical procedure.
   2. Call the HCP to come and speak with her.
   3. Provide some written material about gallbladder disease and options.
   4. Explain general postoperative care, such as coughing and deep breathing exercises.

10. All of these patients must receive their routine morning medications. Which patient should receive his or her medication last?
    1. Ms. H (acute cholecystitis)
    2. Ms. D (bowel obstruction)
    3. Ms. T (ulcerative colitis)
    4. Mr. K (PEG tube)

11. The RN is observing the nursing student perform an abdominal assessment on Ms. D, who was admitted for a bowel obstruction. For which actions will the supervising nurse intervene? **Select all that apply.**
    1. Palpating for abdominal distention with the index fingertip
    2. Auscultating for bowel sounds with the NG tube attached to low wall suction
    3. Performing the physical assessment before asking about pain
    4. Checking the NG collection canister for quantity and quality of drainage
    5. Inspecting for visible signs of peristaltic waves or abdominal distention
    6. Checking for skin turgor over the lower abdominal area

12. The RN is supervising the nursing student in administering Ms. D's (bowel obstruction) medications through the NG tube. When would the nurse intervene?
    1. The student compares the medication administration record with the original prescription.
    2. The student draws up 30 mL of sterile water for flush in a large-bore syringe.
    3. The student performs three checks of the medication names and dosages.
    4. The student crushes tablets and puts all medications in the same cup.

13. The new RN asks the team leader if it is okay to give Ms. D (bowel obstruction) a dose of psyllium using the HCP's standing orders. Ms. D says she feels constipated and takes psyllium on a regular basis at home. What is the team leader's **best** response?
    1. "Call the HCP to see if the standing orders apply to Ms. D."
    2. "Give the psyllium according to the standing orders."
    3. "Laxatives can cause perforation if there is a bowel obstruction."
    4. "The patient can't be constipated because she is NPO."

14. Ms. D (bowel obstruction) reports feeling weak. She seems more confused compared with her baseline. The NG drainage container has a large amount of watery bile-colored fluid. Which laboratory values should be checked **first**?
    1. Blood urea nitrogen and creatinine levels
    2. Platelet count and WBC count
    3. Sodium level, potassium level, and pH of blood
    4. Bilirubin level, hematocrit, and hemoglobin level

15. The nurse reports Ms. D's laboratory results to the HCP, who then prescribes adding potassium to the IV fluid. Based on this prescription, which additional information should the nurse give to the HCP?
    1. Latest blood pressure result
    2. Urinary output per hour

3. Total drainage from the NG tube
4. Report on abdominal assessment

16. Ms. T, who is hospitalized with ulcerative colitis, reports 10 to 20 small diarrhea stools per day, with abdominal pain before defecation. She appears depressed and uninterested in self-care or suggested therapies. What is the **priority** nursing concept to consider when planning interventions?
    1. Elimination
    2. Nutrition
    3. Pain
    4. Adherence

17. Ms. T is discouraged and dispirited about her ulcerative colitis. She is resistant to TPN. Which explanation will encourage Ms. T to allow the TPN therapy?
    1. "It will help you regain your weight."
    2. "It will create a positive nitrogen balance."
    3. "Your HCP has ordered this important therapy for you."
    4. "Your bowel can rest, and the diarrhea will decrease."

18. Drag and Drop

Scenario: The nurse must administer TPN through a central line for Ms. T. To safely administer the therapy the nurse uses the principles of sterile technique and medication administration.

What is the correct order for the steps to safely administer TPN?

Instructions: In the left column are the steps for administering TPN. In the right column write the number to indicate the correct order of the steps, 1 being the first step and 8 being the last step.

Steps for administering TPN	Order of steps
a. Thread the IV tubing through an infusion pump.	
b. Check the solution for cloudiness or turbidity.	
c. Use aseptic technique to insert the connector into the injection cap.	
d. Select and flush the correct tubing and filter.	
e. Set the infusion pump at the prescribed rate.	
f. Confirm the prescription for TPN before administration.	
g. Scrub the hub of the injection cap.	
h. Document the time, procedure, dose, and appearance of central line insertion site.	

19. Which tasks related to the TPN can be delegated to the AP? **Select all that apply.**
    1. Take vital signs every 4 hours.
    2. Notify nurse if the pump alarm goes off.
    3. Check the volume infused every 4 hours.
    4. Weigh Ms. T every day.
    5. Measure and record the intake and output.
    6. Clean the catheter insertion site.

20. The nurse is reviewing the medication administration record for Ms. T (ulcerative colitis). Which situation needs the **most** immediate investigation?
    1. Two tablets of senna were given yesterday morning.
    2. An oral dose of folic acid was given yesterday morning.
    3. An IV infusion of infliximab 5 mg/kg was given yesterday evening.
    4. An IV hydrocortisone 100 mg was given yesterday evening.

21. Ms. T is receiving an oral dose of sulfasalazine 500 mg every 6 hours for treatment of ulcerative colitis. Which assessment finding is cause for **greatest** concern?
    1. Decreased appetite
    2. Nausea and vomiting
    3. Decreased urine output
    4. Headache

22. The AP asks, "Why can't Ms. T (ulcerative colitis) get out of bed and do things for herself? She's only 29 years old." What is the team leader's **best** response?
    1. "The HCP prescribed bed rest for a few days."
    2. "Decreasing activity helps to decrease the diarrhea."
    3. "I see you're frustrated; just do your best to help."
    4. "She is too depressed to get out of bed."

23. Because of Ms. T's (ulcerative colitis) severe diarrhea, the nurse is reviewing the laboratory results. Which laboratory results are cause for **greatest** concern?
    1. WBC count is 11,000/mm³ (11x10⁹/L).
    2. Hemoglobin is 11 g/dl (6.83 mmol/L); hematocrit is 36% (0.36 volume fraction).
    3. Erythrocyte sedimentation (ESR) rate is 22mm/hr.
    4. Sodium is 132 mEq/L (132 mmol/L); potassium is 3.0 mEq/L 3.1mmol/L).

24. While the nurse is teaching Mr. A about dressing changes for his appendectomy wound, he says, "When you live on the street, you can't do everything the way you nurses do in the hospital." What is the **most** important thing to emphasize in helping him to accomplish self-care?
    1. "Change the dressing in the AM and the PM."
    2. "Use the gauze package to make a sterile field."
    3. "Wash your hands before a dressing change."
    4. "Discard any opened packages of unused gauze."

25. Psychosocial assessment reveals that Mr. A (appendectomy) faces several financial and personal problems. Which finding has the **greatest** impact on discharge teaching for wound care and other follow-up issues?
    1. He is homeless and has no family in the city.
    2. He has no money for the prescribed medications.

3. He has no transportation to the follow-up appointment.
4. He cannot read or write very well.

26. Mr. A (appendectomy) will be discharged with prescriptions for pain medication and an antibiotic. What is the **most** important point that the nurse will emphasize about the medications?
    1. "Take the pain medication before the pain becomes severe."
    2. "The pain medication may make you feel drowsy or sleepy."
    3. "All of the antibiotics should be taken, even if you feel good."
    4. "The antibiotics should not be shared with any other person."

27. To provide good continuity of care for Mr. A (appendectomy), who is homeless, which members of the interdisciplinary team should routinely have access to Mr. A's medical records? **Select all that apply.**
    1. The hospital social worker who is helping Mr. A to locate resources
    2. The surgeon who performed Mr. A's appendectomy
    3. An epidemiologist who is collecting data on the homeless
    4. All of the APs who work in the medical-surgical area
    5. The administrator of the shelter where Mr. A frequently stays
    6. The nurse who works at the shelter where Mr. A frequently stays

28. The RN is teaching the nursing student about enteral feedings for patients such as Mr. K, who has a PEG tube. Which assessments must be performed? **Select all that apply.**
    1. Check for residual volume.
    2. Assess for bowel sounds.
    3. Check placement before each feeding.
    4. Monitor for allergic reactions.
    5. Assess for abdominal distention.
    6. Check blood glucose levels.

⚡ **29.** Enhanced Multiple Response _____

Scenario: There are many tasks associated with enteral tube feedings that can be delegated to the AP. However, the nurse must consider when the tube was inserted, the patient's condition, the clinical setting (e.g., hospital vs. home health), and facility policies.

Which tasks related to enteral tube feedings can be delegated to the AP on the medical-surgical unit under the supervision of the nurse?

Instructions: Place an X, in the space provided, or highlight each task that can be delegated to the AP. **Select all that apply.**

1. _____ Assist patient with oral hygiene.
2. _____ Irrigate the NG tube.
3. _____ Maintain the elevation of head of the bed after feeding.
4. _____ Weigh the patient.
5. _____ Clean and assess the skin around a gastronomy tube.
6. _____ Measure and report emesis.
7. _____ Remove the NG tube.
8. _____ Report nausea, vomiting, or diarrhea.
9. _____ Reinforce NPO status as ordered.
10. _____ Measure the external tube length to check position.
11. _____ Assist with ambulation to prevent constipation.

30. Mr. K (PEG tube) needs 1200 kcal/day. The enteral feeding formula provides 1 kcal/mL. After reviewing the feedings that were given yesterday, which action would the nurse take **first**?

Time of yesterday's feedings	Amount
7:00 AM	100 mL
11:00 AM	50 mL
3:00 PM	200 mL
7:00 PM	100 mL

1. Give additional feedings to catch up on nutritional needs.
2. Look at the original prescription to determine frequency and amount.
3. Look at weight trends to see if patient is losing or maintaining weight.
4. Call the nurse who cared for Mr. K yesterday and ask what happened.

31. Because of Mr. K's (PEG tube) advanced age, which complications of enteral feedings may occur? **Select all that apply.**
1. Hyperglycemia
2. Hypotension
3. Aspiration
4. Diarrhea
5. Fluid overload
6. Weight loss

32. In the care of Mr. K (PEG tube), which health care team members are demonstrating the roles and responsibilities that support interprofessional collaboration? **Select all that apply.**
1. The AP tells Mr. K's family that she will be in at 10:00 AM to assist Mr. K with hygiene.
2. The RN gives the AP specific instructions about how to clean around Mr. K's PEG tube.
3. The RN acknowledges that the AP has the best working relationship with Mr. K's daughter.
4. The enterostomal therapist performs care for Mr. K, but staff and family are unsure about follow-up.
5. The nursing student recognizes that dealing with Mr. K's family dynamics exceeds her abilities.
6. The surgeon does mini-grand rounds with the nursing student to explain the purpose of Mr. K's PEG tube.

33. For Mr. K (PEG tube), several new medications and a change in the enteral feeding solution are included in the discharge plan. Which team member is the nurse **most** likely to consult before teaching the patient and family about these new medications and enteral solution?
1. Nutritionist to verify that the calories and other nutrients are sufficient
2. Home health nurse to verify that follow-up teaching will be performed
3. Social worker to verify that the medications and formula are covered by insurance
4. Pharmacist to verify that the medications are compatible with the feeding solution

PART 3 Complex Health Scenarios

 Answer Key for this chapter begins on p. 306

34. The laboratory informs the nurse that the phlebotomist may have mislabeled or drawn the sample for AM blood tests from another patient, not Mr. R (acute pancreatitis). What should the nurse do **first**?
    1. Call the phlebotomist to come back.
    2. Draw a new blood sample and label it.
    3. Report the phlebotomist to his or her supervisor.
    4. Ask the phlebotomist to explain what happened.

35. What instructions will the nurse give to the AP about how to reposition Mr. R to relieve discomfort related to acute pancreatitis?
    1. Place him in a high Fowler position.
    2. Help him to lie in a side-lying "fetal" position.
    3. Lay the bed flat and put the patient's legs on a pillow.
    4. Help him to sit on the edge of the bed and dangle his legs.

36. A labor and delivery (L&D) nurse calls and says, "I heard that Mr. R was hospitalized. He's my ex-husband, so I looked up his medical record. How's he doing?" What should the RN team leader do **first**?
    1. Invite the L&D nurse to come and see Mr. R in person.
    2. Ask Mr. R if he wants information released to his ex-wife.
    3. Report the L&D nurse for violation of patient privacy.
    4. Explain to the L&D nurse that no information can be given out.

37. Mr. R (acute pancreatitis) demonstrates a dry cough. He reports left-sided chest pain when breathing deeply and shortness of breath. He also has a low-grade fever. Which potential complication does the nurse suspect?
    1. Hypovolemic shock
    2. Pleural effusion
    3. Paralytic ileus
    4. Acute respiratory distress syndrome

38. The nurse notes that Mr. R (acute pancreatitis) has a small amount of blood oozing from the IV insertion site, and there is a palm-shaped bruise on his anterior lateral humerus. What action should the nurse take **first**?
    1. Remove the IV line and restart it at a different site.
    2. Remind the AP to handle Mr. R very gently.
    3. Assess for other signs of obvious or occult bleeding.
    4. Obtain an order for coagulation studies.

39. For Mr. R (acute pancreatitis), the calcium level is 7.5 mg/dl (1.875 mmol/L). Which assessment will the nurse perform?
    1. Assess for Cullen sign.
    2. Assess for Grey-Turner sign.
    3. Assess for McBurney sign.
    4. Assess for Chvostek sign.

40. Which information regarding Mr. R (acute pancreatitis) is appropriate to report to the HCP? **Select all that apply.**
    1. Hematocrit has decreased by more than 10%.
    2. Calcium level is 7.5 mg/dl (1.875 mmol/L).
    3. Partial oxygen pressure (Po_2) is less than 60 mm Hg.
    4. Pain is unrelieved by medication.
    5. Blood type is O positive.
    6. NG tube and IV line are intact.

41. Enhanced Multiple Response _____

    Scenario: The HCP has been paged and is en route to see Mr. R for complications related to acute pancreatitis. The patient is increasingly agitated and confused. He pulls out his IV line and NG tube and removes the oxygen nasal cannula. His skin is pale and clammy.

    Vital signs:
    Pulse 140 beats/min
    Respirations 30 breaths/min
    Blood Pressure 140/60 mmHg

    Which emergency actions will the nurse perform while waiting for the HCP to arrive?

    Instructions: Place an X, in the space provided, or highlight each task that the nurse will perform. **Select all that apply.**
    1. _____ Restart the IV line.
    2. _____ Stay with the patient and call for assistance.
    3. _____ Replace the nasal cannula for supplemental oxygen.
    4. _____ Have a coworker gather IV supplies, glucometer, pulse oximeter, and nonrebreather mask.
    5. _____ Check the blood glucose level.
    6. _____ Delegate the AP to take vital signs every 15 minutes.
    7. _____ Prepare the patient for intubation.
    8. _____ Place the patient in a side-lying position with the head of the bed elevated to 45 degrees.
    9. _____ Have IV calcium gluconate at the bedside.
    10. _____ Activate the rapid response team.

42. The HCP arrives while the RN team leader is caring for Mr. R. Because of Mr. R's deteriorating status (refer to questions 37 and 41), the team leader would advocate for which intervention(s)?
    1. Perform additional laboratory tests and continue monitoring.
    2. Prepare Mr. R for emergency surgery.
    3. Prepare Mr. R for transfer to the intensive care unit (ICU).
    4. Reestablish NG suction and apply restraints or use one-on-one observation.

43. Toward the end of the shift, the team leader finds the new RN in the bathroom crying. The new nurse says, "I'm a terrible nurse. I'm so disorganized, and I'm so far behind. I'm going to quit. I hate this job." What is the **best** thing to do?
    1. Have her take a short break off the unit.
    2. Offer to take one of her patients.
    3. Ask the AP to help her.
    4. Calm her down and help her prioritize.

PART 3

Complex Health Scenarios

Answer Key for this chapter begins on p. 306

Answers

1. **Ans: 6** Mr. R has acute pancreatitis and several prognostic factors that increase the risk for death: age older than 50 years, increased WBC count, and an elevated blood glucose level. Shock can occur secondary to bleeding; release of kinins, which cause vasodilation; or release of enzymes into the circulation. He is also at risk for infection and sepsis. Respiratory complications of pancreatitis include pneumonia, atelectasis, pleural effusions, and acute respiratory distress syndrome. **Focus:** Prioritization. **Test-Taking Tip:** This question simulates the information filtering and subsequent decision making that nurses use while listening to the hand-off report. Use the airway, breathing, circulation (ABCs) and determine which patients are at risk for respiratory distress or hemorrhage.

2. **Ans: 1, 2, 4** Ms. H, Ms. D, and Mr. A are in the most stable condition and represent the least complex cases according to the shift report. Mr. R's confusion and belligerence will make pain management especially difficult. Laboratory results and potential complications must be closely monitored. Ms. T is at risk for electrolyte imbalances, especially hypokalemia. She needs repetitive perineal hygiene and skin assessment. TPN and central line management require additional skills. Mr. K is in stable condition, but because of the family dynamics, his care should be handled by an experienced nurse. **Focus:** Assignment.

3. **Ans: 1, 2, 3, 4, 6** Measuring vital signs, performing hygienic care, and transporting (stable) patients are within the scope of the AP's duties. The AP should not remove the dressing. If the dressing needs to be removed, the nurse should remove it, conduct the wound assessment, clean the area, and redress as needed. **Focus:** Delegation.

4. **Ans: 3, 4, 5, 6** The AP can report on changes in vital sign values; giving parameters for notification is better than asking for general reports on any changes. The AP can report that a patient is having pain but is not expected to assess that pain. The AP can report that the family has questions but should not be expected to answer questions about the patient's care. All staff should be aware of when registered patients come and go on the unit and should keep each other advised. (Note: Patients should also be encouraged to tell someone if they are going off the unit.) Judging the response to treatment and evaluating drainage are responsibilities of the RN. **Focus:** Delegation.

5. **Ans: 2** When the shift report is incomplete, the nurse can ask for any type of additional information; however, morning surgery or procedures impact the immediate plan of care for the individual patient and the organization of care for other assigned patients.

HCPs frequently communicate verbally to the nursing staff, but the written notes may be pending, especially if it is an emergency admission or if the HCP is trying to complete rounds or do procedures. Vital sign values and the need for medications can be obtained from the records if the off-going nurse neglects to give that information. A current pain report can and should be obtained directly from the patient. **Focus:** Prioritization.

6. **Ans: 3** An absolute contraindication would be an unsigned consent form. If a patient makes new disclosures about medical history (e.g., untreated conditions or history of untoward affects), these require further investigation before the procedure begins. Nausea and vomiting are not uncommon during acute cholecystitis, and the HCP may order NG tube insertion to decompress the stomach to reduce the risk for aspiration. **Focus:** Prioritization.

7. **Ans 1:** Perforation is the major complication that can occur during any type of endoscopic procedure. The nurse would assess for signs/symptoms, such as abdominal pain, distention, nausea, vomiting, fever, and shock. Pancreatitis is the most common complication; however, the pathogenesis of pancreatitis will develop more slowly. Assessment for pancreatitis will become the priority after the immediate dangers of airway obstruction (return of gag reflex and independent control of airway) and perforation (hemorrhage and peritonitis) are passed. Severe anaphylactic reactions to contrast media would be expected to occur immediately after administration. Delayed reactions may occur but are much less severe. Biliary colic (severe pain, tachycardia, diaphoresis, and prostration) could occur when gallstones are dislodged and move through the ducts; however, biliary colic is not expected after the procedure. **Focus:** Prioritization.

8. **Ans: 4** Severe pain with tachycardia, pallor, diaphoresis, and prostration (exhaustion) are signs and symptoms of severe biliary colic. Keep the patient flat and notify the rapid response team because of the potential for shock. Rebound tenderness and a sausage-shaped mass in the RUQ suggest peritoneal inflammation. Flatulence (gas), dyspepsia (indigestion), and eructation (belching) after eating are commonly reported by patients when they first seek help for gallbladder problems. RUQ pain that radiates to the right shoulder or scapula is reported by some patients in their descriptions of pain patterns. **Focus:** Prioritization.

9. **Ans: 3** Giving written information about gallbladder disease and options will help Ms. H to prepare any questions she might have for the HCP. If diagnostic results are pending, calling the HCP is premature.

Describing the surgical procedure is inappropriate because there is more than one type of procedure, and the one to be used is still undetermined. Explaining postoperative care would be appropriate after the need for cholecystectomy has been verified by the HCP. **Focus:** Prioritization.

10. **Ans: 4** In the provision of routine care and when all patients are stable, patients who need extra time should be left until last so that care for others is not delayed. Mr. K will require more time and assistance because of age and weakness. Also, his medications must be crushed and administered via PEG tube, which is more time consuming. Dealing with Mr. K's family is also more time consuming. Older adult patients and their families typically benefit from and appreciate caregivers who do not act rushed or hurried. **Focus:** Prioritization.

11. **Ans: 1, 2, 3, 6** The flat palmar surface of the hand is better than the fingertips when palpating for distention. If the wall suction is activated, it will interfere with auscultating for bowel sounds. Asking about pain will guide the physical assessment steps. The skin on the anterior chest under the clavicle is a better place to check for turgor than the lower abdomen, especially if abdominal distention is present. Checking the drainage and inspecting for peristaltic waves or distention are correct actions. **Focus:** Supervision. **Test-Taking Tip:** Hypokalemia and paralytic ileus are nonmechanical causes of intestinal obstruction. Physical assessment findings would include abdominal pain and decreased or hypoactive bowel sounds.

12. **Ans: 4** Medications should be given separately because of an increased risk for physical and chemical incompatibilities, increased chance of clogging the tube, and altered therapeutic response. In addition, if the medications are given one-by-one, the nurse knows exactly which medications the patient has received, but if the medications are mixed together and a problem occurs (e.g., vomiting, clogging, allergic reaction), then the amount received for each medication is unknown. The other actions are correct. **Focus:** Supervision.

13. **Ans: 3** Laxatives should not be used for patients with bowel obstructions or fecal impactions because increased peristaltic action can cause rupture and perforation. Assessment for return of bowel function (e.g., passing flatus, hearing bowel sounds) should be performed, and evidence of function should be pointed out to the patient. The patient should be told that being NPO will decrease fecal mass and that an eventual return of function and normalization of bowel pattern are the therapeutic goals. **Focus:** Prioritization, Supervision.

14. **Ans: 3** With continuous NG suction, there is a loss of sodium and potassium. Also, the loss of acid via suctioning will result in an increase in blood pH or metabolic alkalosis. Full assessment of laboratory data is always important when a change in status is noted, but the other values are less relevant to this patient's NG therapy. **Focus:** Prioritization.

15. **Ans: 2** All of this information could be given to the HCP, but validating renal function is a standard action before administering IV potassium. If the blood pressure is very low, the HCP could prescribe a fluid bolus, but potassium would not usually be added to that solution. Drainage from the NG tube would be replaced with IV fluids and electrolytes; therefore the HCP could use this information to adjust the IV rate. Abdominal assessment is part of the evaluation of therapy. **Focus:** Prioritization.

16. **Ans: 1** The immediate problem is controlling the diarrhea. Addressing this problem is a step toward correcting the nutritional imbalance and decreasing the diarrheal cramping. Self-care and adherence with the treatment plan are important long-term goals that can be addressed when the patient is feeling better physically. **Focus:** Prioritization.

17. **Ans: 4** If the bowel is allowed to rest, the cramping will stop. Stopping the diarrhea is a priority for Ms. T. Chronic, frequent diarrhea is demoralizing, and fluid and electrolyte losses cause weakness. The other options also provide accurate information, but the potential resolution of the most disturbing symptom will encourage her to take the TPN. **Focus:** Prioritization.

18. **Ans: f1, b2, d3, a4, g5, c6, e7, h8** The nurse should always check the prescription before administering TPN; generally, each bag is individually prepared by the pharmacist. The solution should not be cloudy or turbid. Prepare the equipment by priming the tubing and threading the pump. To prevent infection, scrub the hub and use an aseptic technique when inserting the connector into the injection cap and connecting the tubing to the central line. Set the pump at the prescribed rate. Document after the procedure is completed. **Focus:** Prioritization.

19. **Ans: 1, 2, 4, 5** Taking vital signs, reporting alarms, weighing the patient, and measuring and recording intake and output are within the scope of practice for the AP. The nurse should take responsibility for periodically checking the volume infused. The rate can be affected by a pump malfunction or catheter problems. Cleaning the catheter insertion site is a sterile procedure; the nurse would be responsible for assessing, cleaning, and redressing the site as needed. **Focus:** Delegation.

20. **Ans: 1** Generally, laxatives should not be given to patients with ulcerative colitis. In Ms. T's situation, controlling her diarrhea is one of the main treatment goals. Senna is a stimulant laxative and will increase peristalsis and cramping. Folic acid is administered when sulfasalazine is prescribed. Infliximab and hydrocortisone (and sulfasalazine) can be used for patients with ulcerative colitis to reduce the inflammation. **Focus:** Prioritization.

21. **Ans: 3** Sulfasalazine is potentially nephrotoxic. The other adverse effects are also possible but are less serious. **Focus:** Prioritization.

22. **Ans: 2** Explaining the physiologic reason helps the AP to understand that rest is part of the therapy.

Following the HCP's orders is important, but it is an inadequate explanation. Acknowledging frustration is appropriate, but a generalized platitude, such as "do your best," does not help the AP understand the goals of therapy. Depression is not an indication for bed rest. **Focus:** Prioritization, Supervision.

23. **Ans: 4** The low potassium (K$^+$) level is the greatest concern because of the potential for cardiac dysthymias. Sodium (Na$^+$) is also lost during diarrhea episodes. The WBC count, C-reactive protein, and ESR rate are likely to be increased because of the inflammatory process of the disease. Low hemoglobin (Hgb) and hematocrit (Hct) can occur because of ulceration and irritation of the intestinal mucosa. **Focus:** Prioritization. **Test-Taking Tip:** For testing purposes and clinical practice, it is worthwhile to memorize normal values for common blood tests. Normal range for Na are 136 to 145 mEq/L (136-145 mmol/L); K 3.5 to 5.0 mEq/L (3.5-5.0 mmol/L); WBC 5000 to 10,000/mm^3 (5-10 X 10^9/L); [female] Hgb 12 to 16 g/dl (7.4-9.9 mmol/L); [female] Hct 37% to 47% (0.37-0.47 volume fraction); [female] ESR 20 mm/hr.

24. **Ans: 3** Washing the hands is the first basic step for a dressing change. Helping Mr. A identify other ways to maintain asepsis would be more useful than stressing strict sterile technique. Changing the dressing in the morning and the evening may be ideal, but this type of dressing change can be done at any time. **Focus:** Prioritization. **Test-Taking Tip:** From fundamentals, recall that hand hygiene is the single most important action to prevent infection.

25. **Ans: 1** Because Mr. A is homeless, he will need instructions for adapting the dressing change procedures because of inconsistent access to hot water, soap, and adequate bathroom facilities. The social worker can be contacted for assistance with financial issues related to medication or transportation. Simplify written material and verbally reinforce it or instruct Mr. A to have a friend read the information to him. **Focus:** Prioritization.

26. **Ans: 3** All of the teaching points are important; however, Mr. A had a ruptured appendix, and it is essential that he complete the antibiotic prescription so that the infection will completely resolve. Recurrent infections can be more difficult to treat because the organisms will develop a resistance. **Focus:** Prioritization. **Test-Taking Tip:** To prevent the development of drug-resistant strains of microbes, patients should always be instructed to complete a prescription of antibiotics.

27. **Ans: 1, 2, 6** Health care staff who provide direct care for the patient have routine access to the patient's medical records. An epidemiologist could access records to gather data at the aggregate level, but this would require special permission. Only the APs who assist in the care of the patient would have access to records, and AP access may be restricted to flow sheets, for recording vital signs, intake and output, and

so on. The administrator of the shelter might be advised about a patient's condition, but the information is likely to come from the nurse or HCP who oversees patient care at the shelter. **Focus:** Prioritization.

28. **Ans: 1, 2, 3, 5, 6** Assessment for tube feedings generally includes checking for residual (except for jejunostomy tubes), assessing for bowel sounds, and checking for placement, abdominal distention, and hyperglycemia. Allergic reactions are not expected, although a history of food or fluid allergies would be assessed for and reported before the selection and preparation of the formula. **Focus:** Prioritization.

29. **Ans: 1, 3, 4, 6, 8, 9, 11** The AP can assist with oral hygiene; maintain the correct position; measure emesis and report nausea, vomiting, and diarrhea; reinforce interventions (e.g., NPO) that have been explained by the nurse; and assist with ambulation. The RN or LPN/LVN would irrigate or remove the NG tube (there is a risk for aspiration) and provide skin care around a gastronomy tube (skin must be assessed during cleaning). Measuring the tube is one method to check placement and this should be performed by a licensed nurse. **Focus:** Delegation.

30. **Ans: 2** First the nurse would look at the original prescription. If the prescribed amount seems insufficient, the nurse could contact the HCP and the nutritionist to have the feeding changed. If the prescribed orders were not followed, the charge nurse should be notified to follow up with all of the nurses who are caring for Mr. K to prevent reoccurrence. Looking at weight trends is part of the routine assessment for patients with feeding tubes and those at risk for nutritional problems. Mr. K only received 450 kcal yesterday, but trying to catch up by overfeeding may cause distention, vomiting, fluid overload, or electrolyte imbalances. **Focus:** Prioritization.

31. **Ans: 1, 3, 4, 5** Older adult patients are especially at risk for hyperglycemia, aspiration, diarrhea, and fluid overload. Hypotension and weight loss should not occur because of enteral feedings. **Focus:** Prioritization.

32. **Ans: 1, 2, 3, 5, 6** The AP informs the family. The RN gives specific instructions. The RN acknowledges the strengths of a team member. The nursing student recognizes her own limitations. The surgeon enhances the student's learning. These team members have filled their roles and responsibilities toward interprofessional collaboration. The enterostomal therapist performs a task but fails to communicate to other team members what is needed for follow-up care. **Focus:** Supervision, Assignment.

33. **Ans: 4** In this circumstance, the nurse is most likely to consult the pharmacist to see if there are any incompatibilities. The nurse is less likely to consult the other team members at this time unless there are specific issues related to insufficient nutrition, a problem with home health care, or inadequate insurance coverage. **Focus:** Prioritization.

34. **Ans: 2** To expedite the blood work, the nurse would draw the specimen. The other options will only delay getting the results. When the nurse has time, tracking down the cause of the error will help to prevent future recurrences. **Focus:** Prioritization, Supervision.

35. **Ans: 2** For patients with pancreatitis, the fetal position or sitting up and holding the knees to the chest will open the retroperitoneal space, which helps to decrease discomfort. For Mr. R, having him lie down is preferable to having him sit because of his mental status and condition. **Focus:** Supervision, Delegation.

36. **Ans: 4** Even if a person is employed by the hospital, only staff members who provide direct care should have access to medical records and patient information. It is inappropriate to invite the L&D nurse to visit the patient. There should be some investigation as to how the L&D nurse found out that the patient was admitted. Health Insurance Portability and Accountability Act violations are very serious. If staff members are giving out information about patients, those employees and the L&D nurse need to be reminded of the consequences (e.g., loss of license or job). Possibly, more safeguards are needed for computer access to records. **Focus:** Prioritization.

37. **Ans: 2** A dry cough, left-sided chest pain when breathing deeply, shortness of breath, and low-grade fever are signs and symptoms of pleural effusion. Patients with acute pancreatitis can develop many complications: pancreatic infection that can lead to septic shock, hemorrhage secondary to necrotizing hemorrhagic pancreatitis, acute kidney failure, paralytic ileus, hypovolemic shock, pleural effusion, acute respiratory distress syndrome, atelectasis, pneumonia, multiorgan system failure, disseminated intravascular coagulation, and type 2 diabetes mellitus. **Focus:** Prioritization.

38. **Ans: 3** First, the nurse would assess for additional evidence of bleeding. Findings would be immediately reported to the HCP because patients with acute pancreatitis have an increased risk for coagulation disorders, such as disseminated intravascular coagulation. Restarting the IV line at a different site will not alleviate the problem. If there is a coagulation disorder, the new insertion site will also bleed. It would be appropriate to initiate interventions for bleeding precautions, such as gentle handling. The nurse anticipates that the HCP will want coagulation studies after assessment findings are reported. **Focus:** Prioritization.

39. **Ans: 4** For a low calcium level (normal range 9.0-10.5 mg/dl [9.0-10.5 mmol/L]), the nurse will assess for Chvostek sign. This is accomplished by gently tapping the facial nerve in front of the ear and observing for contraction of the facial muscles. Hypocalcemia, a complication of acute pancreatitis, can cause tetany, laryngospasm, and seizures. Grey-Turner sign is a bluish discoloration of the flank that occurs with retroperitoneal bleeding of the pancreas. Cullen sign, a bluish discoloration of the periumbilical area, is associated with acute hemorrhagic pancreatitis. Tenderness over McBurney point is a sign for acute appendicitis. **Focus:** Prioritization.

40. **Ans: 1, 2, 3, 4** The low calcium level and the falling hematocrit and Po_2, in combination with the elevated WBC count and his age, are indicators of a high mortality risk. A high level of pain is not a prognostic factor, but severe unrelieved pain should always be reported. Blood type will not affect the HCP's decisions about therapy. Reporting on the NG tube and IV line would be appropriate for a hand-off report, but information about equipment is not reported to the HCP unless there is a specific problem that requires an order or a change of therapy. **Focus:** Prioritization.

41. **Ans: 1, 2, 3, 4, 5, 6, 8, 9, 10** Stay with the patient; call for a colleague to assist in activating the rapid response team and gathering equipment. Reestablish oxygen per nasal cannula. (Note: Check oxygen saturation with nasal cannula in place and replace with nonrebreather mask as needed.) Restart the IV infusion so that emergency fluids or drugs can be given. Check the blood glucose level to rule out a hypoglycemic reaction. Continuously monitor vital signs. A side-lying position with the head of the bed elevated may relieve pain. (If pain is contributing to the agitation, this may help to calm him.) IV calcium should be readily available because hypocalcemia (occurs in severe cases of acute pancreatitis) can cause tetany, laryngospasm, and seizures. Intubation is not needed at this point. If possible, the NG tube would be inserted; however, this is not a life-saving priority and reinsertion attempts may increase the patient's agitation. **Focus:** Prioritization.

42. **Ans: 3** Mr. R has severe life-threatening problems that warrant transfer to the ICU. The HCP is responsible for the decision to transfer Mr. R; however, the nurse must recognize and advocate for patients who are decompensating. Ordering laboratory and other diagnostic testing may be needed, and restraints or one-on-one observation could be suggested to prevent dislodging equipment, but ultimately the patient should be transferred to the ICU. Surgery is unlikely until aggressive medical management measures are exhausted. **Focus:** Prioritization.

43. **Ans: 4** Helping her to prioritize will build skill and confidence. She feels upset, but she has not made any errors that have compromised patient care (the team leader would point this out to her). Sending her off the unit further delays care, leaves her without support, and hinders opportunities to problem solve. Asking the AP to help her or helping her with select tasks is the second-best choice because it demonstrates team support. Taking over one of her patients is not necessary unless care and safety are compromised. **Focus:** Prioritization, Supervision.

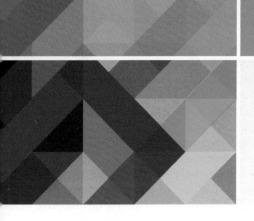

Multiple Patients With Pain

Questions

The RN is the leader of a team caring for patients on a medical-surgical unit. The team includes a newly graduated RN who has recently completed hospital orientation and an assistive personnel (AP). The night shift nurse gives the following report on the six patients that are assigned: (Note to student: Use the information from the hand-off report to make brief notes about these six patients and refer to the notes as you work through the case study.)

- *Ms. R, a 55-year-old woman with rheumatoid arthritis, underwent shoulder arthroplasty 3 days ago. She reports morning stiffness in her joints. Swelling is noted in both wrists and proximal interphalangeal joints.*
- *Mr. L, a 35-year-old man with a history of kidney stones, reports intermittent severe back and right-sided flank pain (rating of 3 to 8 on a scale of 1 to 10). He has had episodic nausea and vomiting. He is urinating but has hematuria and dysuria. Mr. L was admitted through the emergency department (ED) at 10:00 PM. He is using a patient-controlled analgesia (PCA) pump.*
- *Mr. O, an 18-year-old man, sustained a right tibia–fibula fracture in a motorcycle accident 7 hours ago. He has extensive skin abrasions underneath the cast and on the right anterolateral body. Although obvious chest and abdominal trauma were ruled out in the ED, he is being monitored for occult trauma. He is receiving an analgesic via PCA pump. The night shift nurse reports seeing the young man's mother occasionally pushing the PCA pump button.*
- *Mr. H, a 28-year-old man, is currently in the operating room (OR) for an inguinal hernia repair. He should return from the OR later in the shift.*
- *Ms. J, a 65-year-old woman with end-stage multiple myeloma, is receiving hospice care. She has been on the unit for 2 weeks. Her health care provider (HCP) signed the do-not-resuscitate order 3 days ago.*
- *Mr. A, a 55-year-old man, has been on the unit for 3 weeks. He is receiving IV antibiotics for bacterial pneumonia. He has a history of IV drug abuse and chronic back pain and has tested positive for human immunodeficiency virus (HIV) infection. Mr. A's oxygen saturation was decreasing during the night shift.*

1. The team leader decides to do a brief round of all the patients after the shift report to ensure safety and to help determine acuity and assignments. List the order in which the team leader should briefly check in on these patients.
   1. Ms. R (rheumatoid arthritis)
   2. Mr. L (kidney stones)
   3. Mr. O (motorcycle accident)
   4. Mr. H (inguinal hernia repair)
   5. Ms. J (end-stage multiple myeloma)
   6. Mr. A (bacterial pneumonia and HIV positive)

   _____, _____, _____, _____, _____, _____

2. Based on the information that the nurse received during the hand-off report for Mr. A (who has bacterial pneumonia and is HIV positive), which concept is the **priority** to consider in planning care for this patient?
   1. Pain
   2. Gas exchange
   3. Immunity
   4. Cellular regulation

3. The oncoming team leader asks the night shift nurse if anyone spoke to the mother about pushing the PCA button for Mr. O. The night nurse states, "The mother is just concerned about her son and wants him to have pain relief. Besides, the prescribed dose is controlled by the pump." Which action is best?
   1. Report the night nurse to the unit manager for failure to safeguard the patient.
   2. Explain the purpose and function of the PCA delivery system to the mother.
   3. Give the night nurse written information about the dangers of possible overdose.
   4. First talk to the night nurse about the PCA procedure, then talk to the mother.

4. Which of the six patients can be assigned to the new RN? **Select all that apply.**
   1. Ms. R (rheumatoid arthritis)
   2. Mr. L (kidney stones)
   3. Mr. O (motorcycle accident)
   4. Mr. H (inguinal hernia repair)

5. Ms. J (end-stage multiple myeloma)
6. Mr. A (bacterial pneumonia and HIV positive)

5. Which morning tasks can be delegated to the AP? **Select all that apply.**
   1. Assisting Ms. R, who has rheumatoid arthritis, with morning care
   2. Reinforcing to Mr. L, who has a kidney stone, the need to save urine for straining
   3. Preparing Mr. H's room for his return from the OR for hernia repair
   4. Reporting on the condition of Mr. O's skin, resulting from his motorcycle accident
   5. Getting coffee for Ms. J's (end-stage multiple myeloma) family
   6. Checking the pulse oximeter reading for Mr. A, who has bacterial pneumonia

6. Which person is **most** likely to be demonstrating incident pain?
   1. Ms. J (end-stage multiple myeloma) had transdermal fentanyl applied 48 hours ago but now reports unexpected pain.
   2. Ms. R (rheumatoid arthritis) reports having pain when attempting to move her arms/shoulders to put on a blouse.
   3. Mr. A (bacterial pneumonia and HIV positive) reports that the back pain radiates to the back of his thigh and down to his foot.
   4. Mr. O (motorcycle accident) reports that the PCA control is good, but occasionally there is severe pain lasting several minutes.

7. The team leader is talking to Ms. R (rheumatoid arthritis) about discharge plans and follow-up appointments. She begins to cry and says, "I was so active and athletic when I was younger." Which response is **most** therapeutic?
   1. "Your shoulder will get progressively better with time and patience. Don't cry."
   2. "I can see that you are really upset. Is your shoulder hurting a lot right now?"
   3. "I know what you mean. I used to be able to do a lot more when I was younger, too."
   4. "It is difficult to deal with changes. What types of activities did you used to do?"

8. Ms. R (rheumatoid arthritis) tells the nurse, "I really dread doing the postoperative exercises." She seems fearful and grimaces when the nurse suggests that pain medication can be given before the exercises begin. Which member of the health care team would the nurse consult **first**?
   1. Psychiatric clinical nurse specialist to evaluate fears
   2. Occupational therapist to review the goals of therapy
   3. Pharmacist to verify efficacy of pain medication
   4. Surgeon to review the expected progress of healing

9. Which nonpharmacologic pain measure to help Ms. R (rheumatoid arthritis) relieve her early morning stiffness should be delegated to the AP?
   1. Assisting Ms. R to get in a bathtub full of warm water
   2. Sharing some relaxation techniques with Ms. R
   3. Assisting Ms. R to take a warm shower
   4. Evaluating the effectiveness of paraffin therapy

10. For Ms. R (rheumatoid arthritis), which discharge topic is the **most** important to emphasize to prevent a major postsurgical complication?
    1. Activity and movement limitations for the affected shoulder
    2. Continuation of pain medication as prescribed
    3. Possibility of repeat surgery for ongoing disease changes
    4. Expected postsurgical symptoms, such as localized pain

11. Based on the information that the nurse received during the hand-off report for Mr. L (kidney stone), which concept is the **priority** to consider in planning interventions for this patient?
    1. Elimination
    2. Pain
    3. Fluid balance
    4. Infection

12. The new nurse tells the team leader that she cannot find any documentation that shows the time of Mr. L's (kidney stone) last dose of pain medication. Which action would the team leader take **first**?
    1. Help the new nurse look at the chart and medication administration record.
    2. Tell the new nurse to ask the night nurse before she leaves.
    3. Speak to the night shift nurse about the documentation.
    4. Have the new nurse ask Mr. L when he last had medication.

13. Which tasks related to pain management can be delegated to the AP? **Select all that apply.**
    1. Reporting on grimacing seen in unresponsive patients
    2. Asking about the location, quality, and radiation of pain
    3. Reminding patients to report pain as necessary
    4. Observing for relief after medication is given
    5. Asking patients directly, "Are you having pain?"
    6. Determining if a position change relieves pain

PART 3 Complex Health Scenarios

    Answer Key for this chapter begins on p. 316

14. During the shift, the following events occur at the same time. Prioritize the order for addressing these problems.
    1. Mr. L is calling out loudly about right-sided flank pain caused by his kidney stone.
    2. Mr. O, who was in a motorcycle accident, is calling, "The pump tipped over, and it's broken."
    3. Another nurse needs opioid wastage witnessed.
    4. Mr. A, who has bacterial pneumonia, is urinating in the corner of his room.

    _____, _____, _____, _____

15. Mr. L (kidney stone) calls for pain medication. He describes the pain caused by his kidney stone as excruciating. He is crying, diaphoretic, and pacing around the room. What is the **priority** action?
    1. Instruct Mr. L to do deep breathing exercises.
    2. Remind Mr. L to use the PCA pump when he has pain.
    3. Give Mr. L an as needed (PRN) IV bolus dose as prescribed.
    4. Call the HCP immediately to report pain and other symptoms.

16. The team leader is preparing to give Mr. L (kidney stone) pain medication, but the IV site is infiltrated, so the nurse informs him that the IV catheter will have to be reinserted. He yells, "What's wrong with you people?! Can't you do anything right?!" Which response is **best**?
    1. "Let me call the HCP, and we can get you an oral pain medication."
    2. "This is not my fault, but if you will just give me a couple of minutes, I can fix it."
    3. "Let me call the nursing supervisor, and you can talk to her about the situation."
    4. "I know you are having pain. Let me restart your IV line right now."

17. Which nonpharmacologic intervention for pain management is the **most** appropriate for Mr. L (kidney stone)?
    1. Avoid overhydration or underhydration.
    2. Gently massage the lower back.
    3. Darken the room to encourage rest and sleep.
    4. Apply an ice pack to the kidney area.

18. Mr. L (kidney stone) reports that the pain has decreased compared with earlier, but now he is having other symptoms. Which symptom is of **greatest** concern?
    1. Painless hematuria with small clots
    2. Dull pain that radiates into the genitalia
    3. Absence of pain but scant urine output
    4. Sensation of urinary urgency

19. For Mr. O, in addition to pain medication, which action will help the **most** to relieve pain associated with the tibia–fibula fracture caused by his motorcycle accident?
    1. Instruct him to periodically move his toes.
    2. Use diversional therapy.
    3. Elevate the injured leg above the heart.
    4. Instruct him to maintain bed rest.

20. The nurse reinforces teaching about the purpose and correct use of the PCA with Mr. O (tibia–fibula fracture) and his mother. Both express an understanding and willingness to comply. When is the **best** time for Mr. O to activate the PCA to receive a dose of pain medication?
    1. Whenever pain is a 5 on a scale of 0 to 10, with 10 being the worst pain imaginable
    2. 30 minutes after waking up in the morning and 30 minutes before bedtime
    3. As soon as the lockout time expires; if pain is still present, even if it is mild
    4. 10 minutes before a painful procedure such as a dressing change or physical therapy

21. Mr. O (tibia–fibula fracture) is at risk for compartment syndrome because of the cast. Which pain assessment finding **most** strongly suggests compartment syndrome?
    1. Pain on passive motion
    2. Sudden increase in pain
    3. Intense itching sensation
    4. Absence of pain

22. Mr. O (tibia–fibula fracture) reports an increasing pain in the right abdomen. On physical examination, there are hyperactive bowel sounds, a tense abdomen with guarding, and exquisite tenderness with gentle palpation. Which action is the **priority**?
    1. Give a PRN pain medication.
    2. Notify the HCP of findings.
    3. Take a complete set of vital signs.
    4. Assist him to change positions.

23. Mr. H returns from the OR after a hernia repair. He says that he is "afraid to walk because it will make the pain really bad." Which option is **best**?
    1. Pain medication every 4 hours if he needs or wants it
    2. Medication 30 to 40 minutes before ambulation or dressing changes
    3. Around-the-clock pain medication even if he has no report of pain
    4. Talking to the HCP for reassurance about the treatment plan

24. Mr. H (hernia repair) says, "I have several friends who became addicted to drugs, and it totally ruined their lives. I'm afraid to take any kind of addictive drugs." Which response is **best**?
    1. "Your HCP prescribes types of opioids that do not cause addiction."
    2. "You will be given opioids for a very short time, and addiction is unlikely."
    3. "Your friends probably had addictive personalities; you don't need to worry."
    4. "If you become addicted, the HCP will refer you to a drug rehabilitation program."

25. Mr. H (hernia repair) is asking for pain medication, and the HCP has ordered 10 mg of immediate-release oxycodone as needed. The pharmacy has stocked 5-mg tablets of controlled-release oxycodone in the medication cabinet. Which action is the **priority**?
    1. Call the HCP for clarification of the original prescription.
    2. Call the pharmacy and obtain the immediate-release form of the drug.
    3. Ask the patient if the immediate- or controlled-release action is preferred.
    4. Give two of the 5-mg tablets to achieve the correct dose.

26. Mr. H is given a dose of pain medication. One hour later, he is anxious and appears uncomfortable, and he asks, "What's the matter? Is something wrong? I'm still hurting." Which action should be taken **first**?
    1. Call the HCP for a change in medication or dose.
    2. Initiate NPO in case surgery is needed.
    3. Check for bladder distention and last voiding.
    4. Reassure the patient that the hernia is not recurring.

27. Ms. J (end-stage multiple myeloma) is receiving opiates to control her pain. Which side effect is the **major** concern for this patient?
    1. Constipation
    2. Respiratory depression
    3. Nausea and vomiting
    4. Sedation

28. After reviewing Ms. J's (end-stage multiple myeloma) medication list, the nurse is **most** likely to question scheduled doses of which medication?
    1. Naltrexone
    2. Fentanyl
    3. Morphine
    4. Acetaminophen

29. Ms. J (end-stage multiple myeloma) is having severe pain and admits to it; however, she becomes very anxious when certain family members come and go and refuses to take the pain medication. Which adjunct medication would be **most** useful to Ms. J to help her manage these episodes?
    1. Naproxen
    2. Doxepin
    3. Lorazepam
    4. Dicyclomine

30. Ms. J's (end-stage multiple myeloma) son tells the nurse, "My mom is having trouble breathing, and she is having a lot of pain!" On assessment, Ms. J demonstrates rapid shallow breathing and reports pain over the right lateral ribs that increases with movement and breathing. Which action is the **priority**?
    1. Take vital signs with pulse oximeter reading and inform the HCP.
    2. Apply oxygen and raise the head of the bed if patient is not hypotensive.
    3. Obtain an order to start an IV and to give a bolus dose of morphine.
    4. Be calm, stay with the patient, and encourage pursed-lip breathing.

31. Ms. J's (end-stage multiple myeloma) son repeatedly insists that Ms. J is not getting enough pain medication. He threatens to sue. The team leader has used therapeutic communication skills with the son and advocated for the patient with the HCP. The HCP says, "I'll be in tomorrow. Just tell the son not to worry." Which action is **best**?
    1. Call another HCP.
    2. Continue to use the current orders.
    3. Advise the son to call the HCP.
    4. Notify the unit manager.

32. The AP reports that the new nurse is undermedicating the patients. What is the **best** way for the team leader to handle this situation?
    1. Ignore her; the AP is not qualified to judge an RN.
    2. Ask the AP to give specific examples.
    3. Go to the new nurse and question her.
    4. Do an assessment on all of the nurse's patients.

33. One of the staff members is talking about Mr. A, who has bacterial pneumonia, saying, "He complains all the time about pain everywhere. Well, he is going to have pain. He's a drug addict, so what does he expect?" Which response is **best**?
    1. "All patients have a right to care regardless of race or creed."
    2. "I'll take Mr. A; I don't mind taking care of him."
    3. "You should think about how he really feels."
    4. "What can we do to help Mr. A cope with his pain?"

Answer Key for this chapter begins on p. 316

PART 3

Complex Health Scenarios

34. Which tasks related to Mr. A's (bacterial pneumonia) pain management can be delegated to the AP? **Select all that apply.**
    1. Clean the transcutaneous electrical nerve stimulation (TENS) unit.
    2. Notify the nurse about the patient's request for pain medication.
    3. Reinforce the use of a pillow to splint when coughing.
    4. Observe for actions that increase fatigue or anxiety.
    5. Suggest that relatives bring personal comfort items.
    6. Assist the patient to change position every 2 hours.

35. Mr. A (bacterial pneumonia) has a single-lumen peripherally inserted central catheter. The following scheduled medications and IV solutions need to be given now: vancomycin 1.5 g in 250 mL of 5% dextrose over 90 minutes, levofloxacin 750 mg in 150 mL of normal saline over 90 minutes, 5% dextrose and 0.45% saline 1000 mL with 20 mEq (20 mmol) of potassium at 125 mL/hr, and an IV bolus dose of morphine 3 mg. Which action is the **priority**?
    1. Call the HCP and ask if the medication times can be staggered.
    2. Call the pharmacy and inquire about the compatibility of medications and solutions.
    3. Give the bolus dose of morphine because it will take the least amount of time.
    4. Obtain an order to establish an additional peripheral IV site.

36. Mr. A (bacterial pneumonia) reports left-sided anterior chest pain. Which action is the **priority**?
    1. Obtain an order for an electrocardiogram and continuous telemetry monitoring.
    2. Auscultate the lung fields and compare with baseline assessments.
    3. Give a PRN pain medication and reevaluate after 30 minutes.
    4. Ask him to describe the pain and measure all vital signs.

37. Mr. A (bacterial pneumonia) reports, "The chest pain is gone now, but my back really hurts a lot. I need more morphine." Based on the ethical principle of nonmaleficence, which nursing action is the **priority**?
    1. Believe Mr. A's subjective report of pain and give morphine as ordered.
    2. Contact the HCP for an increase in dosage because Mr. A appears to need a higher dose.
    3. Consider the patient's history of addiction and chronic pain, respiratory status, and time of last dose.
    4. Offer nonpharmaceutical measures, such as a position change or distraction.

38. Enhanced Hot Spot _____

Scenario: Mr. A had an opioid overdose 3 years ago. A psychiatrist who managed Mr. A's care after that occurrence sends a document that includes the following history.

Instructions: Underline or highlight factors that increase the patient's risk for future opioid overdose.

Mr. A is a 52-year-old male who was admitted to the acute care psychiatric facility after an overdose of opioid medication. He reports chronic back pain that has persisted for several years after a work-related injury. After the injury, he experienced relief for the acute pain with the prescribed opioid medication. However, he needed continuously larger doses for the chronic pain. This caused him to seek prescriptions from multiple providers and pharmacies and resulted in access to several types of opioid and non-opioid medications. He reports trying nonsteroidal anti-inflammatory drugs (NSAIDs), tramadol, and exercise with some relief, but prefers hydromorphone, "when I can get it." He takes PRN lorazfor anxiety. He denies suicidal intent related to the opioid overdose but does admit to depression. Data from the prescription drug monitoring program indicate that he has received extended-release hydrocodone at doses higher than 90 mme/day.

Based on recently published recommendations from the Center for Disease Control and Prevention for prescribing opioids for chronic pain (excluding active cancer treatment, palliative care, and end-of-life care), which factors place Mr. A at risk for future opioid overdose?

39. It is the end of the shift, and the new nurse is trying to give pain medication to one patient, provide comfort measures for another patient, and redo pain assessments on all of her patients. Her documentation is incomplete. What should the team leader do?
    1. Offer to help her by performing the comfort measures.
    2. Let her struggle through so she can find her own way.
    3. Help her to prioritize and delegate the tasks.
    4. Ask someone from the oncoming shift to help her.

40. At the end of the shift, the opioid count shows that two tablets of oxycodone are unaccounted for. The team leader has spoken to all of the nurses and pharmacists who had access to the medication cabinet during the shift, but no one will admit to removing those two tablets. What should the team leader do? **Select all that apply.**
    1. Inform the staff that no one can leave until the matter is resolved.
    2. Fill out an incident report and include facts about findings and actions.
    3. Interview all of the patients who have orders for oxycodone.
    4. Discuss the matter with the unit manager and review potential problems with the current system.
    5. Review available records of access and medication retrieval for the past 24 hours.
    6. Ask the staff if they saw any other people (e.g., students, HCPs, instructors) who may have accessed the cabinet during the shift.

41. Enhanced Multiple Response _____

Scenario: At the end of the shift, the team leader must ensure that patient needs are met, unit tasks (e.g., restocking, cleaning) are completed and the hand-off report must be prepared to include pertinent data. Some tasks must be performed by the nurses and other tasks can be delegated to AP.

Which end-of-shift tasks can be delegated to the AP?

Instructions: Place an X, in the space provided, or highlight each task that can be delegated to the AP. Select all that apply.
Which end-of-shift tasks can be delegated to the AP? **Select all that apply.**

1. _____ Emptying Ms. J's trash can and placing personal items within reach
2. _____ Checking Mr. A's linens for moisture and soiling and changing as needed
3. _____ Asking Mr. L if he needs a dose of pain medication before shift change
4. _____ Assisting Ms. R to change position in bed to relieve pressure on the joints
5. _____ Ensuring Mr. O's leg is elevated and evaluating comfort
6. _____ Emptying Mr. A's urinal and recording the output
7. _____ Taking a pulse oximeter reading on Mr. A and evaluating respiratory status
8. _____ Restocking the linen cart and tidying up the dirty utility room.
9. _____ Restocking floor stock medications and IV solutions
10. _____ Making sure that soiled linen receptacles have clean bags
11. _____ Organizing patient data for the hand-off report

42. Drag and Drop _____

Scenario: The team leader is giving the end-of-shift report about Ms. R (rheumatoid arthritis) to the oncoming nurse. The team leader knows that an effective report is organized, clear and concise.

What is the order of the information that the nurse will report about Ms. R to the oncoming nurse?

Instructions: In the left column is information that would be included in the report about Ms. R. In the right column write the number to indicate the order of the information, 1 being the first thing to report and 7 being the last.

Information about Ms. R to give to the oncoming nurse.	Order of information
a. "She had shoulder pain (4 of 10) and was reluctant to move around."	
b. "Do you have any questions for me?"	
c. "Ms. R is a 55-year-old woman."	
d. "She had shoulder arthroplasty 3 days ago."	
e. "She received a PRN dose of acetaminophen with codeine, and her pain is now a 1 of 10."	
f. "The physical therapist must speak to Ms. R's daughter, so page him when she arrives."	
g. Discharge teaching was initiated; activity and movement limitations for the shoulder joint should be reinforced.	

 Answer Key for this chapter begins on p. 316

PART 3   Complex Health Scenarios

Answers

1. **Ans: 6, 3, 2, 1, 5, 4** Mr. A's respiratory status (i.e., rate, rhythm, and pulse oximetry reading) should be quickly checked. Mr. O should be checked for shock symptoms, mental status changes, and escalating pain. Mr. L and Ms. R are both in relatively stable condition but need quick pain assessments and reassurance that their needs will be met. Ms. J and her family should be approached last because they need time and patience, and caregivers should not appear rushed. Mr. H is currently in the OR. **Focus:** Prioritization.

2. **Ans: 2** Mr. A has complex problems, but the key points given in the report are the medical diagnosis of pneumonia and the oxygen desaturation during the evening. Also recall that HIV creates a greater risk for sepsis or septic shock. **Focus:** Prioritization.

3. **Ans: 4** The practice of PCA by proxy is not recommended because of the increased risk for oversedation and respiratory depression. The team leader would first talk to the night nurse to remind or educate about the possible dangers. The team leader might also suggest that the night nurse talk to the clinical educator or review the latest literature about PCA usage. It is possible that the night nurse may have seen this practice in a case when the patient was physically incapable of self-administration of PCA and therefore AACA (authorized agent–controlled analgesia) was used, but AACA has strict criteria and the authorized agent must be trained. The team leader would then review the PCA procedure with the mother and emphasize the risks of PCA by proxy. **Focus:** Supervision, Prioritization.

4. **Ans: 1, 2, 4** Ms. R and Mr. L have conditions that require pain medication but are less physiologically complex. Mr. H will be out of surgery later in the shift, but hernia repairs are routine and reasonably predictable; this is a good postoperative case for a new RN. Mr. O will require careful assessment for slowly developing complications such as hemorrhage or peritonitis. Ms. J and her family will need support through anticipated grief and loss and complex decision making for hospice and end-of-life issues. Mr. A's respiratory status must be carefully monitored, and he has complex pain and care issues. **Focus:** Assignment. **Test-Taking Tip:** When considering assignments for new nurses, float nurses, or others who have less experience, the charge nurse would consider the priority concepts that affect patient care. For example, patients with problems with gas exchange or perfusion need closer monitoring. An increased number of concepts also increases the complexity of the care. Patients, such as Ms. J, who have physical pain, breathing problems, and end-of-life issues are best served by experienced nurses.

5. **Ans: 1, 2, 3, 5** Helping with hygienic care and reinforcing instructions that have been explained by the RN are within the scope of practice of the AP. Mr. H should not need any specialized equipment, so the AP can prepare the bed and gather routine equipment, such as devices for measuring vital signs. The AP can get coffee. (Note to student: The nurse may encourage Ms. J's family to take occasional breaks off the floor. Also, sending one of the family members to get things is a way for them to have an active role.) Mr. O's skin care and assessment should be performed by the RN; the problem is extensive, and pain medication may need to be titrated. A nurse should assess Mr. A because his oxygen saturation was decreasing during the night. Decreasing oxygen saturation is a red flag that can indicate actual or impending respiratory failure. In addition, Mr. A is immunocompromised, so he is at risk for sepsis and septic shock. Also, a pulse oximeter is only a tool; many factors can cause inaccurate readings (e.g., cold room temperature, a tight sleeve, position of the sensor); therefore the nurse should check Mr. A's pulse oximeter reading and concurrently assess his respiratory status. **Focus:** Delegation. **Test-Taking Tip:** Analyze the overall intent of the question and the information that is provided. The nurse often delegates performing the pulse oximeter readings to the AP; however, when the patient is critically ill or unstable, the nurse must concurrently check and evaluate vital signs and perform complex assessments.

6. **Ans: 2** Ms. R is having incident pain, which is triggered or related to the movement of the arms and shoulders. Ms. J is having end-of dose failure. Transdermal fentanyl is expected to provide pain relief for 72 hours. Mr. A is describing referred pain; the origin of his pain is in the back and it moves down the leg. Mr. O is describing breakthrough pain. The PCA is generally giving good coverage, but he is experiencing short episodes of pain. **Focus:** Prioritization.

7. **Ans: 4** Acknowledge loss and encourage the patient to talk about the past. During this discussion, the nurse and the patient might find activities that could be adapted to her current situation. Try to avoid giving false reassurance, changing the subject, or switching the focus from the patient's needs to the nurse's concerns. **Focus:** Prioritization.

8. **Ans: 2** The occupational therapist can review the goals, progression, limitations, and overcoming of barriers associated with performing the exercises. If the patient's reluctance continues, other members of the health care team may be consulted as needed. **Focus:** Prioritization.

9. **Ans: 3**   The shower is preferred because patients with arthritis can have trouble getting in and out of a bathtub. An RN should suggest relaxation techniques and evaluate outcomes of therapies. **Focus:** Delegation.

10. **Ans: 1**   The shoulder joint is complex and has many articulation surfaces; therefore partial or complete dislocation is a major potential complication. Excessive force or movement could cause dislocation. **Focus:** Prioritization.

11. **Ans: 2**   Patients with kidney stones usually present to the health care facility because of severe excruciating pain. The pain usually occurs as the stone moves down the ureter. This is not a life-threatening condition, but patients can be in agony. If the patient cannot void, the stone may be lodged; this also causes pain. If the patient cannot pass urine for a prolonged period, then elimination would become the priority concept because of potential damage to the kidneys and inability to eliminate toxic substances. **Focus:** Prioritization.

12. **Ans: 2**   Encourage staff members to deal directly with each other to define and resolve problems. If staff cannot resolve the problem among themselves or if the issue is a chronic problem, then the charge nurse or unit manager should intervene. Helping the new nurse to look at the chart should not be necessary at this point. Asking the patient does not address the problem of the missing documentation. Potentially, the new nurse could look at the PCA pump for a record of self-administered medication, but the machine does not replace good communication among staff members. In addition, the patient's response must be documented even though he is self-administering the medication. **Focus:** Prioritization, Supervision.

13. **Ans: 1, 3, 5**   Because communication is limited in unresponsive patients, all staff members should be watchful for signs. The RN should instruct the AP about specific signs to watch for. Reminding patients that staff are available to help relieve pain is appropriate. If the AP suspects pain, asking the patient a direct "yes-or-no" question is appropriate; then the nurse can be notified. Assessing pain and evaluating outcomes are the responsibilities of the RN. (Note to student: Even if the patient says to the AP, "The position change helps to relieve my pain," the nurse should still follow up and do a pain assessment.) **Focus:** Delegation.

14. **Ans: 2, 1, 4, 3**   It is unlikely that Mr. O's pump will deliver excess medication; however, it is appropriate to discontinue the pump until its functioning can be completely checked. Nevertheless, do not forget to go back soon after and troubleshoot the problem with the pump. Mr. L is probably having ongoing pain issues, but loud calls for assistance must be investigated. Mr. A must be assessed for mental status changes related to hypoxia or encephalopathy. In addition, he needs help to clean up, to get back in bed, and to reposition

the oxygen cannula. The other nurse could ask someone else to witness if necessary. **Focus:** Prioritization.

15. **Ans: 3**   Mr. L is having an exacerbation of pain that is probably related to the movement of the kidney stone. This type of pain is severe but usually transient. If the bolus dose is inadequate, the HCP could be notified for a dosage increase. Deep breathing may help somewhat, but the patient will have trouble focusing. Reminding him to use the PCA pump is not necessary at this point. **Focus:** Prioritization.

16. **Ans: 4**   Use a matter-of-fact tone of voice to acknowledge his underlying problem (pain). Restarting the IV line addresses the immediate issue. Contacting the HCP for oral medications might be considered if no one is able to restart the IV line. Calling the supervisor is a possibility if the patient continues to complain and wants to make a report. Defensive statements such as "It's not my fault" can make the situation worse. **Focus:** Prioritization.

17. **Ans: 1**   Balancing fluids is the best strategy; this makes passage of the stone less painful. **Focus:** Prioritization.

18. **Ans: 3**   Scant output suggests that the stone is lodged and obstructing the outflow of urine. This can result in damage to the kidney. Hematuria with or without pain can occur because the stone has irritated the tissue. Dull pain that radiates into the genitalia and urgency are common with kidney stones. **Focus:** Prioritization. **Test-Taking Tip:** Decreased urine output should always be investigated as a signal of possible dysfunction (in this case, obstruction). Decreased output can also be related to decreased perfusion, which will eventually cause renal failure.

19. **Ans: 3**   Elevating the injured extremity will minimize the swelling. If the leg swells, there is additional pressure on nerves. Moving the toes helps, but Mr. O cannot consistently comply when he is sleeping or fatigued. Diversion therapy is less useful in the acute phase of injury and treatment. The patient does not need to maintain bedrest; however, prolonged activity with the leg in a dependent position would increase swelling and discomfort. **Focus:** Prioritization.

20. **Ans: 4**   Patients are taught to activate the PCA about 10 minutes before painful procedures because this is the approximate time that it takes for the IV morphine to work. Activating the PCA for pain at a level 5 out of 10 may be suitable for some patients, but this level of pain would be excessive for others. Although lockout time should be explained, the nurse should not encourage the patient to focus on it or to take doses based on expiration of lockout time. **Focus:** Prioritization.

21. **Ans: 1**   Pain on passive motion is a sign of possible compartment syndrome. A sudden increase in pain is more associated with arterial obstruction. Itching is a

PART 3   Complex Health Scenarios

frequent problem associated with a cast that can be relieved by blowing cool air under the cast. Absence of pain without medication could be related to maintaining elevation, ice application, and rest. **Focus:** Prioritization.

22. **Ans: 3** Measure vital signs first and then report the findings to the HCP. Mr. O is at risk for occult abdominal trauma, and the findings represent a change of status and could be signs of internal bleeding. **Focus:** Prioritization. **Test-Taking Tip:** Assessment is the first step of the nursing process. In addition, when the nurse calls the HCP, one of the essential parts of the SBAR (situation, background, assessment, recommendation) report is assessment, which always includes vital signs.

23. **Ans: 2** Mr. H is anticipating that the pain is going to be worsened by activity. Giving oral pain medication 30 to 40 minutes before the activity assures him that the pain will be minimized. The second-best option is to reassure him that medication is available if he needs it. Around-the-clock medication and notification of the HCP are not necessary at this point. **Focus:** Prioritization.

24. **Ans: 2** Short-term use of opioids for medical purposes is unlikely to cause any problems. Physical dependency occurs when opioids are abruptly stopped and physical symptoms occur; if dependency does occur, patients can be gradually tapered off opioids. Physical dependency is not the same as addiction. Although there is a small percentage of the population who are prone to addictive behaviors, the majority of patients stop taking opioids when the pain is gone, and there is no addiction. **Focus:** Prioritization.

25. **Ans: 2** Obtain and administer the medication in the dosage and form in which it was prescribed. The nurse can call the HCP if the prescription is not clearly written or if the nurse is trying to get the prescription changed (e.g., the pharmacy does not have the medication). Asking about a preference for immediate- versus controlled-release action is an inappropriate way to phrase the question to the patient. **Focus:** Prioritization. **Test-Taking Tip:** Don't forget to review your fundamentals textbook. Material about medication administration is usually covered in the first semester of the nursing program.

26. **Ans: 3** Mr. H may be experiencing urinary retention because of bladder atony related to the surgical procedure. A distended bladder can mimic hernia pain and cause significant discomfort, and Mr. H may not have the urge to void. Calling the HCP and initiating NPO are premature at this point. Reassurance may be somewhat comforting but does not address the immediate symptom. **Focus:** Prioritization.

27. **Ans: 1** A patient such as Ms. J has taken opiates for a long time. Constipation is the only opioid side effect to which the patient does not develop tolerance. Respiratory depression, nausea, vomiting, and sedation may have occurred when Ms. J was first receiving opioids but are now less of a concern. **Focus:** Prioritization.

28. **Ans: 1** Naltrexone is an opioid antagonist, which would cause opioid withdrawal and result in causing the patient significant pain. It is given if patients have significant respiratory depression caused by opioids. **Focus:** Prioritization.

29. **Ans: 3** Lorazepam is an anxiolytic. Naproxen is a nonsteroidal anti-inflammatory drug. Doxepin is used for depression or neuropathic pain. Dicyclomine is given to reduce smooth muscle spasms. **Focus:** Prioritization.

30. **Ans: 2** The patient needs immediate intervention for relief of dyspnea. Oxygen and elevating the head of the bed are quick actions that the nurse should take immediately. If the patient is hypotensive, there is a possibility of fainting; however, dyspnea usually increases blood pressure because the patient will panic, fight for air, and struggle to sit upright. PRN oral morphine is typically prescribed for hospice patients and those who need end-of-life care. **Focus:** Prioritization.

31. **Ans: 4** Communication skills are important in dealing with the family and the HCP. If the nurse has exhausted this route, the next step is to move up the chain of command. Another HCP is unlikely to get involved, unless he/she is a supervisor of the provider (i.e., nurse practitioners and physician assistants can prescribe, but are supervised by a physician). The nurse should use interdisciplinary collaboration to problem solve rather than shifting the responsibility to the son. The nurse must function under the current prescriptions and use additional nonpharmacologic measures until the issue is resolved. **Focus:** Prioritization.

32. **Ans: 2** Specific examples are more useful than vague generalizations. There may be extenuating circumstances that the AP is misinterpreting. The team leader may decide to talk to the new nurse about the specific circumstances or to assess the patients. Comments about patient care issues should not be ignored; all team members should be encouraged to watch out for the health and safety of patients. **Focus:** Prioritization, Supervision.

33. **Ans: 4** Mr. A has complex needs. Although the staff gets tired of hearing continual complaints, everyone should work together to try to solve the problem. Reminding staff that patients have a right to care is rhetorical and not very useful. Offering to care for Mr. A every day does not help the team to overcome bias or improve patient care. When feedback is given, statements that begin with "You should" should be avoided. **Focus:** Prioritization, Supervision.

34. **Ans: 2, 3, 6** The AP is qualified to help with routine position changes and can reinforce instructions given by the RN. The AP should report a patient's

requests to the nurse. The physical therapist should be consulted about handling the TENS equipment. An RN should assess for fatigue and anxiety. Personal comfort items are permissible, but belongings can get misplaced and the nurse should take responsibility to have this discussion with the family and patient. **Focus:** Delegation.

35. **Ans: 2** First call the pharmacy and ask about compatibilities. If the solutions and medications are compatible, they can be given simultaneously. If there are incompatibilities, the nurse may decide to give the morphine first because this can be administered quickly and will give the patient immediate relief. Then the nurse can call the HCP for a prescription to stagger medication times or to establish a second IV site. (Note to student: Some facilities allow the nurse to independently change medication times or to start a second peripheral IV; however, these interventions generally require a HCP's prescription. Follow policy and procedure manuals and ask charge nurse or supervisor for guidance.) **Focus:** Prioritization.

36. **Ans: 4** Conduct an additional pain assessment with vital sign measurements. This will determine what interventions are needed. **Focus:** Prioritization.

37. **Ans: 3** To exercise nonmaleficence, the nurse must prevent harm to the patient. Mr. A has an extremely complex situation, and the nurse must use clinical judgment and consider multiple factors before offering additional morphine. The nurse recalls that Mr. A was desaturating during the night; therefore respiratory status is the biggest concern. The nurse would not withhold medication because of a history of addiction. Because of addiction, Mr. A is likely to need higher doses to achieve relief. The nurse would review the time of last dose and efficacy of nonpharmaceutical options. Opioids are not typically first-line drugs for chronic back pain; other medication and treatment options are available. **Focus:** Prioritization.

38. **Ans:** Mr. A is a 52-year-old male who was admitted to the acute care psychiatric facility after an **overdose of opioid medication.** He reports chronic back pain that has persisted for several years following a work-related injury. After the injury, he experienced relief for the acute pain with the prescribed opioid medication. However, he needed **continuously larger doses for the chronic pain.** This caused him to seek prescriptions from **multiple providers and pharmacies** and resulted in **access to several types of opioid** and non-opioid medications. He reports trying NSAIDS, tramadol, and exercise with some relief, but prefers **hydromorphone,** "when I can get it." He takes prn **lorazepam for anxiety.** He denies suicidal intent related to the **opioid overdose** but does admit to **depression.** Data from the prescription drug monitoring program indicates that he has received **extended release hydrocodone at doses higher than 90 mme/day.**

Risk factors for opioid overdose and opioid abuse include: chronic pain that is being treated with progressively higher doses of opioids; multiple providers and pharmacies; access to combinations of opioids; potent opioids (hydromorphone), extended release formulations and high doses (greater than 90 mme/day); concurrent use of benzodiazepines (lorazepam); and comorbidities of anxiety and depression. A previous overdose increases the risk for future overdose. **Focus:** Prioritization.

39. **Ans: 3** Help the nurse to prioritize what has to be done and help her recognize what can and cannot be delegated. Offering help is appropriate if patient safety is compromised, and it does contribute to team building; however, it does not help her learn to organize her work. Letting her struggle is one method of learning, but new nurses deserve guidance and support. Help her to determine what tasks can be passed on to the next shift, and then she can discuss this during the shift report. **Focus:** Prioritization Supervision.

40. **Ans: 2, 4, 5, 6** Electronic units are usually very effective in assisting the staff to keep track of dispensed doses; however, users must enter correct data, and most systems have "workarounds" that negate safety measures. Try to gather as much information as possible and discuss the problem with the unit manager. This could be a case of theft, but it may also be a system error that needs to be corrected. It is not appropriate to draw patients into this problem and forcing everyone to stay is pointless if all staff members have already been interviewed. **Focus:** Supervision, Prioritization.

41. **Ans: 1, 2, 4, 6, 8, 10** Emptying the trash; assisting patients with personal items, changing linens, and recording urine as output; restocking linens; tidying the utility room; and making sure that linen receptacles are ready for the next shift are within the scope of duties for the AP. Helping patients such as Ms. R change position in bed is also appropriate. (There may be times when the nurse should change the patient's position if assessments of the skin or mobility are needed.) The nurse should assess Mr. L's back pain and need for additional medication. Mr. O's leg must be assessed by the nurse for perfusion; merely looking to see if the leg is elevated is insufficient. The nurse should assess Mr. A's respiratory status (recall that he had episodes of desaturation). The pharmacist is usually responsible for stocking floor medications and IV solutions. It is the nurse's responsibility to organize patient data for the hand-off report. **Focus:** Delegation.

42. **Ans: 1c, 2d, 3a, 4e, 5g, 6f, 7b** The report should be succinct and organized so that the listener will have a clear idea of who is involved, what the major issues are, what measures were done to address the issues, and what requires follow-up. The listener also needs the opportunity to clarify what has been said. This will increase mutual understanding. **Focus:** Prioritization.

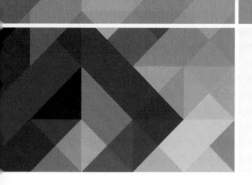

CASE STUDY 11

Multiple Patients With Cancer

Questions

The RN is the leader of a team caring for patients on a medical-surgical oncology unit. In addition to the leader, the team includes an experienced chemotherapy-certified RN, a new assistive personnel (AP), and a first-semester nursing student. The morning hand-off report includes the following information: (Note to student: This case study includes six patients; take notes as though you were listening to the morning report and refer to your notes as you work through the case study.)

- Mr. N, a 68-year-old man, went to see his health care provider (HCP) with fever, weight loss, and painless axillary nodes. After a lymph node biopsy, non-Hodgkin lymphoma was diagnosed. He is receiving chemotherapy and is on neutropenic precautions. He is currently afebrile, in good spirits, and feels reasonably well.
- Mr. L, a 50-year-old man, was transferred 6 days ago from the surgical intensive care unit (ICU) after a tracheostomy and partial laryngectomy. He has a soft, small-bore nasogastric (NG) tube and a tracheostomy tube and is currently receiving chemotherapy. He received radiation therapy before surgery.
- Mr. B, a 59-year-old man, went to his HCP with painless hematuria, and bladder cancer was subsequently diagnosed. He was admitted for intravesical chemotherapy. He received procedure-related teaching before admission. He is alert and conversant, and he independently performs activities of daily living (ADLs).
- Ms. C, a 70-year-old woman, went to her HCP because of rectal bleeding and a change in bowel habits. She underwent a bowel resection and colostomy 5 days ago. She is progressing well but needs and likes companionship at the bedside.
- Ms. G, a 65-year-old woman, was admitted for a right breast lumpectomy; it is scheduled for later in the day. Radiation therapy is planned as part of the follow-up treatment. She appears nervous and tearful and is frequently asking questions.
- Mr. U, a 62-year-old man, has a history of cough, hemoptysis, fatigue, and dyspnea. After bronchoscopy and sputum cytologic analysis, non–small cell lung cancer was diagnosed. He underwent pulmonary resection 5 days

ago and has a chest tube drainage system. He is having significant and continuous pain. A patient-controlled analgesia (PCA) pump is being considered, but Mr. U expresses reluctance to use it.

1. Which **two** patients are the **most** critical and likely to require frequent assessment and skilled care throughout the shift? **Select two.**
   1. Mr. N (non-Hodgkin lymphoma)
   2. Mr. L (tracheostomy and partial laryngectomy)
   3. Mr. B (bladder cancer)
   4. Ms. C (bowel resection and colostomy)
   5. Ms. G (breast lumpectomy)
   6. Mr. U (pulmonary resection)

2. The team leader makes very brief rounds to see each patient before receiving the shift report to ensure patient safety and to help determine acuity and assignments. Which actions will these brief assessments entail? **Select all that apply.**
   1. Asking, "How are you feeling?"
   2. Noting mental status (alert and oriented?)
   3. Measuring vital signs and looking at intake and output
   4. Palpating chest and abdominal areas for pain
   5. Noting the presence and complexity of equipment
   6. Observing ease of respiratory effort

3. The first-semester nursing student tells the team leader that her clinical assignment for the day is to take vital signs and obtain a patient history that will take about 1 or 2 hours to complete. Which patients would the leader recommend that she approach to fulfill her assignment? **Select all that apply.**
   1. Mr. N (non-Hodgkin lymphoma)
   2. Mr. L (tracheostomy and partial laryngectomy)
   3. Mr. B (bladder cancer)
   4. Ms. C (bowel resection and colostomy)
   5. Ms. G (breast lumpectomy)
   6. Mr. U (pulmonary resection)

4. The team leader must assign an AP to help care for Mr. N with non-Hodgkin lymphoma. For this neutropenic patient, which factor is **most** important in making this assignment?
   1. AP is in the first trimester of pregnancy.
   2. AP has had cold symptoms for 3 days.
   3. AP has no experience with neutropenic precautions.
   4. AP has a generalized fear of isolation patients.

5. The nursing student tearfully reports to the leader, "I took some flowers into Mr. N's (non-Hodgkin lymphoma) room to cheer him up, and he told me that he didn't think he was supposed to have flowers. I took them out of the room right away, and then I realized I had made a mistake." What should the team leader do **first**?
   1. Direct the student to read the isolation precautions before entering the room.
   2. Call the nursing instructor and report the student for making an error.
   3. Acknowledge and praise the student for taking responsibility for the mistake.
   4. Write an incident report and have the student and instructor sign it.

6. The team leader is reviewing what the HCP has just prescribed for Mr. N (non-Hodgkin lymphoma). Which order will the team leader question?
   1. Administer filgrastim 5 mcg/kg subcutaneously every day.
   2. Catheterize to obtain a urinalysis specimen.
   3. Flush the IV saline lock every shift.
   4. Monitor vital signs every 4 hours.

7. Mr. N (non-Hodgkin lymphoma) shyly asks, "Do doctors have a special way that they wash their hands? Everybody washes their hands and then rewashes their hands before they touch me or any of my personal items. Everybody—except that one doctor." What is the team leader's **priority** action? the team leader's **priority** action?
   1. Reassure the patient that the HCP probably washed his hands just before entering the room.
   2. Tell the patient that the staff 's actions to protect against infection are based on the latest laboratory results.

   3. Contact the infection control person because the HCP probably needs a review of infection control procedures.
   4. Approach the HCP and explain what the patient noticed and the patient's concerns about the hand washing.

8. The nurse is reviewing Mr. N's (non-Hodgkin lymphoma) medication administration record and sees that the combination therapy aprepitant, dexamethasone, and ondansetron was administered during the last shift. What is the nurse **most** likely to ask to determine the efficacy of the therapy?
   1. "On a scale of 1 to 10, with 1 being the least and 10 being the worst, what number is your pain? Where is the pain located?"
   2. "Have the medications improved your appetite? Are there special foods that you would prefer?"
   3. "Are you having any feelings of nausea right now? When was the last time you vomited?"
   4. "After taking the medications, have you experienced any improvement in your energy level? Do you feel fatigued?"

9. Mr. N (non-Hodgkin lymphoma) reports noticing some transient numbness and tingling in his lower legs with occasional mild burning type pain. What is the nurse most likely to do **first**?
   1. Assess for signs and symptoms of venous thromboembolism.
   2. Check for signs and symptoms of peripheral arterial insufficiency.
   3. Ask the patient to ambulate to stimulate muscles and circulation.
   4. Assess for possible chemotherapy-induced peripheral neuropathy.

Answer Key for this chapter begins on p. 326

10. Enhanced Multiple Response _____

Scenario: The team leader-initiated discharge teaching with Mr. N. The teaching topics are signs and symptoms of infection and what should be reported to the HCP.

Which signs and symptoms would warrant calling the HCP right away?

Instructions: Place an X, in the space provided, or highlight each sign or symptom of infection that warrants calling the HCP. **Select all that apply.**
1. _____ One-time temperature of 99.4°F (37.4°C)
2. _____ Chills and sweats
3. _____ Sore throat
4. _____ Nasal congestion
5. _____ Diarrhea
6. _____ Vomiting
7. _____ Flatulence
8. _____ Burning with urination
9. _____ Stiff neck
10. _____ Insomnia
11. _____ New onset pain
12. _____ Changes in mental status

11. In the early postoperative period, what is the **priority** concern for Mr. L, who has a tracheostomy and partial laryngectomy?
1. Possible infection related to chemotherapy and surgical procedure
2. Poor nutritional intake related to dysphagia and malignancy
3. Difficulty communicating needs because of the tracheostomy tube
4. High risk for aspiration because of secretions and removal of epiglottis

12. Which assessment finding for Mr. L (tracheostomy and partial laryngectomy) would be of **greatest** concern?
1. Pulsation of the tracheostomy tube in synchrony with the heartbeat
2. Increased secretions in and around the tracheostomy
3. Increased coughing, with difficulty in expectorating secretions
4. Presence of food particles in tracheal secretions

13. The team leader is teaching the nursing student about the emergency respiratory equipment that should be available for Mr. L (tracheostomy and partial laryngectomy). Which piece of equipment is the **most** important to show to the student?
1. Adult-sized endotracheal tube
2. Laryngeal scope with blades of several sizes
3. Bag-valve mask with extension tubing
4. Tracheostomy insertion tray

14. Mr. L (tracheostomy and partial laryngectomy) needs to receive a dose of IV chemotherapy during the shift. What is the **most** important action to take to prevent extravasation?
1. Carefully monitor the access site during the administration of the medication.

2. Hold the medication until an implanted port or central line is established.
3. Ensure that a chemotherapy-certified nurse is assigned to care for the patient.
4. Call the pharmacy to find out if the prescribed medication has vesicant properties.

15. Mr. L (tracheostomy and partial laryngectomy) has been receiving 10 mg of IV morphine for pain. The HCP tells the nurse that Mr. L will be switched to oral (liquid) hydromorphone 5 mg. When the nurse checks an equianalgesic dose table, she sees that 10 mg of morphine equals 7.5 mg of hydromorphone. What would the nurse do?
1. Call the pharmacy to double-check that the equianalgesic dose is actually 7.5 mg.
2. Recognize that cross-tolerance is variable and titrating upward is required for safety.
3. Question the HCP because the patient deserves to have adequate pain relief.
4. Give the medication and tell the patient that he is receiving what was prescribed.

16. Mr. B will receive intravesical chemotherapy consisting of bacille Calmette-Guérin (BCG) instillation for his bladder cancer. Place the following steps related to this therapy in the correct order.
1. Clamp the tube distal to the injection port of the catheter.
2. Insert an indwelling urinary catheter.
3. Instill BCG fluid via the catheter.
4. Change the patient's position from side to side every 15 minutes for 2 hours.
5. Direct the patient to drink two glasses of water to flush the bladder.
6. Unclamp the catheter at the end of 2 hours.
_____, _____, _____, _____, _____, _____

Complex Health Scenarios PART 3

17. After the BCG treatment, the team leader delegates disposal of the fluid contents in Mr. B's (bladder cancer) urinary drainage bag to the AP. What instructions should be given to the AP?
    1. "No special handling of the bag or its contents is required."
    2. "Wear a lead apron when you are emptying the drainage container."
    3. "Discard the fluid in the toilet and disinfect the toilet with bleach for 6 hours."
    4. "Wear sterile gloves when you are handling the bag and its contents."

18. Within which time period, after completion of the BCG treatment and removal of Mr. B's indwelling urinary catheter, would the nurse notify the HCP if a normal voiding pattern (e.g., pain free, symptom free) failed to resume?
    1. 6 hours
    2. 12 hours
    3. 3 days
    4. 1 week

19. The nurse sees that Mr. B (bladder cancer) has received docusate for the past 2 days. Which question is the nurse **most** likely to ask to evaluate the effectiveness of the docusate?
    1. "Are you experiencing any burning with urination?"
    2. "Did you have a bowel movement today or yesterday?"
    3. "Has the medication helped to relieve the nausea?"
    4. "Were you able to sleep soundly the last couple of nights?"

20. During the midmorning, the following events occur at the same time. Prioritize the events in the order in which they should be addressed, with 1 being the most urgent and 5 being the least.
    1. Mr. B, who has bladder cancer, reports dysuria.
    2. Mr. U's (pulmonary resection) chest drainage system has tipped over.
    3. Mr. N, who has non-Hodgkin lymphoma, has a fever of 101°F (38.3°C).
    4. Mr. L's (partial laryngectomy) tracheostomy tube needs to be suctioned.
    5. Ms. C, who had a bowel resection, has a red, swollen, tender calf.

    _____, _____, _____, _____, _____

21. Ms. C (bowel resection) repeatedly refuses to perform a return demonstration of any aspect of colostomy care. Despite steady improvement and independent resumption of other ADLs, she protests, "I'm too weak. You'll have to do it for me." At this point, what

is the **priority** nursing concept to consider in planning interventions for Ms. C?
    1. Mobility
    2. Development
    3. Functional Ability
    4. Stress and Coping

22. The nursing staff are making suggestions about how to help Ms. C (bowel resection) overcome her reluctance to perform colostomy care. Which suggestion will the team leader try **first**?
    1. Verbally reexplain the procedure and give her written material.
    2. Have a family member come in and do it for her.
    3. Continue to do it for her until she is ready.
    4. Ask her to hold the clamp while the bag is being emptied.

23. In helping a patient such as Ms. C, who had a colostomy with a bowel resection, which tasks can be delegated to the AP? **Select all that apply.**
    1. Assist Ms. C with perineal care.
    2. Help Ms. C to position the adhesive wafer over the stoma.
    3. Empty the colostomy bag and measure the contents.
    4. Help Ms. C to reapply a new colostomy bag.
    5. Assist Ms. C with selecting dinner items from the menu.
    6. Report that Ms. C has a question about odor from the bag.

24. Ms. C (bowel resection and colostomy) repeatedly calls for help during the shift with various small requests. She is talkative and pleasant, and she does everything she can to get staff members to "stay and chat." What is the **best** response?
    1. "I really like talking to you, but I do have other patients."
    2. "You'll be okay for right now, and I will come back and check on you later."
    3. "I have 10 minutes right now. Later this afternoon, I'll have time to talk."
    4. "Let me call one of the hospital volunteers to come and sit with you."

25. Ms. C (bowel resection and colostomy) is receiving epoetin alfa. Which laboratory result indicates that the HCP should be called to discontinue the medication?
    1. Hemoglobin is 12 g/dl (7.4 mmol/L).
    2. White blood cell (WBC) count is 7,000 mm³ (7 x 10⁹/L).
    3. Potassium level is 3.6 mEq/L (3.6 mmol/L).
    4. Blood glucose level is 85 mg/dl (12 mmol/L).

PART 3   Complex Health Scenarios

    Answer Key for this chapter begins on p. 326

26. The nursing student tells the team leader that Ms. C (bowel resection and colostomy) has just asked her to stay after the shift ends so that she can meet her granddaughter. What is the **best** response?
    1. "What do you think your instructor would tell you to do?"
    2. "What do you think about Ms. C's request?"
    3. "It sounds like you really made a connection with Ms. C."
    4. "Tell Ms. C that you have to go, but you will see her tomorrow."

27. The team leader is working through the preoperative checklist and Ms. G, who has a breast lump, begins to cry. "What do you think about this breast surgery? My friend's arm got really swollen after she had the surgery. Can't I just take medication?" What is the **priority** nursing concept to consider in responding to Ms. G?
    1. Anxiety
    2. Culture
    3. Functional Ability
    4. Adherence

28. Ms. G (breast lumpectomy) continues to be anxious and tearful, and she says that she has changed her mind about the surgery, saying, "I'm going to go home. I just can't deal with everything that is going on right now. I need some time to think about things." What is the **best** response?
    1. "It's okay to change your mind. You have the right to make your own decisions."
    2. "Please reconsider. This surgery is very important, and your health is the priority."
    3. "Would you like me to call your HCP, so you can discuss your concerns?"
    4. "I see you are concerned. What things are you dealing with and thinking about?"

29. The team leader is reviewing the pain management plan for Mr. U. He is having significant pain related to the cancer and the pulmonary resection. Which option would be the **best** for Mr. U?
    1. Mr. U is instructed to ask for pain medication whenever he needs it.
    2. Mr. U should receive around-the-clock fixed doses of opioid analgesics.
    3. Mr. U should be offered the non-opioid medication first to see it if works.
    4. Mr. U has a high risk for respiratory distress, so opioids are not prescribed.

30. For administering pain medication to Mr. U (lung cancer and pulmonary resection), which route is the nurse **most** likely to question?
    1. Oral
    2. IV
    3. Rectal
    4. Intramuscular

31. Emhanced Multiple Response _____

Scenario: The team leader is in the medication area preparing Mr. U's pain medication. Suddenly the student nurse runs up and excitedly says, "Come quick! There's something wrong with Mr. U!" As the nurse enters the room, she notes that Mr. U is gasping for breath and struggling to sit upright. He does not respond to the nurse's question, "Mr. U, what's wrong?" The nurse recognizes that immediate interventions are required.

Which **three** nursing actions will the nurse perform **first**?

Instructions: Place an X, in the space provided, or highlight the three interventions that the nurse will perform first.
1. _____ Assess respiratory effort
2. _____ Take vital signs
3. _____ Position patient in high Fowler
4. _____ Apply oxygen and attach pulse oximeter
5. _____ Assess for pain
6. _____ Call the HCP
7. _____ Call the rapid response team
8. _____ Check chest tube function
9. _____ Help the patient to calm down
10. _____ Assess breath sounds

⚡ **32.** Enhanced Multiple Response _____

Scenario: The nurse notes that Mr. U has tracheal deviation. Tension pneumothorax is suspected because of the sudden onset respiratory distress and the presence of the chest tube, which is a risk factor.

Which signs and symptoms would the nurse expect to observe with a tension pneumothorax?

Instructions: Place an X, in the space provided, or highlight each sign or symptom associated with tension pneumothorax. **Select all that apply.**

1. _____ Severe dyspnea
2. _____ Extreme agitation
3. _____ Decreased or absent breath sounds on the affected side
4. _____ Progressive cyanosis
5. _____ Bradycardia
6. _____ Distended jugular veins
7. _____ Lateral or medial shift in the point of maximum impulse
8. _____ Hemoptysis
9. _____ Profuse diaphoresis
10. _____ Paradoxical chest movement
11. _____ Tachypnea

33. On the figure below locate the tracheal deviation.

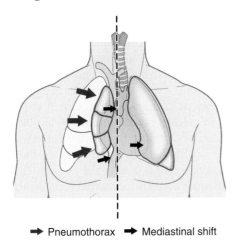

➡ Pneumothorax ➡ Mediastinal shift

34. Mr. U (pulmonary resection) has developed a tension pneumothorax. He is currently receiving high-flow oxygen via a nonrebreather mask but continues to experience respiratory distress. What is the **priority** action?
1. Remove the occlusive dressing around the chest wound.
2. Perform a needle thoracotomy with a 14- to 16-gauge catheter needle.
3. Initiate cardiopulmonary resuscitation (CPR).
4. Call for the crash cart and intubation equipment.

35. The team leader is calling the HCP to report events related to Mr. U's (pulmonary resection complicated by tension pneumothorax) condition. Prioritize the following information according to the SBAR (situation, background, assessment, recommendation) format.
1. "Mr. U is 5 days postoperative for pulmonary resection for non–small cell lung cancer. He has a chest tube that has been draining progressively smaller amounts of dark red blood."

2. "Dr. S, this is Nurse C on the medical-surgical oncology unit. I am calling about Mr. U. About 15 minutes ago, he developed severe respiratory distress, and tracheal deviation was noted. We removed the occlusive dressing at the chest tube insertion site, and his breathing improved. The rapid response team was called and is currently managing the airway. He is receiving 100% oxygen via a nonrebreather mask."
3. "The rapid response team is recommending transfer to the ICU because the exact cause of the tension pneumothorax is undetermined. The radiology department is waiting to do a portable chest radiograph if we could get an order. Would you like us to get an arterial blood gas analysis or do anything else?"
4. "Mr. U is currently alert and anxious, and he is following commands. Blood pressure is 160/96 mm Hg, pulse rate is 110 beats/min, respiratory rate is 32 breaths/min, and pulse oximetry reading is 90% with the patient on 100% oxygen via nonrebreather mask."

_____, _____, _____, _____

36. There are 2 hours left before the shift ends. The new AP tells the team leader that she must leave now because she has a family emergency. What should the team leader do? **Select all that apply.**
1. Ask her what tasks and duties are pending for the next 2 hours.
2. Ask another AP who is scheduled for the next shift to come early.
3. Allow her to leave but remind her that she is still on probation as a new staff member.
4. Call another unit and see if there is an AP who could float to the unit.
5. Ask her to explain the nature of the family emergency so that a decision can be made.
6. Check with the other staff members to see if they will be able to cover her duties.

Answer Key for this chapter begins on p. 326

PART 3 · Complex Health Scenarios

Answers

1. **Ans: 2, 6** Mr L and Mr U have the most critical conditions. Mr. L requires tracheostomy care and frequent suctioning. In addition, he is still learning to cope with impaired communications, changes in breathing, and managing his own secretions. He has tube feedings and is receiving chemotherapy. His energy level will be low, and he needs assistance for most ADLs. Mr. U had major chest surgery. He has a chest tube and requires frequent respiratory assessment. He is having significant pain that is not well controlled. Mr. U is also likely to have little energy to accomplish ADLs and has a risk for post-surgical complications. **Focus:** Prioritization.

2. **Ans: 1, 2, 5, 6** When the patient responds to a question, this provides information about ease of respirations and cerebral perfusion. Noting the presence of complex equipment will help in making assignments, particularly if the staff is inexperienced. Measuring vital signs, checking intake and output, and palpating for pain are not necessary during this brief assessment unless there is reason to suspect that a patient is decompensating. (Note to student: Some nurses briefly palpate the radial pulse to detect irregularities, assess peripheral perfusion, and check skin temperature.) **Focus:** Prioritization.

3. **Ans: 3, 4** Mr. B and Ms. C are patients in relatively stable condition who would be capable of speaking with a nursing student for a prolonged time. Mr. N is also communicative and in stable condition, but limiting the number of people that enter the room is best practice for neutropenic patients. Mr. L has recently been transferred from the surgical ICU. The tracheostomy tube, dealing with the secretions, and the NG tube will make communication very tedious and overwhelming for him and the student. Mr. U needs frequent skilled assessment, and he is likely to be very uncomfortable, exhausted, and possibly dyspneic. Ms. G needs emotional support and preoperative teaching that are beyond the abilities of a first-semester student. **Focus:** Assignment, Supervision.

4. **Ans: 2** Staff and visitors with potentially communicable diseases should not enter Mr. N's protective environment. Pregnancy, inexperience, and fear do not automatically exclude staff members from this assignment. If the team leader has time and options for personnel, then opportunities for duty sharing for pregnant staff members and teaching for the inexperienced and fearful can be explored. **Focus:** Assignment, Supervision.

5. **Ans: 3** Acknowledge the student for taking responsibility for the error. Helping the student to feel comfortable in reporting errors rather than hiding mistakes is essential for patient safety. Notifying the instructor is appropriate so that the student can be counseled and procedures can be reviewed. All involved parties may elect to write separate incident reports. **Focus:** Prioritization, Supervision.

6. **Ans: 2** Catheterizing this patient increases the risk for infection, and the clean-catch method is adequate for a urinalysis. The other interventions would be appropriate for this patient. **Focus:** Prioritization. **Test-Taking Tip:** To reduce catheter associated urinary tract infections (CAUTIs), the nurse must question unnecessary catheterization. For additional evidenced based strategies to reduce CAUTIs, use this link: https://www.nursingworld.org/~4aee34/globalassets/practiceandpolicy/innovation--evidence/clinical-practice-material/cauti-prevention-tool/anacautipreventiontool-guidance-final-5jan2015.pdf.

7. **Ans: 4** The nurse must use a professional and nonaccusatory tone of voice and manner in approaching the HCP. Patient data are communicated to improve patient care. Neutropenic precautions are usually based on laboratory results, but best practices would still include washing hands upon entering the room and then again before touching the patient. The infection control nurse could be contacted if the issue cannot be resolved and the HCP's behavior continues to place patients at risk for infection. **Focus:** Prioritization.

8. **Ans: 3** The combination of medications aprepitant, dexamethasone, and ondansetron is used for high-emetogenic risk for chemotherapy-induced nausea and vomiting. **Focus:** Prioritization.

9. **Ans: 4** Numbness, tingling, and neuropathic pain are reported by patients with chemotherapy induced peripheral neuropathy. For venous thromboembolism, expected signs and symptoms include calf or groin tenderness and pain, and sudden onset of unilateral swelling of the leg and induration (hardening) along the blood vessel and with warmth and edema. Peripheral arterial insufficiency would manifest as pain, pallor, pulselessness, paresthesia, paralysis, and poikilothermy (coolness). Before the patient stands and ambulates, an additional assessment would be performed to prevent falls. **Focus:** Prioritization.

10. **Ans: 2, 3, 4, 5, 6, 8, 9, 11, 12** According to the Centers for Disease Control and Prevention Division of Cancer Prevention and Control, patients who are neutropenic are advised to watch for and immediately report: a fever that is 100.4°F (38°C) or higher for more than one hour or a one-time temperature of 101°F (38.3°C) or higher; chills and sweats; cough or new cough; sore throat or mouth sores; difficulty breathing; nasal congestion; stiff neck; burning, painful, or

increased urination; change in vaginal discharge or irritation; redness, soreness, or swelling in any area; diarrhea; vomiting; new onset of pain and changes in skin, urination, or mental status. Flatulence and insomnia, while troublesome for patients, are not usually associated with infection. **Focus:** Prioritization.

11. **Ans: 4** Increased secretions, difficulty swallowing, and loss of the protective epiglottis put Mr. L at risk for aspiration. The other concerns also apply to this patient but are of lower priority. **Focus:** Prioritization. **Test-Taking Tip:** Use the ABCs (airway, breathing, and circulation) to determine the priorities in the immediate postprocedural or postoperative care of patients who have had invasive procedures or surgery that requires general anesthesia.

12. **Ans: 1** Pulsation would suggest that the tube may be malpositioned and pushing against the innominate artery. This would be considered a medical emergency. The presence of food particles and difficulty with cough or expectoration suggest that cuff pressures should be monitored more closely. Increased secretions are expected in the postoperative period. **Focus:** Prioritization.

13. **Ans: 3** The bag-valve mask (trade name, Ambu bag) is the first thing that is needed if there is a problem with the tracheostomy equipment or with respiratory effort. With a tracheostomy, there should be no need for an endotracheal tube or a laryngoscope. The insertion tray is also probably unnecessary because the site should mature within 72 hours. **Focus:** Prioritization.

14. **Ans: 1** If a very small amount (less than 0.5 mL) of a vesicant (chemical that damages the skin on contact) has leaked into skin, the likelihood of damage is lower. Thus very close monitoring can prevent larger amounts of leakage into the tissues. The chemotherapy-certified nurse has the knowledge to safely administer chemotherapy, but close monitoring is still required. If the medication is a known vesicant, the nurse is more likely to closely monitor the access site, but any infiltration can be uncomfortable and problematic for the patient. Holding the medication is not appropriate, but the nurse may advocate for central line placement. **Focus:** Prioritization.

15. **Ans: 2** The cross-tolerance of opioids can vary. There is a potential that an equal dose could produce a stronger effect, so starting low and titrating upward would be considered safer. **Focus:** Prioritization.

16. **Ans: 2, 1, 3, 4, 6, 5** An indwelling catheter with a drainage bag will be inserted. The tube is clamped distal to the injection port, the BCG fluid is instilled through the catheter, and the catheter remains clamped for 2 hours. During those hours, Mr. B should be reminded to change position from side to side or prone to supine every 15 to 30 minutes. At the end of the 2 hours, the catheter is unclamped, and the fluid is drained. Two glasses of fluid are given to further flush the bladder. **Focus:** Prioritization.

17. **Ans: 3** The toilet should be disinfected for 6 hours after the fluid is discarded. The AP should receive these specific instructions to safely manage this biohazard. Wearing a lead apron offers no protection against this biohazard and wearing sterile gloves is unnecessary. **Focus:** Delegation, Supervision.

18. **Ans: 3** The goal is resumption of normal voiding within 3 days. Immediately after catheter removal and for 1 to 2 days thereafter, Mr. B may experience dysuria, urgency, and frequency. **Focus:** Prioritization.

19. **Ans: 2** Docusate is a stool softener that is given for occasional constipation. **Focus:** Prioritization. **Test-Taking Tip:** Initially, focus your study of pharmacology and medications on the more common medications that are typically used on general medical-surgical units. If you know the purpose of a medication, you can assess for therapeutic effects.

20. **Ans: 4, 2, 3, 5, 1** Mr. L is at risk for aspiration and an immediate airway obstruction if his tracheostomy tube is not suctioned. If a chest drainage system tips over, it is unlikely that anything untoward will occur; however, if the chest tube has been displaced, Mr. U is at risk for an open pneumothorax. The HCP must be notified about Mr. N's fever so that therapy can be changed and cultures ordered to determine the source of infection. Ms. C must be assessed for signs and symptoms of venous thromboembolism. Mr. B needs reassurance that the dysuria is transient and to be expected after intravesical therapy. **Focus:** Prioritization.

21. **Ans: 4** Asking for extra help and delaying independent action is a type of regression that allows Ms. C to cope with the changes in self-image and bodily functions. The nurse should evaluate the situation daily to help Ms. C find alternative coping strategies. **Focus:** Prioritization.

22. **Ans: 4** Have her hold the clamp or do some other small task to engage her in participation. This creates the expectation that she can participate and will eventually handle the equipment. Verbally reexplaining the procedure and providing written material does reinforce the initial teaching, but being told will not help her master the psychomotor aspects. Having a family member or a staff member take over the procedure does not support the goal of eventual independence. **Focus:** Prioritization.

23. **Ans: 1, 3, 6** The AP can assist Ms. C with hygienic care and measuring output. The AP should also report patient's concerns to the RN. The RN should perform the tasks related to changing the colostomy appliance because education and assessment of patient's self-management are necessary. The RN should also assist with the menu selection because some foods increase risk for blockage (e.g., popcorn or seeds) and other foods increase odors (e.g., onions or beans). **Focus:** Delegation. **Test-Taking Tip:** When assigning or delegating tasks remember that the patient's status

PART 3 Complex Health Scenarios

and needs must be considered. In this case, the need for assessment and teaching are beyond the scope of practice for the AP. In other circumstances, such as in the home setting, the AP may be assisting the patient to do many of the routine tasks associated with the colostomy.

24. **Ans: 3** Use 10 minutes to determine if Ms. C has an urgent need, but set some boundaries so that she will know what to expect. Making reference to other patients' needs is not appropriate. Telling her that she is okay minimizes her concerns. Calling a volunteer might be useful after determining that her social needs could be met by a volunteer. **Focus:** Prioritization.

25. **Ans: 1** All values are within normal limits, but if the hemoglobin level exceeds 10 mg/dL (100 g/L), epoetin alfa should be discontinued because of the increased risk for serious disorders, such as hypertension, stroke, and myocardial infarction. Normal range for hemoglobin: female 12 to 16 g/dl (7.4–9.9 mmol/L); WBC count: 5000 to 10,00/mm³ (5–10 x10⁹/L); potassium: 3.5 to 5.0 mEq/L (3.5–5.0mmol/L); blood glucose: 70 to 110 mg/dl (< 6.1 mmol/L). **Focus:** Prioritization.

26. **Ans: 2** This is an opportunity to help the student find her own answer. Help her to work through her own feelings and to identify the boundaries of the nurse–patient relationship. Redirecting the student back to the instructor, acknowledging the student's ability to establish a relationship, and giving direct advice about how to set boundaries are all possible choices in working with students, but they are not as useful as helping students to identify their own best practices. **Focus:** Prioritization, Supervision.

27. **Ans: 1** Ms. G is demonstrating fear and anxiety related to uncertainty of the future. The nurse would first help her to express feelings and decrease anxiety; then information deficits, decision making, and dealing with body image could be dealt with. **Focus:** Prioritization.

28. **Ans: 4** First acknowledge Ms. G's feelings and do additional assessment about "things" in order to design interventions. It is natural for her to be anxious about the surgery, but there may be other issues (e.g., problems with family, money, work). The other options might be appropriate after the situation has been assessed. **Focus:** Prioritization.

29. **Ans: 2** Patients who have continuous pain should be placed on around-the-clock analgesics. Non-opioid analgesics or as needed opioid administration may also be appropriate for situations such as breakthrough pain, but they are not the best solution for continuous pain. Patients should always be monitored for respiratory depression, especially if they are opioid

naïve; however, this patient has advanced cancer, and he is also having postoperative pain, so opioids should not be withheld. **Focus:** Prioritization.

30. **Ans: 4** The intramuscular route is rarely used because it is painful and absorption is uneven. The IV route is frequently used in the immediate postoperative period, especially for patients who are candidates for PCA. The oral route is usually preferred if the patient can swallow. The rectal route is an option for those who cannot swallow. **Focus:** Prioritization.

31. **Ans: 1, 3, 4** In this scenario, there are three key observations that the nurse makes upon entering the room. The patient is gasping for breath. He is struggling to sit upright, and he is not able to answer questions. The nurse immediately does an emergency assessment which includes visually observing for skin color, labored or rapid breathing and listening for wheezing or stridor. Simultaneously, the nurse positions the patient and applies oxygen and pulse oximeter. The patient is using precious oxygen in his efforts to sit upright. Putting him a high Fowler's position is a quick action that helps to improve breathing and will decrease his struggles. If the nursing student knows how to raise the head of the bed, the nurse could delegate this action and perform the second step, which is to apply oxygen and the pulse oximeter; however, a first-year nursing student may not be familiar with the equipment or be able to react quickly in an emergency situation. Once oxygen needs are addressed, the nurse will perform the other interventions. **Focus:** Prioritization. **Test-Taking Tip:** Generally speaking, assessment is the first step of the nursing process. In-depth assessment is deferred if the patient is critically distressed and the question supplies enough information for the nurse to select and perform emergency actions.

32. **Ans: 1, 2, 3, 4, 6, 7, 9, 11** Tension pneumothorax is a medical emergency that occurs when air enters the pleural space, but cannot escape. Pressure builds up on the affected lung, heart, and the great vessels. A mediastinal shift occurs when continued pressure pushes against the unaffected lung and oxygenation and perfusion are further compromised. For Mr. U, the tension pneumothorax is most likely to be associated with the chest tube. Tachycardia, not bradycardia, is expected. Hemoptysis is more likely to occur with a hemopneumothorax. Paradoxical chest movements are associated with flail chest secondary to rib fractures. **Focus:** Prioritization. **Test-Taking Tip:** Learn to recognize the signs and symptoms of life-threatening conditions because interventions need to be immediately initiated.

33. **Ans:** Accumulation of air in the pleural space causes a mediastinal shift. When tracheal deviation is observable, this is considered a late sign.

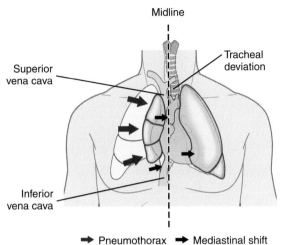

Midline

Superior vena cava

Tracheal deviation

Inferior vena cava

➡ Pneumothorax ➡ Mediastinal shift

34. **Ans: 1** For Mr. U, the tension pneumothorax has most likely been induced iatrogenically by the covering of the chest wound. (For patients without open chest wounds, the priority action is performing a needle thoracotomy.) Initiating CPR is inappropriate at this point. Having the crash cart and intubation equipment nearby is a precaution but should not delay other interventions. **Focus:** Prioritization.

35. **Ans: 2, 1, 4, 3** Using the SBAR format, the nurse first identifies himself or herself, gives the patient's name, and describes the current situation. Next, relevant background information, such as the patient's diagnosis, medications, and laboratory data, is reported. The assessment includes both patient assessment data that are of concern and the nurse's analysis of the situation. Finally, the nurse makes a recommendation indicating what action he or she thinks is needed. **Focus:** Prioritization.

36. **Ans: 1, 2, 3, 4, 6** Determining what tasks and duties are pending and seeking replacement coverage are all appropriate. Because she is new, verbal warnings are appropriate. Any employee could have a personal emergency at any time, so refusing to let her go or expecting disclosure of personal details would only be used if her behavior is repetitive. **Focus:** Supervision, Assignment.

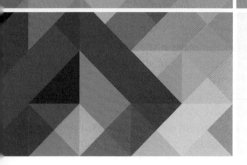

CASE STUDY 12

Gastrointestinal Bleeding

Mr. S, a 50-year-old man, has driven himself to the emergency department (ED) after vomiting a large amount of bright red blood twice within the past 3 hours. He arrives alert and oriented to person, place and time but appears anxious and restless. He is able to provide only a vague history but admits to drink-ing "a few" last weekend. He knows that he is "supposed to stop drinking" and is supposed to take "something for my stomach," but he cannot recall the name of the medication. He reports intermittent dizziness and fatigue that have been worsening over the past 2 days. His skin is pale, cool, and clammy. His abdomen is slightly distended. He reports pain (4 on a scale of 1 to 10) in the midepigastric area and says he is thirsty. Capillary refill is prolonged, blood pressure is 100/90 mm Hg, pulse is weak and thready at 130 beats/ min, respiratory rate is 24 breaths/min, and temperature is 99°F (37.2°C).*

1. Which member of the health care team is the triage RN **most** likely to call for immediate assistance?
   1. Emergency health care provider (HCP) to come to triage and begin treatment
   2. Registration clerk to register Mr. S and place an identification band
   3. Assistive personnel (AP) to get a wheelchair or stretcher for Mr. S
   4. LPN/LVN to triage and assess other patients while the RN assesses Mr. S

2. Enhanced Hotspot

Scenario: Mr. S, a 50-year-old man, has driven himself to the emergency department (ED) after vomiting a large amount of bright red blood twice within the past 3 hours. He arrives alert and oriented but appears anxious and restless. He gives a vague history and admits to drinking "a few" last weekend. He knows that he "should stop drinking" and is supposed to take "something for my stomach," but he cannot recall the name of the medication. He reports intermittent dizziness and noticeable exhaustion that has worsened over the past 2 days. Skin is pale, cool, and clammy. Abdomen is slightly distended. He reports thirst and pain (4 on a scale of 1 to 10) in the midepigastric area. Capillary refill is 4.5 seconds.

Instructions: Underline or highlight the signs and symptoms that indicate that the patient is at risk for hypovolemic shock.

Vital signs:
Temperature 99°F (37.2°C)
Pulse 130 beats/min, weak and thready
Respirations 24 breaths/min
Blood Pressure 100/90 mmHg

Which signs and symptoms indicate to the nurse that risk for hypovs-hock is the focus of the initial assessment?

3. Enhanced Multiple Response _____

Scenario: Mr. S is showing signs and symptoms of hypovolemia and priority collaborative interventions must be implemented. Team members must work together to quickly stabilize his condition.

What are the **priority** collaborative interventions to perform for this patient?

Instructions: Place an X, in the space provided, or highlight each emergency intervention that would be performed to stabilize Mr. S's condition. **Select all that apply.**

1. _____ Prepare for endotracheal intubation.
2. _____ Assist with the central line placement.
3. _____ Check the stool for occult blood.
4. _____ Administer supplemental oxygen.
5. _____ Monitor vital signs and oxygen saturation q 15 min.
6. _____ Insert a large bore nasogastric tube
7. _____ Establish two peripheral IV lines with large-bore catheters.
8. _____ Initiate electrocardiogram (ECG) monitoring.
9. _____ Monitor airway, breathing, and circulation (ABCs).
10. _____ Obtain past medical, surgical, and medication history.
11. _____ Obtain blood for a complete blood count (CBC), clotting studies, and type and cross-match.
12. _____ Administer IV normal saline (NS) fluid bolus 500 mL over 30 minutes.

4. Which immediate (STAT) intervention would the RN perform **first**?
   1. Draw blood for CBC and type and cross-match.
   2. Insert two peripheral IV lines with large-bore catheters.
   3. Insert an indwelling urinary catheter.
   4. Repeat the vital signs and apply the pulse oximeter.

5. Which task would the RN instruct the AP to perform **first**?
   1. Repeat measurement of the vital signs.
   2. Obtain equipment for the stool guaiac test.
   3. Gather and label the patient's belongings.
   4. Clean the skin under the oxygen cannula.

6. The nurse is performing an additional assessment and history taking for Mr. S. Which finding should be immediately reported to the HCP?
   1. Melena stools
   2. History of nonsteroidal anti-inflammatory drug (NSAID) use
   3. Tense and rigid abdomen
   4. Risk factors for human immunodeficiency virus

7. Which action would cause the nurse to intervene?
   1. AP offers the patient a small glass of water.
   2. LPN/LVN inserts an indwelling urinary catheter.
   3. HCP raises the proximal side rails.
   4. Respiratory therapist adds a humidifier to oxygen setup.

8. The results of the initial hematocrit (Hct) and hemoglobin (Hgb) tests, for which the blood was drawn when the patient first arrived in the ED, show that the Hct was 42% (0.42 volume fraction) and the Hgb was 14g/dL (11.2 mmol/L). How does the nurse interpret these results?
   1. The results indicate that there is no active bleeding.
   2. Loss of plasma (fluid) causes artificial high values.
   3. Normal values within the low range indicate chronic bleeding.
   4. The results indicate a need for immediate transfusion of whole blood.

9. The HCP orders a STAT blood transfusion. In an emergency, which type-specific non–cross-matched blood product could be used?
   1. O negative
   2. AB negative
   3. AB positive
   4. A negative

PART 3   Complex Health Scenarios

    Answer Key for this chapter begins on p. 335

10. Drag and Drop _____

Scenario: The nurse is preparing to administer a blood transfusion to Mr. S. To prevent complications and reduce the risk of transfusion reaction, the nurse must perform standard steps and follow protocols for preparing the equipment and monitoring the patient.

Instructions: In the left column are steps to perform for a blood transfusion. In the right column write the number to indicate the correct order of the steps, 1 being the first step and 9 being the last step.

Steps to perform for a blood transfusion	Order of priority
1. Prime the correct tubing and filter with normal saline.	
2. Take vital signs immediately before starting the transfusion.	
3. Transfuse the first 10 mL slowly; monitor the patient closely.	
4. Compare the blood band ID with the tag on the blood bag; this should be performed by two licensed people.	
5. Document outcomes, names of personnel, and starting and ending times.	
6. Repeat vital sign measurement 15 minutes after infusion begins.	
7. Inspect the bag for leaks, clots, or unusual color.	
8. Compare the bag label with the chart and the blood bag forms.	
9. Repeat vital signs every hour until the transfusion is complete	

11. Mr. S's international normalized ratio (INR) value is 2.5. Which action should the nurse take next?
1. Document results as an expected finding related to gastrointestinal (GI) bleeding.
2. The HCP should be notified for possible prescription of fresh frozen plasma (FFP).
3. Laboratory findings should be reevaluated when the treatments are completed.
4. The blood bank should be contacted for more units of packed red blood cells (PRBCs).

12. As part of the medical management for the acute phase of upper GI bleeding, the HCP prescribes an IV loading dose of 40 mg of esomeprazole over 30 minutes. The pharmacy prepares and delivers the infusion. The bag is labeled: 40 mg esomeprazole in 100 mL normal saline. How many milliliters per hour are programmed into the IV pump to deliver the prescribed dose? _____ ml/hr

13. Because of Mr. S's initial comments about "drinking a few" and "supposed to stop drinking," the nurse assesses for risk of alcohol withdrawal syndrome. Which question is the **most** important to ask?
1. "Do you consider yourself to be an alcoholic?"
2. "How much alcohol would you consume in a typical week?"
3. "When was the last time you had a drink?"
4. "Do family or friends express concern about your drinking?"

14. Because Mr. S could be at risk for alcohol withdrawal syndrome, which **early** manifestation will the nurse watch for?
1. Startles easily
2. Paranoid delusions
3. Slurred speech
4. Seizure activity

After emergency treatments are given, Mr. S's vital signs are a blood pressure reading of 130/80 mm Hg, a pulse of 90 beats/min, a respiratory rate of 24 breaths/min, and a pulse oximetry reading of 98% on room air. He has not vomited. Subjectively, he feels "better, but a little nervous." The nurse notes that he is restless and has fine tremors (possible early signs of alcohol withdrawal syndrome). Mr. S is to be admitted to the medical-surgical unit for observation and continued management of acute gastritis with bleeding.

15. The ED nurse must call the receiving nurse on the medical-surgical unit. Prioritize the following information according to the SBAR (situation, background, assessment, recommendation) format.
1. "Mr. S is 50 years old. He admits to drinking alcohol for several days, and he takes medication for his stomach. He had intermittent dizziness and fatigue, which worsened over the past 2 days. He vomited a large amount of bright red blood twice within 3 hours."
2. "This is Nurse X from the ED. I am calling to give a report about Mr. S. He is being admitted for acute gastritis with active bleeding."

3. "Mr. S should be monitored for possible alcohol withdrawal. The HCP is considering an esophago-gastroduodenoscopy (EGD)."

4. "Mr. S is currently alert and oriented. He is nervous and restless and has fine tremors. He was vague about time of last alcohol consumption. BP: 130/80, P: 90 beats/min, RR: 24/min, O2 sat: 98%. Pain is 2 of 10 in the midepigastric area. He has a 16-gauge peripheral IV line in each forearm. He received 500mL of NS fluid bolus and NS is currently infusing at 60 mL/hr in each IV line. He received one unit of PRBCs, one unit of FFP, and a loading dose of 40 mg esomeprazole. He has an indwelling urinary catheter with clear yellow urine. Urinalysis results are pending.

_____, _____, _____, _____

After the SBAR report is completed, Mr. S is prepared for transport to his room on the medical-surgical unit. He is greeted by the medical-surgical nurse who will assume responsibility for this care. The nurse assesses him and orients him to the environment. He is tired but also anxious to see the HCP. The HCP arrives and recommends that Mr. S have an EGD.

16. Mr. S agrees to have the EGD and is being prepared for the procedure. Which instruction will the nurse give to the AP?
    1. Assist Mr. S as needed to the bathroom while he is undergoing bowel preparation.
    2. Help Mr. S to take a shower with the special antibiotic cleaning solution.
    3. Remind Mr. S that he is to have nothing by mouth for 8 hours before the procedure.
    4. Assist Mr. S with undressing and removing all metal objects and then with donning a hospital gown.

17. Which instruction will the RN give to the LPN/LVN related to preparing Mr. S for the EGD?
    1. Have him drink 2 liters of polyethylene glycol solution before the procedure.
    2. Administer the prescribed preoperative medication before he leaves for the procedure.
    3. Spray the back of his throat with a local anesthetic before he leaves for the procedure.
    4. Ask him if he has any allergies or other contraindications for contrast media.

18. During the EGD procedure, Mr. S is given midazolam hydrochloride. What is the **priority** assessment related to this medication?
    1. Monitor for cardiac dysrhythmias.
    2. Assess for adequate pain relief.
    3. Monitor depth and rate of respirations.
    4. Assess for relief of nausea and vomiting.

19. After the EGD procedure, Mr. S returns to the medical-surgical unit. He is drowsy but readily arouses to light stimuli. His vital signs are a blood pressure reading of 110/74 beats/min, a pulse of 82 beats/min, a respiratory rate of 20 breaths/min, and a temperature of 99°F (37.2°C). What is the **priority** intervention?
    1. Offer cool oral fluids for sore throat.
    2. Raise the side rails of the bed.
    3. Apply a small ice pack to the periorbital area.
    4. Assess the presence of the gag reflex.

Hemostasis was achieved during the EGD therapy. The plan is to discharge Mr. S with prescriptions for medications, a follow-up appointment with his primary HCP, and information about alcohol treatment programs.

20. Mr. S's wife visits. They ask for privacy so that they can talk. Later, when the nurse returns to check on him, there is a strong odor of alcohol on Mr. S's breath, and he appears very drowsy. What should the nurse do **first**?
    1. Politely ask the wife to leave and call security to check the room for illicit substances.
    2. Assess the patient's mental status and ask what happened during the visit.
    3. Explain that his behavior is inappropriate and counterproductive to his condition.
    4. Call the HCP for an order for a STAT blood alcohol test and toxicology screen.

21. The nurse is talking to Mr. S about self-care measures that he should take to prevent the recurrence of acute gastritis. For Mr. S, what is the **most** important point to emphasize?
    1. Eat a well-balanced diet that includes protein and carbohydrates.
    2. Avoid drinking excessive amounts of alcoholic beverages.
    3. Use caution in taking aspirin, other NSAIDs, and corticosteroids.
    4. Drink at least eight glasses of noncaffeinated fluid each day.

22. Which medications will the nurse include in the discharge teaching for Mr. S's self-management of gastritis?
    1. H_2-receptor antagonists, proton pump inhibitors, and antacids
    2. Diuretics, beta-blockers, and angiotensin-converting enzyme (ACE) inhibitors
    3. Mucolytics, expectorants, and non-opioid antitussives
    4. HMG-CoA reductase inhibitors (statins) and bile-acid sequestrants

The nurse attempts to give information and do discharge teaching about alcohol treatment programs, but Mr. S believes that he can control his alcohol consumption without entering a treatment program.

Answer Key for this chapter begins on p. 335

PART 3 Complex Health Scenarios

23. Which statement represents the **most** common defense mechanism that is used by people who have problems with alcoholism?
    1. "You would drink, too, if you were married to my wife."
    2. "My wife and I have a couple of beers after work. It's no big deal."
    3. "If you think I drink a lot, you should see my wife put it away."
    4. "I would rather talk to my wife about this situation when I get home."

24. The nurse tells Mr. S that detoxification is safer if performed under medical supervision because alcohol withdrawal can be dangerous. Which problems may result from alcohol withdrawal delirium? **Select all that apply.**
    1. Myocardial infarction
    2. Electrolyte imbalance
    3. Aspiration pneumonia
    4. Anaphylaxis
    5. Sepsis
    6. Suicide

Answer Key for this chapter begins on p. 335

Answers

1. **Ans: 3** The triage RN would instruct the AP to obtain a wheelchair or stretcher so that Mr. S can be moved to a treatment room as soon as possible. The HCP usually does not initiate treatment in the triage area unless the patient is in full cardiac arrest. Registration is important, but this clerical activity could be delayed if the patient is in critical condition or the clerk could go to the bedside to complete the registration process. The LPN/LVN should not be expected to triage patients. The initial assessment and decision making in triage needs to be done by an RN or advanced practice nurse. **Focus:** Delegation.

2. **Ans:** Mr. S, a 50-year-old man, has driven himself to the emergency department (ED) after **vomiting a large amount of bright red blood twice within the past 3 hours.** He arrives alert and oriented but appears **anxious and restless**. He gives a vague history and admits to drinking "a few" last weekend. He knows that he "should stop drinking" and is supposed to take "something for my stomach," but he cannot recall the name of the medication. He reports intermittent **dizziness** and **noticeable exhaustion** that has worsened over the past 2 days. **Skin is pale, cool, and clammy.** Abdomen is slightly distended. He reports **thirst** and pain (4 on a scale of 1 to 10) in the midepigastric area. **Capillary refill is 4.5 seconds.** Vital signs: T 99°F (37.2°C); **P 130 beats/min, weak and thready;** RR 24 breaths/min; **BP 100/90 mm Hg**.

   Losing large amounts of bright red blood in a short time causes hypovolemia and dizziness. Decreased vascular volume results in a lower blood pressure and a weak, thready pulse. Tachycardia is an early compensatory mechanism for decreased volume and typically precedes low blood pressure. The skin becomes pale, cool, and clammy and capillary refill is prolonged (normal: less than 2 seconds) as blood is shunted from the periphery to vital organs. As the fluid volume falls, the osmolality of the blood increases and this triggers thirst. Decreased perfusion and oxygenation causes exhaustion and mental status changes. Restlessness or apprehension are early manifestations. **Focus:** Prioritization.

3. **Ans: 4, 5, 7, 8, 9, 11, 12** The ABCs are used to prioritize care for critical patients. The patient shows no overt signs of respiratory distress; however, there is a high risk for hypovolemic shock, and supplemental oxygen should be given based on the assumption that the patient has already sustained blood loss and therefore has decreased oxygen-carrying capacity. Vital signs and oxygen saturation should be monitored every 15 minutes for all unstable patients. ECG monitoring is initiated because there is a risk for shock; tachycardia is an early sign. In an emergency situation, peripheral IVs are usually established first. Isotonic crystalloids, such as lactated Ringer or normal saline, are administered. Fluid bolus is given to increase vascular volume. Blood samples for CBC and clotting studies guide therapy, and type and crossmatch are done because of the potential need for blood products. The patient does not need endotracheal intubation at this point. Central line placement is a sterile procedure that takes more time and may be delayed, particularly if the patient is actively vomiting. Eventually the stool should be checked for occult blood, but the presence or absence will not affect the emergency treatment decisions. In the past, nasogastric tubes were routinely inserted when patients had active GI bleeding. The HCP may order an NG tube for decompression of the stomach, after the patient is stabilized. Reviewing the patient's history and a description of events leading to the bleeding are deferred until after the life-saving interventions are performed. **Focus:** Prioritization.

4. **Ans: 2** The priority for this patient is fluid loss and potential for hypovolemic shock, so the RN would insert two large-bore peripheral IVs. Drawing blood is important, but this is a lower priority. An indwelling urinary catheter is an important part of the therapy for this patient, but it is not considered a life-preserving measure. Repeat vital signs and application of the pulse oximeter are needed. This can be delegated, but the AP must be instructed to report all values so that the nurse can monitor trends. **Focus:** Prioritization.

5. **Ans: 1** Repeating vital sign measurements falls within the scope of the AP's abilities and is the most important task. Obtaining equipment for the stool guaiac test, gathering and labeling belongings, and providing a comfort measure, such as cleaning the skin, are within the AP's scope of practice, but the AP would be instructed to perform these tasks when other priority interventions are completed. **Focus:** Delegation.

6. **Ans: 3** A tense, rigid abdomen could signal perforation, peritonitis, or a worsening hemorrhage. The other findings are relevant but are less immediately urgent. **Focus:** Prioritization.

7. **Ans 1** It is likely that the HCP will order oral food/fluid restrictions because of vomiting or to facilitate decompression of the stomach for diagnostic testing. The LPN/LVN and the respiratory therapist are performing tasks that are within their scope of practice and both actions would be included in the interdisciplinary treatment plan. If all four siderails are raised, the nurse would ask the HCP to write an order because use of four side rails is considered a form of restraint. **Focus:** Supervision.

8. **Ans 2:** The initial Hct and Hgb values could appear normal but be artificially high because plasma and red blood cells are equally lost during active bleeding. After emergency fluid resuscitation with normal saline or lactated Ringer solution, the nurse would expect the subsequent Hct and Hgb to be much lower. The normal ranges for men are a Hct of 42% to 52% (0.42 to 0.52 volume fraction) and a Hgb of 14 to 18 g/dL (8.7 to 11.2 mmol/L). **Focus:** Prioritization. **Test-Taking Tip:** Don't take laboratory numbers at face value. Results must be interpreted within the context of the patient's condition. Higher Hct and Hgb values would normally accompany dehydration (low vascular volume), whereas lower values would be expected in overhydration (hemodilution).

9. **Ans: 1** In a medical emergency, the patient can receive O-negative blood. An antibody reaction could result if type A or B blood is administered without typing and cross-matching. **Focus:** Prioritization.

10. **Ans: 7, 8, 4, 1, 2, 3, 6, 9, 5** Inspect the bag. If the product appears unusable or if the bag is damaged, contact the blood bank for another unit. Checking bag labels against the blood bank forms is done to prevent administering the wrong blood product. At the bedside, two licensed professionals should compare the bag labels and the identification band. (Note: Priming of the tubing and filter can be done at any time before starting the transfusion. In an emergency situation, equipment preparation can be done while waiting for the blood product to come from the blood bank.) Measuring vital signs immediately before starting the transfusion provides a baseline in case of a transfusion reaction. An acute reaction is most likely to result with transfusion of a small amount of blood (or within 15 minutes). A delayed reaction may occur several days after the transfusion. Frequent measurement of vital signs (according to hospital policy) and complete documentation are standard requirements. **Focus:** Prioritization.

11. **Ans: 2** FFP can be used to replace the coagulation factors. With a history of alcohol abuse, there is a potential for liver disease; the liver produces prothrombin and other blood clotting factors. The INR should be at or below 1.1. A higher than normal INR indicates that blood clotting will be slower than expected. **Focus:** Prioritization. **Test-Taking Tip:** INR has a normal range of 1.1 or less. For patients who are on anticoagulation therapy, recall that the therapeutic range is 2.0 to 3.5 (depending on the purpose of therapy, such as venous thrombosis prophylaxis or prosthetic valve prophylaxis).

12. **Ans: 200mL/hr**
    100mL ÷ 0.5 hr = 200mL
    Focus: Prioritization.

13. **Ans: 3** Any of these questions would be included in the assessment of alcohol use, but early symptoms of alcohol withdrawal syndrome usually occur within a few hours after the last drink. Symptoms will peak within 24 to 48 hours. If there is progression to alcohol withdrawal delirium, this will occur within 3 to 10 days after the last drink. **Focus:** Prioritization.

14. **Ans: 1** Signs of neurologic irritability (e.g., psychological [anxiety, jumpiness, or nervousness] and physical [fine tremors, tachycardia, diaphoresis]) occur earlier. Delusions and seizure are later signs. Slurred speech is more frequently associated with alcohol intoxication. **Focus:** Prioritization. **Test-Taking Tip:** In studying for the NCLEX Examination, make note of the early signs and symptoms of disease processes. Recognizing early symptoms is an important part of ensuring safe care.

15. **Ans: 2, 1, 4, 3** Situation: Identify self, location, and purpose of communication. Background: Include relevant information that provides context for the problems or concerns. Assessment: Include current data that are directly related to care. Recommendations: Suggest actions that are needed for following up and highlight issues that might evolve over time. **Focus:** Prioritization.

16. **Ans: 3** The patient should be NPO for 8 hours before the EGD and the AP can reinforce and remind the patient about information that the nurse has given. Bowel preparation is not required for an EGD. Showering with special cleaning solutions may be part of the skin preparation for certain surgeries. Removing metallic objects is done for magnetic resonance imaging and for some radiology studies. **Focus:** Delegation, Supervision.

17. **Ans 2:** Administering the prescribed preoperative medication is within the scope of practice for the LPN/LVN. Polyethylene glycol solution is part of the bowel prep for a colonoscopy but is not part of the preparation for an EGD. Mr. S. will have a local anesthetic spray, but this will be done just before the insertion of the scope. The RN would assess for contraindications and potential problems; however, contrast media is not used during EGD. **Focus:** Assignment, Supervision.

18. **Ans: 3** Midazolam hydrochloride is commonly used for procedures requiring moderate sedation. Depression of depth and rate of respirations is a possible side effect. **Focus:** Prioritization.

19. **Ans: 4** During the EGD procedure, a local anesthetic is sprayed into the throat. This makes the passage of the tube easier for the patient; however, it also depresses the gag reflex. Food and fluids should be held until the gag reflex returns to reduce the risk of aspiration. A sore throat is expected for a few days and is treated with throat lozenges and cool fluids. The side rails are up during the recovery period but are generally considered a form of restraints. The HCP must prescribe restraints for use on the medical-surgical unit. Periorbital bruising may occur in some patients but should resolve spontaneously after several days. **Focus:** Prioritization. **Test-Taking Tip:** Generally, the priorities for post-procedure care for invasive procedures are based on the ABCs. In this case, assessing for the gag reflex is part of airway management.

20. **Ans: 2** First assess the patient and try to determine exactly what occurred. Based on the assessment findings, the other options may be used. **Focus:** Prioritization.

21. **Ans: 2** All the teaching points are relevant for self-management of gastritis, but based on the patient's history and the possible use of alcohol even in the hospital, it would appear that Mr. S may have the greatest difficulty in decreasing alcohol consumption. **Focus:** Prioritization.

22. **Ans: 1** H_2-receptor antagonists, proton pump inhibitors, and antacids are typical medications used to manage gastritis and other GI disorders that are aggravated by excessive gastric acid. Diuretics, beta-blockers, and ACE inhibitors would be used for hypertension. Mucolytics, expectorants, and non-opioid antitussives are used for symptom relief of allergic rhinitis, cough, or colds. HMG-CoA reductase inhibitors (commonly referred to as statins) and bile-acid sequestrants are used for cholesterol management. **Focus:** Prioritization.

23. **Ans: 2** Denial is the most common defense mechanism seen among substance abusers. Option 1 represents rationalization, or giving reasons for behavior. Option 3 represents projection, which is a transfer of unacceptable behavior onto others. Option 4 represents suppression, which is a conscious awareness of and avoidance of dealing with the problem. **Focus:** Prioritization.

24. **Ans: 1, 2, 3, 5, 6** Death can occur from myocardial infarction, fat embolism, peripheral vascular disease, aspiration pneumonia, electrolyte imbalance, sepsis, or suicide. Anaphylaxis would not ordinarily occur unless the patient was allergic to one of the treatments (e.g., had a drug allergy). **Focus:** Prioritization.

PART 3

Complex Health Scenarios

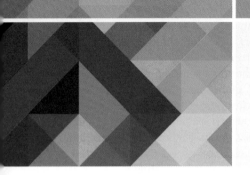

CASE STUDY 13

Head and Leg Trauma and Shock

Questions

Ms. A, a 20-year-old college student who had been drinking at a fraternity party before she fell from a second-floor balcony, has just arrived in the emergency department (ED). A fellow college student who accompanies Ms. A tells the triage nurse, "She was completely knocked out right after the fall. But then she woke up a little, so we thought she was okay—until she stopped moving again."

When the nurse assesses Ms. A, there is no response to commands or to having her name called. Her eyes are shut, and she does not open them even when the nurse applies nail bed pressure. Her pupils are unequal, with the right pupil larger than the left.

Ms. A's blood pressure is 70/30 mm Hg, she is in a sinus bradycardia with a rate of 40 beats/min, and her respiratory rate is 6 breaths/min. Her respirations are irregular, and she has 20-second periods of apnea. She has a large occipital laceration, and her left leg is misaligned.

The paramedics have a cervical collar and backboard in place. A 16-gauge catheter has been inserted at the left antecubital area, and lactated Ringer solution is infusing at 150 mL/hr.

1. Which action by the nurse should be completed **first**?
   1. Administer 100% oxygen by nonrebreather mask.
   2. Administer 500 ml normal saline IV bolus.
   3. Insert a nasopharyngeal airway (NPA).
   4. Direct the paramedic to perform a jaw thrust maneuver.

2. What is the **best** way to clearly document Ms. A's level of consciousness?
   1. Patient is comatose.
   2. Patient is unresponsive.
   3. Patient's Glasgow Coma Scale score is 4.
   4. Patient has a decreased level of consciousness.

3. The nurse notes that Ms. A has abnormal movement when pressure is applied to her nail beds, as shown in the illustration. What is the **best** way to document this finding?

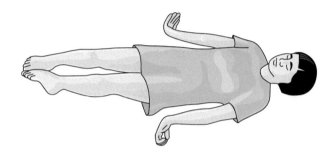

   1. Extensor rigidity
   2. Decorticate posturing
   3. Decerebrate posturing
   4. Traumatic brain injury

4. Based on Ms. A's history, vital signs, and assessment data, the patient is **most** at risk for which types of shock? **Select all that apply.**
   1. Cardiogenic
   2. Hypovolemic
   3. Neurogenic
   4. Septic
   5. Anaphylactic

5. A new medical resident is working in the ED today. Which action by the resident indicates a need for immediate intervention by the nurse?
   1. Assessing for the Babinski sign
   2. Increasing the IV infusion rate to 200 mL/hr
   3. Ordering an electrocardiogram (ECG)
   4. Preparing to perform a lumbar puncture

6. What is the **best** approach by the nurse when communicating concerns about the medical resident's decision making?
   1. Call the medical resident's supervisor about the concerns.
   2. Ask the nursing supervisor to discuss appropriate care with the medical resident.
   3. Advise the medical resident that lumbar puncture could cause brainstem herniation.
   4. Explain that lumbar puncture is not within the medical resident's scope of practice.

7. Which staff member will be **best** to assign to take primary responsibility for Ms. A's ongoing care?
   1. The RN from a temporary agency with extensive previous emergency experience who has been working in this ED for 3 days
   2. The LPN/LVN with 10 years of experience in the ED who is in the last semester of an RN program
   3. The RN who has worked in the ED for the past 5 years after transferring from the mother and baby unit
   4. The RN who has 12 years of intensive care unit (ICU) experience and has floated to the ED today

8. Ms. A suddenly begins to vomit. Which action should the nurse take **first**?
   1. Use the backboard to log-roll Ms. A to her side.
   2. Suction Ms. A's airway with an oral suction device.
   3. Hyperoxygenate Ms. A with a bag-valve mask system.
   4. Insert a nasogastric (NG) tube and connect to low suction.

9. The health care provider (HCP) prescribes these actions. Which action will the nurse take **first**?
   1. Notify family members of Ms. A's admission.
   2. Obtain computed tomography (CT) scan of head.
   3. Clean the occipital laceration and apply a dressing.
   4. Infuse famotidine 20 mg IV every 12 hours.

The results of laboratory tests that were performed when Ms. A arrived in the ED are faxed to the RN. Complete blood count results are as follows:

Hematocrit	42% (0.42)
Hemoglobin level	12.6 g/dL (126 g/L)
Platelet count	200,000/mm^3 (200 × 10^9/L)
White blood cell count	7500/mm^3 (7.5 × 10^9/L)

The metabolic profile shows the following:

Blood urea nitrogen level	13 mg/dL (4.64 mmol/L)
Chloride level	102 mEq/L (102 mmol/L)
Creatinine level	0.7 mg/dL (61.88 μmol/L)
Glucose level	144 mg/dL (7.99 mmol/L)
Magnesium level	1.7 mEq/L (0.85 mmol/L)
Potassium level	4.1 mEq/L (4.1 mmol/L)
Sodium level	133 mEq/L (133 mmol/L)

Arterial blood gas (ABG) results are as follows:

Arterial partial pressure of carbon dioxide (Paco$_2$)	56 mm Hg (7.45 kPa)
Arterial partial pressure of oxygen (Pao$_2$)	65 mm Hg (8.64 kPa)
Bicarbonate (HCO$_3$⁻)	22 mEq/L (22 mmol/L)
O$_2$ saturation	88% (0.88)
pH	7.3

10. Based on the laboratory values, which collaborative intervention will the nurse anticipate **next**?
    1. Type and cross-match for three units of packed red blood cells.
    2. Administer magnesium sulfate 1 g IV over the next 3 hours.
    3. Give insulin aspart dose based on the standard sliding scale.
    4. Obtain an endotracheal intubation tray and assist with intubation.

After being intubated and placed on mechanical ventilation, Ms. A is transported to the radiology department. The CT scans indicate that she has a large epidural hematoma. In addition, chest and left leg radiographs show that she has a left femur fracture and evidence of aspiration pneumonia.

When the nurse reassesses Ms. A, she is flaccid and has no response to verbal or painful stimulation. Her pupils are dilated and nonreactive to light. Vital sign values are:

Blood pressure	190/40 mm Hg
Heart rate	40 beats/min (sinus bradycardia)
O$_2$ saturation	92% (0.92)
Respiratory rate	14 breaths/min (ventilator controlled)
Temperature	96°F (35.6°C) (tympanic)

11. Which complication is the nurse **most** concerned about at present?
    1. Brainstem herniation
    2. Respiratory acidosis
    3. Hemorrhage
    4. Hypothermia

PART 3   Complex Health Scenarios

Answer Key for this chapter begins on p. 342

Ms. A is transported to the operating room, where the epidural hematoma is evacuated, and an open reduction and internal fixation of her left leg fracture is completed. After surgery, Ms. A is transferred to the ICU. She is attached to a cardiac monitor and has an arterial line in place. She is making no spontaneous respiratory effort but is being mechanically ventilated. Ms. A's indwelling urinary catheter is draining large amounts of clear, pale yellow urine. An intracranial monitor is in place. Her vital sign values and intracranial pressure (ICP) are as follows:

Blood pressure	112/64 mm Hg (mean arterial pressure [MAP] of 80 mm Hg)
Heart rate	50 to 56 beats/min (sinus bradycardia)
ICP	22 mm Hg (reference range, 5–15 mm Hg)
O₂ saturation	93% (0.93)
Respiratory rate	20 breaths/min (ventilator controlled)
Temperature	97.4°F (36.3°C) (tympanic)

12. Which of the assessment data listed above requires the **most** immediate nursing action?
    1. Cardiac rhythm
    2. Blood pressure
    3. O₂ saturation
    4. ICP

13. Enhanced Multiple Response

    Question:

    Which of these interventions will be used to meet the goal of maintaining Ms. A's cerebral perfusion pressure (CPP) at 60 mm Hg or more?

    Instructions: Place an X, in the space provided, or highlight each intervention that can be used. **Select all that apply.**
    1. _____ Keep the head of the bed el30 degrees.
    2. _____ Check pupil reaction to light every hour.
    3. _____ Reposition the patient at least every 2 hours.
    4. _____ Perform endotracheal suctionas necessary.
    5. _____ Check the Glasgow Coma Scale score hourly.
    6. _____ Administer mannitol 100 mg IV if ICP is above 20 mm Hg.
    7. _____ Titrate norepinephrine drip to maintain MAP above 80 mm Hg.
    8. _____ Keep the neck midline
    9. _____ Administer acetazolamide 500mg twice a day by mouth

14. The postcraniotomy care plan for the first postoperative day includes these nursing actions. Which actions can the nurse assign to an experienced LPN/LVN working in the ICU?

    1. Checking the gastric pH every 4 hours
    2. Performing a neurologic status examination every 2 hours
    3. Assessing breath sounds every 4 hours
    4. Turning the patient side to side every 2 hours
    5. Monitoring intake and output hourly
    6. Sending a urine specimen to check specific gravity daily
    7. Taking and recording vital signs

15. Which parameter indicates a need for an immediate change in the ventilator settings?
    1. Paco₂
    2. O₂ saturation
    3. HCO₃⁻
    4. Pao₂

16. Using the SBAR (situation, background, assessment, recommendations) format, in which order will the nurse communicate this information about the patient to the HCP?
    1. "I am concerned that Ms. A may develop worsening cerebral hypoxia caused by cerebral vasoconstriction and I would like to decrease the respiratory rate setting on the ventilator."
    2. "This is the nurse caring for Ms. A. The patient's most recent ABGs indicate that her Paco₂ is too low, possibly worsening her cerebral perfusion."
    3. "Her current ventilator respiratory rate is set at 20, and ABGs show the Paco₂ is 25 mm Hg (3.33 kPa), with a pH of 7.54. O₂ saturation is 96% (0.96) with a Pao₂ of 90 mm Hg (11.97 kPa)."
    4. "Ms. A is a 20-year-old woman who had evacuation of an epidural hematoma and has been nonresponsive and ventilator dependent since surgery."

Complex Health Scenarios   PART 3

17. The LPN/LVN reports that Ms. A's output for the past hour was 1200 mL and that her urine is very pale yellow. Which action is best for the nurse to take at this time?
    1. Instruct the LPN/LVN to continue to monitor the urine output hourly.
    2. Send a urine specimen to the laboratory to check specific gravity.
    3. Notify the neurosurgeon and anticipate an increase in the IV rate.
    4. Assess the patient's neurologic status for signs of increased irritability.

18. Ms. A's mother, who has been staying at the bedside, asks the nurse why her daughter is receiving omeprazole, stating that her daughter has no history of peptic ulcers. Which answer is best?
    1. "Omeprazole will lower the chance that she will aspirate."
    2. "Omeprazole decreases the incidence of gastric stress ulcers."
    3. "Omeprazole will reduce the risk for gastroesophageal reflux."
    4. "Omeprazole prevents gastric irritation caused by the orogastric tube."

19. About 20 minutes after Ms. A is positioned on her right side, her ICP has increased to 30 mm Hg. Which action should the nurse take **next**?
    1. Administer the as-needed (PRN) mannitol 100 mg IV.
    2. Assess the alignment of Ms. A's head and neck.
    3. Elevate the head of the bed to 45 degrees.
    4. Check Ms. A's pupil size and response to light.

20. When the nurse assesses Ms. A at 2:00 PM, her left leg is pale, swollen, and very firm to palpation. The left leg pulses are only faintly audible using a Doppler pulse monitor. Which action is **most** appropriate at this time?
    1. Call the orthopedic surgeon to communicate the assessment.
    2. Elevate the left leg on two pillows to decrease the swelling.
    3. Continue to monitor the left leg's appearance and pedal pulses.
    4. Assess the patient for indications of pain, such as restlessness.

21. As the shift ends, the nurse is preparing Ms. A for transfer to surgery for an emergency fasciotomy. What is the best option for obtaining informed consent for the fasciotomy?
    1. Informed consent is not needed for emergency surgery.
    2. Permission for surgery can be given by Ms. A's mother.
    3. Consent for surgery is not required for unconscious patients.
    4. Authorization can be given by the nursing supervisor.

22. Enhanced Multiple Response

Scenario: To prepare the clinical group for postconference, the nurse educator asks the student nurse to compile and explain a list of complications that could ocif an emergency fasciotomy was not carried out on Ms. A.

Instructions: Place an X, in the space provided, or highlight each complication that could occur. **Select all that apply.**
1. _____ Gangrene
2. _____ Loss of the limb
3. _____ Renal failure
4. _____ Cardiac dysrhythmias
5. _____ Contractures
6. _____ Cellulitis
7. _____ Stress fracture
8. _____ Permanent nerve damage
9. _____ Cardiac dysrhythmias

Answer Key for this chapter begins on p. 342

Answers

1. **Ans: 4** National guidelines for the emergency management of traumatic brain injury indicate that the assessment of airway and breathing is the priority action for this patient. Ms. A's slow and irregular respiratory rate is a risk factor for hypoxemia, which would decrease oxygen delivery to the brain as well as other vital organs and tissues. Performance of a jaw thrust maneuver will open the airway and should be used for a patient with C-spine precautions. Once the airway is clear and open, an oral pharyngeal airway can be inserted, oxygen can be applied, and the patient can be prepared for intubation. An NPA should not be inserted at this time because the patient has a head injury and the NPA could penetrate a fractured cribriform plate. IV fluids can be administered after airway and oxygenation issues have been addressed. **Focus:** Prioritization. **Test-Taking Tip:** When prioritizing the order of emergency trauma care, follow, in order, the acronym ABCDE for Airway, Breathing, Circulation, Disability, Exposure.

2. **Ans: 3** The Glasgow Coma Scale offers a standardized and objective way to assess and document neurologic status. Although the other responses also accurately describe the patient's level of consciousness, they do not provide objective data that can be readily used to determine changes in the patient's neurologic status. **Focus:** Prioritization.

3. **Ans: 3** Decerebrate posturing includes stiff extension of the arms and legs, plantar flexion of the feet, and arm pronation and usually indicates brainstem dysfunction. Documenting extensor rigidity alone would be an incomplete description of the patient's assessment. Decorticate posturing involves flexion and internal rotation of the arms. The patient clearly does have a traumatic brain injury, but a clear description of the baseline assessment by the nurse is needed. **Focus:** Prioritization.

4. **Ans: 2, 3** Ms. A's bradycardia and hypotension suggest that she is experiencing neurogenic shock in response to her head injury. It is also important to remember that with any traumatic injury, hypovolemic shock caused by hemorrhage should be considered. In this case, Ms. A should be assessed for blood loss associated with her leg injury and for internal bleeding caused by blunt trauma to her chest and abdomen. There are no indications in the patient's history that she is at risk for cardiac, septic, or anaphylactic shock. **Focus:** Prioritization.

5. **Ans: 4** Lumbar puncture is contraindicated in a patient who may have increased ICP because it increases the risk for herniation of the brainstem through the foramen magnum at the base of the skull. Checking for a positive Babinski sign and obtaining an ECG are not priorities for this patient but would not place the patient at any increased risk. Increasing the IV rate is appropriate based on the patient's blood pressure. **Focus:** Prioritization.

6. **Ans: 3** The Core Competencies for Interprofessional Collaborative Practice indicate that professionals should clearly express knowledge and opinions about patient care to ensure common understanding of information, treatment, and care decisions. In this situation, the nurse needs to rapidly and clearly communicate with the resident to prevent injury to the patient. Calling the resident's supervisor or asking the nursing supervisor to intervene may also be appropriate, but a more direct approach is best in the current situation. The resident will be familiar with medical scope of practice. **Focus:** Prioritization.

7. **Ans: 3** The initial care of patients with traumatic injuries requires the expertise of an RN with extensive ED experience. Neither the agency RN nor the float RN will be familiar with the location of equipment and with the organization of care in the ED. Although the LPN has experience, the LPN/LVN scope of practice does not include the complex assessments and interventions that will be needed in caring for this patient. (The LPN could be assigned to assist the RN in caring for Ms. A, however.) **Focus:** Assignment.

8. **Ans: 1** The most important goal for an unconscious patient who is vomiting is to prevent aspiration. Turning Ms. A to her side (while maintaining cervical spine stability through the use of the backboard and cervical collar) is the best method to ensure that she does not aspirate. Suctioning would also be used but does not clear the airway as well as having the patient positioned on her side. Hyperoxygenation may also be required for this patient but will not protect the airway while she is vomiting. An NG tube is usually not inserted in patients with possible facial fractures. Insertion of an orogastric tube may be indicated but would not protect from aspiration at the present time. **Focus:** Prioritization. **Test-Taking Tip:** Remember that maintenance of the airway and prevention of aspiration will be a priority for any patient who has a decreased level of consciousness.

9. **Ans: 2** National advanced trauma life support guidelines indicate that a CT scan should be done as soon as possible after a closed head injury to determine the extent and types of injury and guide interventions, such as surgery. The other actions are also appropriate for the patient but do not need implementation as rapidly. **Focus:** Prioritization.

10. **Ans: 4** Ms. A's ABG results indicate uncompensated respiratory acidosis and hypoxemia. Because her respiratory drive is suppressed, she will need rapid intubation and ventilation using a mechanical positive-pressure ventilator. She may need surgery, in which case it would be appropriate to have blood available in the blood bank. Although ongoing monitoring of the magnesium level is indicated, the magnesium level is in the low-normal range, so administration of magnesium is not a priority at this time. Insulin would not typically be administered for a small glucose elevation such as this in a nonfasting patient. **Focus:** Prioritization.

11. **Ans: 1** The patient's fixed and dilated pupils, widened pulse pressure, and bradycardia are caused by increasing pressure on the brainstem and indicate that she is at risk for brainstem herniation, which would result in brain death. Immediate surgical intervention is needed to prevent this complication. She is at risk for the other complications, but they are not as life threatening. **Focus:** Prioritization. **Test-Taking Tip:** Although pupil dilation is associated with increases in ICP, remember that this is usually a late sign. You will want to monitor carefully for earlier signs of increased ICP, such as subtle changes in memory, orientation, and responsiveness, and communicate these changes quickly to the HCP.

12. **Ans: 4** Normal ICP is 0 to 15 mm Hg, and CPP should be at least 60 mm Hg or higher. CPP is calculated using the formula MAP − ICP = CPP. Ms. A's CPP is 58 mm Hg (80 − 22 = 58); interventions should be implemented immediately to decrease her ICP and improve CPP. The other data indicate a need for ongoing monitoring but do not require immediate intervention. **Focus:** Prioritization.

13. **Ans: 1, 6, 7, 8** Evidence-based guidelines recommend the use of mannitol in patients who have traumatic brain injury with increased ICP to reduce ICP and improve CPP. In hypotensive patients, cerebral perfusion may also be improved by administering vasopressors to raise arterial pressure. Positioning the head of the bed at 30 degrees also reduces cerebral edema by promoting venous drainage from the cerebral circulation. Keeping the neck midline encourages venous drainage. Although neurologic assessments such as checking the Glasgow Coma Scale score and observing pupil reaction to light are necessary, the stimulation caused by these interventions can increase ICP. Suctioning and repositioning also cause transient increases in ICP. It is important to monitor intracranial and arterial pressures during these procedures and modify care to avoid unnecessary increases in ICP. Administration of acetazolamide may be beneficial however the patient is intubated and should not be given medications by mouth. **Focus:** Prioritization.

14. **Ans: 1, 5, 6, 7** Checking gastric pH, monitoring intake and output, obtaining urine specimens, and taking vital signs are included in LPN/LVN education and scope of practice. An experienced LPN/LVN would be expected to report any changes in patient status to the supervising RN. Usually repositioning a patient would also be included in the LPN/LVN role; however, this patient is at risk for increased ICP during positioning and should be monitored by the RN during and after repositioning. Assessments of breath sounds and neurologic status in critically ill patients should be accomplished by an experienced RN. **Focus:** Assignment.

15. **Ans: 1** Lower-than-normal $Paco_2$ levels cause cerebral vasoconstriction and result in further cerebral hypoxia. The RN should notify the HCP and anticipate a decrease in the ventilator rate. The oxygen percentage being delivered by the ventilator should be evaluated because a lower fraction of inspired oxygen (Fio_2) may be adequate. Nevertheless, the current Pao_2 will not have any adverse effect on cerebral perfusion. The decrease in HCO_3^- reflects a compensatory mechanism for the patient's respiratory alkalosis and will resolve spontaneously when the Pao_2 level rises. **Focus:** Prioritization. **Test-Taking Tip:** When analyzing ABGs, always consider both oxygenation (using Pao_2 and oxygen saturation) and acid-base balance (using pH, $Paco_2$, and HCO_3^-). Even if the patient's oxygenation is adequate, disorders in acid-base balance may lead to poor outcomes.

16. **Ans: 2, 4, 3, 1** Using the SBAR format, the nurse first describes the primary concern (situation) and then provides background information about the patient. Next, the nurse discusses pertinent assessment data. Finally, recommendations for needed changes in the treatment plan are communicated. **Focus:** Prioritization.

17. **Ans: 3** Ms. A's high urine output suggests that she has developed diabetes insipidus, a common complication of intracranial surgery. Because diabetes insipidus can rapidly lead to dehydration in a patient who is unable to take in oral fluids, the priority action needed is to increase the IV rate. Continuing to monitor the output and checking the specific gravity would also be needed but would not correct the risk for hypovolemia and hypotension. Because Ms. A's neurologic status is so poor, it is unlikely that changes in her neurologic status would be helpful in determining the effects of fluid and electrolyte imbalance. **Focus:** Prioritization.

18. **Ans: 2** Gastric stress ulcers are a common complication of head injury unless histamine$_2$ blockers (e.g., famotidine) or proton pump inhibitors (e.g., omeprazole) are administered prophylactically. Administration of omeprazole may decrease the risk of pneumonitis if aspiration occurs, minimize the effects of gastroesophageal reflux, and decrease stomach irritation, but none of the other responses addresses the use of proton pump inhibitors in patients with head injury. **Focus:** Prioritization.

PART 3 Complex Health Scenarios

19. **Ans: 2**   Because the patient has just been repositioned, it is likely that the elevated ICP is caused by poor positioning. The head and neck should be maintained in good alignment because neck flexion can cause venous obstruction and an increase in ICP. Administration of mannitol and further elevation of the head of the bed may be needed if repositioning Ms. A's head and neck is ineffective. These measures should only be used, however, if her MAP is high enough to maintain a CPP of 60 mm Hg. Checking Ms. A's pupils would not offer any additional information, and the stimulation may increase the ICP. **Focus:** Prioritization.

20. **Ans: 1**   The assessment data suggest the development of compartment syndrome, an emergency that can lead to permanent neuromuscular damage within 4 to 6 hours without rapid treatment. Elevation of the leg will further reduce blood flow to the leg. Continuing to monitor the leg without correcting the compartment syndrome will allow the ischemia to persist. Although restlessness may indicate pain in patients with intact neurologic function, Ms. A's neurologic status is severely compromised, and monitoring for restlessness will not be helpful in assessing for ischemic leg pain. **Focus:** Prioritization.

21. **Ans: 2**   When a patient is unable to provide informed consent for a procedure, a close family member (who is likely to be most knowledgeable about the patient's wishes) is able to give permission. Emergency procedures can take place without written consent for an unconscious or incompetent patient when no family or legal representative is available to give permission. The nursing supervisor does not have the authority to consent to surgery for an unconscious patient. **Focus:** Prioritization.

22. **Ans: 1, 2, 3, 4, 5, 8, 9**   Compartment Syndrome is an increase of muscle pressure in an extremity. The increase in pressure is most often caused by trauma (broken bone, burns) that causes bleeding inside the muscle. The bleeding raises the pressure within the muscle and causes muscle and nerve damage. Complications of compartment syndrome include infection. If the infection is not recognized and treated in time, an amputation is likely to prevent gangrene. Contractures can set in if the ischemia is lengthy. Hyperkalemia occurs from electrolytes leaking out of the damaged cells. This can cause life-threatening cardiac dysrhythmias. Damaged muscles also leak proteins (myoglobin) and cause myoglobinuria, which can cause renal failure. Cellulitis is a skin infection, not a complication, and rarely causes a compartment syndrome. Stress fractures are not a complication but can be a cause of compartment syndrome. **Focus:** Assignment.

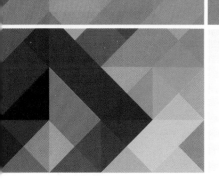

CASE STUDY 14

Septic Shock

Questions

Ms. D, a 54-year-old patient, is brought to the emergency department (ED) by her daughter because of weakness and a decreasing level of consciousness. The daughter says that Ms. D has been reporting nausea, with associated abdominal and back pain. Although Ms. D is usually very alert and oriented, today she has been increasingly lethargic.

Her medical history includes hypertension, atrial fibrillation, and diabetes mellitus type 2.

The initial vital sign values are as follows:

Blood pressure	102/38 mm Hg
Heart rate	102 beats/min
O_2 saturation	76% (0.76)
Respiratory rate	30 breaths/min
Temperature	102.4°F (39.1°C)

1. Based on the initial history and assessment, what is the **first** action of the nurse?
   1. Administer an acetaminophen suppository to lower the temperature.
   2. Start oxygen and maintain oxygen saturation at 90% or higher.
   3. Place the patient on a cardiac monitor.
   4. Initiate intravenous access with normal saline at a keep open rate.

2. Which method of oxygen administration will be best to increase Ms. D's oxygen saturation?
   1. Nasal cannula
   2. Nonrebreather mask
   3. Venturi mask
   4. Simple face mask

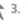 **3.** Enhanced Multiple Response

Case Study and Question

In addition to Ms. D, the nurse is providing care for several other critically ill patients in the emergency room. Available staffing in the ED includes an experienced assistive personnel (AP).

Which actions should the nurse assign to the AP?

Instructions: Read the case study on the left then refer to the case study to answer the question. Circle or highlight the correct answers. **Select all that apply.**
1. Measuring vital signs every 15 minutes
2. Attaching the patient to a cardiac monitor
3. Documenting a head-to-toe assessment
4. Checking orientation and alertness
5. Inserting an IV line
6. Monitoring urine output hourly
7. Obtaining fingerstick blood sugar results
8. Assisting discharged patients to a waiting vehicle
9. Obtaining sutures and a suture tray for the health care provider (HCP)

4. The cardiac monitor shows this rhythm for Ms. D. Routine treatment orders for dysrhythmias are in the ED protocols. Which action should the nurse take **next**?
   1. Continue to monitor cardiac rhythm.
   2. Administer metoprolol 5 mg IV push.
   3. Prepare to perform cardioversion at 50 J.
   4. Administer amiodarone 150 mg IV push.

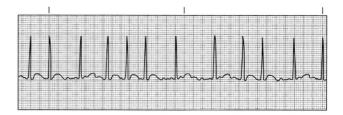

An arterial blood gas (ABG) analysis is performed on Ms. D and the following results are obtained:

Arterial partial pressure of carbon dioxide ($Paco_2$)	62 mm Hg (8.25 kPa)
Arterial partial pressure of oxygen (Pao_2)	50 mm Hg (6.65 kPa)
Bicarbonate (HCO_3^-)	22 mEq/L (22 mmol/L)
O_2 saturation	82% (0.82)
pH	7.23

5. Based on an analysis of the ABG values, which collaborative intervention will the nurse anticipate **next**?
   1. Sodium bicarbonate bolus IV
   2. Endotracheal intubation and mechanical ventilation
   3. Continuous monitoring of Ms. D's respiratory status
   4. Nebulized albuterol therapy

6. When the nurse is preparing to assist with the endotracheal intubation of Ms. D, in which order will these actions be accomplished?
   1. Use capnography to check for exhaled carbon dioxide.
   2. Secure the endotracheal tube in place.
   3. Preoxygenate with the bag-valve mask device at 100% oxygen.
   4. Inflate the endotracheal tube cuff.
   5. Obtain all the needed equipment and supplies.
   6. Insert the endotracheal tube orally through the vocal cords.

   _____, _____, _____, _____, _____, _____

After the successful intubation, the nurse performs a rapid assessment of Ms. D and documents the findings: "Apical pulse irregularly irregular. Face flushed and warm. Extremities cool and mottled. Breath sounds audible bilaterally with crackles present in lung bases. Reports pain with suprapubic palpation. Urine is amber and cloudy, with red streaks. 100 mL urine output when Foley catheter inserted."

The patient's current vital sign values and capillary blood glucose are as follows:

Blood pressure	86/40 mm Hg
Heart rate	102 beats/min
O_2 saturation	93% (0.93)
Respiratory rate	32 breaths/min
Temperature	103°F (39.4°C)
Capillary blood glucose	167 mg/dL (9.27 mmol/L)

7. Which data collected about this patient are **most** important in alerting the nurse to a diagnosis of sepsis? **Select all that apply.**
   1. Hematuria
   2. Atrial fibrillation
   3. Temperature
   4. Apical pulse rate
   5. Blood glucose level
   6. Respiratory rate

8. Based on the assessment data and vital signs, which collaborative actions should the nurse anticipate at this time? **Select all that apply.**
   1. Send specimens for blood and urine culture.
   2. Start norepinephrine infusion at 8 mcg/min.
   3. Give normal saline bolus of 30 mL/kg.
   4. Draw blood for serum lactate level.
   5. Administer vancomycin 1 g IV.
   6. Administer sodium bicarbonate 1 meq/kg IV.

9. When the nurse is infusing the normal saline, which action is **most** important in evaluating for an adverse reaction to the rapid fluid infusion?
   1. Palpating for any peripheral edema
   2. Monitoring urine output
   3. Listening to lung sounds
   4. Checking for jugular venous distention

After infusion of the normal saline bolus, Ms. D's blood pressure is 92/42 mm Hg. Lactate level is elevated at 36.04 mg/dL (4 mmol/L). Norepinephrine infusion is prescribed at 8 mcg/min, and infusion is started through a peripheral IV line.

10. When assessing the norepinephrine infusion site, the nurse notes that the skin around the IV insertion site is cool and pale. Which action should be taken **first**?
    1. Shut off the infusion pump.
    2. Assess for pain at the site.
    3. Notify the HCP about the possible norepinephrine extravasation.
    4. Inject the pale area with phentolamine solution per hospital protocol.

11. The nurse is preparing to transfer Ms. D to the intensive care unit (ICU). Using the SBAR (situation, background, assessment, recommendations) format, in what order will the nurse communicate pertinent information about Ms. D to the ICU nurse?
    1. "Current blood pressure is 92/42, pulse rate is 112, and respirations are 32. Capillary blood glucose is 167 mg/dL (9.27 mmol/L), and lactate level is 36.04 mg/dL (4 mmol/L). Blood and urine cultures are pending."
    2. "The patient has diabetes and chronic atrial fibrillation. She has been experiencing nausea, abdominal pain, and back pain. Today she was noted to be increasingly lethargic."
    3. "Ms. D will need a central line insertion for fluid and vasopressor management, along with titration of norepinephrine and normal saline to maintain mean arterial pressure at 65 mm Hg."
    4. "Ms. D is ready to transfer to intensive care. She has septic shock and is receiving mechanical ventilation, norepinephrine drip, and normal saline infusion through a peripheral line."

    _____, _____, _____, _____

Ms. D is transferred to the ICU, and a two-port central IV line is started at the subclavian site to infuse fluids and norepinephrine.

12. The ICU nurse is working with an experienced LPN/LVN in caring for Ms. D. Which nursing activities included in the care plan should be assigned to the LPN/LVN? **Select all that apply.**
    1. Documenting the hourly urinary output
    2. Monitoring the central line site for signs of infection
    3. Checking capillary blood glucose levels every 2 hours
    4. Completing a head-to-toe assessment every 4 hours
    5. Administering sliding-scale insulin lispro per protocol
    6. Infusing normal saline at 400 mL/hr

After 2 hours, the values for vital signs are as follows:

Blood pressure	104/56 mm Hg
Heart rate	104 beats/min (atrial fibrillation)
O₂ saturation	92% (0.92)
Central venous pressure	3 mm Hg
Respiratory rate	26 breaths/min
Temperature	101.6°F (38.7°C) (rectal)

13. Which information about Ms. D is **most** important for the nurse to communicate rapidly to the HCP?
    1. Decreased blood pressure
    2. Ongoing atrial fibrillation
    3. Low central venous pressure
    4. Continued temperature elevation

14. Which of these actions prescribed by the HCP will be **most** important for the nurse to question?
    1. Increase oxygen flow rate (F_{IO_2}).
    2. Raise normal saline rate to 450 mL/hr.
    3. Administer acetaminophen 650 mg rectally.
    4. Increase norepinephrine infusion rate to 12 mcg/kg.

The nurse quickly reviews Ms. D's latest laboratory test results, which have just arrived on the unit:

Hematocrit	32% (0.32)
Hemoglobin level	10.9 g/dL (109 g/L)
Platelet count	96,000/mm³ (96 × 10⁹/L)
White blood cell count	26,000/mm³ (26 × 10⁹/L)
Blood urea nitrogen level	56 mg/dL (19.99 mmol/L)
Creatinine level	2.9 mg dL (256.36 μmol/L)
Glucose level	330 mg/dL (18.32 mmol/L)
Potassium level	5.2 mEq/L (5.2 mmol/L)
Sodium level	140 mEq/L (140 mmol/L)

15. Which laboratory value requires the **most** immediate action by the nurse?
    1. Creatinine level
    2. Glucose level
    3. Potassium level
    4. Hemoglobin level

16. At the end of the shift, the supervisor consults with the nurse about which of these oncoming staff members should be assigned to care for Ms. D. Which RN will be best to assign to care for this patient?
    1. Travel RN with 20 years of ICU experience who has been working in this ICU for 4 months
    2. Newly graduated RN who worked in the ICU as a nursing assistant and has finished the precepted orientation
    3. Experienced ICU RN who has been called in on a day off to work for the first 4 hours of the shift
    4. RN who has been floated from the post-anesthesia care unit (PACU) to the ICU for the shift

PART 3 Complex Health Scenarios

 Answer Key for this chapter begins on p. 349

17. Cloze

Scenario: The student nurse is assigned a post conference lecture on the Quick Sequential Organ Failure Assessment Score (qSOFA). The student reports that a patient should be evaluated for organ dysfunction if assessment criteria are met. Adults should be assessed for a respiratory rate greater or equal to _____1_____ breaths per minute, altered mental status and a systolic blood pressure less than _____2_____. The sepsis bundle states that within ___3___ hours of suspected sepsis a lactate level should be measured, blood cultures drawn, and broad spectrum antibiotics given. Fluid resuscitation at ___4___ ml/kg should begin if hypotension or a lactate level greater or equal to 4 mmol/L is present.

Instructions: Complete the sentences by choosing the most probable option for the missing information that corresponds with the same numbered list of options provided.

Option 1	Option 2	Option 3	Option 4
18	100	3	20
22	120	2	30
24	90	1	40
30	80	4	10

Answers

1. **Ans: 2** The oxygen saturation indicates that the patient is severely hypoxemic (despite an increased respiratory rate). Because this hypoxia will affect all other body systems, it should be treated immediately. The other orders should also be rapidly implemented, but they do not require action as urgently as the low oxygen saturation. **Focus:** Prioritization. **Test-Taking Tip:** When patients are in critical distress, the ABCs (airway, breathing, and circulation) are usually the best guide to the priority actions, no matter what the patient diagnosis is.

2. **Ans: 2** A nonrebreather mask can provide a fraction of inspired oxygen (FiO_2) of close to 100%, which will be needed for this severely hypoxemic patient. Nasal cannulas deliver a maximum FiO_2 of 44%, simple face masks deliver an FiO_2 of up to 60%, and Venturi masks provide a maximum FiO_2 of 55%. **Focus:** Prioritization. **Test-Taking Tip:** Since administration of oxygen is a common nursing action, you will need to know which type of oxygen administration equipment is needed to achieve a variety of FiO_2 percentages.

3. **Ans: 1, 2, 6, 7, 8, 9** Checking vital signs, obtaining fingerstick blood glucose, and monitoring urine output is included in AP education. Experienced APs will know which patient information to report immediately to the supervising RN. APs working in the ED would also have been trained and know how to establish cardiac monitoring, although dysrhythmia analysis and treatment are the responsibility of the RN. An AP may assist an already discharged patient to the waiting vehicle, and an experienced AP in the ER is able to obtain sutures and a suture tray to assist the HCP. Obtaining and documenting assessments and starting an IV line should be done by the RN. **Focus:** Assignment.

4. **Ans: 1** Although atrial fibrillation at rapid rates can cause a significant drop in cardiac output, the current rate of 100 to 110 beats/min is not a likely cause of the patient's hypotension. Ongoing cardiac rhythm monitoring is necessary, but no treatment of the patient's chronic atrial fibrillation is needed at this time. Cardioversion or administration of antidysrhythmic medications such as amiodarone or metoprolol may be considered if the heart rate increases. **Focus:** Prioritization.

5. **Ans: 2** The ABG values indicate that the patient is hypoxemic (low PaO_2 and oxygen saturation) and has a severe uncompensated respiratory acidosis (low pH and elevated $PaCO_2$). Because she is unable to maintain adequate oxygenation and ventilation independently, intubation and mechanical ventilation are indicated. Sodium bicarbonate is administered only if metabolic acidosis is present. Although the patient will need ongoing respiratory monitoring and may also benefit from albuterol therapy, these therapies are not adequate in a patient with these severe ABG abnormalities. **Focus:** Prioritization.

6. **Ans: 5, 3, 6, 4, 1, 2** All needed equipment and supplies should be obtained before the intubation attempt. To minimize hypoxemia during the procedure, the patient should be preoxygenated for 3 to 5 minutes before the intubation attempt. After the endotracheal tube is inserted by the HCP, inflation of the endotracheal tube cuff is needed for effective ventilation. Checking for exhaled carbon dioxide through continuous wave-form capnography is the most accurate way to assess endotracheal placement. After the initial assessment of endotracheal placement is completed, the tube should be secured. **Focus:** Prioritization.

7. **Ans: 1, 3, 4, 6** The criteria for sepsis is evident in this patient. She has an altered mental status, tachycardia (over 100 beats/min), hypotension (systolic less than 100), temperature over 38.3°C, and a respiratory rate over 22 breaths/min. Ms. D's hematuria (especially with associated suprapubic and back pain) suggests urinary tract infection, pyelonephritis, or both. Atrial fibrillation is chronic for this patient and not an indicator of sepsis. Blood glucose higher than 140 mg/dL (7.77 mmol/L) would suggest sepsis in a nondiabetic patient but is not unusually elevated in this patient who has diabetes. **Focus:** Prioritization. **Test-Taking Tip:** Keep an eye on the Surviving Sepsis guidelines; this important evidence-based information was designed to assist in early detection and rapid treatment of a life-threatening condition. It is likely that these guidelines will be periodically updated throughout your career.

8. **Ans: 1, 3, 4, 5** The initial resuscitation bundle in the Surviving Sepsis guidelines recommends that the measurement of the lactate level, the obtaining of cultures, the administration of broad-spectrum antibiotics, and the infusion of crystalloid solutions such as normal saline be initiated rapidly when sepsis is suspected. Norepinephrine will be indicated if blood pressure remains low after rapid fluid infusion has been accomplished. Even though the pH becomes higher, it is best to treat the cause of the acidosis so sodium bicarbonate is not used to treat acidosis. **Focus:** Prioritization.

9. **Ans: 3** The most common complication of too-rapid IV infusion of fluids is volume overload, leading to fluid overload and heart failure. Although peripheral edema, decreased urine output, and jugular venous distention may be indicators that heart failure is

PART 3 · Complex Health Scenarios

developing, they do not occur as rapidly as the backup of fluids into the pulmonary capillaries and then into the alveoli. **Focus:** Prioritization.

10. **Ans: 1** The first action should be to stop the infusion because pallor and coolness at the site indicate possible extravasation. Assessment for pain, notification of the HCP, and injection of phentolamine at the site to cause vasodilation are also appropriate but should be done after stopping the infusion. **Focus:** Prioritization.

11. **Ans: 4, 2, 1, 3** When using the SBAR format, the nurse initially describes the current situation, then gives appropriate background information, and then the most current assessment data. Finally, the nurse provides recommendations for any anticipated patient needs so that the receiving staff can prepare for patient care. **Focus:** Prioritization.

12. **Ans: 1, 3, 5** LPN/LVNs are educated and licensed to perform tasks such as monitoring and documenting intake and output, monitoring blood glucose at the bedside, and administering insulin under the supervision of an RN. Although LPN/LVNs can collect data about stable patients, head-to-toe and central line assessments of critically ill patients should be done by RNs. LPN/LVNs may be able to administer IV fluids to stable patients (depending on state nurse practice acts and on hospital policy), but infusion of large volumes to unstable patients requires more education and scope of practice and should be done by RN staff members with experience in caring for critically ill patients. **Focus:** Assignment.

13. **Ans: 3** The low central venous pressure indicates that the patient is still hypovolemic and will need an increase in IV fluids. The arterial blood pressure and temperature have improved. The patient has chronic atrial fibrillation, and the rate has remained stable. **Focus:** Prioritization.

14. **Ans: 4** In a hypovolemic patient, increasing the norepinephrine rate will not improve perfusion and may increase the risk for adverse norepinephrine effects such as arrhythmias. The nurse may question the other prescribed actions, but these are not as likely to result in poor patient outcomes. A higher-than-prescribed normal saline infusion rate may be needed to improve volume status, the patient's temperature is already decreasing in response to antibiotic therapy, and oxygen saturation is already at an adequate (though not optimal) level. **Focus:** Prioritization.

15. **Ans: 2** The elevated glucose level will require administration of the ordered insulin lispro using the hospital standard sliding-scale insulin orders. Potassium will move into cells along with glucose as insulin is administered, so the patient's potassium level does not require additional treatment. The other abnormalities indicate the need for continued monitoring but will not require any immediate action at this time. **Focus:** Prioritization.

16. **Ans: 1** The travel RN has the required experience to provide care in this complex case and has been working at the hospital long enough to be familiar with how to obtain supplies, communicate with other departments, and so on. The other nurses either lack experience in caring for critically ill patients (the new graduate and the PACU nurse) or will not be able to offer the continuity of care that is desirable for the patient. **Focus:** Assignment.

17. **Ans: Option 1, 22; Option 2, 100; Option 3, 3; Option 4, 30.** The student nurse is assigned a post-conference lecture on the Quick Sequential Organ Failure Assessment Score (qSOFA). The student reports that a patient should be evaluated for organ dysfunction if two assessment criteria are met. Adults should be assessed for a respiratory rate greater or equal to 22 breaths per minute, altered mental status, and a systolic blood pressure less than 100.
The sepsis bundle states than within 3 hours of suspected sepsis a lactate level should be measured, blood cultures drawn, and broad spectrum antibiotics given. Fluid resuscitation at 30 ml/kg should begin if hypotension or a lactate level greater or equal to 4mmol/L is present.
The clinical presentation of sepsis/septic shock includes an altered mental status, tachycardia, hypotension, dyspnea, fever, and decreased capillary refill. It is imperative to recognize at least two of three qSOFA criteria (respiratory rate greater than 22, altered mental status, and systolic blood pressure less than 100) so that labs, antibiotics and fluid resuscitation can begin. Sepsis is a medical emergency and death will occur if it is not quickly recognized and treated. The mortality rate for septic shock is greater than 50%. **Focus:** Assignment.

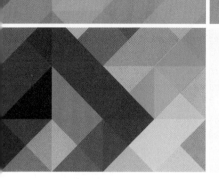

CASE STUDY 15

Heart Failure

Questions

The nurse admits Ms. C, an 81-year-old patient, to the intensive care unit (ICU). Ms. C, who has a history of mitral valve regurgitation and left ventricular failure, came to the emergency department (ED) with symptoms of increasing shortness of breath over the past week. The patient received furosemide 100 mg IV in the ED, and she is receiving oxygen via a nasal cannula at 4 L/min.

When Ms. C arrives in the ICU, she is sitting up in bed at a 60-degree angle. She is pale, with circumoral cyanosis, and her respirations appear labored and rapid. She indicates that she feels very short of breath.

1. What action should the nurse take **first**?
   1. Listen to the breath sounds.
   2. Place the patient on an electrocardiogram monitor.
   3. Check the oxygen saturation.
   4. Raise the head of the bed to 75 degrees and lower the legs.

When the nurse assesses Ms. C, she has crackles audible throughout both lung fields and is coughing up pink, frothy sputum. Her oxygen saturation is 85% (0.85) with the oxygen at 4 L/min per the nasal cannula. The respiratory rate is 38 breaths/min, and she has 3 + to 4 + pitting edema in her feet and up to her midcalf. With the head of the bed elevated to a 75-degree angle, the jugular veins are distended up to the jawline.

2. Based on the patient's history and assessment, the nurse will be **most** concerned about which complication?
   1. Pulmonary edema
   2. Cor pulmonale
   3. Pneumonia
   4. Pulmonary embolus

3. Which action will the nurse take **next**?
   1. Activate the hospital's rapid response team (RRT).
   2. Switch to a nonrebreather mask at a O_2 flow rate of 15 L/min.
   3. Order arterial blood gases (ABGs) and lab work now.
   4. Administer the prescribed morphine sulfate 2 mg IV to the patient.

4. What additional assessment data are **most** important to obtain at this time?
   1. Skin color and capillary refill
   2. Orientation and pupil reaction to light
   3. Heart sounds and point of maximum impulse
   4. Blood pressure and apical pulse

5. Ms. C's blood pressure is 98/52 mm Hg, and her apical pulse is 116 beats/min. The cardiac monitor shows sinus tachycardia at a rate of 110 to 120 beats/min. Which action prescribed by the health care provider (HCP) will the nurse implement **first**?
   1. Give enalapril 2.5 mg PO.
   2. Administer furosemide 100 mg IV.
   3. Obtain a blood potassium level.
   4. Insert a no. 16 urinary catheter.

6. Which prescribed action is best to assign to the experienced LPN/LVN who is assisting with the patient's care?
   1. Give enalapril 2.5 mg PO.
   2. Administer furosemide 100 mg IV.
   3. Obtain a blood potassium level.
   4. Insert a no. 16 urinary catheter.

7. The nurse administers morphine sulfate 2 mg IV to Ms. C. A newly graduated RN who has just started in the ICU asks why morphine is prescribed for this patient. Which responses made by the nurse best answer the newly graduated nurse's question? **Select all that apply.**
   1. "To help prevent chest discomfort."
   2. "To slow Ms. C's respiratory rate."
   3. "To lower Ms. C's anxiety level."
   4. "To decrease venous return to the heart."
   5. "To heighten perception and create a feeling of well-being."
   6. "To increase venous tone."

8. Ms. C's potassium level is 3.3 mEq/L (3.3 mmol/L). The HCP prescribes potassium chloride (KCl) 10 mEq IV. How should the nurse administer the KCl?
   1. Use an infusion pump to give the KCl over 10 minutes.
   2. Dilute the KCl in 100 mL of 5% dextrose in water (D_5W) and infuse over 1 hour.
   3. Administer the KCl by IV push over at least 1 minute using a 10-mL syringe.
   4. Add the KCl to 1 L of D_5W and administer over 8 hours.

9. After infusing the KCl, the nurse administers the furosemide to Ms. C. Which nursing action will be **most** useful in evaluating whether the furosemide is having the desired effect?
   1. Weighing the patient daily
   2. Measuring hourly urine output
   3. Monitoring blood pressure
   4. Assessing lung sounds

10. Ms. C's HCP arrives and, after assessing her status, prescribes nesiritide 100 mcg (2 mcg/kg) IV bolus followed by a continuous IV infusion of 0.5 mcg/min (0.01 mcg/kg/min). Which parameter is **most** important to monitor during the nesiritide infusion?
    1. Heart rate
    2. Blood pressure
    3. Peripheral edema
    4. Neurologic status

11. The nurse is preparing to leave at the end of the shift. Which oncoming nurse is best to assign to care for Ms. C?
    1. Float RN who has worked on the coronary step-down unit for 9 years and has floated to the ICU before
    2. RN from a staffing agency who has 5 years of ICU experience and is orienting to the ICU today
    3. Experienced ICU RN who is already assigned to care for a newly admitted patient with chest trauma
    4. Newly graduated RN who needs more experience in caring for patients with left ventricular failure

A few days later, Ms. C has improved enough to transfer to the step-down unit. Her weight has decreased 4 kg from the admission weight. A systolic murmur is audible at the apex of the heart. She denies shortness of breath and has crackles only at the lung bases. The cardiac monitor shows sinus rhythm with frequent premature ventricular contractions (PVCs). Ms. C reports no dizziness but says that her vision seems "fuzzy." She has 2 + pitting ankle edema. Her vital sign measurements are as follows:

Blood pressure	118/62 mm Hg
Heart rate	86 beats/min
O_2 saturation	95% (0.95), (room air)
Respiratory rate	24 breaths/min
Temperature	97.8°F (36.6°C)

Her medications are the following:
- *Furosemide 40 mg PO twice daily*
- *Aspirin 81 mg PO daily*
- *KCl 10 mEq PO daily*
- *Enalapril 2.5 mg PO daily*
- *Digoxin 0.25 mg PO daily*

12. Which of the assessment findings described earlier are **most** important to report to the HCP?
    1. Crackles and oxygen saturation
    2. Frequent PVCs and fuzzy vision
    3. Apical murmur and pulse rate
    4. Ankle edema and current weight

13. Which current laboratory values for this patient will be **most** important for the nurse to review? **Select all that apply.**
    1. Potassium
    2. Glucose
    3. Magnesium
    4. B-type natriuretic peptide (BNP)
    5. Calcium
    6. Albumin
    7. Creatinine

The laboratory results are:

Laboratory Test:	Result:
Glucose	96 mg/dL (5.33 mmol/L)
Potassium	3.4 mEq/L (3.4 mmol/L)
Magnesium	1.4 mEq/L (0.7 mmol/L)
Calcium	9.1 mg/dL (2.27 mmol/L)
Albumin	3.7 g/dL (37 g/L)
Creatinine	0.96 mg/dL (84.86 µmol/L)
B-type Natriuretic Peptide	194 pg/mL (194 pmol/L)

Answer Key for this chapter begins on p. 354

14. All of Ms. C's medications are scheduled to be given at 9:00 AM. Based on the patient's assessment data and laboratory results, which medications will the nurse hold until after consulting with the HCP? **Select all that apply.**
    1. Furosemide
    2. Aspirin
    3. KCl
    4. Enalapril
    5. Digoxin

15. Using the SBAR (situation, background, assessment, recommendation) format, indicate the order in which the nurse will communicate concerns to the HCP.
    1. "Today her lungs are clear to auscultation, but her potassium level is 3.4 mEq/L (3.4 mmol/L). I am concerned that she may have digoxin toxicity."
    2. "I'd like to obtain a digoxin level and administer additional potassium supplements before giving the prescribed digoxin and furosemide."
    3. "This is the nurse caring for Ms. C; I am calling because she has some PVCs and reports fuzzy vision."
    4. "Ms. C was admitted several days ago with pulmonary edema and dyspnea. She has been receiving digoxin and furosemide daily since admission."

    _____, _____, _____, _____

Ms. C is discharged 2 days later. Her discharge medications are:
- *Furosemide 40 mg PO daily*
- *Aspirin 81 mg PO daily*
- *KCl 10 mEq PO three times daily*
- *Enalapril 2.5 mg PO twice daily*
    In addition, the HCP prescribes a new medication, carvedilol 3.125 mg PO twice daily. A home health referral is also prescribed.

16. Enhanced Multiple Response

Scenario: The nurse is developing a discharge teaching plan for Mrs. C.

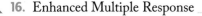

Instructions: Place an X, in the space provided, or highlight the information that the nurse includes when developing the discharge teaching plan for Mrs. C. **Select all that apply**.
1. _____ Avoid nonsteroidal anti-inflammatory drugs (NSAIDS).
2. _____ Weigh yourself every day at the same time.
3. _____ Call the HCP if you feel more short of breath or have weight gain.
4. _____ Drink at least 2500 ml of fluid daily.
5. _____ Make sure you are able to talk during exercise.
6. _____ Avoid cooking with salt or adding salt to food.
7. _____ You will need to make a follow-up appointment to see your HCP soon after discharge.
8. _____ Exercise to maximum heart rate for at least 1 hour every day.
9. _____ Take medications on time as prescribed.

When Ms. C is visited by the home health nurse the next week, she tells the nurse that she is worried because "my pulse rate has been 58 to 62." Her lungs are clear to auscultation, and she has no ankle swelling. Her weight has increased 1 lb (0.45 kg) since hospital discharge.

17. Based on this information, what nursing action is **most** important for Ms. C?
    1. Teach her about the expected effects of carvedilol.
    2. Ask whether she has been taking furosemide daily.
    3. Arrange for transport to the ED.
    4. Remind her that she should not add salt to food.

18. Which additional finding by the home health nurse will be **most** important to communicate to the HCP?
    1. Blood pressure is 108/54 mm Hg.
    2. Apical pulse is 56 beats/min.
    3. Patient states that she takes her daily medications after eating.
    4. Patient reports that she snores when asleep and always feels sleepy.

19. Ms. C's daughter asks the home health nurse if her mother can be cured. What is the best response from the home health nurse?
    1. "A heart transplant is the only potential cure for heart failure, and your mom's age makes that option unlikely."
    2. "Your mother must take her medications and follow the physician orders if she wants to live longer as there is no cure."
    3. "Heart failure is a chronic, progressive, and incapacitating disease. We need to set up a time to talk about advanced directives, so the family understands your mom's wishes about treatments."
    4. "I will leave you some pamphlets explaining the progression of heart failure and a form to fill out for advanced directives to give to your mom's HCP."

PART 3 Complex Health Scenarios

 Answer Key for this chapter begins on p. 354

Answers

1. **Ans: 3** Evidence-based guidelines for the treatment of acute heart failure indicate that oxygen administration to relieve symptoms of hypoxemia is a priority, so the nurse should check oxygen saturation as the first action to determine whether an increase in oxygen delivery is needed. The other actions are also appropriate but not as the initial action. **Focus:** Prioritization.

2. **Ans: 1** The patient's symptoms of hypoxemia and pink, frothy sputum and her history of dyspnea, mitral valve regurgitation, and left ventricular failure suggest pulmonary edema (severe left ventricular failure) as a probable diagnosis. (She also has symptoms of right ventricular failure, but these are not as great a concern.) Her history does not indicate that she has pulmonary hypertension, so cor pulmonale is not a likely concern. Pneumonia will also cause dyspnea and crackles, but sputum is usually thick. Although hypoxemia occurs with a pulmonary embolus, crackles and frothy sputum are not consistent with this complication. **Focus:** Prioritization.

3. **Ans: 2** The patient is hypoxemic, so giving oxygen at the highest level possible is the priority. Activation of the RRT and administration of morphine are also appropriate actions. Lab work and ABGs need to be ordered, but measures should be taken to assist the patient in respiratory distress and the patient should not be left alone to order labs at this time. **Focus:** Prioritization.

4. **Ans: 4** Because cardiac output is frequently decreased in left ventricular failure, monitoring of perfusion with data such as blood pressure and heart rate is essential. The other data may also be useful in determining the adequacy of perfusion, but they are not as important as the blood pressure and pulse rate. **Focus:** Prioritization.

5. **Ans: 3** Although the assessment indicates that a loop diuretic is indicated, it is essential to know the patient's potassium level before administering furosemide. She has already received furosemide in the ED, which can cause hypokalemia. Angiotensin-converting enzyme (ACE) inhibitors can increase potassium levels, so it is also essential to know the potassium level before giving the enalapril. The retention catheter is appropriate for this patient, but the priority is to ensure that her potassium level is within normal limits and then administer the diuretic to decrease volume overload. **Focus:** Prioritization. **Test-Taking Tip:** When administering diuretics, ACE inhibitors, or angiotensin receptor blocking agents, you should be aware of recent electrolyte levels (especially potassium) before giving the medications.

6. **Ans: 4** LPN/LVN education and scope of practice include insertion of urinary catheters. Administering medications to patients in unstable condition is best accomplished by RNs who have experience in caring for critically ill patients. Although some LPN/LVNs may be able to perform venipuncture, obtaining a blood sample could be delegated to the laboratory staff so that the LPN/LVN can insert the catheter. **Focus:** Assignment.

7. **Ans: 2, 3, 4** Although morphine is used to treat angina, this patient has not reported chest pain. Morphine is used in pulmonary edema for its effect as a venodilator (decreases venous tone), which decreases venous return to the heart and reduces ventricular preload. Dyspnea increases tachypnea, which causes hyperinflation. Hyperinflation decreases the inspiration capacity (tidal volume plus inspiration reserve) because of the short expiration cycle. Morphine will decrease the respirations, which will allow for an increase in the inspiration capacity and better gas exchange. Morphine acts on the central nervous system to decrease the patient's anxiety, which also decreases the tachypnea and assists with better gas exchange by increasing inspiration capacity. Morphine alters perception but does not heighten perception. **Focus:** Prioritization. **Test-Taking Tip:** Morphine is one of the most commonly prescribed medications in the hospital. If you were not familiar with the pharmacology of morphine for respiratory applications, look up this information. Also, check out morphine usage for end-of-life patients.

8. **Ans: 2** KCl is infused at a rate no faster than 10 mEq/hr through a peripheral IV line and no faster than 20 to 30 mEq/hr through a central catheter. Infusing KCl too rapidly (over 1 or 10 minutes) is contraindicated because this may cause cardiac arrest. Administering KCl over 8 hours would delay the administration of furosemide. **Focus:** Prioritization.

9. **Ans: 4** Because Ms. C's major problem is pulmonary edema, the most useful information will be changes in her lung sounds. The other data are also helpful in assessing for volume overload but are not as pertinent to the diagnosis of pulmonary edema. **Focus:** Prioritization. **Test-Taking Tip:** Pulmonary congestion caused by fluid overload can occur very suddenly in heart failure but also in other situations, such as IV fluid infusions. Because changes in fluid balance can occur rapidly in acutely ill patients, auscultation of lung sounds is a common and very useful assessment to determine whether changes in treatment need to be considered. You will also need to

monitor other respiratory parameters, such as respiratory effort, respiratory rate, and oxygen saturation.

10. **Ans: 2**   Because nesiritide causes vasodilation and diuresis, hypotension is the most common adverse effect. The other data will also be useful in determining whether the patient's condition is improving or in assessing for adverse effects but are not as important as frequent blood pressure measurement. **Focus:** Prioritization.

11. **Ans: 1**   An RN with experience on a coronary stepdown unit would be familiar with the care of patients with left ventricular failure. There has not been an opportunity to evaluate the knowledge level of the agency RN; in addition, this RN will not be familiar with hospital or ICU policies or the location of supplies. The experienced ICU nurse is caring for a patient whose condition is potentially very unstable, which leaves little time to assess and intervene for Ms. C. The newly graduated RN is not experienced enough to care for a patient like Ms. C, whose condition still may deteriorate. The new graduate could be teamed with a more experienced nurse to learn more about the care of patients with severe left ventricular failure. **Focus:** Assignment.

12. **Ans: 2**   Dysrhythmias and visual disturbances are symptoms of digoxin toxicity, which can lead to fatal dysrhythmias such as ventricular tachycardia and ventricular fibrillation, so measurement of the digoxin level should be ordered. The other findings would not be unusual in a patient with chronic heart failure and mitral valve disease, although ongoing assessments are indicated. **Focus:** Prioritization.

13. **Ans: 1, 3, 4, 7**   Because the patient is receiving diuretic therapy, avoiding hypokalemia and hypomagnesemia is essential. Potassium supplements and ACE inhibitors can increase potassium levels. Diuretic use can impact renal function, so monitoring creatinine is important. BNP levels are used to check for improvement in heart failure. Glucose, calcium, and albumin may also be monitored but are not as important in evaluating for treatment effectiveness or adverse effects of treatment in patients with heart failure. **Focus:** Prioritization.

14. **Ans: 1, 5**   Because the nurse is concerned that the patient may have digoxin toxicity, the digoxin should be held. Hypokalemia can contribute to the risk for digoxin toxicity, and Ms. C is not acutely short of breath, so the furosemide (which causes potassium loss) should also be held until consulting with Ms. C's HCP. There are no indications that the other medications are causing any adverse effects, and they should all be administered. **Focus:** Prioritization.

15. **Ans: 3, 4, 1, 2**   Using the SBAR format, the nurse first identifies himself or herself, gives the patient's name, and describes the current situation. Next, relevant background information, such as the patient's diagnosis and medications, are stated. The assessment includes both pertinent patient data and the nurse's analysis of the situation. Finally, the nurse makes a recommendation indicating what action he or she thinks is needed. **Focus:** Prioritization.

16. **Ans: 1, 2, 3, 5, 6, 7, 9**   National guidelines indicate that discharge instructions for patients with heart failure should address topics such as weight monitoring, low-salt diet, follow-up appointments, medications, activity levels, and what to do if symptoms recur. NSAIDs should be avoided to prevent sodium and fluid retention. Daily weights are an excellent means of monitoring volume status. Fluid should be restricted to 2 liters a day. Patients should stay as active as they can but should not overexert. The patient should be able to talk easily during activity. Not being able to converse during activity or exercise indicates overexertion. Patients should be taught to call the HCP when symptoms first begin to worsen, rather than waiting until they need to be admitted to the hospital. A follow-up appointment should be made to ensure ongoing care and to prevent problems from occurring. **Focus:** Prioritization.

17. **Ans: 1**   Beta-blocker therapy may lead to bradycardia, and the nurse will plan to educate the patient that a slightly low heart rate is not a cause for concern with the carvedilol. If patients are not told to expect side effects such as a slower heart rate, they may discontinue beta-blocking medications. Although the nurse will ask about medication and diet compliance, the patient's clear lungs, minimal weight gain, and lack of peripheral edema indicate that no changes are needed in her self-management at this time. Although worsening heart failure may indicate a need for hospital admission, this patient's assessment indicates a stable condition. **Focus:** Prioritization.

18. **Ans: 4**   Sleep apnea is common in patients with heart failure and can contribute to worsening of heart failure and lead to more frequent hospitalizations. Current heart failure treatment guidelines indicate that sleep apnea should be considered as a cause of fatigue in patients with heart failure. The HCP may want to arrange for sleep studies for this patient. The blood pressure is normal. The patient does have a slight bradycardia, and some medications are better absorbed on an empty stomach, but the assessment data indicate that the current medications are effective, and no changes are needed in the medication regimen. **Focus:** Prioritization.

19. **Ans: 3**   According to the Centers for Disease Control and Prevention, about half of all people diagnosed with heart failure die within 5 years. Heart failure is chronic and debilitating. Death from heart failure can be sudden and without warning. Most transplant centers have a cutoff age of 70 for a heart transplant. Discussing the nature of heart failure, treatments, and advanced directives will prepare the family and the patient on how to act in accordance with the wishes of the patient as the disease progresses. **Focus:** Prioritization.

PART 3 Complex Health Scenarios

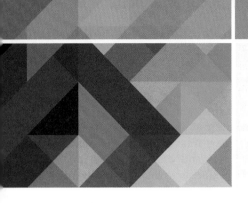

Multiple Patients With Peripheral Vascular Disease

Questions

The RN is the team leader working with an LPN/LVN, an experienced assistive personnel (AP), and a senior nursing student to provide nursing care for six patients in a vascular surgery unit. The patients are as follows:

- *Ms. C, a 38-year-old woman with systemic lupus erythematosus who has developed symptoms of Raynaud phenomenon. She reports numbness, tingling, and cold in her wrists and hands bilaterally.*
- *Mr. R, a 57-year-old man with chronic peripheral arterial disease who reports severe pain from an arterial ulcer on his left great toe.*
- *Mr. Z, a 44-year-old man with Buerger disease who wants to discuss enrolling in a smoking cessation program.*
- *Ms. Q, a 69-year-old overweight woman with chronic hypertension whose blood pressure (BP) at the end of the night shift was 208/96 mm Hg.*
- *Mr. S, a 72-year-old man for whom an abdominal aortic aneurysm (AAA) must be ruled out and who is reporting severe, worsening back pain.*
- *Ms. A, a 65-year-old woman with peripheral venous disease and left calf swelling who is scheduled for venous duplex ultrasonography this morning.*

1. The nurse understands that which conditions are at an increased risk for development when a patient has hypertension? **Select all that apply.**
   1. Gastric ulcers
   2. Kidney disease
   3. Stroke (brain attack)
   4. Emphysema
   5. Myocardial infarction
   6. Parkinson disease

2. After the change-of-shift report, the RN makes rounds on the patients. List the **priority** order for assessing these patients.
   1. Ms. C _____
   2. Mr. R _____
   3. Mr. Z _____
   4. Ms. Q _____
   5. Mr. S _____
   6. Ms. A _____

3. When Mr. S is assessed, which assessment technique would the RN instruct the student nurse to **avoid**?
   1. Auscultating the abdomen for a bruit
   2. Palpating the abdomen to detect a mass
   3. Observing the abdomen for a pulsation
   4. Performing a pain assessment

4. Mr. S continues to report severe back pain. On assessment, the RN detects a bruit and notices pulsation in the left lower quadrant. What is the nurse's best **first** action?
   1. Measure abdominal girth.
   2. Place the patient in a high sitting position.
   3. Notify the patient's health care provider (HCP).
   4. Administer pain medication.

5. All of these interventions for Mr. S are prescribed by the HCP. Which action should the RN assign to the LPN/LVN?
   1. Insert a urinary catheter.
   2. Administer morphine sulfate 2 mg IV push.
   3. Place a second IV saline lock line.
   4. Measure vital signs every 15 minutes.

⚡ **6.** Enhanced Multiple Response

Question

A computed tomography scan reveals that Mr. S has an aneurysm that is 7.5 cm in diameter. Which pre-operative care tasks should the RN delegate to the nursing student under supervision?

Instructions: Circle or highlight all answers that apply.

1. Teaching Mr. S about coughing and deep breathing
2. Assessing all peripheral pulses for postoperative comparison
3. Administering bowel preparation magnesium sulfate orally
4. Drawing blood for the laboratory for typing and screening
5. Discussing the reasons for the surgery
6. Packing Mr. S's belongings in preparation for a postoperative transfer to the surgical intensive care unit (SICU)
7. Reminding Mr. S to take nothing by mouth after midnight.
8. Placing a second IV access in the patient's arm.
9. Checking vital signs before Mr. S is transported to the operating room.

7. At 8:30 AM, the AP reports that Ms. Q, who has chronic hypertension, has a BP of 198/94 mm Hg. Which is the **priority** action and who is the **most** appropriate person to accomplish this action at this time?
   1. Assign the LPN/LVN to give Ms. Q's 9:00 AM furosemide and enalapril now.
   2. Instruct the AP to get Ms. Q back into bed immediately.
   3. Tell the AP to recheck Ms. Q's BP every 15 minutes.
   4. Send the LPN/LVN to recheck Ms. Q's BP to ensure that the reading is correct.

8. The RN is preparing a health teaching plan for Ms. Q. Which key aspects would be included? **Select all that apply.**
   1. Weight reduction strategies
   2. Avoidance of tobacco and caffeine
   3. Drink no more than three alcohol-containing drinks per day.
   4. Exercise 6 to 7 days a week for at least 1 hour.
   5. Use relaxation techniques to decrease stress.
   6. Restrict dietary sodium as recommended by the American Heart Association (AHA).

9. After receiving her morning dose of enalapril, Ms. Q states that she experienced dizziness when getting out of bed to use the bathroom. What is the RN's **priority** action?
   1. Ask the patient about the presence of a nagging cough.
   2. Check the patient's orthostatic BP when lying, sitting, and standing.
   3. Assess the patient for signs of an allergic reaction, such as rashes.
   4. Check the patient's bladder for urinary retention.

10. A nursing concern of chronic pain has been identified for Mr. R, who has chronic peripheral arterial disease (PAD). Which action by the nursing student would cause the RN to intervene?
    1. Administering a narcotic analgesic 45 minutes before an ulcer dressing change
    2. Asking the patient if he has ever tried progressive muscle relaxation
    3. Assessing the patient's response to pain medication administration
    4. Agreeing to hold the patient's docusate at the patient's request

11. Mr. R tells the student nurse that when he walks for only a block or two, he experiences discomfort that is burning and cramping and that is so painful that it makes him stop. The pain goes away with rest. What is the best way for the student to document this finding?
    1. Intermittent claudication
    2. Rest pain
    3. Dependent rubor
    4. Arterial ulcer

12. The RN has assigned the student nurse to teach Mr. R. about foot care related to his PAD. Which teaching points will the RN instruct the student nurse to include? **Select all that apply.**
    1. "Keep your feet clean by washing with a mild soap in room temperature water."
    2. "Wear comfortable, well-fitting shoes except when at home."
    3. "Cut the toenails straight across and keep them clean and filed."
    4. "Apply lubricating lotion to feet to prevent dried and cracked skin."
    5. "Use a heating pad to keep your feet warm, especially at night."
    6. "Avoid extended pressure on your feet and ankles."

PART 3 Complex Health Scenarios

Answer Key for this chapter begins on p. 360

13. At noon, the LPN/LVN goes to cardiopulmonary resuscitation training and is replaced by an RN floated from the pediatric ambulatory care unit (PACU). Which patients should the team leader assign to this floated RN? **Select all that apply.**
    1. Ms. C, who needs teaching about how to avoid exacerbation of symptoms for her condition
    2. Mr. Z, who still needs information about available smoking cessation programs
    3. Ms. Q, whose BP is still elevated and who needs frequent BP monitoring
    4. Ms. A, who is worried because the HCP just told her she has a deep vein thrombosis (DVT)
    5. Mr. S, who reports that his back pain is getting much worse
    6. Mr. R, whose left great toe arterial ulcer continues to be painful even after the student nurse administered his pain medication

14. The nurse is preparing a teaching plan for Ms. C, who has Raynaud disease. Which key points should be included? **Select all that apply.**
    1. "Avoid exposure to cold by wearing warm clothes."
    2. "Nifedipine will help decrease and relieve your symptoms."
    3. "Keep your home at a comfortably warm temperature."
    4. "The problems you experience are caused by the blood vessels in your hands and fingers narrowing."
    5. "Stress reduction techniques can help prevent symptoms."
    6. "Warm beverages such as hot coffee and tea will help decrease symptoms."

15. A nursing concern of poor peripheral perfusion has been identified for Ms. C. Which actions should the RN delegate to the experienced AP? **Select all that apply.**
    1. Assessing for peripheral pulses, edema, capillary refill, and skin temperature
    2. Inspecting the skin for the presence of tissue breakdown and arterial ulcers
    3. Reminding the patient to perform active range-of-motion exercises as tolerated
    4. Reinforcing with the patient the need to take in adequate fluids during the day
    5. Assisting the patient to sit at the bedside and then transfer to a chair
    6. Administering daily oral doses of nifedipine

16. Ms. C asks the student nurse how the drug nifedipine will help with her Raynaud disease. What is the student nurse's **best** response?
    1. "It will slow down your heart rate and decrease your pain."
    2. "It will cause vasodilation and decrease the vasospasms that cause your pain."

    3. "It will lower your blood pressure and decrease the workload of your heart."
    4. "It will help keep your fluids and electrolytes in balance to decrease your pain."

17. What precautions should the RN instruct the student nurse to be sure to teach the patient about taking nifedipine? **Select all that apply.**
    1. "Side effects of this drug can include facial flushing and headaches."
    2. "Be sure to check your respiratory rate before taking this drug."
    3. "When you get out of bed, do so slowly because of the potential for hypotension."
    4. "You should be sure to consume foods rich in potassium such as bananas."
    5. "Avoid grapefruit and grapefruit juice while taking this drug."
    6. "Take over-the-counter calcium tablets every day while on this drug."

18. Ms. A, whose calf is swollen from peripheral venous disease, asks why she must have an injection of low-molecular-weight heparin (LMWH). What is the RN's **best** response?
    1. "LMWH will dissolve the clots in your legs."
    2. "LMWH will prevent new clots from forming."
    3. "LMWH will thin your blood and slow down clotting."
    4. "LMWH will prevent the clots from migrating to your lungs."

19. Ms. A has a nursing concern of increased risk for injury. Which action will the RN delegate to the AP?
    1. Assisting the patient with morning care and repositioning in bed
    2. Monitoring the patient's daily international normalized ratio (INR)
    3. Checking the patient every 4 hours for signs of bleeding
    4. Teaching the patient to call for assistance when getting out of bed

20. Which nursing assessment finding supports the possible diagnosis of a venous thrombosis for Ms. A?
    1. Spasm of her left calf
    2. Shortness of breath
    3. Unilateral swelling of her left calf
    4. Sharp chest pain

21. Ms. A returns from her diagnostic test with a diagnosis of DVT, which is to be treated medically. Which interventions and actions does the nurse expect the HCP to prescribe? **Select all that apply.**
    1. Bed rest
    2. Elevation of the left leg
    3. Compression stockings

4. Daily massage of the left calf
5. Continuation of subcutaneous LMWH
6. Checking of daily INR levels

22. The AP reports to the RN that Mr. Z, who has Buerger disease, awoke from a nap reporting pain in the arch of his left foot. Which actions should the RN take? **Select all that apply.**
    1. Assess the patient's pain.
    2. Administer prescribed nifedipine.
    3. Place the patient in a supine position and elevate the foot.
    4. Lower the room temperature.
    5. Instruct the patient to avoid cold temperatures.
    6. Check the patient's toes for any signs of gangrene or ulcers.

23. The RN is reviewing the lipid profile for Ms. Q, who has been diagnosed with atherosclerosis. Which finding is of **most** concern?
    1. Total serum cholesterol level of 220 mg/dL (5.689 mmol/L)
    2. Triglyceride level of 165 mg/dL (1.863 mmol/L)
    3. Low-density lipoprotein (LDL) cholesterol level of 155 mg/dL (4.008 mmol/L)
    4. High-density lipoprotein (HDL) cholesterol level of 38 mg/dL (0.9827 mmol/L)

24. The RN is teaching the student nurse who is caring for Mr. R how to differentiate peripheral arterial from peripheral venous ulcers. Which characteristics would the RN stress are indications of arterial ulcers? **Select all that apply.**
    1. Claudication is absent.
    2. Rest pain is present.
    3. Ulcers occur at the ends of and between toes.
    4. Brown pigmentation is often present.

5. Pallor is seen when raising the extremity, and dependent rubor is seen when lowering it.
6. Treatment involves damp-to-dry dressing changes.

Three days later, the nursing student returns to complete her clinical rotation on the peripheral vascular unit. To facilitate continuity of care and enhance the student's learning experience about AAA, the student is assigned to assist in the postoperative care and discharge planning for Mr. S.

25. Mr. S underwent surgery 3 days ago and was transferred back to the vascular surgery unit. The student nurse reports that the patient has no bowel sounds present. What does the RN tell the student is the best action?
    1. Check the nasogastric tube for kinks.
    2. Notify the surgeon immediately.
    3. Obtain an abdominal radiograph immediately.
    4. Document the finding in the chart.

26. Mr. S has recovered so the RN and student nurse are preparing for discharge teaching. Which key points would be included in the teaching plan? **Select all that apply.**
    1. Stair climbing is initially strictly limited.
    2. A bedside commode is required even if there is a first-floor bathroom.
    3. Heavy lifting (usually more than 15 to 20 lb [6.8 to 9.1 kg]) must be avoided.
    4. Use caution for activities that involve pulling, pushing, or straining.
    5. Expect to experience abdominal fullness, chest pain, and shortness of breath.
    6. Driving a car will be restricted for several weeks.

  Answer Key for this chapter begins on p. 360

Answers

1. **Ans: 2, 3, 5** Hypertension, or high BP, is the most common health problem seen in primary care settings and can cause stroke, myocardial infarction (heart attack), kidney failure, and death if not treated early and effectively. **Focus:** Prioritization.

2. **Ans: 5, 4, 2, 6, 1, 3** The worsening back pain of Mr. S may signal an AAA that is enlarging, and he is at risk for rupture, which is urgent and immediately life threatening. Ms. Q's hypertension should be assessed next because she is at risk for complications such as stroke. Next, Mr. R, the patient with severe pain, should be assessed and given pain medication. Ms. A is scheduled for Doppler studies and may have questions and need teaching before the procedure. Ms. C, the patient with Raynaud disease, should be assessed next, although the symptoms she is reporting are typical of this problem. Finally, the nurse should see Mr. Z to discuss arranging for someone to talk with him about smoking cessation. **Focus:** Prioritization.

3. **Ans: 2** Palpation of the abdomen must be avoided because the mass may be tender, and there is risk of causing a rupture. Auscultating for a bruit and observing for pulsation are appropriate assessment techniques. Pain assessment is appropriate because such patients typically experience steady, gnawing abdominal, flank, or back pain that is unaffected by movement and may last for hours or days. **Focus:** Supervision, Prioritization. **Test-Taking Tip:** To answer a question like this, the nurse must be aware of assessment techniques that can be dangerous and cause injury to the patient. In this case, palpating the abdomen could cause rupture of the AAA with severe bleeding and risk for death.

4. **Ans: 3** The patient's symptoms and the nurse's assessment findings indicate an AAA that may be expanding, and this places the patient at risk for rupture. This is an urgent situation, and the HCP should be notified immediately. The nurse should not place the patient in a high sitting position because this may place added pressure on the patient's AAA, leading to rupture. **Focus:** Prioritization.

5. **Ans: 1** The patient having surgery for an AAA repair may need a urinary catheter inserted to keep the bladder empty and deflated. LPN/LVN educational preparation includes inserting urinary catheters. In some states, LPN/LVNs can insert IV catheters and administer IV drugs, but this is not true of all states and facilities. To perform these actions, the LPN/LVN would need additional education and training. Check local, state, and facility policies. IV morphine is a high-alert drug, and giving these drugs to unstable patients is best done by an experienced RN. The AP could be delegated to measure the patient's vital signs, with instructions from the nurse about which findings to report (e.g., increased BP or heart rate). **Focus:** Assignment, Delegation, Supervision.

6. **Ans: 1, 2, 3, 6, 7, 9** The nursing student should be able to provide teaching about simple concepts such as coughing and taking deep breaths, perform simple assessments such as measuring peripheral pulses, and administer oral medications, all under the supervision of the nurse. The student could also be assigned to pack Mr. S's personal belongings for postoperative transfer to the SICU. The student can remind Mr. S about what has already been taught and check vital signs. The nurse or someone with special training in performing IV placement and venipuncture should draw blood for the laboratory tests. The patient may have questions about the surgery, so discussion about the reasons for surgery should be carried out by an experienced RN. The nurse could mentor the student, however, by allowing the student to be present during the discussion. **Focus:** Delegation, Supervision.

7. **Ans: 1** Administering the patient's BP medications is aimed at correcting the problem and lowering the patient's BP. Getting the patient back into bed and reassessing the patient's BP are appropriate actions but do not focus on the problem of lowering the patient's BP. **Focus:** Supervision, Delegation, Assignment, Prioritization. **Test-Taking Tip:** To answer a question like this, first the nurse must determine the problem, then the nurse must decide what the best way is to solve the problem. In this case, the problem is that the patient's BP is still fairly high. The best way to solve the problem is to administer medications that will lower the BP.

8. **Ans: 1, 2, 5, 6** The patient is overweight, so weight loss is appropriate as are sodium restriction, avoidance of tobacco and caffeine, and relaxation techniques to reduce stress. A female patient should not consume more than one alcoholic drink per day. Exercise is a good strategy but should be started slowly and is recommended for 3 to 4 days per week for about 40 minutes per day according to AHA guidelines. **Focus:** Prioritization.

9. **Ans: 2** Enalapril is an angiotensin-converting enzyme (ACE) inhibitor drug. These drugs commonly cause dizziness and can increase the patient's risk for falls. The priority action at this time is to check orthostatic BPs. The nurse would also teach the patient to move slowly from lying to sitting and standing positions and to call for help when getting out of bed. A nagging cough is a side effect of these drugs, and the

nurse would want to know about this, but it is not urgent at this time. ACE inhibitors do not cause fluid retention, and dizziness is not a sign of an allergy to the drug. **Focus:** Prioritization.

10. **Ans: 4** The nurse should intervene when the patient asks to have the docusate held because opioids often cause the side effect of constipation. The patient must be taught about the importance of this medication in preventing unwanted side effects. If the patient has a good reason for refusing the docusate (e.g., he has been having episodes of diarrhea), then the nurse may hold the drug (documenting the reason), but the nurse should teach the student about the importance of asking why the patient is requesting that the drug be held. The other actions are appropriate. Giving the pain medication before the dressing change will make the procedure less painful. **Focus:** Assignment, Supervision.

11. **Ans: 1** Most patients with PAD seek medical attention for a classic leg pain known as intermittent claudication (a term derived from a word meaning "to limp"). Usually they can walk only a certain distance before discomfort (e.g., cramping or burning muscular pain) forces them to stop. The pain stops with rest. When patients resume walking, they can walk the same distance before the pain returns. Thus the pain is considered reproducible. As the disease progresses, patients can walk only shorter and shorter distances before pain recurs. **Focus:** Prioritization.

12. **Ans: 1, 3, 4, 6** Comfortable, well-fitting shoes should be worn at all times, even in the home, and heating pads should not be applied to the feet. The other four teaching points are appropriate when teaching a patient with PAD how to care for his or her feet. **Focus:** Prioritization.

13. **Ans: 2, 3** Mr. Z is in stable condition, and the PACU nurse could begin educating him about smoking cessation. The PACU nurse is skilled at BP monitoring and would have no difficulty meeting Ms. Q's needs for care. Ms. A and Ms. C need the care of a nurse who is experienced in caring for and educating patients with peripheral vascular disease to teach and answer questions. Mr. S's worsening back pain may indicate expansion of his AAA, and he should be assigned to an experienced nurse. Mr. R's care should continue to be assigned to the nurse who has been caring for him since the beginning of the shift and is familiar with his case. He will need frequent pain assessments and may need additional pain interventions. **Focus:** Assignment.

14. **Ans: 1, 2, 3, 4, 5** The underlying pathophysiology of Raynaud disease is vasospasm of the arterioles and arteries of the upper and lower extremities, usually unilaterally. Patients with this disorder should avoid caffeinated beverages. All of the other teaching points are appropriate to share with a patient with Raynaud disease. **Focus:** Prioritization.

15. **Ans: 3, 4, 5** The AP can remind about and reinforce nursing care measures that have already been taught by the RN. Assisting patients to get out of bed is also within the scope of practice for APs. Assessing and inspecting the patient require additional education and skills appropriate to the RN's scope of practice. Administering oral medications should be done by licensed nurses. **Focus:** Delegation, Supervision.

16. **Ans: 2** Nifedipine is a calcium channel blocker and a vasodilating drug that will decrease the painful vasospasms that occur and cause the symptoms of Raynaud disease. Nifedipine will decrease heart rate and BP and may impact fluids and electrolytes, but vasodilation is the therapeutic effect when nifedipine is used to treat Raynaud disease. **Focus:** Prioritization.

17. **Ans: 1, 3, 5** When they are taking vasodilating drugs, such as nifedipine, teach patients about side effects such as facial flushing, hypotension, and headaches. Also teach patients taking nifedipine to avoid grapefruit and grapefruit juice to prevent severe adverse effects, including possible death. Nifedipine is a calcium channel blocker, and these drugs do not affect respirations or serum potassium and calcium levels. **Focus:** Prioritization.

18. **Ans: 2** LMWH can be used to treat or prevent DVT. When used for treatment, LMWH prevents new blood clots from forming and prevents existing clots from getting larger. This allows the normal body systems to dissolve the clots that are already formed. This also reduces the risk of pulmonary embolism. The drug does not "thin" a patient's blood or dissolve an existing clot. **Focus:** Prioritization.

19. **Ans: 1** The AP's scope of practice and education includes actions related to assisting patients with activities of daily living, such as morning care and repositioning in bed. Monitoring, assessing, and providing instructions for the patient require additional education and skills and are part of the RN's scope of practice. **Focus:** Delegation, Supervision.

20. **Ans: 3** Classic signs and symptoms of DVT include calf or groin tenderness or pain and sudden onset of unilateral swelling of the leg. Shortness of breath and sharp chest pain are signs of the complication of pulmonary embolus in which a clot dislodges and travels to the pulmonary circulation. **Focus:** Prioritization.

21. **Ans: 1, 2, 3, 5** Bed rest, elevation of the affected extremity, use of compression stockings, and administration of LMWH are strategies to prevent complications of DVT such as pulmonary embolus (PE). The nurse should be aware, however, that some research indicates that ambulation for a patient with DVT does not worsen the risk for PE. Massage of the affected extremity increases the risk for PE. Checking INR or prothrombin time levels is not required when a patient is prescribed a LMWH drug such as enoxaparin or dalteparin. **Focus:** Prioritization.

22. **Ans: 1, 2, 5, 6** Placing the patient in a supine position and elevating his foot places the extremity above heart level, which slows arterial blood flow to the foot and may lead to increased pain. A patient with Buerger disease should avoid the cold and should wear warm clothes. All of the other actions are appropriate for a patient with Buerger disease. Checking the digits for ulcers or gangrene is essential for a patient with this condition. **Focus:** Prioritization.

23. **Ans: 3** Although all of these lipid profile findings are abnormal, the LDL cholesterol ("bad cholesterol") level is much too high. A desirable LDL cholesterol level is less than 130 mg/dL (3.362 mmol/L) for a healthy person or less than 70 mg/dL (1.8102 mmol/L) for a patient with cardiovascular disease or diabetes. The national guidelines for cholesterol management focus on lowering LDL as the primary goal. The other results, including the HDL levels, are of concern and should be attended to, but they are not as excessively abnormal as is the LDL level. **Focus:** Prioritization.

24. **Ans: 2, 3, 5** With PAD, ulcers, claudication, and rest pain are present. Ulcers are deep and occur at the ends of or between the toes. Brown pigmentation occurs with venous ulcers, not arterial. Arterial ulcers are pale when elevated but show dependent rubor when lowered. Treatment of arterial ulcers involves surgical revascularization; for venous ulcers, treatment includes long-term wound care, including Unna boot application and damp-to-dry dressings. **Focus:** Prioritization.

25. **Ans: 4** Postoperatively after AAA repair, bowel sounds are usually absent for 2 or 3 days, and patients have a nasogastric tube in place on low suction until bowel sounds return. The nurse should document the finding only and teach the student that this is to be expected and why. **Focus:** Delegation, Supervision, Prioritization.

26. **Ans: 1, 3, 4, 6** When a patient is discharged to home, stair climbing may be restricted initially, and he or she may need a bedside commode if the bathroom is inaccessible. Teach the patient who has undergone surgical repair about activity restrictions, wound care, and pain management. Patients may not perform activities that involve lifting heavy objects (usually more than 15 to 20 lb [6.8 to 9.1 kg]) for 6 to 12 weeks postoperatively. Advise them to use caution for activities that involve pulling, pushing, or straining. Most patients are restricted from driving a car for several weeks after discharge. Teach patients receiving treatment for hypertension about the importance of continuing to take prescribed drugs. Instruct them about the signs and symptoms that must promptly be reported to the HCP, which include abdominal fullness or pain, chest or back pain, shortness of breath, or difficulty swallowing or hoarseness. **Focus:** Prioritization.

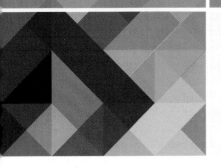

CASE STUDY 17

Respiratory Difficulty After Surgery

Questions

The nurse has just received the change-of-shift report about Mr. E, a 26-year-old man who had a ruptured appendix with an emergency appendectomy 2 days ago. The report included this information about Mr. E's vital signs, assessments, and prescribed therapies:

Vital Signs

Temperature: 101.4°F (38.6°C)
Pulse: 118 beats/min (sinus tachycardia)
Respirations: 28 breaths/min
Blood pressure (BP): 98/56 mm Hg
Oxygen saturation: 90% (0.90) (decreased from 98% [0.98] over the past 4 hours)

Assessment

Respiratory: Fine crackles heard throughout lungs; nonproductive cough
Gastrointestinal: Bowel sounds present, brown purulent drainage from wound drain
Neurologic: Alert and oriented × 3

Therapies

O_2 at 2 L/min per nasal cannula
Antibiotics: Vancomycin and ceftriaxone IV
Arterial blood gases (ABGs), complete blood count (CBC), blood urea nitrogen, electrolytes, and glucose pending
Vancomycin trough level ordered

1. Based on the information in the change-of-shift report on Mr. E, which concept sets a precedent when setting a **priority** for nursing actions?
   1. Infection
   2. Perfusion
   3. Gas exchange
   4. Fluid and electrolytes

2. Mr. E has a dose of vancomycin scheduled at 10:00 AM. At what time will the nurse ask the laboratory to draw blood for determining the vancomycin trough level?
   1. 9:00 AM
   2. 9:45 AM
   3. 12:00 PM
   4. 1:00 PM

When the nurse assesses Mr. E, he is sitting in a chair at the bedside. His respirations appear labored, with a rate of 30 breaths/min. Pulse oximetry readings indicate that his oxygen saturation is 88% to 89% (0.88 to 0.89). He looks anxious and says, "I'm having a little trouble catching my breath." There are fine crackles throughout his lungs.

3. What action will the nurse take **next**?
   1. Assist him back to bed.
   2. Increase the oxygen flow rate to 4 L/min.
   3. Administer the as needed (PRN) morphine IV.
   4. Finish the rest of the head-to-toe assessment.

The ABG analysis is completed, and the results are faxed to the unit:

Arterial partial pressure of carbon dioxide ($Paco_2$)	*30 mm Hg (3.99 kPa)*
Arterial partial pressure of oxygen (Pao_2)	*54 mm Hg (7.18 kPa)*
Bicarbonate (HCO_3^-)	*20 mEq/L (20 mmol/L)*
O_2 saturation	*88% (0.88)*
pH	*7.34*

4. Which action will the nurse take **next** based on the ABG results?
   1. Place Mr. E on oxygen at 15 L/min via a nonrebreather mask.
   2. Obtain an order for sodium bicarbonate 50 mEq (50 mmol) IV.
   3. Support the patient in taking long, slow breaths to decrease the respiratory rate.
   4. Continue to monitor Mr. E's respiratory status and vital signs.

5. The CBC results are now also available. Which result is of **most** concern to the nurse?
   1. Hematocrit of 37% (0.37)
   2. Hemoglobin level of 10.5 g/dL (105 g/L)
   3. White blood cell (WBC) count of 24,000/mm3 (24 × 109/L)
   4. Platelet count of 120,000/mm3 (120 × 109/L)

Because Mr. E's condition is unstable, the nurse's other assigned patient (Ms. O) for the shift will need to be reassigned to another staff member. Ms. O has diabetes and was admitted yesterday with pyelonephritis and hyperglycemia. She is receiving a regular insulin infusion using the hospital's standard insulin sliding-scale protocols and needs to have blood glucose monitoring every hour. Her temperature has decreased from 102°F to 100.6°F (38.9°C to 38.1°C) since antibiotics were started yesterday.

6. Which staff member is best to assign to care for Ms. O?
   1. RN who has 10 years of experience on the pediatric unit and has floated to the step-down unit for the day
   2. Newly graduated RN who has finished a 3-month orientation and is scheduled for the first day without a preceptor
   3. On-call RN with 5 years of experience on the step-down unit who will be able to arrive in about 1 hour
   4. Experienced RN from a staffing agency who is on orientation to the unit today in preparation for a 6-month assignment

7. The nurse is considering Mr. E's history of a ruptured appendix, current vital signs, assessment data, and laboratory results. After 15 minutes of oxygen administration using the nonrebreather mask, Mr. E's pulse oximeter still indicates that the oxygen saturation is 88% to 89% (0.88 to 0.89). Which complication is **most** likely?
   1. Aspiration pneumonia
   2. Acute asthma attack
   3. Spontaneous tension pneumothorax
   4. Acute respiratory distress syndrome (ARDS)

8. Using the SBAR (situation, background, assessment, recommendation) format, indicate the order in which the nurse will communicate the concerns about Mr. E to the health care provider (HCP).
   1. "His pulse oximetry reading is only 88% to 90% (0.88 to 0.90), although he is receiving high-flow oxygen by a nonrebreather mask. I am concerned he may have sepsis and be developing ARDS."
   2. "This is the nurse caring for Mr. E. I'm calling because the patient has increasing hypoxemia, as well as elevated WBC count, hypotension, and tachycardia."
   3. "I think that you need to come and evaluate this patient as soon as possible; he may need mechanical ventilation."
   4. "Mr. E had an emergency appendectomy 2 days ago and has had purulent abdominal drainage and a fever, but he has not had any respiratory difficulty until today."

   _____, _____, _____, _____

9. The HCP assesses Mr. E and prescribes these actions. Which action should the nurse implement **first**?
   1. Place the patient on bilevel positive airway pressure (BiPAP) ventilation.
   2. Arrange to transfer the patient to the intensive care unit (ICU).
   3. Administer nebulized albuterol every 4 hours as needed for dyspnea.
   4. Obtain blood, urine, and abdominal drainage samples for culture.

With the BiPAP, Mr. E's oxygenation improves only slightly. He is transferred to the ICU and intubated.

10. Which is the best way to confirm correct placement of the endotracheal (ET) tube?
    1. Check the pulse oximetry level.
    2. Observe for chest rise with ventilation.
    3. Auscultate bilateral breath sounds.
    4. Use continuous waveform capnography.

Mr. E's ET tube is secured, with the 23-cm mark on the tube at the level of Mr. E's teeth. Mr. E is connected to a positive-pressure ventilator with the following settings:

Fraction of inspired oxygen (FIO_2)	70% (0.70)
Mode	Assist control ventilation
Positive end-expiratory pressure	10 cm
Respiratory rate	30 breaths/min
Tidal volume (V_T)	500 mL

The following ABG values are obtained 30 minutes after Mr. E is placed on the ventilator:

HCO_3^-	20 mEq/L (20 mmol/L)
O_2 saturation	95% (0.95)
$Paco_2$	47 mm Hg (6.25 kPa)
Pao_2	65 mm Hg (8.64 kPa)
pH	7.31

11. Which ventilator change will the nurse anticipate based on analysis of the ABG values?
    1. Increasing the tidal volume to 600 mL
    2. Changing the rate on the ventilator to 35 breaths/min
    3. Decreasing the Fio_2 to 60% (0.60)
    4. Changing to continuous mandatory ventilation (CMV) mode

The nurse assists with the insertion of a central IV line for monitoring of the central venous pressure and for fluid administration. A nasogastric (NG) tube is also inserted.

When the nurse reassesses Mr. E, he has scattered crackles throughout both lung fields. He is restless and needs frequent reminders not to pull on the ET or NG tubes. His urine output over the past 2 hours has been 50 mL of clear amber urine. Bowel sounds are slightly hypotonic but are audible in all four abdominal quadrants. The abdominal drainage is unchanged. The following vital signs and central venous pressure values are obtained:

BP	100/46 mm Hg
Heart rate	124 beats/min (sinus tachycardia)
O_2 saturation	90% (0.90)
Central venous pressure	3 mm Hg
Respirations	24 breaths/min
Temperature	102.1°F (38.9°C)

12. Based on the vital signs and assessment data, which collaborative interventions will the nurse anticipate at this time? **Select all that apply.**
    1. Increase the IV rate to 150 mL/hr.
    2. Administer furosemide 40 mg IV.
    3. Start norepinephrine infusion.
    4. Give diltiazem 15 mg IV.
    5. Administer high-calorie enteral feeding at 25 mL/hr.
    6. Obtain a portable x-ray to assure correct placement of nasogastric tube

13. Although his oxygen saturation remains at 90% (0.90), Mr. E continues to be restless and needs frequent reminders to not pull at the ET tube. Which method to reduce his anxiety and decrease the risk for accidental extubation will the nurse try **first**?
    1. Obtain an order to restrain his hands and apply soft wrist restraints.
    2. Administer neuromuscular blockade medications and sedatives.
    3. Have a family member stay at Mr. E's bedside and reassure him.
    4. Remind Mr. E frequently that he needs the ET tube to breathe.

14. A student nurse is assigned to the ICU and is preparing to suction Mr. E. Which action by the student requires that the nurse intervene immediately?
    1. Increasing the Fio_2 to 100% (1.00) for 5 minutes before suctioning
    2. Using an open-suction technique to perform the suctioning
    3. Administering morphine 2 mg IV per standing order before suctioning
    4. Applying suction to the catheter while inserting it into the ET tube

15. Which actions will the nurse use to decrease Mr. E's risk for developing ventilator-associated pneumonia (VAP)? **Select all that apply.**
    1. Avoid sedating the patient when possible.
    2. Change the ventilator tubing and humidifier daily.
    3. Assist the patient with exercises several times daily.
    4. Keep the head of the bed elevated to at least 30 degrees.
    5. Provide oral care several times daily with antibacterial solution.
    6. Monitor residual gastric volumes and hold feedings for volumes of 50 mL or more.

16. All of these activities are included in the plan of care for patients with ARDS. Which activities can be assigned to an experienced LPN/LVN? **Select all that apply.**
    1. Provide oral care every 4 hours.
    2. Place the patient in the prone position for 10 hours daily.
    3. Assess breath sounds every 4 hours.
    4. Check axillary or tympanic temperature every 4 hours.
    5. Suction the ET tube as needed.
    6. Teach the patient and family about routine nursing care.

Answer Key for this chapter begins on p. 367

The nurse hears the ventilator high pressure alarm and finds that Mr. E appears very agitated, with a respiratory rate of 40 breaths/min. The continuous pulse oximeter indicates an oxygen saturation of 81% (0.81). Mr. E's cardiac monitor shows a sinus tachycardia with a rate of 142 beats/min.

17. What action should the nurse take **first**?
    1. Listen to Mr. E's breath sounds.
    2. Increase the Fio_2 setting to 100% (1.00).
    3. Check the ventilator settings and readouts.
    4. Suction Mr. E's ET tube after hyperoxygenating him.

18. No breath sounds are audible over Mr. E's right side, and the right side does not expand much with inspiration. The ET tube is still at the 23-cm mark at the patient's teeth. What complication of mechanical positive-pressure ventilation is **most** likely?
    1. Aspiration pneumonia
    2. Inadvertent extubation
    3. Tension pneumothorax
    4. ET tube displacement

19. Which action should the nurse take **next**?
    1. Notify the HCP about the patient's respiratory distress.
    2. Gather the equipment needed for chest tube insertion.
    3. Offer reassurance and explanations to the patient.
    4. Give the prescribed lorazepam 1 mg IV PRN for agitation.

20. The HCP inserts a chest tube into the right anterior chest at the second intercostal space. After connection of the chest tube collection device, which finding by the nurse is **most** important to report to the HCP?
    1. The patient indicates that he has pain with every ventilator-assisted inspiration.
    2. A large number of air bubbles appear in the water-seal chamber during expiration.
    3. Continuous bubbling occurs throughout the respiratory cycle in the suction control chamber.
    4. 100 mL of blood drains into the collection chamber immediately after the chest tube insertion.

21. Just before the change-of-shift report to the oncoming RN, the nurse reviews Mr. E's other laboratory test results for today. Which information is **most** important to communicate to the HCP?
    1. Blood glucose level of 140 mg/dL (7.7 mmol/L)
    2. Potassium level of 5.1 mEq/L (5.1 mmol/L)
    3. Sodium level of 134 mEq/L (134 mmol/L)
    4. Blood urea nitrogen level of 52 mg/dL (18.56 mmol/L)

22. Cloze

Scenario: Mr. E's persistent hypoxemia was the cardinal feature that indicated ___1___. Mr. E's condition most likely occurred because of (a/an) ___2___. Specific management of Mr. E's condition included mechanical ventilation. Another treatment to promote gas exchange might include ___3___. Recent research shows that ___4___ is the best way to maintain fluid balance.

Instructions: Complete the sentences by choosing the most probable option for the missing information that corresponds with the same numbered list of options provided.

Option 1	Option 2	Option 3	Option 4
pulmonary edema	systemic inflammatory response	decreasing positive expiratory end pressure (PEEP)	aggressive fluid therapy
acute respiratory distress syndrome	fluid overload	administration of Nitrous Oxide	conservative fluid therapy
pneumonia	infection	prone positioning	colloidal intravenous therapy
refractory hypoxemia	high tidal volumes	maintaining the supine position	total parenteral nutrition

Answers

1. **Ans: 3** The increase in respirations and the marked decrease in oxygen saturation over the past few hours indicate that Mr. E is developing respiratory complications that will require immediate nursing action. The other information also calls for assessment and possible intervention but not as urgently as the change in his respiratory status. **Focus:** Prioritization. **Test-Taking Tip:** Even when vital signs and oxygen saturation are still in the normal range, rapid or sudden changes in temperature, heart rate, BP, respiratory rate, or oxygen saturation are a red flag for an acute underlying process and require further assessment or intervention. When prioritizing nursing actions, think ABCs: Airway, Breathing, and Circulation.

2. **Ans: 2** Samples for measurement of antibiotic trough levels are drawn just before the next scheduled dose. Drawing the blood at 9:00 AM will give a slightly inaccurate trough level. Obtaining blood at 12:00 PM or 1:00 PM would be appropriate for assessing the peak vancomycin level, which should be obtained 1 to 2 hours after the IV dose is infused. **Focus:** Prioritization.

3. **Ans: 2** Oxygen saturations of less than 90% (0.90) indicate hypoxemia, so the most important action is to improve oxygenation. The general rule is that every liter of oxygen after the first liter that increases the F_{IO_2} by 3%, increases the F_{IO_2} by 4%. Rates above 5L can cause discomfort and nosebleeds. Sitting in a chair usually improves gas exchange because the lungs can expand more easily. Mr. E's anxiety is because of hypoxemia, so morphine (which may suppress respiratory drive) is not an appropriate intervention to decrease anxiety. The assessment should be completed after interventions to improve oxygenation have been implemented. **Focus:** Prioritization.

4. **Ans: 1** The ABG results indicate that Mr. E is hypoxemic and has metabolic acidosis because of a cellular shift to the anaerobic metabolic pathway. These abnormalities should be corrected by increasing the Pao_2 level. The nonrebreather mask is capable of delivering F_{IO_2} levels of close to 100% (1.00). He is hyperventilating in response to hypoxemia, so administering morphine is not indicated. Although the nurse will continue to monitor this patient's respiratory status, monitoring alone is not enough at this time. **Focus:** Prioritization.

5. **Ans: 3** The increase in WBC count is an indicator of infection, a major concern in a patient who has had a ruptured appendix. A change in antibiotic therapy may be needed. The nurse should also assess for other data that might indicate developing sepsis in this patient. The abnormalities in the other parameters indicate

that ongoing monitoring of the CBC is necessary, but they do not require any acute interventions. **Focus:** Prioritization. **Test-Taking Tip:** Because not every abnormal laboratory value indicates a need for immediate action by the nurse, good prioritization requires you to recognize which values indicate critical illness or need to be corrected quickly.

6. **Ans: 1** An RN with experience in caring for pediatric patients would be familiar with the care of patients with infection and hyperglycemia, including blood glucose monitoring and administration of insulin. The newly graduated RN does not have enough experience to care independently for a patient who is still in somewhat unstable condition. Ms. O will require an assessment and interventions before the on-call RN will be able to arrive. The agency RN will not be familiar with the location of supplies or with hospital policies, such as the standard sliding-scale insulin protocol. **Focus:** Assignment.

7. **Ans: 4** The patient's history of a ruptured appendix, elevated temperature and WBC count, tachycardia, elevated respiratory rate, and worsening hypoxemia even with increases in supplemental oxygen are most consistent with ARDS associated with sepsis. The other complications may also cause hypoxemia but are not supported by the data for this patient. Aspiration pneumonia usually occurs in patients who are not alert or are unable to protect their airway. Wheezes caused by bronchoconstriction are heard with asthma attacks, and breath sounds are absent on one side with pneumothorax. **Focus:** Prioritization.

8. **Ans: 2, 4, 1, 3** Using the SBAR format, the nurse first introduces himself or herself and then indicates the current patient situation that requires intervention. The nurse then gives pertinent background information about the patient. Next, the current pertinent assessment data and analysis of the patient's problem are communicated. Finally, the nurse makes a recommendation for the needed action. **Focus:** Prioritization.

9. **Ans: 1** Rapidly improving Mr. E's oxygenation is the priority. BiPAP provides noninvasive positive-pressure ventilation, which can decrease the work of breathing and rapidly improve gas exchange. Transfer to the ICU is appropriate but does not need to be done before BiPAP is initiated. Administering a bronchodilator may be needed and specimens for culture will be sent, but these should be done after starting BiPAP ventilation. **Focus:** Prioritization.

10. **Ans: 4** Current guidelines indicate that monitoring for carbon dioxide exhalation by continuous waveform capnography is the best choice for confirmation and ongoing monitoring of ET placement. Other actions performed after intubation are listening for bilateral

breath sounds, observing for symmetrical chest wall movement with ventilation, and obtaining a chest radiograph. Monitoring of oxygen saturation is useful in assessing response to treatment, but it is not the best indicator of correct ET placement, especially in severely hypoxemic patients. **Focus:** Prioritization.

11. **Ans: 3** Current evidence-based guidelines for mechanical ventilation in ARDS suggest a Pao_2 of 55 to 80 mm Hg as a goal; the Fio_2 should be decreased because exposure to high oxygen levels causes alveolar damage. Although the $Paco_2$ is slightly elevated, mild hypercapnia is acceptable according to the most current research. Raising V_T will increase the chance for complications such as pneumothorax. The CMV mode is generally used for patients who are unconscious or paralyzed because it allows the patient no control of respirations and is very uncomfortable. **Focus:** Prioritization.

12. **Ans: 1, 5, 6** The central venous pressure and urine output suggest that Mr. E is hypovolemic, so increasing his IV fluid intake is essential. Nutritional interventions are important in critically ill patients. Enteral feeding is the preferred method for administering nutrition because the patient has bowel sounds. Correct placement of the NG tube should be confirmed with an X-ray. Furosemide administration would lead to further dehydration. Because the patient's hypotension and tachycardia are most likely caused by hypovolemia, norepinephrine and diltiazem are not appropriate. **Focus:** Prioritization.

13. **Ans: 3** Having a family member at the bedside will decrease the sense of isolation and anxiety that occurs in the intensive care environment, especially in patients who cannot easily communicate because of intubation. Reminding the patient frequently not to pull at the tube may also be helpful. The other methods listed may also be used, although restraints, anti-anxiety medications, and paralytic medications all have potential adverse effects. Restraints are sometimes needed in agitated or confused patients, although the need for restraints must be re-evaluated frequently. Many patients do benefit from the use of anti-anxiety medications, but excessive sedation should be avoided. The use of neuromuscular blockade or paralysis is avoided unless it is necessary to improve ABG values. **Focus:** Prioritization. **Test-Taking Tip:** Remember that the least restrictive means for avoiding injury should be used when there is a concern that patients may pull at tubes or other equipment. Less restrictive means usually include environmental controls, including observation by staff or family. More restrictive means include physical restraints or sedative medications.

14. **Ans: 4** The applying of suction causes hypoxemia and trauma to the tracheal mucosa. Suction should only be applied to the catheter while it is being withdrawn to minimize these problems. Hyperoxygenation

is necessary before performing suction for a patient who is at risk for hypoxemia, although 5 minutes of hyperoxygenation is usually not necessary. Use of a closed-suction technique helps decrease the cost of suction catheters and is preferred for patients receiving positive end-expiratory pressure ventilation, but an open-suction technique may also be used. Some patients may require sedatives or analgesics before suctioning, although these are not routinely given. **Focus:** Prioritization.

15. **Ans: 1, 3, 4, 5** Current evidence-based recommendations for prevention of VAP include avoiding sedation so that the patient's ability to ventilate independently can be evaluated more frequently, mobilizing the patient to avoid muscle loss, keeping the head elevated to 30 to 45 degrees to help prevent aspiration, and providing oral care with chlorhexidine solution. Current research does not support the need for changing ventilator tubing every 24 hours. Research suggests that small residual gastric volumes in patients who are receiving enteral feedings do not increase aspiration risk and that stopping feedings unnecessarily adversely affects nutritional status. **Focus:** Prioritization.

16. **Ans: 1, 4** LPN/LVN education includes skills such as providing oral care and taking temperatures. Although assistive personnel may also be able to do some of these activities in a stable patient, more education is needed to provide oral care or take temperatures in a patient who is intubated and receiving mechanical ventilation. An experienced LPN/LVN would know which patient data need to be reported to the supervising RN immediately. Positioning a patient is also included in LPN/LVN education; however, placing a patient with an ET tube and central IV line in a prone position requires multiple staff members and should be supervised by the RN caring for the patient. ET tube suctioning may be delegated to an experienced LPN/LVN in some settings, but in a patient in unstable condition, suctioning should be done by the RN. Respiratory assessment of critically ill patients should be done by the RN. Education of the critically ill patient and family requires RN-level assessment and planning. **Focus:** Assignment.

17. **Ans: 1** When an alarm sounds, the initial action should be to assess the patient. In this situation, the assessment of breath sounds, chest movement, and respiratory effort will help determine which respiratory complication the patient is experiencing. Depending on the assessment findings, the other actions may also be necessary. **Focus:** Prioritization. **Test-Taking Tip:** Because the plan of care is determined by patient assessment data, remember to question whether more data are needed before deciding which actions the nurse should take.

18. **Ans: 3** The absence of breath sounds on the right and the high pressures needed to ventilate the patient suggest a tension pneumothorax caused by

barotrauma associated with positive-pressure ventilation and the use of positive end-expiratory pressure. Displacement of the ET tube into one side or extubation also may lead to decreased breath sounds, but the ET tube position would change with these complications. Aspiration pneumonia is a common complication but does not present with a sudden onset and absent breath sounds. **Focus:** Prioritization.

19. **Ans: 1**   Because the data indicate a likely pneumothorax, a chest tube will need to be inserted by the HCP to allow re-expansion of the lung on the affected side. This should take place quickly because the patient's gas exchange will be adversely affected by pneumothorax. The other actions are also appropriate, but the initial action will be notification of the HCP so that the pneumothorax can be rapidly treated. **Focus:** Prioritization.

20. **Ans: 4**   With a tension pneumothorax, there are usually only a few milliliters of blood in the collection chamber because there is no blood or fluid trapped in the pleural space. The presence of 100 mL of blood indicates that there may have been trauma to the lung during the chest tube insertion. The other data are expected with chest tube insertion and pneumothorax. The air leak should be monitored, and analgesics should be used to control the pain Mr. E is experiencing. **Focus:** Prioritization.

21. **Ans: 4**   Mr. E has multiple risk factors for acute kidney injury, including sepsis, dehydration, and use of the potentially nephrotoxic antibiotic vancomycin. Acute kidney injury is one of the common complications of ARDS. The other laboratory values are also abnormal but do not indicate a need for a change in therapy at present. **Focus:** Prioritization.

22. **Ans: Option 1, acute respiratory distress syndrome; Option 2, systemic inflammatory response; Option 3, prone positioning; Option 4, conservative fluid therapy.**   Mr. E's persistent hypoxemia was the cardinal feature that indicated acute respiratory distress syndrome. Mr. E's condition most likely occurred because of (a/an) systemic inflammatory response. Specific management of Mr. E's condition included mechanical ventilation. Another treatment to promote gas exchange might include prone positioning. Recent research shows that conservative fluid therapy is the best way to maintain fluid balance. The hallmark feature of ARDS is persistent hypoxemia despite increasing oxygen administration. ARDS occurs after an acute lung injury, which can occur in people without an actual injury to the lung. Systemic inflammatory response is the initiating cause of ARDS. There is evidence and clinical trial data that support using prone positioning to improve gas exchange for patients with moderate to severe ARDS. The use of conservative over liberal or aggressive fluid therapy along with diuretic therapy improves lung function by limiting the damage to the already fluid-filled alveoli. Early recognition of patients at risk and scrupulous infection control methods are nursing priorities to prevent acute respiratory distress syndrome. **Focus:** Priority.

PART 3   Complex Health Scenarios

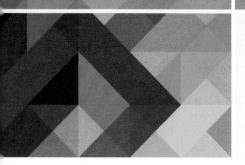

Questions

The RN is the nursing supervisor for the evening shift at a 30-bed long-term care facility (nursing home). The staff for the evening includes an LPN/LVN and three assistive personnel (APs). During the change-of-shift report, the following information is given on these six patients: *Mr. B is a 79-year-old man who underwent hip replacement surgery 3 days ago. He needs help getting out of bed, getting dressed, and ambulating. He was admitted yesterday from the hospital for rehabilitation. Ms. R is an 86-year-old woman who has heart failure and type 2 diabetes and is recovering from a recent myocardial infarction. She has an indwelling urinary catheter. She is usually alert and oriented, but she has become confused over the past 12 hours. Mr. K is a 53-year-old man with a diagnosis of amyotrophic lateral sclerosis. He is totally dependent when it comes to activities of* daily living (ADLs) and has a percutaneous endoscopic gastrostomy tube through which he receives intermittent feedings every 4 hours. He is incontinent of urine and stool. He has a living will requesting that no heroic measures be used to prolong his life.

Ms. L is an 81-year-old woman with diagnoses of hypertension and Alzheimer disease. She is confused, wanders off the unit when not watched, and needs reminders for ADLs. Mr. W is a 68-year-old man who has chronic kidney disease, coronary artery disease, and chronic obstructive pulmonary disease (COPD). He is currently reporting shortness of breath and is receiving oxygen at 2 L/min via nasal cannula. He is lying in bed with his head elevated. He needs help with ADLs. Ms. Q is a 95-year-old woman with a diagnosis of os-itis. She needs help getting out of bed, bathing, dressing.

1. Enhanced Multiple Response

Scenario: Using information from the hand over report, the nurse applies principles of delegation and assignment to ensure that patients receive care from staff members who are functioning within scope of practice.

Which patients could receive **most** of their necessary care from the APs under the supervision of the RN or LPN?

Instructions: Place an X, in the space provided, or highlight each patient that could receive most of their care from the APs. **Select all that apply.**

1. _____ Mr. B
2. _____ Ms. R
3. _____ Mr. K
4. _____ Ms. L
5. _____ Mr. W
6. _____ Ms. Q

2. Which patient will the RN assess **first?**
   1. Ms. R
   2. Mr. K
   3. Mr. W
   4. Ms. Q

3. Which baseline information is the **most** important to obtain from the off-going nurse?
   1. Ms. L's last blood pressure
   2. Mr. B's subjective reports of hip pain
   3. Mr. W's oxygen saturation trends
   4. Ms. R's last blood glucose level

4. Drag and Drop _____

Scenario: The RN supervisor has the responsibility for ensuring that all aspects of patient care are performed and is also responsible for correctly assigning and delegating tasks according to the abilities and experience of each staff member.

Which team member should be assigned or delegated to the tasks listed below?

Instructions: Staff members are listed in the left column. In the right column, in the space provided, write in the letter for the best staff member for each task. Note that all responses will be used and may be used more than once.

Staff members	Tasks
a. RN	1. _____ Assisting Mr. B to ambulate in the hallway
b. LPN/LVN	2. _____ Administering Mr. K's evening tube feeding
c. AP	3. _____ Reminding Ms. L to use the bathroom every 4 hours
	4. _____ Assessing Mr. W's oxygenation status
	5. _____ Giving Ms. R the evening dose of metformin
	6. _____ Evaluating Ms. R's change of mental status
	7. _____ Performing hygiene for Mr. K after incontinence
	8. _____ Assessing Ms. Q's pain and need for medication
	9. _____ Talking to Mr. K's mother about his living will
	10. _____ Assisting Mr. W with oral hygiene after dinner

5. Mr. W continues to report shortness of breath. When the RN assesses him, bilateral crackles are heard with auscultation, and the patient has a productive cough with thick greenish sputum. He is diaphoretic. What would the RN check **next**?
1. Oxygen saturation
2. Blood pressure
3. Heart rate
4. Urine output

6. The nurse suspects a respiratory infection and asks the AP to take Mr. W's temperature. Which instructions would be **best** to give to the AP?
1. Place the thermometer probe in the armpit with arm snugly at side for at least 5 minutes.
2. Wait 30 minutes after foods/fluids, then hold the oral probe under tongue for 3 minutes.
3. Wipe forehead of perspiration, then swipe the forehead using a temporal artery thermometer.
4. Gently pull the earlobe back and insert the probe snugly into the ear canal; push the button.

7. What is the **priority** nursing concern for Mr. W?
1. Thermoregulation
2. Anxiety
3. Infection
4. Gas exchange

8. Mr. W's arterial oxygen saturation (SaO_2) by pulse oximetry is now 89%. Which action would the nurse perform?
1. Increase his oxygen flow rate to 10 L/min via nasal cannula.
2. Attempt to suction the patient's airway by the nasotracheal route.
3. Assist the patient to lie down in bed.
4. Notify the health care provider (HCP).

The RN has received the following orders from Mr. W's HCP:
- *Obtain a sputum sample for culture and sensitivity testing.*
- *Have the patient use the incentive spirometry every 2 hours while awake.*
- *Check pulse oximeter oxygen saturation (SpO_2) every 4 hours.*
- *Administer levofloxacin 250 mg PO twice daily.*

9. To which staff member would it be appropriate to assign carrying out all of these orders from the HCP?
1. Experienced AP
2. Experienced LPN/LVN
3. AP with medication certification
4. RN supervisor

PART 3

Complex Health Scenarios

    Answer Key for this chapter begins on p. 374

10. Enhanced Hot Spot

Scenario: Ms. R is an 86-year-old woman with heart failure and type 2 diabetes. She is recovering from a recent myocardial infarction. Ms. R is usually alert and oriented, but today she is anxious and fearful and does not recognize familiar staff or know where she is at. She has been incontinent with liquid stool for the past 2 days. She has an indwelling urinary catheter. Her urine is dark with a strong foul odor.

Instructions: Underline or highlight the factors or assessment findings that indicate UTI and risk for urosepsis.

Vital signs:
Temperature 97°F (36°C)
Pulse 100 beats/min
Respirations 20 breaths/min
Blood pressure 130/80 mmHg

Which risk factors and current assessment findings indicate that the patient has a urinary tract infection (UTI), that could lead to urosepsis if left untreated?

11. Drag and Drop

Scenario: The RN supervisor notifies Ms. R's HCP about the assessment findings. The HCP prescribes therapies, and the RN plans additional nursing interventions. The RN supervisor must delegate and assign the orders and interventions that are listed below to provide quality care for Ms. R.

Which HCP orders and nursing interventions would be delegated to the AP and which would be **more** appropriately assigned to the LPN/ LVN?

Instructions: Staff members are listed in the left column. In the right column, in the space provided, write in the letter to indicate whether the task would be delegated to the AP or assigned to the LPN/ LVN. Note that all responses will be used and may be used more than once.

Staff members	HCP prescriptions and nursing interventions
A.LPN/LVN	1. _____ Obtain a urine sample for culture and sensitivity testing.
B. AP	2. _____ Administer diphenoxylate 5 mg PO every 6 hours until liquid stools resolve.
	3. _____ Give ciprofloxacin 250 mg PO every 12 hours for 3 days.
	4. _____ Place a clock and calendar where the patient can easily see them.
	5. _____ Check the patient for liquid stools at least every 2 hours.
	6. _____ Obtain a stool sample for ova and parasite testing.
	7. _____ Perform catheter care every shift.
	8. _____ Measure and record intake and output.
	9. _____ Auscultate bowel sounds and assess abdomen.
	10. _____ Observe for deterioration of mental status.

12. The AP informs the nurse that Mr. K has developed redness on his buttocks and that his incontinence pad has been changed very frequently. Which condition is **most** likely?
    1. Stage 1 pressure injury
    2. Incontinence-associated dermatitis (IAD)
    3. Skin lesion development
    4. Skin tears from mechanical shearing force

13. The RN nursing supervisor is creating a care plan for Mr. K. Which key points should be included? **Select all that apply.**
    1. Clean the affected area gently with minimal friction after each episode of incontinence.
    2. Use regular soap and warm water to clean the patient.
    3. Gently dry after each cleansing.
    4. Apply a skin protectant to all skin that could come into contact with urine or stool.
    5. Check skin protectant ingredients to be sure the patient is not allergic or sensitive.
    6. Alternate use of alkaline and acidic skin protectants for rapid skin improvement.

14. Which instruction would the RN give to the AP about moving and repositioning Mr. K in bed?
    1. Turn and reposition Mr. K every 4 hours.
    2. Place Mr. K in a supine position for napping.
    3. Keep the head of the bed (HOB) elevated at least 90 degrees while Mr. K is awake.
    4. Use a draw (pull) sheet to avoid friction skin tears.

15. The RN reassesses Mr. W. He reports that his breathing is better. The AP tells the RN that his latest pulse oximetry reading is 90%. What is the RN's **best** action?
    1. Notify the HCP.
    2. Decrease the oxygen flow.
    3. Document the findings as the only action.
    4. Instruct the night shift AP to wake Mr. W every hour for incentive spirometry.

16. At 5:30 PM, the AP reports that Mr. B, who had hip replacement surgery 3 days ago, refuses to get out of bed to walk in the hall as prescribed. What is the RN's **first** action?
    1. Ask the LPN/LVN to administer as needed (PRN) pain medication.
    2. Tell the AP that Mr. B must get up to prevent pneumonia.
    3. Remind the AP that Mr. B has the right to refuse.
    4. Talk to Mr. B about why he does not want to get up.

17. Mr. B tells the RN that he was taking a nap when the AP woke him to get up and walk. He reports that he did not sleep well last night and was angry at being awakened. What are the RN's **best** actions at this time? **Select all that apply.**
    1. Ask Mr. B if he is willing to get up and walk now.
    2. Remind Mr. B that there are 30 patients who need care.
    3. Offer Mr. B PRN pain medication before he gets up to walk.
    4. Instruct the AP never to wake a patient from a nap.
    5. Discuss strategies to help Mr. B achieve good rest at night.
    6. Teach Mr. B the importance of preventing respiratory problems.

18. Ms. Q, who has osteoarthritis, refuses to take her evening dose of calcium because it makes her stomach upset. What is the **priority** teaching that the RN will give to the LPN/LVN about the calcium?
    1. Tell the LPN/LVN that Ms. Q must take her calcium because she is at risk for fractures.
    2. Suggest rescheduling the dose time so that Ms. Q receives the calcium with food.
    3. Remind the LPN/LVN that calcium is best absorbed on an empty stomach.
    4. Instruct the LPN/LVN to hold the dose and notify the HCP.

19. Ms. L, who has Alzheimer disease, wanders into Mr. K's room. The LPN/LVN finds her disconnecting Mr. K's tube feeding. Ms. L says, "Hello, dearie, I was just cleaning this up for you." What is the **best** action for the LPN/LVN to take at this time?
    1. In a loud and stern voice, tell Ms. L that this is not her room.
    2. Ask the AP to escort Ms. L back to her room and keep her there.
    3. Gently reorient Ms. L and reconnect Mr. K's tube feeding.
    4. Remind Ms. L that she is a patient and should not perform care for other patients.

20. Mr. K's mother comes running out of his room, yelling, "He's dying! Call 911! Hurry, hurry!" What is the RN's **best** action at this time?
    1. Call the emergency squad because the mother's wishes supersede Mr. K's.
    2. Call the HCP and ask for orders to give emergency interventions.
    3. Begin cardiopulmonary resuscitation and continue until help arrives.
    4. Assess Mr. K's status, provide emotional support, and respect his wishes.

    Answer Key for this chapter begins on p. 374

PART 3 Complex Health Scenarios

Answers

1. **Ans: 1, 4, 6** Although some aspects of care for all six patients could be delegated to the AP, Mr. B, Ms. L, and Ms. Q need assistance with ADLs. Routine assistance with ADLs is within the scope of practice of the AP. Ms. R's change in level of consciousness needs to be assessed because this is a change from her baseline and the care plan may need revision. Many aspects of Mr. K's care can be assigned to an AP, but his tube feeding must be done by a licensed nurse. Mr. K also needs ongoing assessment and support for emotional needs. Mr. W's difficulty with breathing also requires assessment from a licensed nurse because this is a change from his baseline. Based on assessment findings, the nurse may instruct the AP to modify assistance with ADLs or defer select activities until Mr. W is feeling better. **Focus:** Delegation.

2. **Ans: 3** Mr. W is having difficulty breathing. He may need immediate life-saving interventions. Ms. R needs to be assessed second. New onset confusion is a change of mental status for her. Urinary tract infection is common among older persons in long-term care; however, there are many causes that must be considered, such as: diabetes, electrolyte imbalances, medication side effects, decreased cardiac output, decreased oxygenation, stroke or head injury. **Focus:** Prioritization.

3. **Ans: 3** Mr. W is having problems breathing; therefore the nurse needs to be aware of trends of oxygen saturation. Baseline information is always valuable, but it is most useful in situations where the patient's condition changes over the course of the shift. **Focus:** Prioritization.

4. **Ans: 1c, 2b, 3c, 4a, 5b, 6a, 7c, 8b, 9a, 10c** Tube feeding, medication administration, and assessment of chronic pain are within the scope of practice of an LPN/LVN. The scope of practice of an AP includes assisting with ambulation, toileting, and hygiene. The RN would assess acute conditions such as Mr. W's oxygenation status and Ms. R's change of mental status. Talking to relatives about legal, ethical, and emotionally laden issues such as a living will should also be done by the RN. **Focus:** Assignment, Delegation.

5. **Ans: 1** Checking oxygen saturation via pulse oximetry will give the RN important information about Mr. W's oxygenation status and a possible reason for why he is experiencing difficulty breathing. Although checking blood pressure, urine output, and heart rate are important, they are not the priority at this time. **Focus:** Prioritization.

6. **Ans: 4** For Mr. W, the tympanic method is the best choice. All methods of measuring temperature have advantages and disadvantages. The tympanic method is quick and easy for the patient and the caregiver. Cerumen in the canal can affect results. In this case, irrigating the ear is inappropriate; it is time consuming, and the focus of the care should be on resolving the breathing problem. Axillary temperatures are generally the least favored by HCPs because they tend to be the least accurate, possibly because the full 5 minute time length is not always performed as it should be. Oral temperatures are traditional, but patients with dyspnea are likely to be mouth breathing (which lowers the oral temperature) and may be unable or unwilling to keep the thermometer probe in place for 3 minutes. Temporal artery thermometers are accurate and easy for the patient and the caregiver; however, dyspnea (and fever) usually causes perspiration and wiping or drying the forehead is insufficient because the cooling mechanism of perspiration will still create a falsely low skin temperature. **Focus:** Prioritization. **Test-Taking Tip:** Don't forget to go back and review your fundamentals textbook. Information about how to take vital signs was covered in the first semester of nursing school and you have studied many topics since then.

7. **Ans: 4** The priority concern for Mr. W is gas exchange. Thermoregulation and infection underlie the problem. Anxiety often accompanies dyspnea, but this should abate after the gas exchange is corrected. **Focus:** Prioritization.

8. **Ans: 4** Mr. W has crackles, a productive cough, and decreased gas exchange. The HCP needs to be notified because these signs and symptoms may indicate a respiratory infection that needs to be treated. Patients with COPD should receive low-flow oxygen (3 L/min or less) because their stimulus to breathe is a low oxygen level. The patient is already having shortness of breath, which may be worsened with attempts to suction or to lay the patient flat in bed. **Focus:** Prioritization.

9. **Ans: 2** All of the nursing responsibilities associated with the HCP's orders are within the scope of practice of an LPN/LVN. Because Mr. W is experiencing changes, an experienced LPN/LVN would be preferred to an AP with medication certification. The nurse supervisor would direct the LPN/LVN to give regular updates about Mr. W's condition. **Focus:** Assignment.

10. **Ans:** Ms. R is an **86-year-old woman** with **heart failure** and **type 2 diabetes**. She is recovering from a **recent myocardial infarction**. Ms. R is **usually alert and oriented**, but today she is **anxious and fearful**

and **does not recognize familiar staff or know where she is at.** She has been **incontinent with liquid stool** for the past 2 days. She has an **indwelling urinary catheter.** Her **urine is dark with a strong foul odor.** Vital signs: Temperature 97°F (36°C); **Pulse 100/min;** Respirations 20/min; Blood pressure 130/80 mmHg. Older age, female sex (a shorter urethra increases the risk for urinary infections), and chronic health conditions, such as heart failure and diabetes, are risk factors. Diabetes increases the risk for infection, and recovering from a myocardial infarction would affect the immune system. An indwelling urinary catheter is invasive; in combination with incontinence of liquid stool, the catheter is a route for fecal contamination to move up into the urinary system. The color and odor of the urine suggest that a UTI is in progress. She does not have a fever, but older people may not have elevated temperatures with infection. She does have a sudden and unexplained change in mental status. Her pulse suggests an increase in metabolic activity and physiological or psychological distress. **Focus:** Prioritization. **Test-Taking Tip:** Urinary tract infections and pneumonia often occur in institutionalized or bedridden older adults. Typical infection signs, such as fever or inflammation, may not occur.

11. **Ans: 1B, 2A, 3A, 4B, 5B, 6B, 7B, 8B, 9A, 10A**   Much of the care that occurs in long-term care facilities is within the scope of practice of an AP. In this case, medication administration is done by a licensed nurse. The LPN/LVN would also assess the abdomen because diphenoxylate was administered for liquid stools. The LPN/LVN would observe for and immediately report deterioration of mental status to the RN. **Focus:** Assignment, Delegation, Supervision. **Test-Taking Tip:** In some states, long-term care facilities employ medication APs. These APs must complete a special state-approved program and must demonstrate competency to take a pulse and measure blood pressure. The licensed nurse is still responsible for knowing the purpose and dealing with the side effects of medications that are administered by the APs. Be sure to check the scope of practice limits for your specific state and facility.

12. **Ans: 2**   IAD describes the skin damage associated with exposure to urine or stool. It causes considerable discomfort and can be difficult, time consuming, and expensive to treat. It is an irritant contact dermatitis (inflammation) often found in patients with urinary or stool incontinence. IAD appears as erythema and can range from pink to red. Patients with IAD are at an increased risk for skin infections, especially candidiasis. **Focus:** Prioritization.

13. **Ans: 1, 3, 4, 5**   Principles of cleaning to prevent and manage IAD include cleansing daily and after every episode of stool incontinence; using gentle technique with minimal friction and avoiding rubbing or scrubbing of skin; avoiding standard (alkaline) soaps; choosing a gentle, no-rinse liquid skin cleanser or premoistened wipe (designed and indicated for incontinence care), with a pH similar to normal skin; using a soft, disposable nonwoven cloth; and gently drying skin if needed after cleansing. Principles of skin protectant use to avoid or manage IAD include applying the skin protectant at a frequency consistent with its ability to protect the skin and in line with the manufacturer's instructions, ensuring the skin protectant is compatible with any other skin care products (e.g., skin cleansers that are in use), and applying the skin protectant to all skin that comes into contact with or potentially will contact urine or stool. **Focus:** Prioritization.

14. **Ans: 4**   Friction occurs when surfaces rub the skin and irritate or tear fragile epithelial tissue. Such forces are generated when the patient is dragged or pulled across bed linen. Use of a pull or draw sheet when moving a patient in bed helps prevent this type of skin injury. Patient turn schedules should be every 2 hours but also should be individualized based on needs. The supine position is not appropriate for a patient with a feeding tube because of an increased risk for aspiration. Ninety-degree HOB elevation is likely to be too high for comfort for most patients. **Focus:** Delegation, Supervision. **Test-Taking Tip:** If patients are already at risk for injury related to the loss of skin integrity, actions such as turning and repositioning can contribute to the problem. The nurse is responsible to give the AP specific instructions about how to prevent injuries.

15. **Ans: 3**   Mr. W is much improved. A pulse oximetry reading of 90% is acceptable for a patient with COPD, and the oxygen flow does not need to be changed. Waking the patient every hour for incentive spirometry is counterproductive because the patient will not get the rest he needs. **Focus:** Prioritization. **Test-Taking Tip:** When a patient is much improved and assessment findings are within normal limits, the RN's main responsibility is to document the changes.

16. **Ans: 4**   The first priority is assessing to gather more information. Pain may be the reason for Mr. B's refusal, but that is not known until the patient is assessed. Patients do have the right to refuse treatment, but the purpose of Mr. B's admission is rehabilitation so that he can go home, and early ambulation is important in the prevention of respiratory complications. **Focus:** Prioritization.

17. **Ans: 1, 3, 5, 6**   Mr. B does need to get up and walk. Administering his PRN pain medication may facilitate this. It is important to be attentive to the underlying problem and to strategize how to ensure that he receives appropriate rest, which will aid his recovery. If he is unaware of the respiratory risks associated with failing to ambulate, this is a teaching opportunity. It is not appropriate to belittle Mr. B's concerns by reminding him of the other patients' needs. Although the RN may want to talk with the AP about getting

PART 3   Complex Health Scenarios

more information and allowing patients to rest, there may be times when it is important to awaken patients from naps. **Focus:** Prioritization.

18. **Ans: 2**   A fairly common side effect of calcium therapy is gastrointestinal upset with nausea and vomiting, and giving this drug with food can minimize or eliminate this side effect. Although Ms. Q is at risk for fractures, this answer does not focus on the problem. Giving the drug on an empty stomach will most likely make the nausea and vomiting worse. Holding the dose does not focus on the problem. **Focus:** Prioritization.

19. **Ans: 3**   Ms. L is confused and should respond better to a gentle reorientation than to a loud, stern reprimand. The priority is ensuring that Mr. K's tube feeding is restarted; then the LPN/LVN could escort Ms. L back to her room or delegate this to the AP. When Ms. L is being reoriented, the LPN/LVN should remind her that she is a patient, but rather than scolding her, give her a positive response that would redirect her to an alternative activity (e.g., "You are a patient and you are invited to an interesting activity in the day room."). **Focus:** Prioritization, Assignment.

20. **Ans: 4**   Mr. K's living will is a legal document and must be respected. The nurse should assess his status and check his advance directive document to make sure it is current and then respect his wishes. The nurse would call the HCP with notification of the patient's death. The nurse should take his mother into a quiet room, calmly remind her of his wishes, have someone stay with her, and ask if there is someone who can be called for her (e.g., a spiritual advisor or another family member). **Focus:** Prioritization.

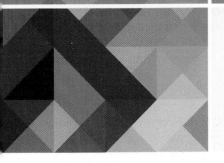

CASE STUDY 19

Pediatric Patients in Clinic and Acute Care Settings

Questions

The charge nurse is working in a large urban pediatric walk-in clinic that offers well-baby care, provides immunizations, and is an educational resource for child health topics. In addition, the clinic also accommodates walk-in patients and offers basic diagnostic testing and emergency care. The staff includes a pediatrician, a graduate student who is working toward an advanced practice nursing (APN) degree, an experienced RN, an experienced LPN/LVN, a pediatric social worker, a graduate nurse (GN), and an assistive personnel (AP). This morning, in addition to scheduled appointments, there is an immunization clinic. The charge nurse receives two phone calls, and there is one walk-in patient.

1. To ensure efficient workflow of the clinic and maximize available expertise, which task should be assigned to the experienced LPN/LVN?
   1. Perform triage for walk-in patients.
   2. Perform physical assessment of walk-in patients.
   3. Give routine immunizations.
   4. Obtain weight and height measurements.

2. A mother brings her 12-month-old child to the clinic for an influenza vaccination. The RN tells the mother that the child is also due for doses of measles-mumps-rubella, varicella, and hepatitis A vaccines. The mother declines the nurse's advice because "he has already had enough of those." What is the **priority** action?
   1. Encourage a follow-up appointment and notify Child Protective Services (CPS).
   2. Assess the mother's concerns and current level of knowledge about immunization.
   3. Emphasize the benefits of immunization; explain the purpose and schedule.
   4. Respect the mother's decision and alert the pediatrician to the situation.

3. A 9-month-old child arrives at the health center with his mother for immunizations. The child is fussy with rhinorrhea and has an axillary temperature of 100.4°F (38°C). The pediatrician has determined that the child has nasopharyngitis. What is the **priority** action?
   1. Administer half of the immunizations and reschedule a subsequent appointment for the other half.
   2. Advise the mother that fever is a contraindication for immunization and reschedule the appointment.
   3. Administer acetaminophen to reduce fever and apply an anesthetic cream to the injection site.
   4. Advise the mother that the child will likely need an antibiotic and reschedule the appointment.

4. A parent calls in for advice because her 18-month-old toddler has stumbled and bumped his head on the coffee table. Which symptom is cause for the **greatest** concern?
   1. A swelling the size of a golf ball that is tender to the touch
   2. Two episodes of vomiting a small amount of undigested food
   3. Continuous crying for 2 hours, unrelieved by familiar comfort measures
   4. Gaping 1.5-inch (4-cm) laceration on the forehead, with bleeding controlled by pressure

5. A parent calls in for advice because "Missy is 5 years old, and she just won't sleep in her own bed. For the past 4 months, she wakes and comes to sleep with me and my husband. She cries and cries if we take her back to her own room." What is the **priority** action?
   1. Send the mother a brochure of things she can try to assist the child to sleep independently.
   2. Advise the mother that this is a normal behavior that will eventually pass with time.
   3. Suggest that the child be put back into her own bed and allowed to cry herself to sleep.
   4. Schedule an appointment with the APN student for assessment and management.

6. Six-year-old Billy woke last night with dyspnea, restlessness, wheezing, and cough. Mother and child spent the night in a reclining chair. His mother declares, "He is having an asthma attack. We are both exhausted. I'm tired of waiting forever to see the doctor!" What is the **priority** nursing concern?
   1. Billy's poor sleep quality and restlessness
   2. Billy's ongoing shortness of breath
   3. Mother's report of feeling exhausted
   4. Mother's frustration with health care system

7. As the nurse approaches Billy, which presentation would be of **most** concern and require immediate intervention?
   1. Alert and irritable, lying recumbent on the examination table
   2. Awake and nervous, sitting upright and crying, skin pale and dry
   3. Agitated, sweating, and sitting upright with shoulders hunched forward
   4. Asleep in a side-lying position breathing through open mouth

8. Which assessment finding for Billy is the **most** urgent and requires immediate intervention and notification of the pediatrician?
   1. Sudden increase in respiratory rate and decreased breath sounds
   2. Rattling cough productive of frothy, clear, gelatinous sputum
   3. Crackles auscultated on inspiration in the lower lung fields
   4. Restlessness and wheezing auscultated at the end of expiration

9. Drag and Drop

Scenario: The nurse is aware that Billy requires close monitoring and emergency interventions that can be accomplished in the clinic. However, Billy's condition is serious and to prevent complications, he will have to be transferred to a hospital setting.

What is the sequence of implementing the following prescribed actions?

Instructions: In the left column are the prescribed therapies and actions. In the right column write the number to indicate the correct sequence. 1 being the first action and 8 being the last action.

Prescribed Actions	Order of sequence
a. Administer IV methylprednisolone.	
b. Contact the hospital about admission.	
c. Give nebulized albuterol now and every 30 minutes.	
d. Teach about measuring peak expiratory flow rate to determine personal best.	
e. Obtain a chest radiograph and a complete blood count (CBC).	
f. Administer humidified oxygen to maintain saturation above 90%.	
g. Schedule a radioallergosorbent (RAST)	

10. Billy is to be transferred from the clinic to the hospital for his asthmatic condition. Which tasks are RN responsibilities and should not be delegated or performed by another member of the health care team? **Select all that apply.**
    1. Give a report to the attending pediatrician at the receiving hospital.
    2. Give a report to the charge nurse at the receiving hospital.
    3. Help the parent and child to collect and bag up personal items.
    4. Determine that the patient's condition is stable enough for transport to the hospital.
    5. Assess the response to treatment and document the patient's condition.
    6. Assist the patient when transferring to the ambulance stretcher.

11. Drag and Drop

Scenario: In the afternoon, several patients come to the clinic for walk-in care. The nurse must prioritize the following patients in the order in which they should be seen to ensure safe care and efficiently manage patient load.

What is the order for patients to receive care?

Instructions: In the left column are the patients who need care. In the right column write the number to indicate the order for patients to receive care. 1 being the first and 4 being the last.

Walk-in patients who need care	Order of care
A. Daisy is 4 years old; she is alert and irritable with pale, sweaty skin. An older neighbor who was temporarily watching Daisy reports that she was running around and playing, and then she got "grumpy." Daisy has diabetes, but the neighbor "was not sure how to give her the insulin."	
B. Sarah is 11 months old; she is dirty and crying, and her right arm is swollen and red. Sam is Sarah's 2-year-old brother; he is dirty and hungry and reaches out to be picked up. Ms. A, their mother, is 19 years old and single. She is thin and disheveled and seems somewhat confused. She is having trouble answering the nurse's questions. Ms. A says, "Those kids play too rough! The older one is always pushing the baby off the bed	
C. Terry is 7 months old; he rubs at both of his ears, acts fussy, refuses to suck, and has a temperature of 101.2°F (38.4°C). He has had three episodes of otitis media in the past. Social history includes night bottle-feeding and parents who smoke cigarettes.	
D. James is 3 years old. He woke last night with a sore throat, difficulty swallowing, and a fever. He is flushed, anxious, and drooling. The nurse observes a thick, muffled quality to his voice and slow, quiet breathing. The nurse notes that James looks sick.	

12. What is the **priority** concern for James (refer to question 11)?
1. Fever
2. Drooling
3. Sore throat
4. Flushing

13. What is the **priority** action for James (refer to question 11)?
1. Visually inspect the throat with a tongue blade and auscultate the lungs.
2. Administer humidified oxygen and have the child sit upright on a parent's lap.
3. Notify the pediatrician and prepare intubation equipment.
4. Reassure the parents the symptoms will resolve with breathing of cool moist air.

14. The APN student and the pediatrician are at James' bedside. Which two additional team members would be the **best** combination to provide the initial care for James (refer to question 11)?
1. The experienced RN and the experienced LPN/LVN
2. The experienced RN and the AP
3. The experienced RN and the GN
4. The experienced LPN/LVN and the GN

15. The pediatrician examines James and determines that he should be taken immediately to the Children's Hospital emergency department (ED). The child is breathing slowly and quietly; humidified oxygen is being administered. What is the **priority** action?
1. Instruct the parents to drive the child to the hospital immediately and call the ED.
2. Contact a private ambulance service and prepare the patient for transport.
3. Call 911, ask for advanced emergency medical services (EMS), and monitor the child.
4. Assist the pediatrician to intubate the child and then arrange for transport.

16. Daisy (refer to question 11) has type 1 diabetes. She is currently alert but irritable. She looks pale and her skin is clammy. What is the **priority** action for Daisy?
1. Locate the mother to obtain a history and permission to treat.
2. Administer supplemental oxygen, alert the pediatrician, and establish IV access.
3. Ask the child to describe how she feels and use simple questions to obtain a history.
4. Perform blood glucose testing and then give the child a carton of milk.

Answer Key for this chapter begins on p. 382

PART 3   Complex Health Scenarios

17. Daisy's mother arrives at the clinic, and she is relieved to find Daisy happy and smiling, but the mother bursts into tears and begins to yell at her neighbor and the nursing staff for "not taking care of her!" What is the best way to handle her anger and tears?
    1. Remind the mother that the child is okay and that the neighbor was doing what she thought was best based on the information that she had.
    2. Allow the mother to express her feelings and then take the neighbor aside and explain that the mother is just temporarily upset.
    3. Teach the mother about ways to communicate the child's needs to all caregivers and help her make a list of specific instructions.
    4. Direct the mother to a private area and encourage her to ventilate feelings; then gently assess how she typically manages Daisy's diabetes.

18. What is the **priority** nursing concern for Terry, who is rubbing at his ears, acting fussy, refusing to suck, and has a temperature of 101.2°F (38.4°C)?
    1. Pain
    2. Poor nutrition
    3. Recurrent ear infections
    4. Elevated temperature

19. For 7-month old Terry (refer to question 11), which task would be appropriate to assign to the LPN/LVN?
    1. Teach parents that passive smoking and night bottles contribute to ear infections.
    2. Explain the concept of "watchful waiting" for 72 hours for uncomplicated otitis.
    3. Administer ordered dose of acetaminophen and apply a warm moist compress to pinna.
    4. Prepare the child for a myringotomy and assist the pediatrician during the procedure.

20. The GN is preparing to give an antibiotic tablet to 7-month-old Terry. She checks a drug reference book, crushes the tablet, and then mixes it into 3 oz (85 grams) of applesauce. As the supervising nurse, what is the **priority** action?
    1. Accompany her into the room and observe while she administers the drug.
    2. Allow her to proceed independently and ask her to report on the outcome.
    3. Suggest that she consider again the patient's circumstances and developmental needs.
    4. Suggest that she recheck the drug reference book before administering the drug.

21. What is the **priority** nursing concern in caring for the A family? (Refer to question 11 for a description of the A family's circumstances.)
    1. Hygiene
    2. Safety
    3. Development
    4. Growth

22. Which tasks related to the care of Sarah, Sam, and Ms. A can be delegated to the AP? **Select all that apply.**
    1. Assist the toddler to eat an age-appropriate meal.
    2. Apply a supportive splint to the infant's arm.
    3. Report any behavioral signs of child abuse.
    4. Report any findings to CPS if appropriate.
    5. Assist by holding one child while the other is being examined.
    6. Accompany the infant to the radiology department.

23. The pediatric social worker has just informed Ms. A that CPS has been notified and that a representative will arrive shortly to speak with her about the family's situation. Ms. A starts to cry and threatens to leave. What is the **priority** action?
    1. Obtain an "against medical advice" (AMA) form and have her sign it.
    2. Notify the pediatrician of the mother's intent to leave.
    3. Inform the mother that the police will be notified if she leaves.
    4. Encourage Ms. A to remain and to express feelings and fears.

Rebecca is a 6-year-old girl with cystic fibrosis. She arrives at the pediatric cystic fibrosis clinic for her routine 3-month appointment. The nurse obtains and calculates the following growth parameters: Weight, 33 lbs (15 kg) (< 5%); height, 42 in. (106 cm) (5%); and body mass index (BMI), 13 (< 5%). Her parents report specks of blood in her sputum after chest physiotherapy. Her forced expiratory volume in 1 second (FEV_1) has decreased 25% from her last visit 3 months ago. Rebecca has clubbing of both her finger and toe nails.

24. How would the nurse best interpret Rebecca's decreased FEV_1?
    1. Decreased oxygenation
    2. Increased obstruction
    3. Presence of infection
    4. Pulmonary remodeling

25. What is the **most** likely cause of the specks of blood in Rebecca's sputum?
    1. A sign of pulmonary infection
    2. A sign of bronchial remodeling
    3. A sign of gastric irritation
    4. A sign of gastrointestinal bleeding

26. The nurse establishes that Rebecca has poor airway clearance. Which intervention is **most** important for the nurse to implement for this problem?
    1. Increased fluid requirements
    2. Inhaled corticosteroids
    3. Oxygen therapy
    4. Flutter valve with huffing

27. The nurse reviews Rebecca's growth chart and determines her weight and BMI have consistently remained below the 5th percentile. Which collaborative intervention is the nurse **most** likely to anticipate when planning teaching?
    1. Preparing the child and family for potential gastrostomy tube placement
    2. Focusing on increasing the child's intake of protein and calories
    3. Suggesting an increased dosage of pancreatic enzymes
    4. Preparing the child and family for potential total parenteral nutrition

28. Which laboratory value is consistent with the clubbing of Rebecca's finger and toe nails?
    1. Elevated white blood cell (WBC) count
    2. Elevated red blood cell (RBC) count
    3. Decreased hematocrit
    4. Decreased mean corpuscular volume

Four-year-old Bobby is admitted to the pediatric unit with Kawasaki disease. Today is the seventh day of fever. Laboratory studies reveal a C-reactive protein level of 3.1 mg/dL (29.5 mmol/L) and a WBC count of 17,000 mm³ (17 × 10⁹/L).

29. Which nursing assessment is a **priority**?
    1. Obtain a rectal temperature.
    2. Auscultate the lungs.
    3. Obtain a blood pressure.
    4. Auscultate the heart.

30. Which pharmacologic intervention should the nurse anticipate at this time?
    1. IV methylprednisolone
    2. IV immunoglobulin
    3. IV ibuprofen
    4. IV infliximab

31. After a 14-day hospitalization, Bobby is discharged home on a regimen of long-term aspirin therapy. What advice should the nurse provide regarding influenza vaccination?
    1. The influenza vaccine is indicated for children 4 months to 18 years of age.
    2. The influenza vaccine should be postponed for 11 months after treatment.
    3. The influenza vaccine is indicated for children receiving long-term aspirin therapy.
    4. The influenza vaccine should be postponed in children receiving long-term aspirin therapy.

Eight-year-old Charlie had a laparoscopic appendectomy. During surgery, the appendix perforated. Charlie arrives on the pediatric unit from the operating room. His weight on admission was 46 lbs (21 kg). He has a peripheral IV line in the left basilic vein with D₅W and 20 mEq/L (20 mmol/L) of KCl running at 70 mL/hr. A nasogastric tube (NG) is attached to low suction.

32. Which assessment should be **most** concerning to the nurse?
    1. Oral temperature of 100.4°F (38°C)
    2. Decreased bowel sounds in all quadrants
    3. Urine output of 160 mL over 4 hours
    4. Respiratory rate of 15 breaths per minute

33. Charlie's parents ask the nurse if the NG tube can be removed because it is irritating Charlie's nose. What is the nurse's **best** response?
    1. "The NG tube is necessary to prevent aspiration of the stomach contents into the lungs."
    2. "The NG tube is necessary because Charlie will need to have feedings through it."
    3. "The NG tube is necessary to keep Charlie's stomach empty, allowing the intestines to rest."
    4. "The NG tube is necessary to prevent swallowed air from building up in the stomach."

34. The nurse performs a pain assessment. Charlie rates his pain as 4 of 10 on the Wong-Baker FACES® Pain Rating Scale. Which intervention should the nurse implement?
    1. Administer 200 mg of ibuprofen.
    2. Administer 5 mg of hydrocodone.
    3. Administer 100 mg of acetaminophen.
    4. Administer 10 mg of codeine.

35. At the change of shift, the nurse reassesses Charlie. His NG tube is patent and drained 120 mL over 12 hours. His oral temperature is 99.5°F (37.5°C), heart rate is 80 beats/min, and respiratory rate is 17 breaths/min. Charlie appears groggy and confused. Charlie's muscle strength is 3 of 5 in his upper and lower extremities. Laboratory tests are ordered. Which results are **most** consistent with Charlie's clinical presentation?
    1. K⁺, 3.3 mEq/L (3.3 mmol/L); Cl⁻, 95 mEq/L (95 mmol/L); pH, 7.55
    2. K⁺, 3.3 mEq/L (3.3 mmol/L); Cl⁻, 110 mEq/L (110 mmol/L); pH, 7.55
    3. K⁺, 5.2 mEq/L (5.2 mmol/L); Cl⁻, 110 mEq/L (110 mmol/L); pH, 7.20
    4. K⁺, 3.3 mEq/L (3.3 mmol/L); Cl⁻, 95 mEq/L (95 mmol/L); pH, 7.20

 Answer Key for this chapter begins on p. 382

Answers

1. **Ans: 3**   LPN/LVN skills are appropriate for giving routine immunizations; the RN or GN could also give injections, but in a busy clinic the RN should perform triage and initial physical assessments and mentor the GN in these tasks. Obtaining height and weight should be delegated to the AP. The pediatrician will perform physical assessments of all walk-in patients and supervise the APN student, who can perform physical assessments and triage. **Focus:** Assignment.

2. **Ans: 2**   First the nurse should assess the mother's decision and her level of knowledge. She may not understand the pharmacology of immunizations, or the child may have had a problem with previous immunizations. She has agreed to immunizations in the past, but now something has changed her mind. Other options may be appropriate depending on the assessment findings. **Focus:** Prioritization.

3. **Ans: 3**   Acetaminophen will reduce the child's fever, and an anesthetic cream will reduce pain at the injection site. By taking this action, the nurse is preparing to give the child the recommended immunizations. Fever and minor illnesses are not contraindications for immunizations. Nasopharyngitis is a common cold that is caused by a virus, and antibiotics are not indicated for viruses. Additionally, antibiotics are not a contraindication for immunizations. Splitting immunizations is not recommended because it would result in immunization delay. The scheduling of immunizations is such that it protects children at times when they are most vulnerable to morbidity and mortality related to the natural diseases. Delayed immunization places the child at risk for vaccine-preventable diseases. **Focus:** Prioritization.

4. **Ans: 3**   Inconsolable crying for 2 hours is excessive, prolonged, and abnormal and may be a sign of increased intracranial pressure (ICP). Instruct the parent to call 911. The swelling can be treated with ice packs. Vomiting can be a sign of increased ICP, but fewer than three episodes is usually associated with minor injuries. A laceration on the forehead needs suturing, which should be done within several hours to prevent infection and reduce scarring, but the more pressing issue is to reaffirm with the caller that the bleeding is controlled. **Focus:** Prioritization.

5. **Ans: 4**   Additional psychosocial and physical assessment is needed to intervene properly. The other three options may be appropriate after the initial assessment is completed. **Focus:** Prioritization.

6. **Ans: 2**   The priority is the child's ongoing dyspnea, which indicates poor control of his asthma and possible hypoxemia. Additionally, restlessness is a clinical manifestation of impending respiratory failure. This requires rapid intervention. The mother's exhaustion should improve with treatment for the asthma attack. The mother's frustration with Billy's health care is important to address, but this is not immediately life threatening. **Focus:** Prioritization.

7. **Ans: 3**   Agitation and sweating are signs of severe respiratory distress. In addition, the child is attempting to maximize the thoracic cavity and to oxygenate more effectively by sitting upright and hunching forward. **Focus:** Prioritization.

8. **Ans: 1**   An increased respiratory rate and decreased breath sounds are ominous signs of airway obstruction. Respiratory arrest is imminent. A productive cough warrants close observation because the patient is at risk for mucus plugs and bronchial spasm, which can cause an obstruction. Restlessness and wheezing are characteristic clinical manifestations of an asthma exacerbation and require attention but are not urgent. Crackles are suggestive of pneumonia and need to be monitored but are not the priority in this scenario. Respiratory arrest is the life-threatening event that the nurse must address. **Focus:** Prioritization.

9. **Ans: a3, b5, c1, d6, e4, f2, g7**   Dyspnea and restlessness are clinical manifestations of impending respiratory failure. Wheezing and cough indicate bronchoconstriction. This requires rapid intervention. The onset of action of nebulized albuterol is 5 to 7 minutes. Administering albuterol first results in bronchodilation, which is essential for oxygen to actually reach the airways. Humidified oxygen can then be administered because albuterol results in bronchodilation, which allows oxygen to enter the lungs. In acute exacerbations of asthma, short-acting beta$_2$ agonists are given followed by corticosteroid therapy. The onset of action for methylprednisolone is 1 to 2 hours. A chest radiograph and CBC are appropriate to determine underlying pathology such as infection that may contribute to the episode. Arrangements should be made to transfer the patient to the hospital after the patient's condition has been stabilized. Measuring peak flow rates to determine personal best is part of long-term management and patient education. RAST can be scheduled on an outpatient basis. **Focus:** Prioritization. **Test-Taking Tip:** Understanding both the action and the onset of action of medications facilitates prioritization.

10. **Ans: 2, 5**   The RN must give the nursing report to the receiving nurse and assess response to treatment and document the patient's condition. The pediatrician must give the physician-to-physician report and determine if the patient is stable enough for transfer. The RN can delegate to the AP: collecting of

personal items and helping the patient to transfer. The RN must supervise and know that the AP has had proper training to handle patient belongings and in transfer techniques to prevent injury to self or patient. **Focus:** Supervision, Assignment, Delegation.

11. **Ans: 4, 1, 2, 3** James's condition is the most critical. He has airway compromise that could suddenly turn into a complete airway obstruction. Daisy is the next in priority. Although she is conscious, she cannot be allowed to continue unattended for a long period. At a minimum, delegate performing a blood glucose check to the LPN/LVN (or AP if appropriate training has been given) with instructions that the results be reported to the RN immediately. Sarah, Sam, and Ms. A have complex social circumstances that will be very time consuming to address; however, this family is a flight risk. Quickly check on the A family and alert all staff members about the need to support this family. Terry has a treatable ear infection; treatment and education are relatively straightforward. Then go back and do an in-depth assessment of the A family. **Focus:** Prioritization.

12. **Ans: 2** James has symptoms of epiglottitis and is at high risk for an airway obstruction. Drooling is a classic symptom of epiglottitis and indicates that airway obstruction may be imminent. The other data are relevant and support the epiglottitis diagnosis but do not indicate a need for immediate action. **Focus:** Prioritization. **Test-Taking Tip:** Be able to differentiate between clinical manifestations that are characteristic of a disease and those that indicate a severe consequence of a disease. In the case of epiglottitis, drooling indicates airway obstruction.

13. **Ans: 2** The child has an immediate need for oxygen. An upright position facilitates breathing, and parental comfort minimizes agitation and crying, which would increase oxygen consumption. Inspecting the throat is contraindicated because the procedure could exacerbate airway obstruction. Intubation equipment should always be available but is not needed yet; however, the pediatrician should be made aware of the child's drooling. (Note: If the clinic were attached to a hospital, the nurse could alert the operating room about the need for a potential emergency intubation, tracheostomy, or both.) Reassuring the parents that the condition will resolve spontaneously is inappropriate. **Focus:** Prioritization.

14. **Ans: 3** In addition to the APN student and the pediatrician, the best combination would be the experienced RN and GN. The child is acutely ill and may require immediate intervention for airway management. This is an opportunity for the experienced RN to closely supervise and mentor the GN. In the initial care of this child, there are few tasks that can be delegated to the AP, and the expertise of the LPN/LVN is best used to monitor and assess other patients in more stable conditions. **Focus:** Supervision, Assignment.

15. **Ans: 3** In a clinic setting, calling 911 is the best and safest option. Directing the parent to drive would be considered dangerous malpractice. There is a wide variation in skill set among ambulance drivers, but advanced EMS paramedics that respond to 911 calls are routinely trained to intubate. Although the pediatrician is qualified to intubate, this is not a typical task in a clinic setting, and prophylactically intubating the child at this point would be inappropriate. **Focus:** Prioritization.

16. **Ans: 4** Based on the available information, the nurse would suspect and confirm hypoglycemia and then give food or fluids to prevent complications. According to the American Diabetes Association, milk is better than juice because the body's blood glucose level is stabilized by the lactose, fat, and protein. The mother should be notified and advised to come to the clinic; however, emergency treatments would not be delayed if she cannot be located. Asking the child to describe how she feels is appropriate, but taking time to elicit details of history from a 4-year-old child with hypoglycemia is not a good use of time in the immediate situation. The pediatrician should be alerted about the child's condition; however, oxygen is not needed, and it is unlikely that IV access is required at this time. **Focus:** Prioritization.

17. **Ans: 4** The mother is very emotional, and she must be allowed to express her feelings first. In addition, accusing others of "not taking care of her" suggests that the mother may be using the defense mechanism of projection (transferring feelings and inadequacies of self onto others). Her anger and fear may be related to guilt for not appropriately informing the neighbor about the child's health condition. The nurse could consider using the other three options after allowing the mother to express herself and further assessing the situation. **Focus:** Prioritization.

18. **Ans: 1** Acute otitis media is painful, and the child is demonstrating behaviors indicative of pain. Symptoms are relieved with acetaminophen and the application of a warm, moist towel to the outer ear. Poor nutrition and lack of fluid intake are concerns, but relief of pain will likely improve the child's willingness to suck and improve oral intake. The other concerns are pertinent but less urgent. **Focus:** Prioritization.

19. **Ans: 3** The LPN/LVN can administer medication and apply warm compresses for comfort. Teaching the parents about the impact of passive smoking and night bottles should be done by the RN. "Watchful waiting" is not usually done for infants of this age with bilateral otitis media but would certainly require teaching by the RN about what type of symptoms indicate that further treatment is needed. A myringotomy (surgical opening of the eardrum) would be performed after antibiotic treatment, if pain and infection did not resolve. **Focus:** Assignment.

20. **Ans: 3** Remind the GN the infant is refusing to suck. Administering a crushed tablet in applesauce requires that the infant chew or suck and swallow. The GN can request that the pharmacy provide a liquid preparation of the medication. When administering liquid medication to an infant, the nurse positions the syringe toward the inside of the cheek and the back of the throat. The infant only needs to swallow the liquid. Mixing medication with applesauce is appropriate in some circumstances, but for this patient, the volume of 3 oz (85 grams) is excessive. In addition, applesauce may or may not have been introduced into the diet, and it is inappropriate to introduce new foods during an illness. **Focus:** Supervision, Assignment.

21. **Ans: 2** Data suggest that Sarah may have an arm injury such as a fracture or sprain that will need intervention. Additionally, this type of injury is not consistent with Sarah's level of development, which raises the question of abuse or neglect. The other concerns also need to be addressed for the long-term benefit of this family, but the most immediate concern is the acute injury to Sarah's arm. **Focus:** Prioritization.

22. **Ans: 1, 3, 5, 6** The AP can hold one child, accompany the infant to radiology, and assist the toddler to eat. All caregivers should observe for and report signs of abuse. The AP will have less formal training in this area, but his or her input is still valuable. Any caregiver can contact CPS; however, in this case, the social worker is present and is the most appropriate person. If a social worker were not available, then the RN should assume this responsibility. The RN should apply the splint and assess for the 6 Ps (pain, pulse, paresthesia, paralysis, pallor, and poikilothermia [temperature control]) before and after the splint application. **Focus:** Delegation.

23. **Ans: 4** Try to use therapeutic communication first. An AMA form is not appropriate in this situation because the mother's ability to make good judgments and to care for her children is a concern. The pediatrician should be notified because the mother may respond to the pediatrician's advice if she will not listen to anyone else; however, therapeutic communication should be the first intervention. Threatening to call the police is likely to increase the mother's agitation and fears. **Focus:** Prioritization. **Test-Taking Tip:** In stressful situations, be aware of behaviors that reflect emotional turmoil. Providing the opportunity to express emotions is therapeutic and can also diffuse a potentially volatile situation.

24. **Ans: 2** FEV_1 measures the amount of air expired after 1 second of forced expiration. Thus a decrease in FEV_1 indicates obstruction. As a result of obstruction, the child may have decreased oxygenation and carbon dioxide retention; however, FEV_1 reflects obstruction and not oxygenation. FEV_1 is not a method of determining pulmonary infection or pulmonary remodeling. **Focus:** Prioritization.

25. **Ans: 1** Hemoptysis (the specks of blood in Rebecca's sputum) is a sign of pulmonary infection. Pulmonary infection erodes the pulmonary blood vessels, resulting in hemoptysis. Although there may be bleeding with gastric irritation, the presence of dark brown or black-colored blood suggests that hydrochloric acid in the stomach is breaking down RBCs and changing the appearance (denaturing) of the blood. **Focus:** Prioritization.

26. **Ans: 4** Forced expiration and huffing is an effective method to clear the airways. Children with cystic fibrosis do not have increased fluid requirements. The use of inhaled corticosteroids has not been demonstrated to improve pulmonary function in children with cystic fibrosis. Oxygen therapy is administered for impaired oxygenation. **Focus:** Prioritization.

27. **Ans: 1** Lower BMI in children with cystic fibrosis is associated with poor pulmonary function. The need for increased calorie consumption and malabsorption characteristic of cystic fibrosis can often make it difficult for children to consume adequate calories for growth. This child has consistently been below the 5th percentile for both weight and BMI. In this case, alternative feeding routes such as gastrostomy tube feedings are considered. Total parenteral nutrition is not suitable for long-term management of nutritional deficits. **Focus:** Prioritization.

28. **Ans: 2** Clubbing occurs with chronic arterial desaturation. Chronic arterial desaturation can result in polycythemia (increased RBCs). This would result in increased hematocrit, not a decrease. Increased WBCs are indicative of infection. Decreased mean corpuscular volume is associated with diseases that may affect formation of the RBCs such as microscopic anemia resulting from iron deficiency. **Focus:** Prioritization.

29. **Ans: 4** Kawasaki disease is one of the most common causes of vasculitis in children and may result in cardiac complications. Early indications of cardiac involvement include tachycardia out of proportion to fever and a gallop rhythm; therefore auscultating the heart is the priority. It has already been established that this child has a fever; thus obtaining a rectal temperature is not a priority. Respiratory changes are not characteristic of complications of Kawasaki disease. Although shock is a complication of Kawasaki disease, hypotension is a late and ominous sign of shock in children. In fact, tachycardia is an earlier sign of shock in children, which further validates the need to auscultate the heart. **Focus:** Prioritization.

30. **Ans: 2** IV immunoglobulin is the first line of treatment for children with Kawasaki disease because it has been demonstrated to reduce the incidence of coronary artery aneurysms (which are life threatening). Methylprednisolone and infliximab are indicated for refractory Kawasaki disease. Ibuprofen may be administered for fever, which is a symptom of Kawasaki disease, but does not decrease the incidence of coronary

aneurysm. Additionally, it usually is not administered intravenously. **Focus:** Prioritization.

31. **Ans: 3**   Children older than 6 months of age who are receiving long-term aspirin therapy should receive the influenza vaccine to prevent the risk of Reye syndrome. The influenza vaccine is not approved for children younger than 6 months of age. There is no need to postpone the vaccine. Immune globulin administration can decrease the effectiveness of live-virus vaccines; however, influenza is a conjugate vaccine and not a live-virus vaccine. Conjugate vaccines stimulate the immune response by introducing a piece of the pathogen. **Focus:** Prioritization.

32. **Ans: 4**   The respiratory rate is low and indicates possible postoperative atelectasis. It is expected that after a perforated appendix, the patient may have a slightly elevated temperature and decreased bowel sounds. A urine output of 160 mL over 4 hours is normal based on 1 to 2 mL/kg/hr. **Focus:** Prioritization.

33. **Ans: 3**   Charlie has decreased bowel sounds and a perforated appendix, which place him at risk for ileus. Insertion of an NG tube is recommended for gastric decompression. **Focus:** Prioritization.

34. **Ans: 1**   Charlie is experiencing moderate pain for which 200 mg of ibuprofen is appropriate. The recommended dose of ibuprofen is 4 to 10 mg/kg/dose.

Charlie weighs 21 kg, so the therapeutic dose range would be 84 mg to 210 mg; 200 mg is within the therapeutic range. Hydrocodone is for severe pain. Additionally, an adverse effect of hydrocodone is decreased gastrointestinal motility. Charlie is at risk for ileus, and administering hydrocodone will increase the risk. Although acetaminophen could also be administered for mild to moderate pain, the dose is too low. The therapeutic dose of acetaminophen is 10 to 15 mg/kg/dose. The therapeutic dose range based on Charlie's weight will be 210 to 315 mg per dose. Current recommendations by the American Academy of Pediatrics advise against codeine for pain. Codeine is metabolized in the liver to morphine. There is genetic variability in the activity of the hepatic enzyme (CYP2D6) that converts codeine to morphine; therefore, some children may have no effect from codeine, and some children may be highly sensitive to codeine. **Focus:** Prioritization.

35. **Ans: 1**   NG suctioning can result in metabolic alkalosis, hypokalemia, and hypochloremia. Charlie's low respiratory rate, grogginess, and confusion are indicative of metabolic alkalosis. Metabolic alkalosis is further evidenced by increased pH. Muscle weakness is a sign of hypokalemia. **Focus:** Prioritization.

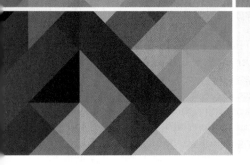

CASE STUDY 20

Multiple Patients With Mental Health Disorders

Questions

Note: In this case study, the term psychiatric nursing assistant (PNA) is used rather than the more familiar assistive personnel (AP). Different facilities and localities will use different titles for APs. The key point to remember in assigning tasks or making patient assignments is that APs who routinely work on a medical-surgical unit will have different skill sets compared with PNAs, who usually work on a psychiatric unit.

The RN is the charge nurse caring for psychiatric patients on an acute admission unit. The team includes an experienced male RN, a female RN who has floated from a medical-surgical unit, an experienced female LPN/LVN, and two experienced PNAs. There is also a male nursing student on the unit today. The morning hand-off report includes the following information about the patients. (Note to student: This case study includes seven patients and simulates some events that could occur over the course of one shift. Take notes as though you were listening to the morning report. This will give you practice in identifying important information. Refer to your notes and use critical thinking to respond to the questions.)

- *Ms. G, an 82-year-old woman, has a history of dementia and depression. She has been admitted because her daughter believes that "Mom is getting more depressed and confused." She is oriented to self and believes it is 1985. She is continuously trying to "find my coat so I can go to work." She is ambulatory with an unsteady gait and can perform self-care with step-by-step coaching. Her daughter would like her transferred to a long-term geropsychiatric unit.*
- *Ms. B, a 32-year-old woman, has borderline personality disorder and a history of frequent admissions to the psychiatric unit. Five days ago, she was admitted for suicidal gesture after self-infliction of cuts to the posterior forearm. She tries to manipulate others, and she is extremely flirtatious with males. She can independently perform activities of daily living (ADLs) but will dress in an excessively provocative manner.*

- *Mr. D, a 58-year-old man, has a long history of major depression. He appears lethargic and disinterested in the environment and in others. He responds appropriately when asked a direct question but does not initiate any social interaction. He requires verbal prompting for all ADLs, which he can perform himself; however, he says, "I would rather not."*
- *Mr. S, a 38-year-old homeless man, has disorganized schizophrenia and was found wandering naked on a busy street. He has been on the unit for 7 weeks with minimal improvement, but he has not been aggressive toward anyone. He frequently giggles to himself, and if allowed, he weaves bits of garbage into his hair. He demonstrates word salad (schizophasia) and looseness of associations. He requires repetitive coaching to perform all ADLs.*
- *Mr. V, a 62-year-old man, voluntarily committed himself 2 days previously for recurrent thoughts of suicide since the death of his wife several months ago. He reports frequently sitting at her graveside with a gun and a bottle of whiskey. He is alert and oriented × 3 (e.g., knows who he is, where he is, and what day and year it is) and answers questions appropriately, but he is preoccupied with thoughts of death. He is on one-to-one suicide precautions.*
- *Ms. M, a 40-year-old woman, is diagnosed with manic phase of bipolar disorder. She was admitted after a verbal altercation in an expensive department store when her credit cards were declined because she was over the $10,000 limit. She is talkative, grandiose, and emotionally labile. She can accomplish ADLs but will change her clothes repeatedly throughout the day.*
- *Mr. P, a 20-year-old man, has paranoid schizophrenia and was admitted yesterday through the emergency department after causing a disturbance on a public bus. He appears disheveled and acts suspicious. He has been refusing to eat or sleep because he believes that "those guys have been trying to kill me because I know who they are!"*

1. Which **two** patients are the most acute and have the **highest** risk for danger to self or others? **Select two**.
   1. Ms. G (older patient with dementia)
   2. Ms. B (borderline personality)
   3. Mr. D (major depression)
   4. Mr. S (disorganized schizophrenia)
   5. Mr. V (suicidal thoughts)
   6. Ms. M (manic phase bipolar disorder)
   7. Mr. P (paranoid schizophrenia)

2. Which **two** of the seven patients would be **best** to assign to the nurse who has floated from the medical-surgical unit? **Select two**.
   1. Ms. G (older patient with dementia)
   2. Ms. B (borderline personality)
   3. Mr. D (major depression)
   4. Mr. S (disorganized schizophrenia)
   5. Mr. V (suicidal thoughts)
   6. Ms. M (manic phase bipolar disorder)
   7. Mr. P (paranoid schizophrenia)

3. As the charge nurse is completing handover activities, organizing assignments, and instructing team members, Ms. M (bipolar manic phase) approaches the desk and demands attention from the person in charge. Which action will the charge nurse use **first?**
   1. Tell Ms. M that she has to go to her room until shift change activities are complete.
   2. Instruct the PNA to accompany Ms. M to the gift shop and let her shop for one hour.
   3. Remind Ms. M that interruptions are rude and that she needs to wait her turn.
   4. Inform Ms. M that there will be time to listen to her concerns at 10:30 AM.

4. A medical-surgical AP is being temporarily floated to the unit for 2 hours to assist with morning hygiene. Which patient would be **best** to assign to the AP for hygienic care?
   1. Ms. B (borderline personality)
   2. Mr. P (paranoid schizophrenia)
   3. Mr. S (disorganized schizophrenia)
   4. Mr. D (major depression)

5. The nursing student tells the charge nurse that his clinical assignment for the day is to obtain a patient history and perform a mental status examination that will take about 1 or 2 hours to complete. Which patient would be **best** to suggest to the student?
   1. Ms. M (manic phase bipolar disorder)
   2. Mr. V (suicidal thoughts)
   3. Ms. G (older patient with dementia)
   4. Mr. D (major depression)

6. The charge nurse is receiving a report from a relatively new night shift nurse. She says that Ms. G (dementia) was confused during the evening and kept getting out of bed. Because of this, an as-needed (PRN) sedative was administered, and a temporary chest restraint was placed to prevent falls. What is the charge nurse's **priority** action?
   1. Report the night nurse to the supervisor for violating the patient's rights.
   2. Assess the patient and obtain additional information about the incident.
   3. Advise the night nurse to seek out the unit manager and discuss the incident.
   4. Call the health care provider (HCP) to obtain prescriptions for medication and restraints.

7. The nursing student is assisting Ms. G (older patient with dementia). The supervising nurse would intervene if the student performed which action?
   1. Made a seasonally appropriate decoration to hang on the patient's wall.
   2. Cleaned and rearranged the patient's room and put personal items in the closet.
   3. Checked the patient's armband and asked the patient to state her name.
   4. Displayed current pictures of the patient's family on the bedside table.

8. Fluoxetine, a selective serotonin reuptake inhibitor (SSRI), is prescribed for Ms. G (dementia) to treat depression. Which instruction related to the fluoxetine is the charge nurse **most** likely to give to the PNA?
   1. "Watch for and report mild nausea."
   2. "Assist patient to stand for orthostatic hypotension."
   3. "Offer fluids and oral hygiene for dry mouth."
   4. "Perform hygiene in the afternoon because of morning sedation."

9. Ms. G's (dementia) daughter says, "I'm tired of waiting for my mother to be transferred to a geropsychiatric unit. I'm taking her home today!" What is the **priority** action?
   1. Obtain an "against medical advice" (AMA) form, explain the consequences to the daughter, and have her sign the form.
   2. Call the HCP about the situation and encourage the daughter to call the HCP directly.
   3. Encourage the daughter to wait and reassure her that the transfer to the geropsychiatric unit will occur soon.
   4. Verify the unit's AMA policies and check on the status of the patient's transfer and explain findings to the daughter.

 Answer Key for this chapter begins on p. 393

Complex Health Scenarios   **PART 3**

10. A psychiatric social worker is conducting a community meeting; all the patients are in attendance. The nurse is the co-leader. Ms. M (manic phase bipolar disorder) continuously and loudly interrupts, "Ms. B (borderline personality) stole my lipstick. Look at her lips!" What is the nurse's **best** response to this situation?
    1. Walk over to Ms. M and quietly escort her out of the meeting.
    2. Allow the psychiatric social worker to control the patients' behaviors.
    3. Instruct Ms. B to give an honest response to Ms. M's accusations.
    4. Tell Ms. M that thefts are investigated and to please not interrupt.

11. The HCP verbally directs the charge nurse to seclude Ms. M (manic phase bipolar disorder) for several hours because "she was belligerent and argumentative" during an interview. The nurse requests this be written, but the HCP declines because "it is just temporary, and I already explained the consequences of the behavior to the patient." What is the **best** approach in dealing with this situation?
    1. Assess the patient for signs of aggressive or dangerous behavior and discuss findings and concerns with the HCP.
    2. Refuse to follow the verbal order because there is a violation of the patient's rights if there are no written orders.
    3. Recognize that setting limits and enforcing consequences are part of the treatment plan, so seclude and monitor accordingly.
    4. Document the situation; seclude the patient; and continue to provide patient care, safety, and emotional support.

12. Which laboratory result causes the **most** concern for Ms. M (manic phase bipolar disorder), who is receiving lithium?
    1. Serum chloride level of 100 mEq/L (100 mmol/L)
    2. Serum sodium level of 125 mEq/L (125 mmol/L)
    3. Serum potassium level of 5 mEq/L (5 mmol/L)
    4. Serum glucose level of 140 mg/dL (7.8 mmol/L)

13. What is an **early** sign that alerts the nurse that Ms. M (manic phase bipolar disorder) may be having lithium toxicity?
    1. Demonstrates fine hand tremors as she reaches for a spoon.
    2. Appears heavily sedated at a time of day when she is usually alert.
    3. Has very scant amounts of urine output for the past 16 hours.
    4. Displays gait abnormalities and loss of muscle control.

14. Ms. M (manic phase bipolar disorder) is very happy to see her family, but she starts crying. The daughter says, "Mom, please, if you would just stay on your medication, you wouldn't have to keep coming back here." What should the nurse do **first** to promote medication adherence?
    1. Explain the purpose of the medication and reassure that addiction is not an issue.
    2. Tell the family to assume responsibility for medication adherence.
    3. Give Ms. M and her family written instructions about dosage and frequency.
    4. Ask Ms. M to outline the steps she uses when she takes the medication.

15. Ms. B (borderline personality disorder) says that the male nursing student was flirting and trying to kiss her and touch her breasts. The student denies the accusation but says, "She asked me if I thought she was attractive, and I said yes." What is the **best** way to handle this situation?
    1. Advise the student that this type of behavior is typical for Ms. B but suggest that he contact the instructor and fill out an incident report.
    2. Tell the student that this is a learning experience, but he should remember to carefully consider the impact of casual comments when working with psychiatric patients.
    3. Go with the student to confront Ms. B so that the details of the incident can be clarified and then write an incident report.
    4. Tell the student that the incident will have to be reported to the board of nursing but that nothing is likely to come of it.

16. Ms. B (borderline personality disorder) tells the nurse that her stepfather raped her several times in the past and that she plans to "buy a gun and shoot him the next time I see him coming at me!" What is the **best** approach in responding to this information?
    1. Recognize that this is the patient's attempt to gain sympathy and gently but firmly set limits.
    2. Spend additional time with the patient and gather more information about the incident and her feelings.
    3. Acknowledge feelings of anger and powerlessness and tell her that the conversation must be reported to the psychiatric team.
    4. Assess the patient for any physical evidence, offer to contact a rape crisis counselor, and provide support group information.

17. Mr. D has major depression, and in addition to receiving pharmacologic and milieu therapy, he is to start electroconvulsive therapy (ECT). Which tasks related to the ECT can be delegated to the PNA? **Select all that apply.**
    1. Before the procedure: Reinforce that the patient is NPO for 6 to 8 hours.
    2. Before the procedure: Remove jewelry and devices such as dentures and hearing aids.
    3. During the procedure: Monitor the heart rate.
    4. After the procedure: Measure and report vital sign values.
    5. After the procedure: Reorient the patient and assess for short-term memory loss.
    6. After the procedure: Help the patient to eat a meal.

18. Mr. D's (major depression) wife comes to visit. As she is leaving, the nurse notices that she is crying. She says, "He's not getting any better. He's been here 3 weeks, and he actually seems a little worse." What is the nurse's **best** response?
    1. "You seem very upset; that's understandable. Come back in a few days. I'm sure he'll be better."
    2. "Medication therapy may take 4 to 8 weeks to be effective, and the ECT was just started this week."
    3. "Your husband really is getting the best treatment possible, and you just have to be patient and optimistic."
    4. "If you would like to talk to the HCP, I would be glad to contact him for you. He can explain what's happening."

19. The nurse is talking to Mr. S, who has disorganized schizophrenia with obvious thought disorder. The patient says, "I am God Jesus God. I will pray, pray, say pray, say pray say day a pray for you." What is the **most** therapeutic response?
    1. "Thank you, Jesus, I need all the prayers I can get."
    2. "Praying is a good thing to do, but you are not Jesus."
    3. "Let's talk about something else right now."
    4. "Your offer to pray for me is kind and generous."

20. The nursing student asks, "How do I start therapeutic communication with a patient like Mr. S who has schizophrenia? With his thought disorder, word salad (schizophasia), inappropriate giggling, and the loose associations, I can't understand him." Which option would the nurse recommend as the **best** option for the student to use with this patient?
    1. "Come and join us in a card game. We would enjoy your company."
    2. "My name is _____. I am a nursing student. What is your name?"
    3. "I have 15 minutes. Would you like to sit down and talk for a while?"
    4. "I heard you were walking down the street. What do you remember about that?"

21. Clozapine is prescribed for Mr. S (disorganized schizophrenia). Which laboratory tests are the **most** important to monitor in relation to this medication?
    1. White blood cell (WBC) and absolute neutrophil counts
    2. Fasting blood glucose and hemoglobin A1c test
    3. Cholesterol and triglyceride levels
    4. Cardiac enzymes and troponin 1 and troponin T

22. The nursing student tells the charge nurse that he needs information about the side effects of antipsychotic medications, such as the clozapine that is prescribed for Mr. S (disorganized schizophrenia). Which action would the charge nurse take **first**?
    1. Recommend that the student purchase a drug reference book.
    2. Teach the student how to access electronic drug information.
    3. Ask the student how he usually researches drug information.
    4. Give the student the pharmacist's contact information.

23. The medication nurse tells the charge nurse that Mr. S (disorganized schizophrenia) is attempting to "cheek" his medication, and medicating him is progressively more time consuming. "He wants water, then juice, then water, then a different juice, then new paper cups; then he walks away to the bathroom, and it starts all over again." What suggestion would the charge nurse tell the medication nurse to try **first**?
    1. Continue to spend extra time giving medications and observing him because he is in the acute phase of illness.
    2. Be kind and firm and tell Mr. S that he must take the medication and that all of the paper cups and fluids are safe.
    3. Consult the pharmacist and HCP to see if a sublingual tablet, such as asenapine, would be appropriate for Mr. S.
    4. Talk to Mr. S and explain that taking medication is essential and ask him if he would prefer an injection.

24. Mr. V is a quiet and cooperative patient; however, he is on suicide precautions with one-to-one observation because "my [dead] wife told me in a dream how I could be with her." Which tasks, under the appropriate supervision, can be delegated to the PNA? **Select all that apply.**
    1. Assist Mr. V with hygiene while he shaves his face and takes a shower.
    2. Evaluate mood, statements, and behavior every 15 to 30 minutes.
    3. Explain the need for one-to-one observation.
    4. Use good communication techniques, such as active listening.
    5. Go through the patient's belongings and remove potentially harmful objects.
    6. Maintain an arm's length distance from Mr. V at all times.

Answer Key for this chapter begins on p. 393

PART 3 Complex Health Scenarios

25. Mr. V (suicidal thoughts) is prescribed fluoxetine. What is the **most** important nursing intervention related to this medication?
    1. Monitor for initial weight loss followed by long-term weight gain.
    2. Inform patient about high probability for sexual dysfunction.
    3. Assess for self-harm behavior because medication increases risk.
    4. Observe for headaches, nausea, or sensory disturbances.

26. Mr. V (suicidal thoughts), who was admitted 2 days ago, develops agitation, confusion, disorientation, anxiety, and poor concentration. Which adverse medication effect related to the prescribed fluoxetine does the nurse suspect?
    1. Neuroleptic malignant syndrome (NMS)
    2. Withdrawal syndrome
    3. Extrapyramidal side effects
    4. Serotonin syndrome

27. Mr. P (paranoid schizophrenia) is screaming at the medication nurse, "You are trying to poison me!" The medication nurse is gently trying to calm him down, but the patient is yelling, "It's the wrong pill! It's wrong!" What is the charge nurse's **priority** action?
    1. Support the medication nurse's efforts to administer the medication.
    2. Advise the medication nurse to double check the HCP's prescription.
    3. Advise that the medication be held and then notify the HCP.
    4. Try to get Mr. P to take the medication by handing it to him.

28. Mr. P (paranoid schizophrenia) is pacing in the day room. His fists are clenched, he appears tense and suspicious, and he periodically yells at an empty chair. What is the **priority** action?
    1. Quickly step between Mr. P and any other patients who are nearby.
    2. Gather several staff members for a show of force and unity.
    3. Administer an PRN anxiolytic to Mr. P.
    4. Use a calm, clear tone of voice to give simple, concrete instructions.

29. The medication nurse asks the charge nurse if the HCP should increase or change Mr. P's (paranoid schizophrenia) antipsychotic medication "because he is pacing and agitated." What is the **best** rationale for conducting further assessment before calling the HCP for a prescription change?
    1. The charge nurse would collect complete data for the SBAR (situation, background, assessment, recommendation) format before calling the HCP for a prescription change.
    2. Akathisia (pacing and squirming) is a side effect of antipsychotic medication; a dosage increase could worsen side effects.
    3. Mr. P was just recently started on medication, so there has been insufficient time to evaluate the efficacy of the current dosage.
    4. Other nonpharmacologic therapies should be attempted before medication is changed or the dosage is increased.

30. Mr. P (paranoid schizophrenia) is at risk to harm himself or others because of his fear and paranoid behavior. Which task can be delegated to the PNA?
    1. Observing his interactions and behavior toward the other patients
    2. Following him around the day room to prevent occurrences of aggression toward other patients
    3. Serving his food tray and pointing out that all items are wrapped and sealed in original packaging
    4. Checking all his personal belongings for items that are potentially dangerous

31. Mr. P (paranoid schizophrenia) tells the charge nurse, "No information should be released to anybody in my family. Not while I am in the hospital or after I am released!" What should the nurse do **first**?
    1. Tell Mr. P that his request will be respected but the health care team must allow the family to express their concerns.
    2. Listen to Mr. P and document his request but let the HCP decide if Mr. P is mentally able to withhold consent.
    3. Try to get Mr. P to change his mind by explaining how vital it is to have the family's help and support.
    4. Do not argue with Mr. P but gently redirect him toward another activity because he won't remember his request.

32. Drag and Drop

Scenario: The following events are happening at the same time in the day-room. The charge nurse must delegate or assign care to various members of the mental health team to ensure safety and meet the patients' needs.

Under supervision, and with instructions, which member of the team would be **best** to assign or delegate to each patient situation?

Instructions: Staff members are listed in the left column. In the right column, in the space provided, write in the letter for the best staff member to assign or delegate each patient situation. **Note that all responses will be used and may be used more than once**.

Staff members	Patient Situations
A. Experienced female LPN/LVN B. Experienced female PNA C. Experienced male RN D. RN charge nurse	1. _____ Ms. B (borderline personality disorder) blocks the bathroom door and yells, "I'll drown myself in the toilet!" 2. _____ Mr. D (depression) has fecal incontinence in the day room and makes no effort to clean himself 3. _____ Ms. M (mania) is outside in the courtyard removing her clothes 4. _____ Mr. S (disorganized schizophrenia) needs his routine medication and must be observed for "pouching." 5. _____ Mr. V (suicidal thoughts) is sitting at a table and writing letters to his family and friends 6. _____ Ms. G (dementia) is looking for her coat and trying to get out the front door 7. _____ Mr. P (paranoid schizophrenia) is standing at the nurse's station demanding to talk to the HCP 8. _____ The HCP needs to relay information regarding Ms. G's transfer to the long-term geropsychiatric facility

33. The charge nurse is giving an SBAR (situation, background, assessment, recommendation) report to the HCP about Ms. B (borderline personality disorder), who locked herself in the bathroom and threatened to drown herself in the toilet. Place the following information about the incident in the correct order using the SBAR format.
1. "Ms. B was admitted 4 days ago for self-inflicted cuts to the arms and has a diagnosis of borderline personality disorder. She voluntarily opened the door; her clothes, face, and hair were completely dry. She did not verbalize suicidal intent, but this morning she had a verbal disagreement with another patient over a lipstick and claimed that a nursing student made sexually inappropriate advances toward her."
2. "Dr. S, this is Nurse J from the acute psychiatric unit. I am calling about Ms. B. At 3:15 PM, she locked herself in the bathroom and threatened to drown herself in the toilet."
3. "She is currently alert, conversant, and uninjured. Her blood pressure is 120/80 mm Hg, pulse rate is 82 beats/min, and respiratory rate is 16 breaths/

min. She is apologetic about causing a commotion, but she refuses to sign a no-suicide contract for safety, and she says that she'll probably try something else."
4. "She is in her room, and we placed her on one-to-one observation. I would like to continue the observation. And is there anything else you would like us to address at this time?"

_____, _____, _____, _____

34. It is 6:30 PM, and the charge nurse receives a call from a newly hired nurse who is scheduled to work at 7:00 PM. She tells the charge nurse that she is sick and will not be able to come in. What should the charge nurse do **first**?
1. Tell her that 30 minutes is insufficient for a call-in; ask if she understands the call-in policy.
2. Instruct her that she must call around and find someone to work for her or come in herself.
3. Document in her file that she failed to give adequate notice for calling in sick.
4. Tell the oncoming charge nurse that there was a call-in, so staffing will be short for the evening.

Answer Key for this chapter begins on p. 393

PART 3 · Complex Health Scenarios

35. Enhanced Multiple Response

Scenario: The charge nurse assigns tasks to the PNAs to provide comfort and ensure safety for the patients at the end of the shift. Completing end-of-shift task facilitates a smooth transition and contiof care for the oncoming shift.

Instructions: Place an X, in the space provided, or highlight each task that could be delegated to the PNAs. **Select all that apply**.

Which end-of-shift tasks would be delegated to the PNAs? **Select all that apply**.

1. _____ Assisting Ms. G (dementia) in changing her soiled blouse before evening visitors arrive
2. _____ Accompanying Ms. B (borderline) to the bathroom to prevent a repeat of blocking the door
3. _____ Encouraging Mr. D (depression) to finish a glass of water for the allotment of the shift
4. _____ Accompanying Mr. S (disorganized schizophrenia) to the gift shop before it closes
5. _____ Maintaining one-to-one observation with Mr. V (suicidal) until the oncoming shift takes over
6. _____ Assisting Mr. P (paranoid schizophrenia) in straightening his room and picking up his belongings
7. _____ Supervising Ms. M (manic phase bipolar) when performing personal hygiene before dinner time
8. _____ Searching Ms. B's (borderline) belongings for objects that are potentially harmful to self or others

36. Enhanced Multiple Response

Scenario: Part of the charge nurse's role is to ensure continuity of care from one shift to the next. Tasks must be prioritized and essential information from health care staff, other departments, patients, and family members must be collated, organized, and communicated to the oncoming staff.

Instructions: Place an X in the space provided, or highlight each task that should be completed before leaving at the end of the shift. **Select all that apply**.

Which end-of- shift tasks would the charge nurse complete? Select all that apply.

1. _____ Initiate a patient assignment sheet for the onshift.
2. _____ Take brief information (from the admitting office) on a new patient who will be admitted from the emergency department.
3. _____ Call social services to search for the family of Mr. S (homeless, found wandering).
4. _____ Check with the PNA who is performing one-to-one observation with Mr. V (suicidal thoughts).
5. _____ Thank the ancillary staff for their help.
6. _____ Talk to each RN and LPN/LVN about their concerns related to assigned patients.
7. _____ Prepare a hand-off report to give to the oncharge nurse.
8. _____ Verify with the medication nurse that the HCP was contacted about any medication changes for Mr. S and/or other patients.

Complex Health Scenarios · PART 3

Answers

1. **Ans: 5, 7** Mr. V and Mr. P are the most acute. Mr. V is actively suicidal; he requires one-on-one observation and frequent assessment for escalating thoughts of self-harm. Mr. P, who has paranoid schizophrenia, is newly admitted. His suspicious and paranoid behavior are barriers to establishing a trusting nurse-patient relationship. His fear and anxiety increase the risk for defensive and aggressive behavior. **Focus:** Prioritization.

2. **Ans: 1, 3** Ms. G (dementia and depression) and Mr. D (major depression) require physical care and verbal coaching. The medical-surgical nurse would be most familiar with the mental health conditions of these two patients because depression often accompanies chronic health problems and older patients with confusion or dementia are frequently admitted to the medical-surgical units for comorbid conditions. **Focus:** Assignment.

3. **Ans: 4** Giving Ms. M a specific time is the best way to establish boundaries. If she approaches again, she can be reminded about the 10:30 AM time slot. Sending her (or threatening to send her) to her room is a violation of her rights. From a patient's point of view, "until shift change activities are complete" is a vague answer. Going to the gift shop is generally regarded as a privilege and the charge nurse would not reinforce intrusive behaviors with a reward. Gentle reminders about previously discussed behaviors are usually part of the treatment plan, but "waiting your turn" is a social construct that will be difficult for Ms. M to process during the acute manic phase. **Focus:** Prioritization.

4. **Ans: 4** Mr. D (depression) needs assistance and encouragement to meet his hygienic needs, and he can understand and follow instructions. He would be the best patient to assign to the medical-surgical AP. Ms. B (borderline personality disorder) and Ms. M (manic phase bipolar disorder) can accomplish their own hygienic care, but specific boundaries may need to be set about dressing appropriately. Mr. P (paranoid schizophrenia) could be easily provoked because of his paranoia. Mr. S (disorganized schizophrenia) has severe communication barriers that the AP may not understand. Mr. V (suicidal thoughts) is on suicide precautions. Ms. G (dementia) could also be assigned to the AP; however, patients with dementia do better if they have the same caregiver whenever possible. **Focus:** Assignment.

5. **Ans: 1** For students, this type of assignment is generally easier to complete with patients who are willing and able to carry on a reasonably coherent conversation.

Ms. M (manic behavior) is a good choice because she is likely to seek out new people who enter the unit and initiate a conversation. Mr. V (suicidal thoughts) might benefit from the attention that a student could give him, but the assigned PNA and the student must be aware that the patient is on continuous one-to-one observation and that the presence of the student does not replace the observations made by the staff. Mr. D (depression) could answer questions appropriately, but his energy will not sustain a prolonged interview. Ms. B (borderline personality disorder) is likely to seek out the student; however, special attention from a young man is not likely to be part of her treatment plan. Mr. P (paranoid schizophrenia) is likely to refuse an interview or will have a low tolerance for interaction. Mr. S (disorganized schizophrenia) provides an interesting opportunity for observing symptoms, but he is not a good historian, and chart data may be limited. Ms. G (dementia) would be an interesting choice for a mental status examination; however, she is not a good historian, and prolonged questioning is likely to increase her restlessness and agitation. **Focus:** Prioritization, Supervision.

6. **Ans: 2** First, assess the patient for current mental status and for safety and comfort related to the use of restraints. The chest restraint is a particularly dangerous choice for this confused patient because of the risk for strangulation. Additional information is necessary to validate the need for medications and restraints and to determine if other interventions were tried before resorting to chemical or physical restraints. Based on the assessment of the patient and situation, the other three options may be appropriate. **Focus:** Prioritization, Supervision. **Test-Taking Tip:** Use the principles of the nursing process and the concept of safety to determine priorities. Assessment is the first step of the nursing process. The safety of the patient precedes any investigation of this inappropriate use of restraints.

7. **Ans: 2** Although minimizing clutter is important, rearranging furniture and belongings can increase confusion. Seasonal decorations, patient identification, and family pictures are appropriate interventions to use with a patient who has dementia. **Focus:** Supervision. **Test-Taking Tip:** There is a focus on care for older patients, so it is likely that the NCLEX® Examination will include these types of questions. Recall that older patients need more time and patience to accomplish tasks; patients with dementia benefit from adherence to routines and familiar surroundings, objects, and caregivers.

PART 3   Complex Health Scenarios

8. **Ans: 1**   The most common side effects of SSRIs include sexual dysfunction, mild nausea, headache, nervousness, insomnia, and anxiety. Sedation, orthostatic hypotension, anticholinergic effects, and cardiotoxicity are not expected side effects of SSRIs; these side effects are more associated with tricyclic antidepressants or monoamine oxidase inhibitors. **Focus: Delegation.**

9. **Ans: 4**   AMA policies may vary, and transfer to specialty facilities can be complex and time consuming. Explain to the patient and family that leaving AMA may actually delay geropsychiatric placement because the patient's place on waiting lists may be lost or a relationship may have to be established with another referring provider. The HCP writes the order for transfer but is usually not involved in making the administrative arrangements. False reassurance to placate the daughter is not the best approach. After the AMA policy has been verified, the daughter can be assisted in filling out the appropriate AMA forms if she still wants to take her mother home. **Focus: Prioritization.**

10. **Ans: 4**   Support the therapeutic milieu by demonstrating to all the patients that the psychiatric unit has social norms. Instructing Ms. M to stop interrupting is a concrete direction that delineates expected group behavior. Escorting her out may be the easiest solution, but parameters for behavior (e.g., "Raise your hand if you want to speak") and consequences (e.g., "If you interrupt one more time, you will have to leave") should be clarified first. If the social worker is not able to control Ms. M, the co-leader could assist with individual behavioral management while the leader keeps the group on task. Ideally, these roles are discussed beforehand. Encouragement of confrontation could be used in a small group therapy session to teach patients to directly express and respond to one another; however, in this community meeting, having Ms. B defend herself is likely to lead to a loud and unproductive public argument. **Focus: Prioritization.**

11. **Ans: 1**   Assess the patient for behaviors that would warrant seclusion (e.g., danger to self or others) and then discuss concerns with the HCP. If seclusion is punitive, there is a potential for violation of rights regardless of whether the order is verbal or written. Although patients do need limit setting and clear boundaries, the health care team must intervene in the "least restrictive" manner. After additional assessment, documentation, seclusion, and continued care are options. Going up the chain of command to prevent future similar incidents is also an option. **Focus: Prioritization.**

12. **Ans: 2**   When the sodium level (normal range 136–145 mEq/L or 136–145 mmol/L) is low, the body retains lithium, so there is an increased risk for lithium toxicity. The chloride (normal range 98–106 mEq/L or 98–106 mmol/L) and potassium (normal range 3.5–5.0 mEq/L or 3.5–5.0 mmol/L) levels are within normal limits. The glucose level (normal fasting range

70–110 mg/dL or < 6.1 mmol/L) would be considered elevated if the patient had not eaten within the past several hours. **Focus: Prioritization.**

13. **Ans: 1**   Even when lithium levels are still within the therapeutic range, there can be some mild, early responses, such as fine hand tremors, nausea, vomiting, diarrhea, polyuria, lethargy, slurred speech, and muscle weakness. Excessive sedation, decreased urinary output, gait abnormalities, and loss of muscle control are later signs that are associated with higher plasma levels of lithium. **Focus: Prioritization.**

14. **Ans: 4**   First, assess for successful attempts with medication adherence. This is a way to give positive feedback and to identify factors that contributed to success; then barriers to adherence could be reviewed to develop a plan. After assessment, the other options could be used, although the family is generally encouraged to assist rather than assume responsibility for medication adherence. **Focus: Prioritization.**

15. **Ans: 1**   Have the student contact the instructor. An incident report should be filed so that a detailed record is available for review. The instructor can debrief the student, who is likely to be upset, and there may be unintentional elements of his behavior that triggered Ms. B's response. Ms. B should have an opportunity to talk about the incident also, but the charge nurse must avoid taking sides. The charge nurse should write an incident report that is separate and independent from the student's account. The incident is unlikely to be reported directly to the board of nursing, but it could go to peer review if the student's behavior appears to be questionable. **Focus: Prioritization, Supervision.**

16. **Ans: 3**   Acknowledging feelings is therapeutic; at the same time, this does not necessarily confirm or deny the veracity of Ms. B's statements. Explain that any verbalizations of potential harm must be shared with the HCP and psychiatric team. Rather than spend additional time with Ms. B, gently inform her that the appropriate team members must be contacted for follow-up. Physical assessment will not provide any evidence of rape, but a rape crisis counselor could be contacted for long-term follow-up. **Focus: Prioritization.**

17. **Ans: 1, 2, 4, 6**   Under appropriate supervision, a PNA can assist patients with preparing for the procedure by reinforcing foods and fluid restrictions, and removing and storing personal items. PNAs can also take vital signs and assist with meals. The RN, anesthetist, or physician should monitor the heart rate and rhythm on the cardiac monitor. The RN should assess for short-term memory loss, which is expected, and concurrently reorient the patient. **Focus: Delegation.**

18. **Ans: 2**   Antidepressant medication does not give immediate relief. Generally, the HCP will prescribe an antidepressant and evaluate the efficacy for 4 to 8 weeks before any changes are made. Vague reassurance or empty platitudes are not useful to the wife. The

nurse would contact the HCP if the wife continued to have questions or needed additional information about the treatment plan. **Focus:** Prioritization.

19. **Ans: 4** Acknowledge the underlying "healthy" intent and express appreciation for the gesture. The patient is expressing a delusion of grandeur and religiosity with clang associations. Addressing the patient as Jesus supports the delusion, whereas contradicting the delusion is thought to have a reinforcing effect. Redirecting to concrete, here-and-now topics is appropriate after acknowledging the underlying feelings. Redirection is also appropriate when the patient is repetitive with delusional content. **Focus:** Prioritization.

20. **Ans: 2** With thought disorder patients, use short, simple questions that are easy to understand and respond to. If this particular patient can state his name in response to the question, it would be a therapeutic accomplishment because of his severe thought disorder. The other options show interest in the patient, but it is unlikely that this patient could sustain the concentration required to play cards, to sit for 15 minutes, or to recall the events preceding hospitalization. **Focus:** Prioritization.

21. **Ans: 1** One of the most dangerous adverse effects of clozapine is life-threatening agranulocytosis; therefore WBC and absolute neutrophil counts must be within normal limits before starting the medication, and weekly monitoring is required until the HCP opts to decrease the frequency of monitoring. Weight gain also increases the risk for diabetes and dyslipidemia, so glucose and lipid levels would also be monitored. Adverse cardiac effects are rare, but possible, so chest pain, palpitations, and dyspnea should be immediately reported. **Focus:** Prioritization.

22. **Ans: 3** The charge nurse would first assess how the student usually acquires new information. Based on the student's preferred learning style, the nurse may elect to use the other options. Some students use a personal drug reference book that can be flagged or highlighted. Other students find that electronic sources are faster. Some students are auditory learners, and they retain more information by listening and talking. **Focus:** Prioritization, Supervision.

23. **Ans: 3** If the pharmacist and HCP agree that asenapine would be acceptable, sublingual tablets, such as asenapine are ideal for patients who "cheek or pouch" because placing the tablet in the buccal space allows the medication to be absorbed as intended. The medication nurse has been spending extra time, and this strategy is not working. Recall that Mr. S has severe thought disorders associated with schizophrenia; he may or may not benefit from the underlying intent of limit setting and verbal reassurance. Offering sealed containers of fluid would be a better option. Mr. S could view an injection as more threatening, and the suggestion could cause fearful or aggressive behavior. **Focus:** Prioritization.

24. **Ans: 1, 4, 6** The PNA can assist with hygiene. All team members should use good communication techniques. The RN can delegate one-to-one observation to the PNA but must supervise and give specific instructions. The RN retains responsibility for frequent assessment. The RN is responsible for teaching and explaining safety measures. Searching the patient's belongings should not be delegated; the task requires clinical judgment about the potential for self-harm. **Focus:** Delegation.

25. **Ans: 3** Antidepressants increase the risk of suicide, although the greatest risk is seen in children, adolescents, and young adults; however, this is also the priority intervention for Mr. V because he is already manifesting suicidal thoughts. Fluoxetine may also cause sexual dysfunction and initial weight loss with weight gain after long-term treatment. Headaches, nausea, sensory disturbances, tremor, anxiety, and dysphoria may occur if the drug is abruptly discontinued. **Focus:** Prioritization.

26. **Ans: 4** Signs and symptoms of serotonin syndrome include agitation, confusion, disorientation, anxiety, poor concentration, and hallucinations. These usually begin 2 to 72 hours after an SSRI is started. Symptoms should resolve when the medication is discontinued. Symptoms of NMS include fever, altered mental status, muscle rigidity, dysrhythmias, and autonomic instability. NMS is more likely to occur with the first-generation antipsychotics, such as haloperidol or loxapine. Withdrawal syndrome occurs when an SSRI is abruptly discontinued. Symptoms include dizziness, headache, tremor, nausea, sensory disturbance, anxiety, and dysphoria. SSRIs can cause extrapyramidal side effects, but the incidence is low, and restlessness and agitation are the most common manifestations. **Focus:** Prioritization.

27. **Ans: 2** Although Mr. P is paranoid, psychiatric patients may be able to recognize their own medications. As with any patient, double check the HCP's original prescription to see if there has been an error. Compare the prescription with the medication reconciliation list (if it is available) to see if the current prescription matches what the patient has taken in the past. The other options could be used after the medication prescription is clarified. **Focus:** Prioritization. **Test-Taking Tip:** Always pay attention to patients' comments about their own medications. Whenever there is any doubt about the medications, check the original prescription.

28. **Ans: 4** The patient is in the pre-assaultive stage. Use a calm tone of voice and explain what he is expected to do. This will help him to gain control and conveys respect for his ability to participate in his own behavior control. A show of unity or anxiolytic medications may be necessary if verbal intervention is insufficient. If at all possible, avoid sudden or quick actions, which

PART 3 Complex Health Scenarios

could be interpreted as physical aggression. **Focus:** Prioritization.

29. **Ans: 2** If the observed behavior is a side effect of the medication, a dosage increase would worsen the symptoms. For protection of the patient, the nurse would not initiate a potentially harmful change. The other options also play a part in the charge nurse's decision to perform additional assessment before calling the HCP to request any changes in prescription medications. **Focus:** Prioritization.

30. **Ans: 3** Give the PNA specific instructions to point out that the food is wrapped and sealed. This should help to decrease anxieties related to fear of poisoned or tainted food. Following him around the day room is not a good strategy because it is likely to increase his suspicions and make him more anxious. Observing his interactions and checking his belongings for dangerous items should be performed by the RN. **Focus:** Delegation.

31. **Ans: 1** All competent adult patients have the right to decide how their medical information is handled. If there is a danger to self or others, this could change; otherwise, the health care team would respect the patient's wishes. It is a good idea to inform Mr. P that the health care team will listen to the family because he may see them talking to the staff. If the nurse is unsure about a patient's mental competency, then it is appropriate to consult the HCP, but the HCP would then inform the patient about the need to share information with the family. The nurse may try later to get Mr. P to give consent for sharing information but not while he is in an agitated or argumentative state. Mr. P does not have dementia, so redirecting him and anticipating that he will not remember the request is not the best action. **Focus:** Prioritization.

32. **Ans: 1D, 2B, 3B, 4A, 5C, 6B, 7C, 8D** The PNA would be instructed to first redirect Ms. G away from the door. The PNA can assist Mr. D with hygienic care and help Ms. M to don clothing, but the follow-up therapeutic intervention of setting boundaries and linking immediate behavior to consequences should be done by the LPN/LVN assigned to care for Ms. M. Administering oral medications is within the scope of practice of the LPN/LVN. Psychiatric patients are routinely observed for "pouching" pills in the buccal area. The experienced male RN is assigned to care for Mr. V and Mr. P. Mr. P needs assessment and intervention for escalating aggression. Mr. V needs assessment for suicidal thoughts. Writing letters could be a positive and therapeutic activity; however, letters may also contain evidence of final goodbyes. The charge nurse would assume care of Ms. B, who was originally assigned to the LPN/LVN, because threat of suicide increases the acuity and requires the skills of an RN. The patient must be assessed and suicide precautions with one-to-one observation must be

initiated. The HCP must be notified, and the incident must be documented. The charge nurse should speak to the HCP about Ms. G's transfer; information must be conveyed to the patient and family members. The admissions office and the receiving nurse must be notified. Arrangements need to be made for transportation. There is extensive documentation for a transfer that must be initiated and completed as soon as possible. **Focus:** Delegation, Assignment.

33. **Ans: 2, 1, 3, 4** Using the SBAR format, the nurse first identifies himself or herself, gives the patient's name, and describes the current situation. Next, the nurse gives relevant background information, such as the patient's diagnosis, medications, and laboratory data. The assessment includes both patient assessment data that are of concern and the nurse's analysis of the situation. Finally, the nurse makes a recommendation indicating what action he or she thinks is needed. **Focus:** Prioritization.

34. **Ans: 1** First give a verbal warning; the new hire must acknowledge that she understands the call-in parameters. Explain that this type of behavior jeopardizes her probation status and that next time, the incident will go into writing. Forcing an employee to come in during illness is not good for the other employees or the patients. The oncoming nurse must be informed about the short staffing, but the acting charge nurse would try to find a replacement. Working short staffed is not safe or pleasant for anyone. **Focus:** Supervision, Assignment.

35. **Ans: 1, 2, 3, 5, 7** Helping patients to change clothes, perform hygiene or toileting and encouraging fluids, as specified in the care plan, are tasks that can be delegated to the PNAs. Patients with disorganized schizophrenia are allowed to go off the unit when there is sufficient improvement for them to benefit from the experience, but Mr. S is currently too disorganized. For patients with paranoid schizophrenia, belongings should not be touched until anxiety and suspicions are better controlled, unless there is a safety issue. Searching belongings for harmful objects should be done by an experienced RN, who can analyze the potential for harm. **Focus:** Assignment.

36. **Ans: 1, 2, 4, 5, 6, 7, 8** Initiating an assignment sheet, preparing brief information about new admissions, documenting specific patient issues expressed by staff, and preparing a hand-over report are necessary tasks to provide a thorough shift-change report and facilitate a smooth handover. Thanking staff should be done routinely for team building and morale. Discussions about complex situations, such as family support or discharge for Mr. S, should be left for the next business day, when social services personnel will be available to assist the nursing staff and the patient with these issues. **Focus:** Prioritization.

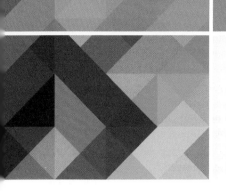

CASE STUDY 21

Childbearing

Questions

Ms. N is a 20-year-old gravida 1, para 0 (G1P0) woman who begins her prenatal care today at 24 weeks' gestation. She says that she didn't know she was pregnant until now. Her pre-pregnancy body mass index was 23. She has gained 30 lb (13.6 kg) so far. She admits that she eats poorly and smokes a half-pack of cigarettes daily but uses no other substances. She lives with her boyfriend and has no immediate family in the area. She reports no significant medical, surgical, or family history. The RN is taking her history and drawing samples for laboratory work today on this first prenatal visit.

1. Which would be the **priority** topics in patient teaching today? **Select all that apply.**
   1. Smoking cessation methods
   2. Recommendation of a flu shot (if flu season)
   3. Danger signs during pregnancy
   4. Basics of nutrition
   5. Pain relief options in labor and birth

Ms. N returns for her second prenatal appointment 1 week later. Her laboratory results include the following abnormal findings: 1-hour glucose tolerance test, 190 mg/dL (10.5 mmol/L); chlamydia test, positive for the organism. The health care provider (HCP) has written orders for a 3-hour glucose tolerance test, and has provided a prescription for azithromycin 1 g by mouth. Ms. N has increased her smoking to 1 pack a day because of stress.

2. Which information would be the **priority** for the nurse to provide Ms. N about the positive chlamydia test result?
   1. By taking the medication now and having her partner treated, she can help avoid complications in the pregnancy and delivery.
   2. Some medications used to treat chlamydia infections are not safe in pregnancy, and she should use condoms until she can be treated postpartum.
   3. Chlamydia infection may recur despite treatment.
   4. Chlamydia infection may harm the baby at delivery, but treatment will prevent this harm.

3. Which other education would the nurse provide to the patient today?
   1. Instruct Ms. N not to fast for the 3-hour glucose tolerance test because it is hard to do so in pregnancy.
   2. Refer Ms. N to a social worker because her increased stress can be a risk factor for preterm birth.
   3. Remind Ms. N that she has increased the risks to her infant by smoking more at this time.
   4. Instruct Ms. N not to have intercourse with her partner as he was likely the source of her chlamydia infection.

Later that evening Ms. N calls the clinic and reports vaginal bleeding and cramping. The nurse advises her to go to the emergency department (ED) and tells the patient that her HCP and the RN in the ED will be notified.

4. Using the SBAR (situation, background, assessment, recommendation) format, in which order will the nurse communicate information in the report to the ED RN?
   1. "The patient is coming to the ED for evaluation for possible preterm labor and bleeding."
   2. "She has multiple high-risk pregnancy factors, including an elevated 1-hour glucose level and a positive chlamydia test. She's had only two prenatal visits and no ultrasound yet. The patient smokes cigarettes; reports a lot of stress; and is single, unemployed, and with little support."
   3. "The patient is a 20-year-old G1P0 at 24 weeks' gestation who reports vaginal bleeding and cramping starting this evening."
   4. "Please be sure she also gets a social work consult and ensure that she has taken the prescribed azithromycin 1 gram to treat the chlamydia infection."
   ———, ———, ———, ———

Ms. N arrives in the obstetrics triage area crying and accompanied by an agitated man who is speaking angrily to the patient.

5. Indicate the order in which the RN should take the following actions at this time.
   1. Apply a fetal monitor and measure vital signs.
   2. Obtain a thorough history from the patient.
   3. Notify the HCP.
   4. Instruct the man to wait in the waiting area and notify security.
   5. Call a social worker for a consult.

   _____, _____, _____, _____, _____

Ms. N relates that when she told her partner about the positive chlamydia test result, he became violent and began hitting her in the face and abdomen. Upon examination, Ms. N's cervix is found to be 2 cm dilated and 50% effaced, she is contracting every 6 minutes, and she has a small amount of vaginal bleeding. Her ultrasound findings are normal and show no placenta previa. She is admitted to the hospital for treatment of preterm labor. The HCP has prescribed the following medications:
- *Nifedipine 30 mg PO followed by 10 mg PO every 4 hours*
- *Betamethasone 12 mg intramuscularly (IM) every 24 hours × 2 doses*

6. Which information would be the **priority** to give Ms. N at this time about the treatment?
   1. Nifedipine effectively treats angina.
   2. Glucose testing cannot be done after administration of betamethasone.
   3. Betamethasone helps the infant's lungs to mature.
   4. Nifedipine is a calcium channel blocker that reduces blood pressure.

After treatment, Ms. N's contractions stop, and there is no further cervical dilation. After 1 day of observation, Ms. N is being discharged today. Her discharge medications are as follows:
- *Prenatal vitamin PO 1 daily*
- *Ferrous sulfate 325 mg PO 1 daily*

7. Which task to prepare for Ms. N's discharge could be delegated to assistive personnel (AP)?
   1. Teaching Ms. N the signs of preterm labor
   2. Discussing nutrition, smoking cessation, and stress reduction
   3. Calling the prenatal clinic to schedule the next prenatal appointment within 1 week
   4. Calling a social worker to discuss a plan of care given the history of domestic violence

8. A student nurse is helping the nurse prepare for Ms. N's discharge. Which statement made to Ms. N by the student would require the nurse to intervene and correct the information given?
   1. "Iron may cause constipation."
   2. "Iron should be taken daily with milk."
   3. "Iron may cause darkening of the stools."
   4. "Iron does not take the place of a high-iron diet, which should also be followed."

Ms. N is now at 32 weeks' gestation, and her pregnancy is going well. The nurse midwife has prescribed the Tdap (tetanus, diphtheria, pertussis) vaccine to be administered today. Ms. N and her mother decline the vaccine as they would prefer that Ms. N not get a vaccine in pregnancy.

9. Which response by the nurse would be best?
   1. Explain to the patient and her mother that the vaccine can be given at any time and that she can plan to receive it after the baby is born if she prefers.
   2. Explain to the patient and her mother that the vaccine is optional, and if the patient does not want it, it will not be given.
   3. Explain to the patient and her mother that the rationale for giving the vaccine in late pregnancy is to provide whooping cough immunity for the baby.
   4. Explain to the patient that the vaccine is important and that the nurse midwife has prescribed it at this time, so it must be given today.

The patient recalls that she received the Tdap vaccine in the ED a few years ago after accidentally injuring her foot with a piece of dirty glass on the street. She wonders why she should get the vaccine again.

10. Which response by the nurse to the patient's question is **best**?
    1. Explain to the patient that the vaccine in the ED would have only covered tetanus but that the currently recommended vaccine also covers whooping cough or pertussis.
    2. Explain to the patient that the currently recommended vaccine is indicated specifically to provide immunologic protection for the baby she is now carrying and that a vaccine given a few years ago would not deliver the same protection to her unborn baby.
    3. Thank the patient for providing that information and ask her if she can provide documentation of that vaccine so that the nurse can reevaluate the need for the current vaccine based on this information.
    4. Educate the patient that the Tdap vaccine is needed again at this time to provide immunologic protection to the baby so that the baby will not need to receive dangerous vaccines after he or she is born.

11. The patient's mother mentions that the nurse midwife told her that she should also get the Tdap vaccine. The patient's mother states she got all her childhood vaccines, so she doesn't need any more now. What is the best explanation the nurse can provide regarding the recommendation for the Tdap vaccine for the patient's mother?
    1. Explain to the mother that if all of the adults caring for the infant are also vaccinated against whooping cough (pertussis), it reduces the risk of whooping cough in the newborn and that childhood vaccines would not be sufficient to provide this protection.
    2. Advise the patient's mother to check her vaccination records and if she received the vaccine in childhood, she should be fine.
    3. Advise the patient's mother that receiving Tdap at this time will ensure that she is up to date with tetanus vaccine recommendations and would be protected from this disease.
    4. Explain to the patient's mother that the Tdap vaccine at this time reduces the risk of diphtheria to both herself and the newborn baby. Her childhood vaccines are not sufficient to provide this protection.

Ms. N's pregnancy continues uneventfully. She separates from her boyfriend and begins counseling, which she says makes her feel stronger and calmer. She has decreased her smoking to 1 to 2 cigarettes per day. Her mother comes from out of state to live with her and cooks healthy foods. She is now at 38 weeks' gestation and calls the RN to report that she has had uterine contractions for 6 hours.

12. What would be **priority** data for the RN to obtain before giving Ms. N advice by phone? **Select all that apply.**
    1. Did she take her vitamin and iron today?
    2. What are the frequency and intensity of the contractions?
    3. Is there vaginal bleeding?
    4. Did her water break?
    5. How far does Ms. N live from the hospital?
    6. Has she felt the baby moving?

13. Which response by Ms. N would prompt the RN to notify the HCP and advise Ms. N to go straight to the hospital?
    1. "The contractions are extremely painful."
    2. "I have vaginal bleeding that soaks about a pad an hour."
    3. "I have vaginal bleeding that is mixed with a lot of mucus."
    4. "My baby is moving a lot today."

Ms. N arrives at the hospital at 38 weeks' gestation in active labor. Her membranes are intact. Her contractions are every 3 minutes. Her mother is at the bedside assisting her with breathing and relaxation. A vaginal examination reveals that the cervix is 5 cm dilated and 100% effaced, with the fetal head at −1 station. Her vital sign values are as follows:

Blood pressure	140/90 mm Hg
Heart rate	88 beats/min
Respiratory rate	24 breaths/min
Temperature	98.6°F (37°C)

The fetal heart rate is 140 beats/min. There is average variability. Accelerations are present, and no decelerations are noted.

14. Based on Ms. N's vital sign measurements, which are the **priority** questions that the RN would ask? **Select all that apply.**
    1. Is she having headaches?
    2. Is she having pain with urination?
    3. Is she having epigastric pain?
    4. Is she experiencing visual changes?
    5. Has her water broken?
    6. Are the contractions very consistent?

The RN takes Ms. N's blood pressure a few more times and is careful to measure it in between contractions. All of the subsequent blood pressure values are normal, and Ms. N is admitted to the labor and delivery unit. She chooses not to receive pain medication at this time, and her mother continues to assist her with relaxation and breathing. She goes into the shower to help with the back pain she is feeling. When she comes out, there is a gush of vaginal fluid from the patient, and the RN notes that the fluid is green.

15. Indicate the order in which the following nursing actions should be accomplished at this time.
    1. Prepare the infant bed for possible tracheal suctioning or intubation of the newborn.
    2. Assess the fetal heart rate.
    3. Notify the HCP.
    4. Assess the contraction pattern and Ms. N's coping abilities.

    _____, _____, _____, _____

Ms. N is now moaning with her contractions, perspiring profusely, feeling nauseous, and experiencing an urge to push. A vaginal examination reveals that the cervix is 9.5 cm dilated and 100% effaced, and the fetal head is at +1 station.

 Answer Key for this chapter begins on p. 403

16. A student nurse is working with Ms. N. Which is an inappropriate action by the student at this time that would require the nurse's intervention?
    1. Discussing with Ms. N the option of butorphanol for pain relief
    2. Reassuring Ms. N and her mother that these are normal reactions near the end of labor
    3. Applying firm pressure on Ms. N's lower back
    4. Encouraging Ms. N to continue breathing with her contractions and to refrain from pushing if possible

Ms. N is experiencing increased pain and the HCP is at the bedside. The cervix has still not dilated fully, and Ms. N is urgently asking for pain relief. The HCP explains the option of nitrous oxide. The patient would like to use this inhalation method of pain relief at this time, and the HCP orders it.

17. The RN remembers hearing at a recent meeting that nitrous oxide has now been approved at this hospital for pain relief in labor, but has not yet scheduled a required training session on how to safely administer and evaluate the medication. How would the nurse proceed?
    1. Inform the patient and the HCP that she has not yet been trained on this method and so cannot safely administer it.
    2. Ask the HCP to remain in the room and guide in the administration of the nitrous oxide.
    3. Quickly request the consultation and presence of the charge nurse to ascertain who on the unit has been trained and can administer the nitrous oxide.
    4. Inform the student nurse that the method should not be prescribed until every nurse is trained.

Ms. N's cervix is now completely dilated, and she pushes effectively and has a normal spontaneous delivery of a 7-lb male infant. She has a small first-degree perineal laceration, which is repaired under local anesthesia. The neonatologist is present to evaluate the infant because of the presence of meconium. The infant is initially limp and pale at birth. His heart rate is 90 beats/min, and he is not breathing.

18. Indicate the order in which the following actions should be taken with this newborn.
    1. Provide positive-pressure ventilation to the infant.
    2. Provide the infant warmth.
    3. Open the infant's airway.
    4. Provide tactile stimulation to the infant.
    5. Suction the infant's mouth and nose if excessive mucus or fluids are present.

    _____, _____, _____, _____, _____

The newborn responds quickly to resuscitation, and by 3 minutes of age is breathing, is crying spontaneously, and has good color and tone. The neonatologist leaves, and the RN continues to assess the newborn.

19. Which finding would prompt the RN to call the neonatologist back to evaluate the infant further?
    1. Cyanosis of the hands and feet
    2. Heart rate of 160 beats/min
    3. Respiratory rate of 55 breaths/min
    4. Central cyanosis

20. Indicate the order in which the following nursing actions would be performed in the immediate care of a healthy normal newborn in the delivery room.
    1. Place identification bracelets on the mother and infant.
    2. Administer vitamin K to the infant.
    3. Assess the infant's airway and breathing.
    4. Perform bulb suctioning if excessive mucus is present.
    5. Assess the infant's heart rate.

    _____, _____, _____, _____, _____

21. Ms. N plans to breastfeed her infant. Which actions would the RN take in the delivery room to enhance the success of breastfeeding? **Select all that apply.**
    1. Place the infant on the warming bed until his temperature is stable, then bring the infant to the mother and assist in breastfeeding.
    2. Place the infant skin to skin with the mother as soon as possible after birth.
    3. Assist the mother to breastfeed in the first hour of life.
    4. Allow the mother to rest and give a first feeding of sterile water to assess infant sucking and swallowing, then assist with breastfeeding at the next feed.
    5. Instruct Ms. N to breastfeed for 5 minutes on each side.

22. After the placenta is delivered, Ms. N is noted to be bleeding profusely. Oxytocin 20 units in 1000 mL of lactated Ringer solution is infusing. The HCP also prescribes carboprost 250 mcg IM. Which finding would be a relative contraindication to administering carboprost?
    1. Temperature of 101°F (38.3°C)
    2. Blood pressure of 148/96 mm Hg
    3. History of asthma
    4. Allergy to penicillin

23. Which nursing actions are **most** important at this time to prevent further hemorrhage? **Select all that apply.**
    1. Monitor vital signs.
    2. Assess and massage the uterine fundus every 15 minutes.
    3. Ensure that the maternal bladder is emptied.
    4. Assist Ms. N into a left lateral position.
    5. Provide a lunch tray with high-iron foods.
    6. Ensure that the IV with oxytocin remains patent and infusing as ordered.

24. The nurse is preparing to transfer Ms. N to the postpartum unit. Which statement by the patient is **most** indicative of a need for further assessment before transfer?
    1. "My nipples are very sore."
    2. "I feel something gushing."
    3. "I feel dizzy if I walk."
    4. "I have bad cramping in my abdomen."

25. The RN receiving Ms. N on the postpartum unit is aware of her postpartum hemorrhage. Which would be the **first** clinical sign of hypovolemia related to postpartum hemorrhage?
    1. Hypotension
    2. Tachycardia
    3. Mental status changes
    4. Decreased urine output

Ms. N is now on day 2 postpartum. Her vital signs are: a temperature of 103°F (39.4°C), a pulse of 100 beats/min, and respirations of 20 breaths/min. Her physical examination findings are breasts filling, nontender, and nipples intact. The abdominal examination reveals tenderness with palpation of the uterine fundus. She has a slight cough. The HCP has ordered a chest x-ray examination, which was done and the results were negative, and a urine culture, which is in progress. The HCP has placed orders for clindamycin 900 mg IV every 8 hours and gentamycin 80 mg every 8 hours. The presumptive diagnosis is endometritis.

26. Which statements to the patient by the student nurse working with Ms. N today would require the nurse to intervene and correct the information given to the patient? **Select all that apply.**
    1. Endometritis is an infection of the uterus.
    2. The reason for the antibiotics is to kill the bacteria causing the infection.
    3. Because of your fever, the baby will need to be moved to the nursery.
    4. The baby will be fed formula while away from you.
    5. The antibiotics that you are receiving are not recommended during breastfeeding.

27. What signs and symptoms related to endometritis should the nurse monitor? **Select all that apply.**
    1. The patient's temperature
    2. The amount of vaginal bleeding
    3. Feelings of hopelessness
    4. The presence of erythema on the breasts
    5. Tenderness on palpation of the uterine fundus
    6. The color of the colostrum

Ms. N is now doing well and states she feels fine and is not experiencing pain. She has been afebrile for 36 hours and antibiotics have been discontinued. She is preparing for discharge with her infant. Her discharge orders are: Prenatal vitamins 1 daily PO, Ferrous sulfate 325 mg 1 daily PO, ibuprofen 600 mg q 6 hours as needed (PRN) for pain, hydrocodone bitartrate 5mg/acetaminophen 325 mg (Norco) 1 to 2 tablets q 4 to 6 hours PRN PO for pain, and to make a follow-up appointment in 4 to 6 weeks with her HCP.

28. Which order would the nurse discuss with the HCP?
    1. Prenatal vitamins
    2. Ferrous sulfate
    3. Ibuprofen
    4. Hydrocodone bitartrate

29. Which part of the discharge process could be appropriately delegated to the AP working with the nurse today?
    1. Teaching the patient the signs of postpartum depression
    2. Teaching the patient the signs of dehydration in the newborn
    3. Ordering a breast pump for the patient
    4. Doing the final physical assessment of the patient before discharge

Ms. N has now brought her breastfed newborn to the pediatric clinic for newborn follow-up with the nurse. He is 5 days old.

30. Which finding will be **most** important for the pediatric nurse to report to the pediatric provider?
    1. The baby's umbilical cord stump is still attached.
    2. The baby's stools are unformed and yellow.
    3. The baby has lost 5% of his birth weight.
    4. The baby had two wet diapers yesterday.

PART 3   Complex Health Scenarios

Answer Key for this chapter begins on p. 403

31. The nursing student who has two children of her own whom she breastfed is assigned to provide further education to the patient about breastfeeding. Which information given by the nursing student would require the nurse to intervene?
    1. "Breastfeeding helps to prevent infections in the infant."
    2. "Breastfed babies are less likely to develop allergies."
    3. "When I breastfed, I felt tired a lot. Have you noted this?"
    4. "When I breastfed, my babies gained weight from the beginning and were never sick."

Ms. N is now at her 6-week follow-up visit. The nurse is interviewing her and learns that she is breastfeeding successfully and has a new sexual partner who she describes as a great guy who is helpful to her and her baby. She would like to discuss birth control.

32. Which of the following is a concern when considering oral contraceptives (OCs) for Ms. N? **Select all that apply.**
    1. OCs need to be taken at the same time daily.
    2. Lactation could be affected by the use of OCs.
    3. Ms. N is also taking an iron supplement.
    4. Ms. N got pregnant while taking OCs in the past.
    5. Ms. N's new partner is a smoker.
    6. Ms. N has not had a menstrual period since her baby was born.

Ms. N decides that she would like to use the subdermal hormonal contraceptive implant etonogestrel 68 mg. She is happy to learn that it lasts for 3 years.

33. Which statement by the nursing student giving instruction to Ms. N about the contraceptive implant is incorrect and would require the nurse to intervene to correct the information?
    1. "It does not prevent sexually transmitted infections, so condoms should also be used."
    2. "It is compatible with breastfeeding."
    3. "Irregular vaginal bleeding is common with this method."
    4. "The implant is associated with a delayed return to fertility after removal."

34. Ms. N states that her new sexual partner is bisexual and also has male sexual partners. Which information would be the **priority** for the nurse to communicate to Ms. N today?
    1. Explain that multiple sexual partners increase the risk for sexually transmitted diseases (STDs); offer full STD testing and counsel on safer sexual practices.
    2. Advise her that she should stop seeing her partner because of his dangerous sexual practices.
    3. Inform her of where she can get free condoms.
    4. Explore her feelings about her partner's bisexuality and infidelity and how it will affect her and her child.

35. Ms. N comes back for a follow-up visit 6 months after delivery. She had noted painful genital lesions and the HCP has diagnosed her with genital herpes and prescribed valacyclovir. Which education should be provided to Ms. N today? **Select all that apply.**
    1. Genital herpes is a sexually transmitted infection (STI) that can be managed with medication.
    2. Screening for all STIs would be recommended.
    3. Condoms are helpful in preventing the spread of STIs.
    4. Ms. N will need to stop breastfeeding with this diagnosis.
    5. Ms. N may safely use valacyclovir while breastfeeding.
    6. The valacyclovir will cure the herpes infection.

36. Ms. N also states that her partner wants her to have her contraceptive implant removed. How would the nurse respond?
    1. Explain how to set up an appointment to remove the implant.
    2. Explore what Ms. N thinks would be best for her in regard to the implant.
    3. Inform Ms. N that the device lasts for 3 years and should be kept for that long.
    4. Inform Ms. N that since her baby is only 6 months old, she should keep the implant in as it is too soon to get pregnant again.

Answers

1. **Ans: 1, 2, 3, 4** Ms. N began prenatal care late at 24 weeks. She needs to know the danger signs and how to contact her HCP if they occur. She should be offered assistance with smoking cessation because smoking is a known risk factor for prematurity, low infant birth weight, perinatal infant death, and sudden infant death syndrome. Undertaking interventions now can help the pregnant woman to quit or reduce smoking and impact outcomes. Educating on the basics of nutrition is also a high priority because Ms. N is 24 weeks' pregnant, admits to a poor diet, and has gained excess weight in her pregnancy. Getting a flu shot in flu season is recommended for pregnant women. Pain relief would not be considered a priority topic because the patient is only at 24 weeks' gestation and has higher priority issues to address at this time; pain relief education can be addressed later. **Focus:** Prioritization.

2. **Ans: 1** Chlamydia infection is associated with preterm labor and birth and with neonatal infection and thus should be treated in pregnancy. Azithromycin is safe in pregnancy; although some alternate treatment medications are not, this would not be priority information. Telling the patient that chlamydia may recur is true, but the primary reason for recurrence is reinfection and not treatment failure. If the patient is free from chlamydia at the time of birth, no chlamydia related neonatal complications would occur; however, the nurse should not link treatment and a guarantee of no neonatal complications as reinfection is possible. **Focus:** Prioritization.

3. **Ans: 2** Stress has been linked to preterm delivery and low birth weight of infants and should be addressed by the nurse as a serious risk factor. Seeking a consultation with a social worker would be the appropriate action. A 3-hour glucose tolerance test requires fasting even in pregnancy. The patient can be counselled to bring a sandwich or healthy snack to eat right after the test is completed. A teaching that merely increases the patient's sense of guilt is not effective in smoking cessation. Advising the patient simply not to have intercourse with her partner is not an effective way to prevent reinfection. Appropriate education would include treatment of the partner. Sometimes this can be provided along with the patient's treatment using expedited partner treatment protocols. Education would also include prevention of reinfection. **Focus:** Prioritization.

4. **Ans: 3, 2, 1, 4** Using the SBAR format, the nurse first indicates the current patient situation that requires intervention. The nurse then provides pertinent background information about the patient. Next, the current pertinent assessment data and an analysis of the patient's problem are communicated. Finally, the nurse makes a recommendation for needed actions. **Focus:** Prioritization.

5. **Ans: 4, 1, 3, 2, 5** This ordering is based on patient and staff safety. The agitated and angry man is a safety threat to the patient and possibly to the staff, and dealing with him needs to be the first priority. The nurse must always be alert to the risk of violence and notify the security team as soon as possible when a potentially volatile situation is noted. The woman's report of bleeding and cramping are a safety threat to the fetus and so must be assessed quickly by measuring vital signs and applying a fetal monitor. The HCP should be notified so that an examination can be performed promptly. After the immediate safety of the mother and fetus are ensured, it would be appropriate to obtain a more thorough history. A social work consult would be indicated but should be deferred until after the assessment is complete. **Focus:** Prioritization.

6. **Ans: 3** Betamethasone administration is an evidence-based intervention that has been shown to decrease many neonatal complications such as respiratory distress, neonatal death, necrotizing enterocolitis, and cerebral vascular hemorrhage in the case of preterm delivery. This practice supports the Perinatal Core Measure of increasing the percentage of women at risk of preterm delivery who are given antenatal steroids. Nifedipine is used in this situation as a tocolytic to reduce uterine contractions. It is also a treatment for hypertension and angina, but that is not the purpose of the medication in this case. Glucose testing can be done after administration of betamethasone, but some sources recommend waiting 1 week to do glucose testing because the steroid may cause the glucose levels to be temporarily higher. **Focus:** Prioritization. **Test-Taking Tip:** You must be familiar with Core Measures that are related to various practice areas. For additional information, see The Joint Commission's website: https://www.jointcommission.org/core_measure_sets.aspx.

7. **Ans: 3** Scheduling a follow-up appointment is within the scope of practice of an AP. Options 1 and 2 are important patient education tasks that the RN must perform. Option 4 requires professional collaboration between the RN and the social worker. **Focus:** Delegation.

8. **Ans: 2** Ferrous sulfate should be taken with water or juice. Milk can slow the absorption of iron. The other statements are appropriate. **Focus:** Supervision.

9. **Ans: 3** The question asks how the nurse can help the patient understand the rationale for the timing of the vaccine. Option 3 explains the exact purpose of the vaccine at this time. The Tdap is recommended in the third trimester of pregnancy to provide initial protection of the newborn from pertussis until the baby's own vaccines are completed. Option 1 does not explain the purpose of giving the vaccine in the third trimester of

PART 3 Complex Health Scenarios

pregnancy. Options 2 and 4 do not offer education to help the patient understand the rationale for the timing of the vaccine. The nurse should always consult the Centers for Disease Control and Prevention for the most current vaccine recommendations as these recommendations may change over time. **Focus:** Prioritization.

10. **Ans: 2**   Option 2 correctly and clearly provides the rationale for repeating the vaccine at this time. Option 1 assumes that tetanus only was given without verifying information, and also misses the point that the pertussis component is the focus here. Option 3 also focuses on the specifics of the vaccine received a few years ago. These specifics would not change the recommendation for the Tdap vaccine in pregnancy, and advising the patient to try to obtain records would put a burden on her that would make no difference in the recommendation. Option 4 gives the nurse's opinion that vaccines are dangerous, which is inappropriate and erroneous information. **Focus:** Prioritization.

11. **Ans: 1**   Option 1 correctly and clearly summarizes the rationale for vaccination of the patient's mother. Option 2 considers the mother's childhood history of vaccine, which would not change the recommendation. Options 3 and 4 place the focus on the tetanus and diphtheria components of the vaccine, which are not the primary goal of the Tdap vaccine for adults who will be caring for newborn infants. **Focus:** Prioritization.

12. **Ans: 2, 3, 4, 5, 6**   These are all necessary data for the RN to have before recommending that the patient either wait at home or come to the hospital. The RN must consider the patient's history; current symptoms; presence of fetal movement; and practical matters, such as distance to the hospital, available transportation, and traffic conditions before giving guidance. Whether the patient took her vitamin and iron today would not be priority information at this time. **Focus:** Prioritization.

13. **Ans: 2**   Options 1, 3, and 4 do not represent abnormal conditions in labor. Option 2, however, indicates more bleeding than normal in labor. It could be a sign of placental abruption or placenta previa and the nurse would communicate to the patient the need to come into the hospital promptly and would notify the HCP of the potential problem and the action the nurse has taken. **Focus:** Prioritization. **Test-Taking Tip:** By becoming familiar with the stages of labor and the normal clinical findings in each stage, you can then identify a symptom or finding that is clearly abnormal.

14. **Ans: 1, 3, 4**   The elevated blood pressure could be a sign of preeclampsia, stress due to pain, or anxiety about labor and hospitalization. This would prompt the RN to ask follow-up questions regarding symptoms of preeclampsia. The symptoms in Options 1, 3, and 4 are characteristic of preeclampsia. Options 2, 5 and 6 are not. **Focus:** Prioritization.

15. **Ans: 2, 3, 1, 4**   After rupture of the membranes, it is a priority to assess fetal heart tones because the intrauterine contents shift, and the umbilical cord may be compressed or in rare circumstances may prolapse. The green color of the fluid indicates the presence of meconium in the fluid, which may indicate fetal hypoxia and thus also indicates the need for assessment of fetal heart tones. After heart tones are assessed, the HCP should be notified of the presence of meconium in the fluid. The infant bed should be prepared in anticipation of a possible need for suctioning or intubation of the neonate at delivery because of the presence of meconium. Finally, Ms. N should be assessed to determine what the contraction pattern is and how she is coping because the contractions may become more intense after rupture of the membranes. **Focus:** Prioritization. **Test-Taking Tip:** The prioritization is based on patient safety and requires you to know the implications of meconium-stained fluid and to anticipate changes in the plan of care because of it.

16. **Ans: 1**   Because Ms. N's labor is progressing rapidly and she is nearing delivery, an opioid would not be an optimal choice at this time. Although butorphanol is associated with less respiratory depression than other opioids, if it is given close to delivery, it can cause respiratory depression in the neonate at birth. This medication would be more appropriately used earlier in labor if desired. The other choices are appropriate nursing actions for the pain and distress of this stage of labor. **Focus:** Supervision.

17. **Ans: 3**   Nitrous oxide is an inhalation, patient-administered analgesia that is being increasingly used in labor in hospitals around the country. It is short acting and so can be used in any stage of labor. The nurse is aware that it has been approved for use in her hospital, but has not yet received training in the method. The correct option is for the nurse to move quickly, seek consultation, and have a trained nurse administer the medication. An effective unit encourages consultation among nurses with the goal of safe and satisfying care to patients and safe clinical practice for the nurses. The patient's nurse would stay in the room to observe the procedures and the patient's response to the medication together with the trained nurse. This option not only provides the patient with the medication that has been appropriately ordered for her but also protects patient safety and the nurse's liability. Option 1 would represent a nurse obstructing a viable option for the patient. Option 2 would not be recommended, because the hospital has recommended training for the nurse to ensure safe use of the method, and the nurse would be taking risks with her own professional status as well as the safety of the patient if she administered the method without the recommended training. Option 4 does not accomplish the goal of safe administration of an appropriate treatment to a patient, and it also denies an opportunity for the student nurse to observe important professional collaboration and adherence to safe care. **Focus:** Assignment.

18. **Ans: 2, 3, 5, 4, 1**   The American Academy of Pediatrics and the American Heart Association publish guidelines for neonatal resuscitation that are updated regularly. The first action with this newborn is to move him to

a prewarmed table in the delivery room. Provision of warmth avoids the added challenge of cold stress for the newborn. The airway is opened by placing the infant in a supine position with the head very slightly extended. The mouth and nose can be gently suctioned if excessive fluids or mucus are present. After suction, the infant is stimulated by gently slapping the soles of the feet, rubbing the back, or both. If the infant remains apneic or with a heart rate of less than 100 beats/min, positive-pressure ventilation with bag and mask is initiated. The steps of resuscitation should be done rapidly and in the correct order. All resuscitation equipment should be prepared for each delivery in case of need. Gloves should be worn and all equipment should be clean or sterile as indicated to support the Perinatal Core Measure of reducing health care–associated bloodstream infections in newborns. **Focus:** Prioritization.

19. **Ans: 4**   The heart rate, respiratory rate, and findings of peripheral cyanosis are normal in the first hour of life. Central cyanosis, however, may suggest a cardiac or respiratory abnormality and must be evaluated. **Focus:** Prioritization.

20. **Ans: 3, 4, 5, 1, 2**   The first assessment is of the airway and respirations. Next, suctioning is performed if indicated. The heart rate is then assessed. Placement of identification bands is important for newborn security, but assessing and ensuring the physical stability of the infant in a systematic way is the first priority. IM administration of vitamin K is recommended for the newborn, but this can be done after the initial assessments and proper identification of the newborn. **Focus:** Prioritization. **Test-Taking Tip:** You should keep in mind the basic ABCs (airway, breathing, and circulation) as the critical priority components of newborn assessment and care at birth. After these are assessed and any necessary resuscitation is done, the other tasks can be completed.

21. **Ans: 2, 3**   Early skin-to-skin contact and early breastfeeding are associated with breastfeeding success. This supports the Perinatal Core Measure of increasing the percentage of newborns who are fed breast milk only. It is not recommended to give sterile water to a breastfeeding infant or to limit nursing time. **Focus:** Prioritization.

22. **Ans: 3**   Asthma is a relative contraindication to the use of carboprost because of its potential to cause bronchospasm. There are other appropriate drugs for postpartum hemorrhage that can be used in place of carboprost, such as misoprostol. **Focus:** Prioritization.

23. **Ans: 2, 3, 6**   Assessing and massaging the uterine fundus help to prevent further hemorrhage by contracting the uterus firmly, which decreases the rapid blood loss present with uterine atony. If the maternal bladder is full, it can prevent effective contraction of the uterus, leading to uterine atony and continued blood loss. The nurse should encourage the mother to void frequently, and if she is unable to do so, bladder catheterization would be indicated. Ensuring that

the IV with oxytocin is infusing as ordered helps the uterus to maintain contraction. Checking vital signs and providing a high-iron diet are appropriate but do not stop the bleeding. Maternal position is unrelated to hemorrhage. **Focus:** Prioritization.

24. **Ans: 2**   The statement that something is "gushing" would prompt the RN to assess immediately for further postpartum hemorrhage. The other reported symptoms are nonemergent and can be evaluated on the postpartum unit. **Focus:** Prioritization.

25. **Ans: 2**   Tachycardia is an early sign of possible hypovolemia from hemorrhage. Hypotension, mental status changes, and decreased urine output are later signs. The relative hypervolemia in pregnancy allows the mother to tolerate normal blood loss at delivery with relatively little change in vital signs. The RN must be alert to early signs of hypovolemia and assess promptly for excessive blood loss. **Focus:** Prioritization.

26. **Ans: 3, 4, 5**   The student nurse is correct in explaining endometritis and the rationale for antibiotics. It is not recommended that an infant be separated from the mother with the diagnosis of endometritis because it is not communicable to the baby with normal contact. Breastfeeding is considered acceptable with both clindamycin and gentamycin. Changes to the intestinal flora of the nursing infant can occur, however, so the infant should be monitored for diarrhea and other gastrointestinal symptoms. The student nurse should also be praised for thinking of the effects of medications on the nursing infant but instructed to always consult an evidence-based source and consult with the nurse before giving advice that could jeopardize the success of breastfeeding. **Focus:** Assignment.

27. **Ans: 1, 2, 5**   Resolution of the patient's fever would be an indication that the antibiotic treatment of endometritis is effective. The amount of vaginal bleeding should be monitored carefully because if the uterus is infected as in endometritis, it may not contract effectively and therefore may allow increased vaginal bleeding. Tenderness with palpation of the uterine fundus is a sign of endometritis and will resolve with successful treatment. Feelings of hopelessness relate more to emotional status. Erythema of the breasts may be a sign of mastitis but is not related to endometritis. Colostrum is the first breast milk and the color would not be significant in the assessment of endometritis. **Focus:** Prioritization.

28. **Ans: 4**   All members of the health care team should work diligently to reduce the unnecessary use of opioids. In this scenario, the patient is not having pain and perhaps the HCP orders the hydrocodone bitartrate/acetaminophen routinely for all postpartum patients. The nurse would call the HCP and express concern about the use of an opioid in a patient who is not experiencing pain. The young woman in the case study has a history of nicotine dependence, is socially at risk, and is entering the emotionally difficult postpartum period. These factors could contribute to a risk of developing opioid

dependency. The nurse's careful analysis of the patient's situation, her need for pain relief, and the risk of opioid medication use is crucial at this time. The nurse should also take follow-up action and convene a discussion among the team about routine orders for opioids to ensure appropriate use of pain medications in all patients. The other orders are appropriate. The nurse could educate the patient on effective use of ibuprofen if the patient experiences pain after discharge. **Focus:** Prioritization.

29. **Ans: 3** The AP could order the breast pump for the patient. Options 1 and 2 involve teaching the patient, and although the AP can always assist with giving information to patients, the nurse remains responsible for the teaching process, which involves assessing a patient's readiness to learn, obstacles to learning, delivery of information, and demonstration of patient understanding of the teaching. Option 4 is the final assessment before discharge and should be done by the nurse to be sure that the discharge is safe and appropriate for this patient at this time. **Focus:** Delegation.

30. **Ans: 4** A newborn at 4 to 5 days of life should have at least six wet diapers per day. The mother's report of only two should be explored. It could be that the mother is not noting small voids in very absorbent diapers, or it could be a sign of inadequate intake. Option 1 is a normal finding as the umbilical cord usually falls off at 7 to 14 days. Option 2 represents the normal stool of a breastfed infant. Option 3 is a finding of weight loss within the normal range for age. Birth weight should be regained by 7 to 14 days of life. **Focus:** Prioritization.

31. **Ans: 4** Options 1 and 2 are correct facts about breastfeeding that may encourage the mother to see the benefits of breastfeeding. Option 3 shares some personal information but with the focus of encouraging the mother to discuss the possible challenges she may be having with breastfeeding. Option 4 shares personal information without putting the focus on the patient. The statement also sets up the patient for feelings of inadequacy because her baby lost some weight. An appropriate action would be for the nurse to privately speak with the student about how to use personal experiences in a therapeutic way and always keep the focus on the patient and her well-being. The student could then return to the patient and clarify the normal weight changes in the patient's infant. **Focus:** Assignment, Supervision.

32. **Ans: 1, 2, 4, 6** Options 1 and 4 address the concern that OCs are a highly reliable method only if the user is highly reliable in the way she takes the pill. Most pregnancies that occur on the pill are the result of user error. Ms. N now has a busy life with a new baby. The nurse would need to explore with the patient if she believes she could be a reliable pill user at this time. Option 2 refers to the estrogen component of the OCs, which can reduce the milk supply. There is, however, a progestin-only OC that is more appropriate for the lactating woman. Option 6 states that Ms. N has not had a menstrual period since her delivery. This can be completely normal in

a breastfeeding woman, but the nurse would need to ask Ms. N if she has had any unprotected intercourse and if so, a pregnancy test would be needed before beginning oral contraception. Options 3 and 5 would not affect Ms. N's use of an OC. **Focus:** Prioritization.

33. **Ans: 4** Options 1, 2, and 3 are accurate information regarding the implant and provide useful and important information to the patient. Option 4 is an inaccurate statement about this contraceptive. After removal of the implant, the serum level of etonogestrel is often undetectable by 7 days. Pregnancies have been known to occur 7 to 14 days after removal. The nurse must ensure that the patient does not leave the clinic with the idea that the device is associated with this complication because this may undermine her ability to choose a highly effective method. The nurse can take the student aside and explain the correct information and then return to the patient together and correct the information clearly. **Focus:** Prioritization.

34. **Ans: 1** Option 1 is the priority information for Ms. N. It clearly delineates the risks that she has and offers her appropriate testing and information about prevention of STDs. Option 2 is directive and does not acknowledge that Ms. N is happy in her relationship at this time. Option 3 is appropriate information but does not also include the education component, which is vital. Option 4 is appropriate discussion content for the nurse and patient but is not the priority information that the nurse must communicate to the patient at this time. **Focus:** Prioritization.

35. **Ans: 1, 2, 3, 5** A diagnosis of herpes can be very upsetting to a patient and the nurse would need to communicate accurate information to her regarding herpes being a manageable condition with medication. Because Ms. N is still breastfeeding, clear information should be given that neither the diagnosis of genital herpes, nor the prescribed medication would interfere with breastfeeding. The fact that herpes is an STI means that screening for all STIs should be offered to see if there are any concurrent infections. Condom use should be discussed with the patient as STI prevention. Valacyclovir will not cure herpes, but it will reduce symptoms and if taken continually can reduce the frequency of outbreaks. **Focus:** Prioritization.

36. **Ans: 2** Whenever a patient reports that her partner is wanting her to discontinue her contraceptive method, the nurse would need to explore the possibility of partner coercion. This type of coercion is a form of control and can be associated with intimate partner violence. The nurse would need to ascertain what the patient herself wants to do and why and to screen for intimate partner violence. Option 1 does not demonstrate professional analysis of the patient's comment, but just tells her how to accomplish the removal. Options 3 and 4 would not be correct information. A patient always has the right to have her contraceptive device removed after appropriate counseling. **Focus:** Prioritization.

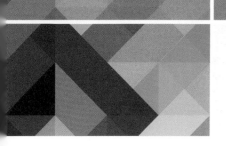

Illustration Credits

Chapter 1
43. From Gray Morris D: *Calculate with confidence*, ed 6, St. Louis, 2014, Mosby.

Chapter 2
41. From Ignatavicius D, Workman ML: *Medical-surgical nursing*, ed 8, St. Louis, 2016, Elsevier.

Chapter 6
3. From Ignatavicius DD, Workman ML, Rebar CR, Heimgartner NM: *Medical-surgical nursing*, ed 9, St. Louis, 2018, Elsevier.

Chapter 7
29. From Ignatavicius D, Workman ML: *Medical-surgical nursing*, ed 8, St. Louis, 2016, Elsevier.
38. From Mulholland JL, Turner S: *The nurse, the math, the meds: drug calculations using dimensional analysis*, ed 3, St. Louis, 2015, Mosby.

Chapter 9
1. From Ignatavicius D, Workman ML: *Medical-surgical nursing*, ed 8, St. Louis, 2016, Elsevier.

Chapter 10
20. From Ignatavicius D, Workman ML: *Medical-surgical nursing*, ed 8, St. Louis, 2016, Elsevier.

Chapter 11
1. From Harding MM, Kwong J, Roberts D, Hagler D, Reinisch C: *Lewis's Medical-surgical nursing*, ed 11, St. Louis, 2020, Elsevier.
33. From Ignatavicius D, Workman ML: *Medical-surgical nursing*, ed 8, St. Louis, 2016, Elsevier.

Chapter 12
43. From deWit SC, O'Neill P: *Fundamental concepts and skills for nursing*, ed 4, St. Louis, 2013, Saunders.

Chapter 13
32. From Ignatavicius D, Workman ML: *Medical-surgical nursing*, ed 8, St. Louis, 2016, Elsevier.

Chapter 14
34. From Ignatavicius D, Workman ML: *Medical-surgical nursing*, ed 8, St. Louis, 2016, Elsevier.

Chapter 15
24. From Ogden SJ, Fluharty L: *Calculation of drug dosages: a work text*, ed 10, St. Louis, 2016, Elsevier.

Chapter 16
39. From Ignatavicius D, Workman ML: *Medical-surgical nursing*, ed 9, St. Louis, 2018, Elsevier.

Case Study 1
19. From Ignatavicius D, Workman ML: *Medical-surgical nursing*, ed 9, St. Louis, 2018, Elsevier.

Case Study 5
23. From Lewis SL, Bucher L, McLean Heitkemper M, Harding MM: *Medical-surgical nursing*, ed 10, St. Louis, 2017, Elsevier.

Case Study 11
33. From Harding MM, Kwong J, Roberts D, Hagler D, Reinisch C: *Lewis's Medical-surgical nursing*, ed 11, St. Louis, 2020, Elsevier.

Case Study 13
3. From Ignatavicius D, Workman ML: *Medical-surgical nursing*, ed 8, St. Louis, 2016, Elsevier.

Case Study 14
4. From Ignatavicius D, Workman ML: *Medical-surgical nursing*, ed 8, St. Louis, 2016, Elsevier.

DEFINITIONS

Prioritization: Deciding which needs or problems require immediate action and which ones could tolerate a delay in action until a later time because they are not urgent.[a]

Delegation: Transferring to a competent individual the authority to perform a selected nursing task in a selected situation. The nurse retains the accountability for the delegation.[b]

Assignment: The distribution of work that each staff member is responsible for during a given shift or work period.[c]

THE FIVE RIGHTS OF DELEGATION[b,d]

Right circumstances
Right task
Right person
Right direction and communication
Right supervision

THE FOUR Cs OF COMMUNICATION

Instructions and ongoing direction must be:
Clear
Concise
Correct
Complete

PRINCIPLES FOR IMPLEMENTATION OF PRIORITIZATION, DELEGATION, AND ASSIGNMENT[d,e]

- The RN should always start with the patient's and family's preferred outcomes in mind. The RN is first clear about the patient's purpose for accessing care and his or her picture for a successful outcome.
- The RN should refer to the applicable state nursing practice statute and rules as well as the organization's job descriptions for current information about the roles and responsibilities of RNs, LPNs/LVNs, and unlicensed assistive personnel.
- Student nurses, novices, float nurses, and other infrequent workers will also require variable levels of supervision, guidance, or support.
- The RN is accountable for nursing judgment decisions and for ongoing supervision of any care that is delegated or assigned.
- The RN cannot delegate the nursing process (in particular the assessment, planning, and evaluation phases) or clinical judgment to a non-RN. Some interventions or data-gathering activities may be delegated based on the circumstances.
- The RN must know as much as practical about the patients and their conditions, as well as the skills and competency of team members, to prioritize, delegate, and assign. Decisions must be specifically individualized to the patient, the delegatees, and the situation.
- In a clinical situation, everything is fluid and shifting. No priority, assignment, or delegation is written indelibly and cannot be altered. The RN in charge of a unit, a team, or one patient is accountable to choose the best course to achieve the patient's and family's preferred results.

---

[a]Silvestri L: *Saunders comprehensive review for the NCLEX-RN® Examination*, ed 7, St Louis, 2017, Saunders.
[b]National Council of State Boards of Nursing: Delegation: concepts and decision-making process, *Issues,* December, pp. 1-4, 1995.
[c]National Council of State Boards of Nursing: *Business book: NCSBN annual meeting: mission possible: building a safer nursing workforce through regulatory excellence,* 2005.
[d]Hansten R, Jackson M: *Clinical delegation skills: a handbook for professional practice,* ed 4, Sudbury, MA, 2009, Jones & Bartlett.
[e]Hansten R: *Relationship and results oriented healthcare™* planning and implementation manual, Port Ludlow, WA, 2008, Hansten Healthcare PLLC.